MW00617913

ALGORITHMIC AND ARTIFICIAL INTELLIGENCE METHODS FOR PROTEIN BIOINFORMATICS

Wiley Series on

Bioinformatics: Computational Techniques and Engineering

A complete list of the titles in this series appears at the end of this volume.

ALGORITHMIC AND ARTIFICIAL INTELLIGENCE METHODS FOR PROTEIN BIOINFORMATICS

Edited by

YI PAN
Georgia State University

JIANXIN WANG
Central South University, China

MIN LI
Central South University, China

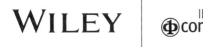

Library of Congress Cataloging-in-Publication Data:

Algorithmic and AI methods for protein bioinformatics / [compiled by] by Yi Pan, Jianxin Wang,
 Min Li.
    pages cm
  ISBN 978-1-118-34578-8
1. Proteins–Analysis–Mathematics. 2. Bioinformatics. 3. Artificial intelligence. I. Pan, Yi,
1960- editor of compilation. II. Wang, Jianxin, 1969- editor of compilation. III. Li, Min,
1978- editor of compilation. IV. Title: Algorithmic and artificial intellingence methods for protein
bioinformatics.
  QP551.A4335 2012
  572′.6–dc23

                                                                        2012040076

Printed in the United States of America

10 9 8 7 6 5 4 3 2 1

CONTENTS

III PROTEIN STRUCTURE ALIGNMENT AND ASSESSMENT

IV PROTEIN–PROTEIN ANALYSIS OF BIOLOGICAL NETWORKS

V APPLICATION OF PROTEIN BIOINFORMATICS

PREFACE

Proteins are any of a group of complex organic macromolecules that contain carbon, hydrogen, oxygen, nitrogen, and usually sulfur and are composed of one or more chains of amino acids. Proteins are fundamental components of all living cells and include many substances, such as enzymes, hormones, and antibodies, which are essential for the proper functioning of an organism. *Protein bioinformatics* is a newer name for an already existing discipline. It encompasses the techniques and methodologies used in bioinformatics that are related to proteins. Proteins can be described as a sequence, a two-dimensional (2D) structure, or a three-dimensional (3D) structure. In addition, interactions among proteins can be described as a network or a graph. Hence, many traditional algorithmic techniques such as graph algorithms, heuristic algorithms, approximate algorithms, parameterized algorithms, and linear programming can be applied to analyze protein interaction networks. On the other hand, because of the large amount of data available from wet labs and experiments with proteins, traditional algorithmic methods may not be sufficiently powerful and intelligent to be applied. Hence, we can use many mature machine learning or artificial intelligence (AI) methods to analyze protein data such as predicting protein structures based on existing databases or datasets. These AI techniques include support vector machines (SVMs), hidden Markov models (HMMs), neural networks, decision trees, reinforcement learning, genetic algorithms, pattern recognition, clustering, and random forests. Combinations of traditional algorithms such as graph algorithms, statistical methods, and AI techniques such as SVM have been used in protein structure prediction and protein interaction networks, and many good results have been achieved. The objective of this book is to promote collaboration between computer scientists working on algorithms and AI and biologists working on proteins by presenting cutting-edge research topics and methodologies in the area of protein bioinformatics.

This book comprises chapters written by experts on a wide range of topics that are associated with novel algorithmic and AI methods for analysis of protein data. This book includes chapters on analysis of protein sequences, structures, and their interaction networks using both traditional algorithms and AI methods. It comprehensively summarizes the most recent developments in this exciting research area. Protein bioinformatics plays a key role in life science, including protein engineering via designing tailor-made proteins, drug design based on finding docking molecules to kill disease cells, and improvement of protein effectiveness through modifying biocatalysts. Because of the many advantages of protein bioinformatics compared to traditional wet lab experiments, applications of protein bioinformatics are also described in this book. The important work of some representative researchers in protein bioinformatics is brought together for the first time in one volume. The topic is treated in depth and is related to, where applicable, other emerging technologies such as data mining and visualization. The goal of the book is to introduce readers to the most recent work and results in protein bioinformatics in the hope that they will build on them to make new discoveries of their own. It also arms the readers with the analysis tools and methods used in protein bioinformatics to enable them to tackle these problems in the future. The key elements of each chapter are briefly summarized below.

This is the first edited book dealing with the topic of protein bioinformatics and its applications in such a comprehensive manner. The material included in this book was carefully chosen for quality, coverage, and relevance. This book also provides a mixture of algorithms, AI methods, data preparation, simulation, experiments, evaluation methods, and applications, which provide both qualitative and quantitative insights into the rich field of protein bioinformatics.

This book is intended to be a repository of case studies that deal with a variety of protein bioinformatics problems and to show how algorithms and AI methods are used (sometimes together) to study the protein biological data and to achieve a better understanding of the data. It is hoped that this book will generate more interest in developing more efficient and accurate methodologies and solutions to protein bioinformatics problems and applications. This should enable researchers to handle more complicated and larger protein data once they understand the theories of the algorithms and AI methods described in this book and how to apply them. Although the material contained in this book spans a number of protein bioinformatics topics and applications, the chapters are presented in such a way that makes the book self-contained so that the reader does not have to consult external sources. This book offers (in a single volume) a comprehensive coverage of a range of protein bioinformatics applications and how they can be analyzed and used through the use of algorithms and AI methods to achieve meaningful results and interpretations of the protein data more accurately and efficiently.

The goal of this edited book is to provide an excellent reference for students, faculty, researchers, and people in the industry in the fields of bioinformatics, computer science, statistics, and biology who are interested in applying algorithms and AI methods to solve biological problems. This book is divided into five parts: (I) From Protein Sequence to Structure, (II) Protein Analysis and Prediction, (III) Protein Structure Alignment and Assessment, (IV) Protein–Protein Analysis of Biological Networks, and (V) Application of Protein Bioinformatics. The chapters are briefly summarized as follows:

- Chapter 1 discusses scaling of similarity sensitivity in remote homology modeling on yeast species and how the candidate genes are searched; these studies are important for different stages of embryogenesis of model plant species *Arabidopsis thaliana* in light of the concept of *dynamical patterning modules*.

- Understanding the biological term *sequence motif* is an important task in modern bioinformatics research, and these motif patterns may be able to predict the structural or functional area of other proteins. Protein sequence motif discovery is discussed in Chapter 2.

- Chapter 3 introduces methods for identifying calcium binding sites in proteins. Three methodologies for predicting calcium binding sites in proteins are reviewed and compared using different algorithms and AI methods.

- Chapter 4 proposes an imbalance learning method for protein methylation prediction using ensemble SVMs. It focuses on computational predictions of a particular posttranslational modification (PTM)–protein arginine methylation.

- Chapter 5 studies the prediction of protein posttranslational modification sites. By taking advantage of the large magnitude of experimentally verified PTM sites and utilizing a comprehensive machine learning method, a useful bioinformatics software system for PTM site prediction is provided.

- Chapter 6 describes an effective and a reliable tool using data mining and machine learning techniques for predicting local protein structure.

- In Chapter 7, a novel effective approach for predicting the boundaries of protein structure elements instead of individual residues structures using SVM is proposed.

- The states of the art of different machine learning-based RNA binding site prediction methods are overviewed in Chapter 8.

- In Chapter 9, many sequence-based and mass spectrometry data-based frameworks for determining disulfide bonds are presented.

- Chapter 10 gives the most recent update on protein contact order prediction. A new contact order web server is described that can predict the contact order by structure and sequence homology contrarily to the existing servers.

- Chapter 11 surveys about 15 computational methods for cysteine oxidation state prediction developed since the early 1990s.

- Chapter 12 addresses the computational methods in cryoelectron microscopy 3D structure reconstruction and its multilevel parallel strategy on the GPU platform.

- Chapter 13 gives a brief introduction to the biological, mathematical, and computational aspects of making pairwise comparisons between protein structures.

- To discover protein structures for optimal structure alignment, methods for using vector space model and suffix trees for efficient string matching and querying and how to index 3D protein structure are explained in Chapter 14. Furthermore, a protein similarity algorithm is explained in detail.

- Chapter 15 discusses several issues of structural alignment and methods that are implemented for sequence-order-independent structural alignment at both the global and local surface levels.
- Chapter 16 describes the methods used to study the prediction of protein structure classes and functions and measures, such as physicochemical features of amino acids, Z-curve representation, and the chaos game representation of proteins.
- Chapter 17 describes a new machine learning algorithm that uses a support vector machine (SVM) technique that understands structures from the Protein Databank (PDB) and, when given a new model, predicts whether it belongs to the same class as the PDB structures.
- The characteristics, strengths, and shortages of many network algorithms for clustering biological networks are discussed in Chapter 18. It includes various algorithms to cluster on protein–protein interaction networks (PPINs) based on the features of PPINs.
- Chapter 19 describes different algorithms applied to identify protein complexes, including methods based solely on PPIN data, methods combined with multiple information sources, and new trends in prediction of protein complexes on dynamic networks.
- To detect functional modules from protein–protein interaction networks, an ant colony optimization (ACO)-based algorithm with the topology of the network for the functional module detection is proposed and discussed in Chapter 20.
- Chapter 21 gives a brief overview of current state of the art in metabolic pathway/network alignment and how it can be used in automatic data curating.
- Chapter 22 starts by providing some background information on how PPI networks can be modeled on different PPI network alignments, and then focuses on local PPI network alignment algorithms and global PPI network alignment algorithms. Coarse-grain comparison is also addressed in that chapter.
- Among many machine learning techniques proposed for quantitative structure–activity relationship (QSAR) analysis and drug activity comparison, Chapter 23 focuses on the design and results of SVMs used for protein-related drug activity comparison.
- The main goal of Chapter 24 is to analyze how the general problem of finding repetitions in biological data evolved from sequences to networks data, by focusing on the open challenges and specific applications in biological networks.
- Chapter 25 gives a brief overview of an online resource and prediction server named MeTaDoR that provides comprehensive structural and functional information on membrane targeting domains.

- Chapter 26 gives a brief review of network-based identification and integration of gene signature of complex disease. In particular, it focuses on breast cancer gene signature in protein interaction networks using graph centrality.

We would like to express our sincere thanks to all authors for their effort and important contributions. We highly appreciate the reviews and corrections done by Ms. Tammie Dudley, which have improved the manuscript tremendously. We would also like to extend our deepest gratitude to Simone Taylor (senior editor) and Diana Gialo (editorial assistant) from Wiley for their guidance and help in finalizing this book. Finally, we would like to thank our families for their support, patience, and love. Without the collective effort of all of the above mentioned individuals, this book might be still in preparation. We hope that our readers will enjoy reading this book and give us feedback for future improvements.

YI PAN
Department of Computer Science, Georgia State University, Atlanta, Georgia, USA
Email: pan@cs.gsu.edu

JIANXIN WANG
School of Information Science and Engineering, Central South University, Changsha, China
Email: jxwang@mail.csu.edu.cn

MIN LI
School of Information Science and Engineering, State Key Laboratory of Medical Genetics,
Central South University, Changsha, China
Email: limin@mail.csu.edu.cn

CONTRIBUTORS

AJITH ABRAHAM, Machine Intelligence Research Labs, MIR Labs (Global Network)

GULSAH ALTUN, University of California, San Diego (UCSD), CA 92037

VO ANH, School of Mathematical Sciences, Queensland University of Technology, Brisbane, Australia

ANAMIKA BASU, Assistant Professor, Gurudas College, Kolkata, India

PIOTR BERMAN, Department of Computer Science, Georgia State University, Atlanta, GA 30303

NITIN BHARDWAJ, Department of Bioengineering, University of Illinois at Chicago, IL 60607

CURTIS HARRISON BOLLINGER, Computer Science Department, C.S. Bond Life Sciences Center, University of Missouri, Columbia, MO 65211

MARK BRANDT, Department of Chemistry and Biochemistry, Rose-Hulman Institute of Technology, Terre Haute, IN 47803

BERNARD CHEN, University of Central Arkansas, Conway, AR 72032

GANG CHEN, School of Information Science and Engineering, Central South University, Changsha 410083, China

LUONAN CHEN, Key Laboratory of Systems Biology, SIBS-Novo Nordisk Translational Research Centre for PreDiabetes, Shanghai Institutes for Biological Sciences, Chinese Academy of Sciences, Shanghai, China

QIONG CHENG, Department of Computer Science, Georgia State University, Atlanta, GA 30303

ANJUM CHIDA, Georgia State University, Atlanta, GA 30303

WONHWA CHO, Department of Chemistry, University of Illinois at Chicago, IL 60607

BHASKAR DASGUPTA, Department of Computer Science, University of Illinois at Chicago, IL 60607

HAI DENG, Sigma-Aldrich Bioinformatics, St. Louis, MO 63103

ZEJIN DING, Georgia State University, Atlanta, GA 30303

AIGUO DU, Dow Chemical Company, 2301 N. Brazosport Blvd, Freeport, TX 77541

JOSEPH DUNDAS, Department of Bioengineering, University of Illinois at Chicago, IL 60607

VALERIA FIONDA, Free University of Bozen-Bolzano, Italy

JIANJIONG GAO, Computer Science Department, C.S. Bond Life Sciences Center, University of Missouri, Columbia, MO 65211

ROBERT W. HARRISON, Department of Computer Science, Georgia State University, Atlanta, GA 30303

JIEYUE HE, Southeast University, China

ALLEN HOLDER, Department of Mathematics, Rose-Hulman Institute of Technology, Terre Haute, IN 47803

MORTEN KÄLLBERG, Department of Bioengineering, University of Illinois at Chicago, IL 60607

TIMOTHY LEE, San Francisco State University, San Francisco, CA 94132

XIUJUAN LEI, Shanxi Normal University, Shanxi, China

MIN LI, School of Information Science and Engineering, Central South University, Changsha 410083, China; State Key Laboratory of Medical Genetics, Central South University, Changsha 410078, China

JIE LIANG, Department of Bioengineering, University of Illinois at Chicago, IL 60607

GUOHUI LIN, Department of Computing Science, University of Alberta, Edmonton, Canada

HUI LIU, Computer Science Department, Missouri State University, Springfield, MO 65897

ZHI-PING LIU, Key Laboratory of Systems Biology, SIBS-Novo Nordisk Translational Research Centre for PreDiabetes, Shanghai Institutes for Biological Sciences, Chinese Academy of Sciences, Shanghai, China

ZHIYONG LIU, Institute of Computing Technology, Chinese Academy of Sciences, Beijing, China

Hui Lu, Department of Bioengineering, University of Illinois at Chicago, IL 60607

William Murad, San Francisco State University, San Francisco, CA 94132

Tomáš Novosád, Department of Computer Science, VSB—Technical University of Ostrava, Ostrava 70833, Czech Republic

Suely Oliveira, Department of Computer Science, University of Iowa, Iowa City, IA 52242

Yi Pan, Department of Computer Science, Georgia State University, Atlanta, GA 30303

Xiaoqing Peng, School of Information Science and Engineering, Central South University, Changsha 410083, China

Simona E. Rombo, Universitá degli Studi di Palermo, Department of Mathematics, Computer Science Section, 90123 Palermo, via Archirafi 34, Italy

Anasua Sarkar, Assistant Professor, Government College of Engineering and Leather Technology, Kolkata, India

Lei Shi, State University of New York at Buffalo, NY 14214

Yi Shi, Department of Computing Science, University of Alberta, Edmonton, Canada

Yosi Shibberu, Department of Mathematics, Rose-Hulman Institute of Technology, Terre Haute, IN 47803

Rahul Singh, San Francisco State University, San Francisco, CA 94132

Václav Snášel, Department of Computer Science, VSB—Technical University of Ostrava, Ostrava, 70833, Czech Republic

Phang C. Tai, Georgia State University, Atlanta, GA 30303

Xiaohua Wan, Institute of Computing Technology and Graduate University, Chinese Academy of Sciences, Beijing, China

Jianxin Wang, School of Information Science and Engineering, Central South University, Changsha 410083, China

David S. Wishart, Department of Computing Science, University of Alberta, Edmonton, Canada

Dong Xu, Computer Science Department, C.S. Bond Life Sciences Center, University of Missouri, Columbia, MO 65211

Jack Y. Yang, Harvard University, Cambridge, MA 02140

Jian-Yi Yang, Center for Computational Medicine and Bioinformatics, University of Michigan, Ann Arbor, MI 48109

QIUMING YAO, Computer Science Department, C.S. Bond Life Sciences Center, University of Missouri, Columbia, MO 65211

ZU-GUO YU, Hunan Key Laboratory for Computation and Simulation in Science and Engineering, Xiangtan University, Hunan, China; Key Laboratory of Intelligent Computing and Information Processing, Ministry of Education of China, Xiangtan University, Hunan, China; School of Mathematical Sciences, Queensland University of Technology, Brisbane, Australia

ALEXANDER ZELIKOVSKY, Department of Computer Science, Georgia State University, Atlanta, GA 30303

AIDONG ZHANG, State University of New York at Buffalo, NY 14214

FA ZHANG, Institute of Computing Technology, Chinese Academy of Sciences, Beijing, China

YAN-QING ZHANG, Georgia State University, Atlanta, GA 30303

WEI ZHONG, University of South Carolina Upstate, Spartanburg, SC 29303

JIANJUN ZHOU, Department of Computing Science, University of Alberta, Edmonton, Canada

SHAO-MING ZHU, Hunan Key Laboratory for Computation and Simulation in Science and Engineering, Xiangtan University, Hunan, China

PART I

FROM PROTEIN SEQUENCE TO STRUCTURE

CHAPTER 1

EMPHASIZING THE ROLE OF PROTEINS IN CONSTRUCTION OF THE DEVELOPMENTAL GENETIC TOOLKIT IN PLANTS

ANAMIKA BASU and ANASUA SARKAR

The diversity in land plants due to size, shape, and form is the combined result of different developmental processes for adult plant formation from the zygote and their evolution. The ancestral patterning toolkit designed by Floyd [1] for land plants was constructed by using developmentally important gene families that are responsible for flowering plant growth, patterning, and differentiation. In this chapter we search for the candidate genes, which are important for different stages of embryogenesis of the model plant species *Arabidopsis thaliana* in light of the *dynamical patterning modules* concept. This is a novel idea that Newman [2] applied to build a *developmental genetic toolkit* by using a set of genes that mobilize the physical processes that are important in metazoan development. In this chapter we focus on a small number of gene families, which are related to physical characteristics, such as turgor pressure, asymmetric cell division, asymmetric distribution of cellular components, anisotropic expansion, and dynamics in merstemic cell maintenance and finally establish their evolutionary developmental (evo-devo) roles in land plant development with a functional/biological analysis.

1.1 INTRODUCTION

In the evolutionary history of the plant kingdom, the plants evolved through increasing levels of complexity, from a freshwater green alga, through bryophytes, lycopods, ferns, and gymnosperms to the complex angiosperms of

Algorithmic and Artificial Intelligence Methods for Protein Bioinformatics. First Edition.
Edited by Yi Pan, Jianxin Wang, Min Li.
© 2014 John Wiley & Sons, Inc. Published 2014 by John Wiley & Sons, Inc.

today. Between about 480 and 360 million years ago (mya), from a simple plant body consisting of only a few cells, land plants (liverworts, hornworts, mosses, and vascular plants) evolved to an elaborate two-phase lifecycle with complex organs and tissue systems [3]. As mentioned above, the diversity of plant kingdom due to size, shape, and form is the combined result of different developmental processes for adult plant formation from the zygote, which evolved progressively [4].

Identifying the genes, which act in the developmental pathways and consequently in determining how they are modified during evolution, is the focus of the field of evolutionary developmental (evo-devo) biology. The fundamental aspects of the plant body plan have been found to be remarkably consistent within the plant kingdom irrespective of vast diversification [5]. Graham et al. [5] identified nine fundamental body plan features that originated during radiation of algae and were inherited by the plant kingdom. In light of these fundamental features, we analyze the evo-devo roles of embryogenesis in plants. In this chapter we select some candidate genes to construct a genetic toolkit for land plants, and establish their biological/functional significances with an evolutionary analysis.

1.2   EVOLUTIONARY DEVELOPMENTAL (EVO-DEVO) ROLES IN EMBRYOGENESIS OF PLANTS (IN DEVELOPMENTAL PLANT GENETIC TOOLKIT FORMATION)

To explore the evo-devo biology of embryogenesis in plants, we select some candidate genes and relate them to their physical properties to depict the developmental genetic toolkit of land plants, following studies by Newman [2]. Table 1.1 shows the candidate genes, their physical principles, and their relevant evo-devo roles.

1.3   PHASES IN EMBRYOGENESIS IN *Arabidopsis Thaliana*

In *embryogenesis*, a multicellular organism forms from a single cell. In *Arabidopsis thaliana*, embryogenesis is a continuous process that can be divided into three major phases, described as early, mid, and late. In this section, we review all these phases starting from the early phase of embryogenesis.

The early phase consists of pattern formation, morphogenesis, defining the axes of the plant body plan, and forming the organ systems. Embryogenesis involves three basic steps: (1) cell growth, (2) cell differentiation, and (3) morphogenesis. The embryo grows up to certain limit, and then differentiates into cells that differ from their mother cell in structure and function. Thus different morphological structures such as stem, root, or flower are formed, enabling the formation of a total plant.

TABLE 1.1   Relationship between Candidate Genes and Their Physical Properties and Evolutionary Developmental (Evo-Devo) Roles

Characteristic Molecules	Physical Principles	Evo-Devo Roles
Expansin	Turgor pressure	Cell wall expansion and organ initiation
Extensin	Turgor pressure	Growth initiation by cell plate formation
GNOM	Asymmetric cell division	Apical–basal axis formation
TORMOZ	Longitudinal cell division	Pattern formation
PIN	Asymmetric distribution	Tissue polarization
ACTIN	Anisotropic expansion	Cellular polarity determination
G proteins	Dynamics in meristem maintenance (differential cell division)	Lateral organ formation
NPH4 TF	Differential cell expansion	Aerial tissue formation
AGO10	Complementary sequence binding	Adaxial–abxaial polarity formation
FT protein	Signaling	Floral morphogenesis
LEAFY	Intercellular communication through gradient formation	Flower patterning

1.3.1   Cell Growth Phase

The growth in plants is defined as an irreversible increase in cell mass [6]. Since the cell mass value factors both in cell volume and cell number, there are two processes relevant to the plant growth: (1) an irreversible increase in cell size, known as *cell elongation*, and (2) an increase in cell number, defined as *cell division*.

1.3.1.1   Cell Elongation Phase   Cell expansion, driven by the turgor pressure, mediates the plant growth. During this process, cells increase manyfold in volume and become highly vacuolated. The cell membrane and the cell wall surround the plant cell, whereas for an animal cell, only cell membrane is present. Since the structure of the cell wall is more rigid than that of the cell membrane, the cell growth mechanism differs in plants and animals. Because of the presence of the rigid cell wall, no cell migration occurs during plant development. During embryogenesis, the zygote elongates 3 times before cell division as a result of the extension of the cells along the sidewalls. Before cell division, the cell nucleus moves to the position of the new cell walls to be formed [7]. Two cells are formed from the zygote following the asymmetric cell division: a small apical cell and a larger basal cell with different cell contents. The dense cytoplasm is present in the apical cell and in most of the basal cell vacuole (see Fig. 1.1).

The steps listed below (1–6) in generation of the embryo proper and the suspensor from the apical and the basal cell, respectively, are shown in Figure 1.2a:

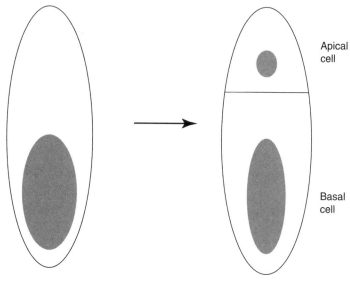

Elongated zygote

Figure 1.1   Asymmetric cell division of the zygote.

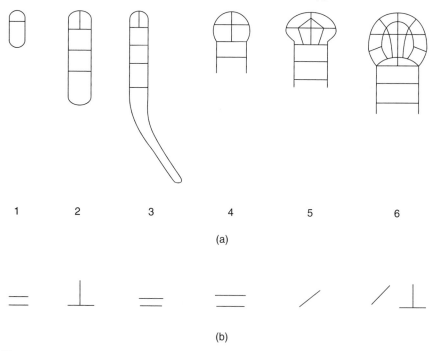

Figure 1.2   Generation of the embryo proper and the suspensor: (a) the steps involved in formation of the embryo proper and the suspensor; (b) the plane of cell division in each step: horizontal —, longitudinal ⊥, and transverse /.

1. The zygote undergoes a cell division along the horizontal axis, producing a smaller apical cell (1) and a larger basal cell.
2. The apical cell undergoes a cell division along the longitudinal ⊥ axis to form the embryo proper, and the basal cell develops the suspensor by cell division along the horizontal axis.
3. Cell expansion occurs in the suspensor.
4. The embryo proper divides by another horizontal division, perpendicular to the plane of the previous division. The basal portion of the suspensor is not shown.
5. The four quadrants of the embryo proper have divided by transverse divisions to produce an eight-cell embryo proper.
6. The cells of the embryo proper have divided by some transverse and two longitudinal cell divisions to form a 16-cell embryo proper.

The topmost cell of the suspensor has divided transversely to produce the hypophysis.

The zygote cell initially divides along apical–basal axis. Then the cell growth or expansion occurs. By a few successive cell divisions along different planes, the apical cell and the basal cell, respectively, form the embryo proper and the suspensor. In the embryo proper, eight cells are formed by two vertical and one horizontal cell divisions, whereas the basal cell divides along vertical axis only. The embryo proper will form most of the mature embryo, which are cotyledons, shoot meristem, hypocotyl regions, and part of the radical (or embryogenic) root. From the basal cell, the suspensor and the hypophysis are formed. The hypophysis contributes to the root meristem. *Thus, cell growth and expansion in a specific direction and selection of a division plane, all play important roles in plants morphogenesis.*

The irreversible increase in cell volume and surface area, as in the cell wall, are determinants of plant cell growth. Both intrinsic and extrinsic factors are required for cell growth. Both light and gravitational forces act as extrinsic factors, whereas the turgor pressure and many other biomolecules are intrinsic factors. Turgor pressure can be generated by water uptake of growing cells in their vacuoles. Since this pressure is homogeneous and multidirectional, the cell wall expands uniformly over the whole cell. Cell wall expansion consists in two processes: (1) stretching of the cell wall resulting from turgor pressure and (2) deposition of new material by the cell membrane in a specific direction. These two processes are related. During cell growth, the cell wall is stretched by turgor pressure because interpolymeric bonds in the wall naturally break and re-form. Thus the polymers forming cell wall, under tension from the turgor pressure, tend to slip past each other irreversibly to enlarge the cell wall. When the cell wall is stretched (normally 10–100-fold), it does not become thinner because new material is deposited to resist the strain of turgor pressure [8]. So the growing cell secretes substances to form a polymeric structure of crystalline cellulose microfibrils, embedded in a hydrophilic matrix, which are composed of hemicelluloses and pectins.

1.3.1.1.1   Role of Expansin and Extensin Proteins in Cell Elongation   Cosgrove [9] proposed the role of protein *expansins* in cell wall expansion by slippage or rearrangement of matrix polymers. Plant cell wall expansion occurs more rapidly at low pH. This event is known as *acid growth*. The primary cell wall of plant is composed of xylans (homopolymers of xylose), xyloglucans (heteropolymers whose backbone consists of glucose and sidechains with xylose), and mixed linked glucans (homopolymers of glucose). Xlycan (polysaccharide) molecule are present in the cell wall. They can stick to each other, as well as connect the cellulose microfibrils to each other. Expansins disrupt both types of bonding: between xlycans and between xlycan and cellulose. In presence of turgor pressure, expansins cause the displacement of wall polymers and a slippage occurs at the point of polymer adhesion. In shoot apical meristem, the expansins are expressed, and these proteins are present in primordium forming cells. During leaf initiation, the cell wall is altered by expansins. Thus, in presence of the turgor pressure, the cell wall of meristem expands in a specific direction; For example, it may bulge outward to form primodium. This is the regulatory role of the cell wall protein (expansin) in leaf initiation (plant morphogenesis) [10].

Extensins are a family of hydroxyproline-rich glycoproteins (HRGPs), which are found in the cell walls of higher plants. They play important roles in determining the cell shape and formation of the division plane during cell division. In dicots, extensins have a repeated pentapeptide Ser–(Hyp)$_4$ structure. It has been proposed that a positively charged extensin scaffold reacts with acidic pectin to form extensin pectate. This can act as the template for a newly synthesized cell plate during cell division. Thus extensins play an essential role in growth initiation of plants.

The *RSH* gene is a lethal mutant in *Arabidopsis* embryogenesis that encodes extensin AtEXT3, a structural glycoprotein located in the nascent cross wall or "cell wall" and also in mature cell walls. *RSH* is essential for the correct positioning of the cell plate during cytokinesis in cells of the developing embryo. *RSH* is detected in the first asymmetric cell division of the zygote [11]. In the *RSH* mutant, both apical and basal cells are formed, but the position of the plane of the newly synthesized cell wall is different, which may be compared to that of wild types. As a result, this event forms either same sized apical and basal cells or larger apical cells. This type of mutant also affects embryonic development in later stages, such as the globular stage. Cell division occurs during this stage, but the specific plane of division, as shown in Figure 1.2b, is not maintained. Therefore, cell divisions occur randomly. These stop the normal bilateral symmetry of embryogenesis.

The major component of the plant cell wall is polysaccharides (80% present in *Arabidopsis*). Pectin and hemicellulose are the main polysaccharides. In the mature cell wall, pectin is present in middle lamella, which adheres two adjacent plant cells to each other. Hemicellulose is involved in cell expansion, cell growth, and thus in cell shape formation. Both pectin and hemicellulose are synthesized and modified in Golgi complex. After packing into different vesicles (specific for each component), they are targeted to different domains of the cell wall. This type of physical segregation of components of cell wall is important for the normal growth and the development of plants. Extensin proteins, as mentioned earlier, are modified in *cis*-Golgi network and through secretary vesicles delivered to *trans*-Golgi network and ultimately to cell wall. Thus cell growth occurs. This explains the importance of selecting expansin and Extensin proteins in the genetic toolkit for plant cell elongation.

1.3.1.2 *Cell Division Phase* After elongation in a specific direction, cell division occurs in a specific plane, so that cell partition occurs along its longest axis. This is observed in the first cell division of the zygote, where apical–basal axis is formed by an asymmetric cell division.

1.3.1.2.1 Role of GNOM for Normal Cell Division From the very first cell division, Shevell et al. [12] observed that orientation of the plane of cell division, the rate of cell division, and GNOM gene products control the direction and amount of cell expansion. In the GNOM mutant, instead of asymmetric cell division in the zygote, two nearby equal-sized cells are formed. As a result of the distorted orientation of the plane of cell division, an altered octant embryo is formed with twice the number of cells found in the wild type. No cotyledonary primodia forms from apical cell. The root development is inhibited in the GNOM mutant because the basal cell fails to form the hypophysis. Very little elongation occurs in mutant cells with abnormal vacuoles [12]. In dark, wild-type hypocotyls elongate in the longitudinal direction. But for the dark-grown GNOM mutant, expansion occurs in both horizontal and longitudinal directions [12]. Thus, in the GNOM mutant, regulation on the direction of cell elongation is absent. Another important observation is that GNOM mutant cells can be separated easily from one another. This may be due to the inappropriate deposition of pectin or its derivatives in cell wall. From these observations, we can conclude that GNOM is essential for normal cell division, cell expansion, and cell adhesion in *Arabidopsis*.

ARF (ADP ribosylation factor) proteins are small guanine–nucleotide binding proteins. They are interconverted between two forms, such as GTP-bound ARFs and GDP-bound ARFs, by guanine–nucleotide exchange factors (GEFs) and by GTPase activating proteins (GAPs), respectively [13]. GNOM is a guanine–nucleotide exchange factor of ARF class proteins. It is present in the cytosolic face of endosomes. Generally ARFs are responsible for formation of vesicle coats, which are necessary for the formation of transport vesicles from donor compartments (i.e., vesicle budding) and cargo selection for transmembrane proteins. Here, GNOM proteins are involved in coat recruitment to endosomes for PIN1 protein targeting. PIN1 is a transmembrane protein, which is responsible for auxin hormone transport. GNOM proteins, as a regulator of intracellular vesicle trafficking, controls the rapid cycling of PIN1 proteins between the basal domain of plasma membrane and the endosomal compartments. Thus the embryos lacking the GNOM protein fail to establish the coordinated polar localization of the auxin–efflux regulator PIN1. This explains our selection of GNOM protein for the evolutionary–developmental (evo-devo) role of cell division in the plant genetic toolkit.

1.3.2   Cell Differentiation Phase

The term *differentiation* with respect to the plant cell refers to the property of plant cells to form quantitatively different specialized cell groups. During this phase, a number of cells that are derived from a single progenitor cell or a group of cells are qualitatively different in their contents and are specialized for different functions [6].

Several different mechanisms are involved in plant cell differentiation:

1. Signaling through cell wall–associated determinants (e.g., PIN)
2. Polarity by F-actin
3. Asymmetric cell division
   a. Differential cell division by G protein
   b. Asymmetric cleavages in different cell planes by TORMOZ
   c. Differential expansion rate by NPH4 transcription factor
4. Micro-RNA regulation by ZWILLE

In the next section, for each of these mechanisms, we evaluate the importance of associated proteins, to form the plant genetic toolkit.

1.3.2.1   *Role of PIN for Signaling through the Cell Wall (Associated Determinants)*   Cell polarity is an asymmetric distribution of the cellular components with respect to an arbitrary axis inside the cell [14]. An important example of plant polarity is the apical–basal polarity of the PIN family of auxin efflux facilitators, which forms the organization of the entire plant body. In plants, the matured embryo contents a main axis of polarity, with the shoot meristem flanked by the cotyledons (embryonic leaves) at the top end and separated by hypocotyl (embryonic stem) and root from the root meristem at the opposite pole [15]. This is due to tissue polarization (in addition to cell polarization) during plant development, which is necessary for organogenesis. Auxin hormone as a key regulator of tissue polarization controls its own polar transport in response to internal factors (various transcription factors) and external factors (light, gravity). Thus auxin is distributed asymmetrically along matured embryo.

Auxin is a multifunctional phytohormone that controls various developmental processes, such as cytoskeleton organization, intracellular membrane trafficking, cell polarity and morphogenesis, cell division, cell expansion, cell differentiation, organ formation and growth (lateral organ and root hair production), organization of plant architecture (phyllotaxis), and tropic growth [16]. The asymmetric distribution of auxin depends on polar transport of auxin by different transporter proteins such as PIN and AUX1, which facilitate the auxin efflux out of the cells and influx toward the cells, respectively.

In *Arabidopsis* the PIN (PINFORMED) family consists of eight members, which are distributed asymmetrically on different sides of various cells. According to the chemiosmotic model of auxin biology, the direction of intercellular auxin movement within the fields of cells is controlled by the position of efflux carriers at one side of the transporting cells. Thus auxin mediates the tissue and organ polarity. During the apical–basal axis formation of embryo, the polar localization and coordinated functions of PIN1, PIN2, PIN3, PIN4, and PIN7 are shown in Table 1.2 (see also Fig. 1.3).

Dhonukshe et al. [19] proposed a two-step mechanism for PIN polarity generation:

1. PINs are first targeted to the plasma membrane without apparent asymmetry (as shown in Table 1.2 in two-celled embryo for PIN1 protein).
2. Then they attain polarity by subsequent endocytic recycling.

In step 2, the clathrin-dependent endocytosis is crucial to establish polarity. The polar PIN localization is dynamic. PIN proteins continuously undergo cycles of clathrin-dependent endocytosis and ARF-GEF-(guanine–nucleotide exchange factors for ADP ribosylation factor GTPases)-dependent recycling such as the GNOM-depedent pathway for PIN1. The internal factor, the Ser/Thr kinase PINOID (PID) [20], plays a central role in the control of apical–basal PIN targeting [15]. The PID phosphorylates Ser337 and/or Thr340 in the central hydrophilic

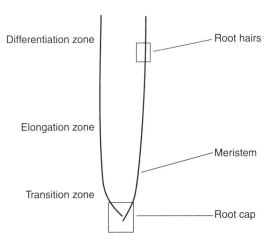

Figure 1.3 Matured root with different developmental regions.

TABLE 1.2   Tabulation Indicating Direction of Auxin Flow and Localization of PIN Proteins on Plasma Membrane during Four States of Embryogenesis

Stage of Embryogenesis	PIN Protein	Localization of PIN Proteins on Plasma Membrane	Direction of Auxin Flow and Developmental Output in Plant
Early two-celled stage	PIN1	In a nonpolar manner at inner cell boundary	Auxin accumulates in the proembryo through PIN7-dependent transport and triggers apical pole specification
	PIN7	*Apical* side of suspensor cells	
Middle globular stage	PIN1	*Basal* region in provascular cells	Auxin produced in the apical part and transported towards basal part of the embryo. Auxin accumulation causes root meristem specification.
	PIN7	*Basal* region of suspensor cells (relocalization)	
Early heart stage	PIN1	*Apical* surface of proembryo (relocalization)	Auxin accumulated symmetrically in position 2, triggering embryogenic leaves generation; auxin accumulation in hypophysis causing root pole specification
	PIN4	In central root meristem	
Matured root (Fig. 1.3)	PIN1	*Basal* end of vascular cells mainly and weakly in epidermis and cortex	Establishment of proper auxin transport route in root
	PIN2	*Apical* face in epidermal and lateral root cap cells and *basal* in cortical cells	
	PIN3	In nonpolar manner in tiers 2 and 3 of columella cells, *basal* side of vascullar cells, and *lateral* side of pericycle cells of elongation zone	
	PIN4	*Basal* surface in provascular cells and around the quescent centre and its surrounding cells	
	PIN7	*Lateral* and *basal* side of provascular cells in meristem and elongation zone and in columella cells	

Sources: Firml et al. [15], Blilou et al. [17], Feraru et al. [18].

loop of PIN proteins and PP2A phosphatase antagonizes this action. It has been observed that when PIN is in dephosphorylated form, basal PIN polar targeting occurs, and in phosphorylated state apical trafficking is preferred [21]. Thus the phosphorylaion acts as an internal signal for PIN polarization. PIN polarity forms auxin gradient by controlling the direction of auxin flow, resulting in organ formation in the plants. Furthermore, intact actin cytoskeleton plays an important role in interphase PIN trafficking, whereas this trafficking depends on microtubule during the cell divison phase [22].

1.3.2.2 Role of F-Actin in Cell Polarity (Determinant)

In the plant cell, the cytoskeleton, which is composed of microtubules and actin filaments, mediates cell growth. This cytoskeleton plays an important role in cell division, cell shape determination, cell expansion, and organelle movement. Specifically, three-dimensional (3D) networks of actin filaments are responsible for organelle and vesicle transport. Actin disrupting drugs can alter PIN1 positioning in plasma membrane because actin cytoskeleton controls the cycling of PIN1 between the endosomes and the cell membrane [22]. In columella cells, PIN3 targeting changes from the basal position toward the lateral side of the plasma membrane when the actin cytoskeleton is disrupted. This evokes a bending response in the root [23]. In shoots, actin disruption inhibits polar auxin transport. So, the auxin transport in plant is facilitated by dynamics of actin. It has been observed that intracellular motility of actin filaments will be decreased by stabilized actin in presence of auxin [24]. The bundling of actin causes reduced longitudinal transport of auxin and consecutively hampers root growth in the presence of gravitational force. The opposite result is observed with exogenous auxin addition by restoring normal actin network [25]. Thus it can be concluded that auxin controls its own efflux via actin cytoskeleton.

Phytohormone auxin is the central element for axis formation and pattern formation in plants. Auxin transport inhibitors (ATIs) establish the role of actin cytoskeleton in auxin polar transport. 2,3,5-Triidobenzoic acid (TIBA) and 2-(1-pyrenoyl) benzoic acid (PBA) are two ATIs. They stabilize the actin network by bundling of actin [19]. Thus the actin dynamics is inhibited in the plant. This stabilization hampers actin-dependent trafficking of auxin, causing a disturbance in the endocytosis, vesicle motility, and thus in the auxin transport. As a result, the plant development will be affected, since TIBA and PBA can disturb actin network in plant, by disrupting subcellular trafficking of PIN.

Actin proteins are present in two forms: (1) G-actin or globular subunit and (2) F-actin or filament actin. Both F-actin and actin filaments are polymeric form of monomeric G-actin. Actin binding proteins bundle actin filaments. Bundling of actin is the close alignment of F-actins, in either parallel or antiparallel orientation. These bundles are often aligned with the long axis of the cells. The actin network is composed of complicated configuration of filaments and bundles surrounding nucleus. There are 10 actin genes in the *Arabidopsis* genome. Among them, eight functional genes can be divided, according to their patterns of expression in plant, into two groups:

1. *Vegetative*—ACT2, ACT7, and ACT8
2. *Reproductive*—ACT1, ACT3, ACT4, ACT11, and ACT12

These five reproductive genes are expressed predominantly in reproductive organs such as in pollen tubes, but also in some vegetative tissues. Several different cellular processes are controlled by actin proteins:

1. *Cell Shape and Polarity.* These properties are established and maintained through auxin transport
2. *Tip Growth.* During cell growth, anisotropic expansion may result from continuous remodeling of the actin network [24]. Tip growth in root hair cells and pollen tubes is dependent on actin cytoskeleton [26]. Reduced cell elongation or expansion occurs as a result of actin cytoskeleton defects, as actin filaments are used as tracks for the transport of post-Golgi vesicles filled with cell wall components.
3. *Cytoplasmic Streaming.* The active movement of vesicles and organelles through the cytoplasm [46] have been identified by a mutant, substituting lysine with Glu272 in hydrophobic loop of ACT8. This position is very important for polymerization of G-actin. In mutants, the dynamics of Golgi stacks and mitochondria were disrupted. This proves the role of actin filaments in organelle transport.
4. *Cell Division.* The position of cell plate between two daughter cells during cell division is determined by the location of actin by formation of the preprophase band.

Arabidopsis-related protein 7 (ARP7) is an essential gene and is required for normal embryogenesis in *Arabidopsis*. For mutant embryo, the growth is stopped at the heart or torpedo stage [27]. ACT11 is the only *Arabidopsis* actin gene expressed at significant levels in ovule, embryo, and endosperm. The ACT11 isovariant plays distinct and required roles during *Arabidopsis* development [28].

1.3.2.3 *Role of TORMOZ in Asymmetric Cleavages in Different Cell Planes*

During development of the *Arabidopsis* embryo, the cell fate is determined in a position-dependent manner, since cell migration does not occur in the plant body. To obtain distinct cell types from a single progenitor cell, the asymmetric cell division is a common method. When a plant cell divides, a new cell wall forms between the daughter cells. The positioning of new walls has significant effects on development. By partitioning the cell into unequal parts with differing environments and differing contents, the site of the division plane influences subsequent cell fate. The selection of division plane or orientation of cell division is an important aspect in plant tissue organization and overall organ formation, including morphogenesis. Actin filaments accompanied by microtubules guide the formation of new cell wall during cytokinesis.

During embryogenesis in *Arabidopsis*, the first few successive cell divisions occur mostly perpendicular to previous divisions as shown in Figure 1.2.

The *TORMOZ* (*TOZ*) gene encodes a nucleolar protein. The mutation of the *TORMOZ* (*TOZ*) gene yields embryos with different cell division planes with abnormal patterns. Longitudinal division planes of the proembryo are changed mainly to transverse divisions and sometimes to oblique divisions. Again, divisions of the suspensor cells, which divide only transversely, appear generally unaffected [29]. Thus, TOZ function is to direct longitudinal cell divisions in the *Arabidopsis* embryo in the plant developmental gene toolkit.

1.3.2.4 *Role of G Protein in Differential Cell Division*

In animal the kingdom, heterotrimeric G proteins containing α, β, and γ subunits play important roles in different signaling pathways. Similarly, these types of plants proteins are important for various response reactions for hormones, drought, pathogens, and different developmental processes such as lateral root formation, hypocotyl elongation, and leaf expansion. Cell division is one of several biological processes that can be regulated by G-protein complex. *Arabidopsis* Gα (GPA1) and *Arabidopsis* Gβ (AGB1) subunits are more strongly expressed in roots than in shoots in young seedlings. Stem cells of the root apical meristem (RAM) generate different types of cells through cell division, followed by cell elongation. Root growth is a total process, the combined effect of maintenance of cells of root apical meristem (RAM) in the undifferentiated state and lateral root formation. The GTP-bound form of GPA1 accelerates cell division in the RAM. In the apical meristem, the GTP-bound form of the Gα subunit role is a positive modulator for cell proliferation. Lateral root production requires meristem formation by the founder pericycle cells. The *β* subunit of the *Arabidopsis* G protein negatively regulates cell division. The G*βγ* dimer inhibits cell division in the pericycle founder cells [30]. It was observed that the null alleles of *Arabidopsis* Gα (*gpa1*) have a reduced number of lateral root primordia, whereas the null alleles of *Arabidopsis* Gβ (*agb1*) have enhanced the cell division in roots, resulting in excessive lateral roots [31]. These results suggest that *Arabidopsis* heterotrimeric G-protein subunits have differential cell division in roots. Therefore, we select a G-protein subunit to include in the cell division phase of the developmental plant genetic toolkit.

1.3.2.5 *Role of NPH4 Transcription Factor in Differential Expansion Rate*

The unequal cellular growth in one position of an organ relative to an opposing position is observed in response to the environmental signals This is known as *differential growth*. Auxin modulates plant growth by regulating the transcription of specific mRNAs that encode proteins necessary for the growth control, such as α expansins.

The NPH4 gene of *Arabidopsis* is required for auxin-dependent differential growth responses of aerial tissues for both phototropism and gravitropism [32]. NPH4 gene encodes the auxin-regulated transcriptional activator ARF7. Auxin has been proposed to modulate gene expression through modification of ARF activity by auxin-dependent ARF–ARF and ARF–Aux/IAA dimerization. The dissociation–association state of NPH4/ARF7, whether it is present alone or as a complex with MSG2/IAA19 [33], determines the tropic responses of the hypocotyl. Tatematsu et al. [33] proposed a simple regulatory feedback loop for the control of auxin-dependent tropic responses, in which the transcriptional activity of NPH4/ARF7 is controlled by the Aux/IAA repressor protein MSG2/IAA19 via action of IAA-amido synthetases. When auxin accumulates, the ability of NPH4/ARF7 to function as a transcriptional activator is expected to be highest, and cell elongation is stimulated. In response to this event, the gravitropic or phototropic stimuli in hypocotyls two expansin genes, *EXPA1* and *EXPA8*, are upregulated only in the section where the cell elongation occurs [34]. These two tropic stimulus-induced genes, *EXPA1* and *EXPA8*, encode enzymes involved in cell wall extension. This response is essential for the differential growth leading to curvature. It was observed that before the macroscopic curvature *EXPA1* and *EXPA8* mRNAs expression was increased and cell expansion should be enhanced by the increased expansin delivery at the cell wall in response to auxin. Thus *EXPA1*- and *EXPA8*-encoded proteins are directly involved in differential growth response through the activity of NPH4 transcription factor in the developmental gene toolkit in plants.

1.3.2.6   *Role of ZWILLE as a Micro-RNA Regulation*   Posttranscriptional gene silencing is another method for plant cell differentiation. The small noncoding RNAs play an important role in the gene regulation in association with a unique class of proteins called argonautes [35]. When they are bound with small regulatory RNAs such as short interfering RNAs (siRNAs), or micro-RNAs (miRNAs), argonaute proteins can control protein synthesis by affecting messenger RNA stability.

Arabidopsis contains 10 Argonaute (AGO) proteins. *AGO10* is a member of the AGO family. This protein is required to establish the central–peripheral organization of the embryo apex. An empty apex, or a pinlike structure or the solitary leaf in place of the apex was observed in the mutants of *AGO10* gene, known as *pinhead* (*pnh*) or *zwille* (*zll*). *AGO10* plays another role in the formation of leaf adaxial–abaxial polarity to specify the leaf adaxial identity in plants [36]. AGO10 does both SAM maintenance and formation of leaf polarity by repressing miR165/166. Micro-RNAs (miRNAs) are ~21-nucleotide noncoding RNAs. Here two miRNAs, miR165 and miR166, differ in only one nucleotide in their mature RNA sequences. Because *PHB, PHV, and REV* have a complementary sequence of miR165 and miR166, so they can act as target sites for the cleavage activity of these two miRNAs cleavage activity. In earlier experiments it was shown that abnormally increased miR165/166 levels could result in a severe reduction of HD-ZIP III transcripts such as *REV,PHB*. The genes, which belong to HD-ZIP III transcription factor family such as *PHABULOSA (PHB)*, *PHAVULOTA (PHV)*, and REVOLUTA (REV), control vascular bundle development and adaxial–abaxial axis formation in leaves. Therefore the plant miRNAs (miR165/166) control the developmental pattern by downregulating important developmental transcription factors in the developmental genetic toolkit.

1.3.3 Plant Morphogenesis Phase

Plant morphogenesis is the development of plant form or shape and structure by coordinated cell division and growth. It is one of the three fundamental aspects of developmental biology along with the control of cell growth and cellular differentiation. The process controls the organized spatial distribution of cells during the embryonic development of an organism. Morphogenesis may be concerned with the whole plant, with a plant part, or with the subcomponents of a structure.

Since the cardiovascular system is absent in plants, plants have evolved specialized transport pathways to distribute signals and nutrients for coordination among different organs of the whole plant as well as different parts of an organ. There are two transport mechanisms: vascular system and intercellular transport pathways for plants. Two vascular networks, the phloem and the xylem, are primarily responsible for longdistance transport. The plasmodesmata, which form a meshwork of plant-specific cytoplasmic tunnels, play major role for intercellular transport.

Several different molecules are related to plant morphogenesis:

1. Long-range signaling through low-molecular-weight substances (FT protein)
2. Short-range signaling via transcription factor transfer (LEAFY)
3. Tissue identity maintenance signals (BEL1)
4. Signaling through extraembryonic and/or cell wall–associated determinants

1.3.3.1 Role of FT Protein in Longrange Signaling through Low-Molecular-Weight Substances
FLOWERING LOCUS T (FT) is a small globular protein of 20 kDa that serves as a long-range developmental signal in the plants. This mobile signal FT is expressed in the phloem tissues of cotyledons and leaves. It travels from the leaves to the shoot apex, through phloem companion cells, and triggers floral morphogenesis. The long-distance signal, called *florigen*, initiates flower formation that induces flowering in response to daylength. FT protein in *Arabidopsis* is an important part of florigen. It has been shown that full FT action in the leaf is dependent on the flowering time gene *FD*. Environmental factors such as temperature and light intensity, can change the timing of the transition to flowering not only by modifying *FT* transcript levels but also by modifying FT activity [37]. CONSTANS(CO) gene mediates transcriptional activation of *FT* under inductive daylength conditions. This gene itself regulates by a complex interplay of signals in the photoperiod pathway.

There are two types of mechanisms for regulation of FT gene expression:

1. Highly conserved sequence blocks in the 5-kb upstream promoter region, which are essential for *FT* activation by CONSTANS(CO) [38].
2. Binding of chromatin-associated proteins throughout the *FT* locus required for *FT* upregulation [38]. The *FD* gene, a bZIP transcription factor, identified as *AtbZIP14* (At4g35900), is preferentially expressed in the shoot apex. FD and FT are interdependent partners through protein interaction. FT is

likely to affect transcription of select genes, which together initiate a cascade of events leading to FT-dependent transcriptional changes in hundreds of genes within the shoot apex.

The FT protein acts in the shoot apex to induce target meristem identity genes such as *APETALA1* (*AP1*) and initiates floral morphogenesis [39]. Therefore FT and FD together act redundantly with the floral integrator LEAFY (LFY) to activate *AP1* transcription, because a plant containing mutations in both FT and LFY completely lacks floral structures and *AP1* expression [37].

1.3.3.2 *Role of LEAFY in Shortrange Signaling via Transcription Factor Transfer*

For intercellular communication, plants have evolved cytoplasmic bridges, called *plasmodesmata*, which act as a link of the fluid cytoplasm between adjacent cells. Many transcription factors can move between cells through plasmodasmata. Not all transcription factors move freely in the plant, because there are active mechanisms that regulate transcription factor movement [40]. Shoot apical meristem (SAM) consists of three tissue layers: the outermost layer (L1), the subsurface layer (L2), and the inner layer (L3). Within floral meristems LEAFY is expressed as mRNA in cells of L1 layer. Previously, LEAFY protein was found in a gradient that extended into several interior cell layers [47]. Not only LEAFY can undergo cell-to-cell transport into the underlying L2 and L3 layers, but it also retains its biological activity after transport as a DNA binding transcription factor [41].

The plant-specific transcription factor LEAFY (LFY) has central, evolutionarily conserved roles, both in the formation of the first flower during the meristem identity (MI) transition from vegetative growth and later in flower patterning in angiosperms probably since the origin of flowering plants [42,43]. LEAFY (LFY) is found in all land plants, which evolved during the past 400 million years, including both flowering and nonflowering plants [44]. But their role in nonflowering plants is not well understood. It has been proposed that LFY homologs have an ancestral role in regulating cell division and arrangement [43]. In flowering plants LFY protein provides only a redundant mechanism to ensure complete conversion of a meristem into a flower by movement of the protein to adjacent cells. During the floral transition, *AP1* expression is directly activated by LFY and by a complex consisting of FT and FD [45]. AP1 binds to promoter and regulates the expression of flowering time genes SVP, SOC1, and AGL24. This establishes the significance of LEAFY proteins in the role of short-range signaling via transcription factor transfer in the plant developmental genetic toolkit.

1.4 ANALYSIS

We analyze the candidate genes of the developmental genetic toolkit by using PLAZA 2.0, which integrates structural and functional annotation of 23 plants: 11 dicots, 5 monocots, 2 (club)mosses, and 5 algae. PLAZA is an access point for plant comparative genomics centralizing genomic data produced by different genome sequencing initiatives. It integrates plant sequence data and comparative genomic methods and provides an online platform to perform evolutionary analyses and data mining within the green plant lineage (viridiplantae).

The explicit phylogenetic framework existing in PLAZA framework depicts the early key events and evolution of land plants. Figure 1.4 exhibits a morphological evolution of land plants, consecutively descending from green plants, land plants, vascular plants (monocots), angiosperms, eudicots, and rosids to fabids. For analyzing our embryogenesis toolkit on land plants, we follow another simplified version of phylogenetic species tree, as illustrated in Figure 1.5.

Historically the "plant" phylum implies an association with certain traits, such as multicellularity, cellulose, and photosynthesis. In the evolutionary phylogenetics, *green plants* are also known as *viridiplantae*, *viridiphyta*, or *chlorobionta* [48]. This clade also includes the land plants plus Charophyta (i.e., stoneworts), and Chlorophyta (i.e., other green algae such as sea lettuce). The Viridiplantae clade encompasses a group of organisms that possess chlorophyll *a*, *b*, that have plastids that are bound by only two membranes and are capable of storing starch, and have cellulose in their cell walls. The multicellular land plants, called *embryophytes*, include the vascular plants, such as plants with full

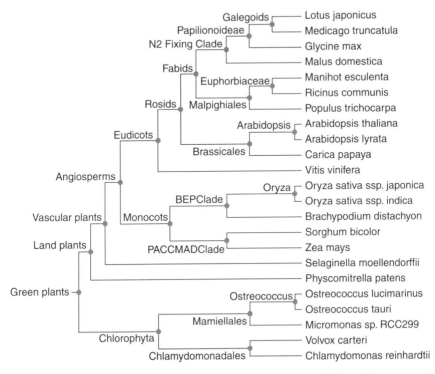

Figure 1.4 Phylogenetic relationships among different plants as inferred from state-of-the-art molecular and morphological phylogenetic analysis (PLAZA, web page).

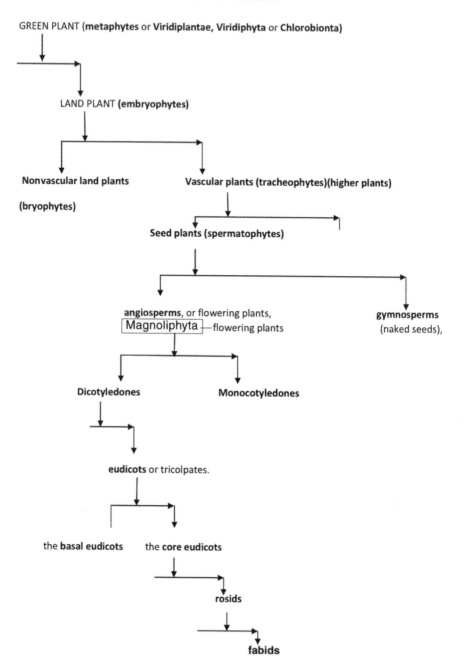

Figure 1.5   Phylogenetic tree of the evolution of land plants.

systems of leaves, stems, and roots. Consequently, early seed plants are referred to as *gymnosperms* (naked seeds) and angiosperms, representing the flowering plants.

Descending further in the evolutionary history, the *dicotyledons*, also known as *dicots*, are a group of flowering plants whose seed typically has two embryonic leaves or cotyledons. There are around 199,350 species within this group [49]. Flowering plants that are not dicotyledons are monocotyledons, typically having one embryonic leaf. Descending from this clade, the vast majority of "dicots" do form a monophyletic group called the *eudicots* or *tricolpates*. The term *eudicots* has been widely adopted to refer to one of the two largest clades of angiosperms (constituting >70% of all angiosperms); monocots constitute the other. Eudicots can be divided into two groups: basal eudicots and the core eudicots [49]. The term *basal eudicots* is an informal name for a paraphyletic group. The core eudicots are a monophyletic group. Within the core eudicots, the largest groups are the *rosids*, which are a large clade of flowering plants, containing about 70,000 species, [50] more than a quarter of all angiosperms [51]. This group is divided into 16–20 orders, depending on circumscription and classification. These orders, in turn, together comprise about 140 families [52]. The rosids and the asterids are by far the largest clades in the eudicots.

Considering this pattern of phylogenetic history as the baseline for the genetic systems evolution among plants, we further synthesize the phylogenetic relationships of the functions of our chosen developmental genes and their roles in hypothesizing the ancestral land plant developmental toolkit. Figures 1.6–1.16 illustrate the *cladograms*, which depicts relationships of our chosen orthologous developmental genes in land plants inferred from PLAZA 2.0 [54]. In each figure, the known gene names are labeled next to the lineages on the right side. The labels near each event indicate the clade for descendant lineages mapped onto the simple land plant phylogeny. The labels next to the branches indicate the branch length of the specific plant clade.

The following proteins and genes are analyzed here:

Expansin. The ATEXP1 family protein provides a more general role in embryogenesis inferring turgor pressure. This expansin family protein AT1G69530 has been implicated in expansion of cell wall and organ initiation. To assess the phylogenetic distribution of ATEXP1 gene family representing AT1G69530 gene, in Figure 1.6 we found that the orthologous genes of expansin genes are first present in eudicots. Therefore, introducing expansin for embryogenesis was a novel function acquired by the AT1G69530 gene in eudicot ancestors. Subsequently, ATEXP1 orthologous genes are expressed in the rosids, fabids, *Arabidopsis*, Euphorbiaceae, and then to Papilionoideae lineages. So expansin gene is included in developmental toolkit for plants.

Extensin. The leucin-rich ATEXT3 repeat family protein provides a more general role in embryogenesis inferring ancestral states from land plants. This extensin family protein AT1G21310 have been implicated in structural

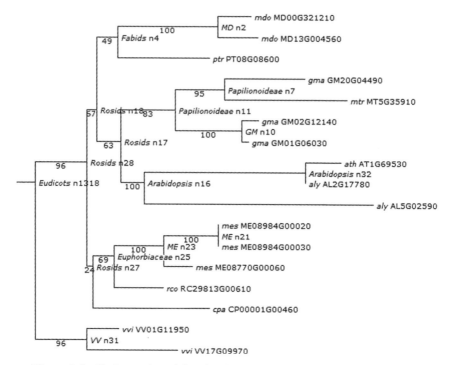

Figure 1.6   Phylogenetic and functional evolutionary history of ATEXP1 genes.

constituents of cell wall and protein binding, located in plant-type cell walls. The results for the ATEXT3 family protein in PLAZA are not satisfactory. Therefore, to verify the phylogenetic relationship of ATEXT3, we further analyze it using PHYTOZOME [53]. The results are depicted in Figure 1.7. The gene AT1G21310.1 is present in tracheophyte (~420 mya). These genes represent the most recent common ancestor of selaginella (spikemoss) and the angiosperms.

GNOM. Similarly, in Figure 1.8 the cladogram for GNOM gene (AT1G13980) is shown, which is responsible for asymmetric cell division in apical–basal axis formation. We find that GNOM gene was first present in all green plants. Not only in land plants, three genes from chlorophyta clade are also orthologous to the AT1G13980 gene of *A. thaliana* according to analysis using PLAZA 2.0. The phylogenetic branch length according to our PLAZA results is 100 for chlorophyta and angiosperm clades. This establishes the existence of the GNOM gene phylogenetically from green plants in plant evolutionary history.

TORMOZ. The TORMOZ gene is responsible for longitudinal cell division in pattern formation. Our phylogenetic analysis of orthologous genes of

7 families found

SEARCH CRITERIA *revise your search*
Search term: **peptidename:AT1G21310.1**
Search target: **families**
Member filtering: none
Search type: **Symbols/Identifiers/Deflines**

	NODE	DESCRIPTION	M. esculenta	R. comunis	P. trichocarpa	M. truncatula	G. max	C. sativus	P. persica	A. thaliana	A. lyrata	C. papaya	V. vinifera	M. guttatus	A. coerulea	S. bicolor	Z. mays	S. italica	O. sativa	B. distachyon	S. moellendorffii	P. patens	C. reinhardtii	V. carteri
296	Tracheophyte	LTPL116 - Protease inhibitor/seed storage/LTP family protein precursor, expressed	15	12	16	13	36	11	10	28	14	7	7	5	23	22	22	11	26	14	4	-	-	-
291	Embryophyte	Hypothetical gene (#27070060)	12	6	24	9	42	9	10	41	17	7	7	5	11	24	8	6	27	15	11	-	-	-
275	Viridiplantae	Hypothetical gene (#27074571)	6	3	24	8	42	7	10	41	13	5	7	5	8	24	8	6	28	16	11	1	2	-
35	Angiosperm	Hypothetical gene (#27054628)	2	-	3	-	7	-	2	9	2	-	1	-	3	1	-	2	3	-	-	-	-	-
8	Core Eudicot	Hypothetical gene (#27053935)	-	-	-	3	-	1	4	4	-	-	-	-	-	-	-	-	-	-	-	-	-	-
8	Rosid	Hypothetical gene (#27046853)	-	-	-	3	-	1	4	-	-	-	-	-	-	-	-	-	-	-	-	-	-	-
1	Arabidopsis thaliana columbia	ATEXT3 (EXTENSIN 3); structural constituent of cell wall	-	-	-	-	-	-	-	1	-	-	-	-	-	-	-	-	-	-	-	-	-	-

Figure 1.7 Phylogenetic analysis of extensin genes in PHYTOZOME.

23

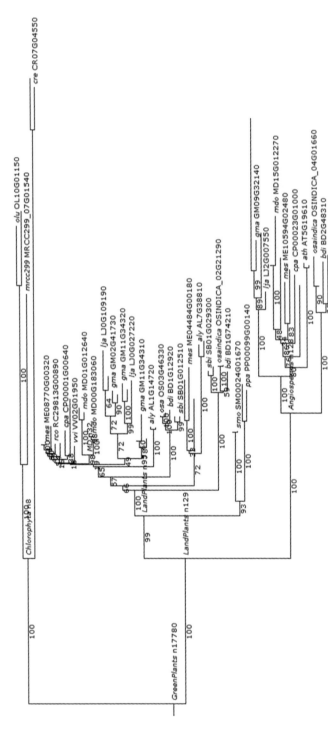

Figure 1.8 Phylogenetic and functional evolutionary history of GNOM genes.

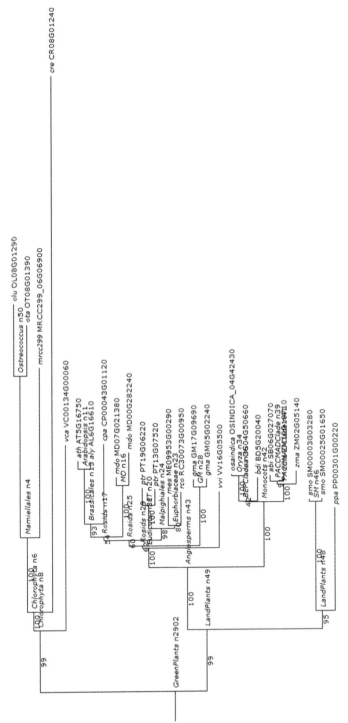

Figure 1.9 Phylogenetic and functional evolutionary history of TORMOZ genes.

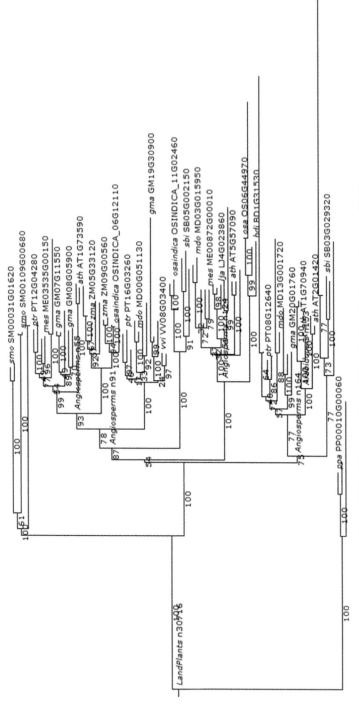

Figure 1.10 Phylogenetic and functional evolutionary history of PIN genes.

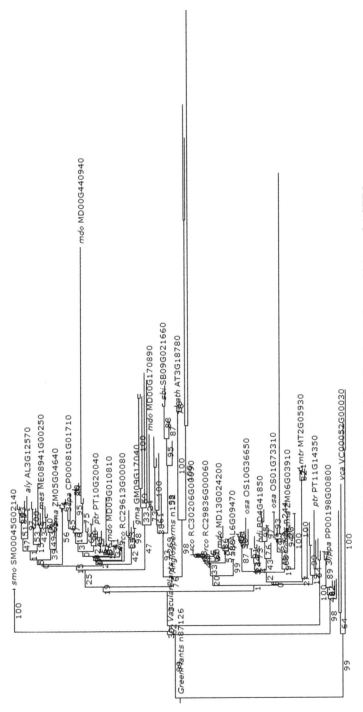

Figure 1.11 Phylogenetic and functional evolutionary history of ACTIN genes.

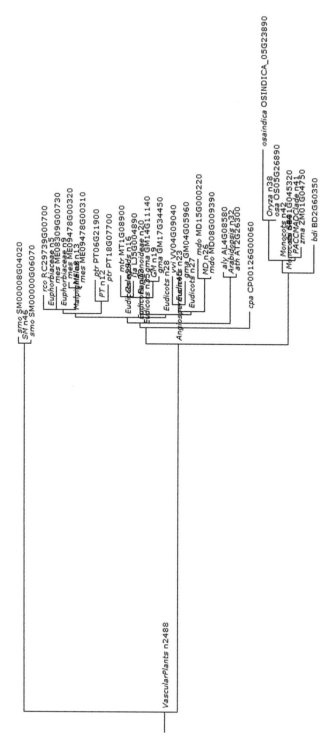

Figure 1.12 Phylogenetic and functional evolutionary history of G proteins.

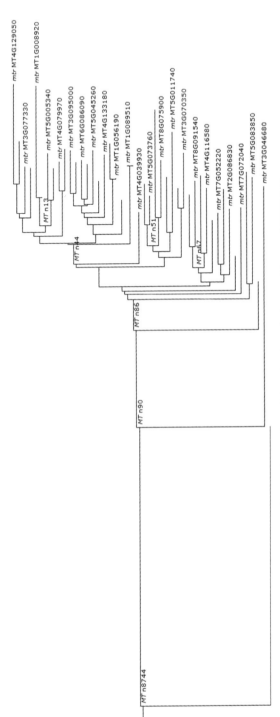

Figure 1.13 Phylogenetic and functional evolutionary history of NPH4TF.

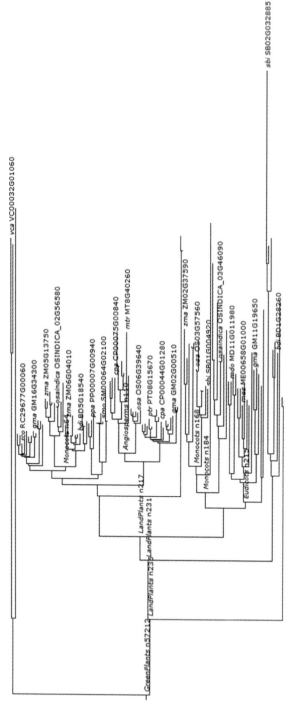

Figure 1.14 Phylogenetic and functional evolutionary history of AGO10.

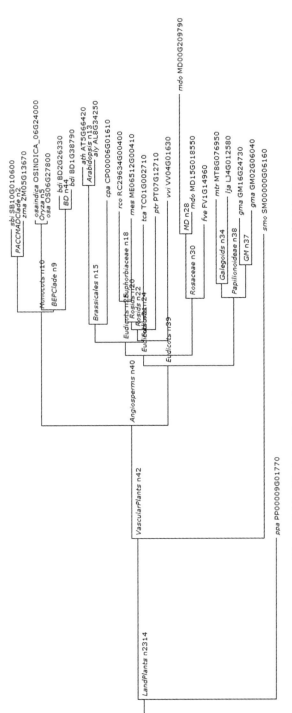

Figure 1.15 Phylogenetic and functional evolutionary history of LEAFY.

31

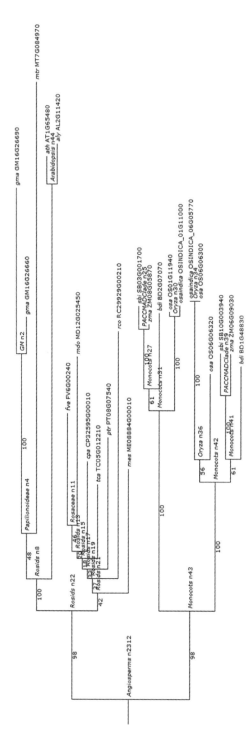

Figure 1.16 Phylogenetic and functional evolutionary history of FT protein.

TORMOZ family protein produces a gene tree that does not conflict with the organismic evolution tree in land plants. The orthologous genes of AT5G16750 TORMOZ gene, are identified in chlorophyta, land plants, angiosperms, eudicots, and rosids as shown in Figure 1.9. The topology suggests that diversification occurs following the divergence of green plants and descends to the major lineages of land plants.

PIN. Similarly, the ATPIN1 gene in the Pin protein family is responsible for asymmetric distribution in tissue polarization. In an attempt to assess the phylogenetic distribution of the ATPIN1 gene family representing the AT1G73590 gene, we observed the orthologous genes of the ATPIN1 gene to be initially present in land plants (Fig. 1.10). Subsequently, ATPIN1 orthologous genes are expressed in the angiosperms and *Arabidopsis*. Thus the ATPIN1 gene is included in the developmental toolkit for plants.

ACTIN. The ACT11 gene in *A. thaliana* AT3G12110 performs the function of anisotropic expansion for cellular polarity determination. To assess the phylogenetic distribution of the ACT11 gene family representing the AT3G12110 gene, we found that the orthologous genes of actin genes are initially present in all green plants (Fig. 1.11). Therefore, introducing actin for embryogenesis was a novel function acquired by the AT3G12110 gene in green plants ancestors, as one gene from S*elaginella moellendorffii* species is orthologous to the AT3G12110 gene of *A. thaliana* according to analysis using PLAZA 2.0. The *S. moellendorffii* species is a member of an ancient vascular plant lineage that first appeared in the fossil record some 400 mya. These lycopsids lack true leaves (having microphylls instead) and roots and thus represent an important node on the plant evolutionary tree. The presence of orthologous genes ACT11 in such ancient plant species as well as in comparatively younger vascular plants and angiosperms strongly suggest that ACTIN genes should be included in the developmental toolkit for plants.

G proteins. G proteins are responsible for dynamics in meristem maintenance with differential cell division, which results in lateral organ formation. Figure 1.12 shows that the ATGPA1 gene (AT2G26300) phylogenetically was initially present in all vascular plants, as two genes, SM00008G4020 and SM0000G06070 of S*elaginella moellendorffii* species, are orthologous to AT2G26300 gene of *A. thaliana* species.

NPH4 TF. Similarly, NPH4TF genes are responsible for the differential cell expansion in aerial tissue formation. However, phylogenetic analysis revealed this gene to be the smallest encompassing phylogenetic clade for this gene family as galegoids as shown in Figure 1.13. Although galegoids are mostly temperate and include clover, favabean, and the model legumes, which occupy a very small portion of the total plant kingdom, but these genes are included in developmental genetic toolkit for all plants because of their important functional characteristics.

AGO10. Consequently, the same quest for the phylogenetic evolution for AGO10 gene reveals its existence from all green plants as shown in Figure 1.14. The AGO10 gene is responsible for the complementary sequence binding in adaxial–abaxial polarity formation. This is possible for the existence of the orthologous gene VC00032G01060 in *Volvox carteri*. Each *Volvox* species is composed of numerous flagellate cells similar to *Chlamydomonas*, on the order of 10003000 in total, interconnected and arranged in a glycoprotein-filled sphere (coenobium). The cells swim in a coordinated fashion, with a distinct anterior–posterior configuration, or since *Volvox* resembles a small planet, with "north" and "south" poles. Following the phylogenetic tree, this gene is also present in ancestor clades such as land plants, angiosperms, monocots, and eudicots. This pattern reveals its selection for the phylogenetic toolkit.

LEAFY. The LEAFY protein acts in the intercellular communication through gradient formation for flower patterning. The existence of the PP00009G01770 gene in *Physcomitrella patens* in Figure 1.15 also proves the existence of LEAFY proteins in land plants in the phylogenetic evolution. Evidence for the existence of LEAFY protein is also revealed in vascular plants, angiosperms, eudicots, monocots, BEPClade, Euphorbiacae, Rosacae, Papilionoidae clades, and so on. Therefore, the LEAFY protein is included in the developmental genetic toolkit of plants.

FT Protein. Phylogenetic analysis for FT protein also shows its existence from all angiosperms. It is responsible for the signaling in floral morphogenesis. The orthologous genes of AT1G65480 in *A. thaliana* in Figure 1.16 are also present in monocots, rosids, Papilionoideae, and Rosaceae clades, so we include this gene in our plant developmental toolkit.

1.5 CONCLUSIONS

The plant kingdom includes familiar organisms such as trees, herbs, bushes, grasses, vines, ferns, mosses, and green algae. About 350,000 species of plants, defined as seed plants, bryophytes, ferns, and fern allies, are estimated to exist currently. As of 2004, approximately 287,655 species had been identified, of which 258,650 are flowering plants, 16,000 bryophytes, 11,000 ferns, and 8000 green algae. Despite the vast diversity of the plant kingdom in terms of size, shape, and form, nine fundamental body plan features originating from algae have been inherited by all members of the kingdom [5]. The 12 types of biomolecules mentioned in this chapter, are significant for three plant developmental processes such as cell growth, cell differentiation, and morphogenesis. The same molecules have been observed to be related to the nine fundamental body plan features. The relationships between features and types of biomolecules are described as follows:

1. Cellulosic cell wall—expansins
2. Cytokinetic phragmoplast—F-actin
3. Plasmodesmata—LEAFY
4. Apical meristematic cell—None found
5. Apical cell proliferation (branching)—extensins
6. Tissue differentiation—NPH4
7. Asymmetric cell division—TORMOZ, G proteins, and GNOM
8. Cell specialization capacity—FT proteins

All these biomolecules, discussed above, play important roles in plant pattern formation. At the same time, these molecules are well conserved along plant evolutionary history (see Table 1.3).

TABLE 1.3 Important Biomelecules and their Biological Roles in Evolutionary History

Characteristic Molecules	Physical Principles	Evo-devo Roles	Smallest Encompassing Phylogenetic Clade for This Gene Family
Expansin	Turgor pressure	Cell wall expansion and organ initiation	Vascular plants
Extensin	Turgor pressure	Growth initiation by cell plate formation	Land plants
GNOM	Asymmetric cell division	Apical–basal axis formation	Green plants
TORMOZ	Longitudinal cell division	Pattern formation	Green plants
PIN	Asymmetric distribution	Tissue polarization	Land plants
ACTIN	Anisotropic expansion	Cellular polarity determination	Green plants
G proteins	Dynamics in meristem maintenance (differential cell division)	Lateral organ formation	Vascular plants
NPH4 TF	Differential cell expansion	Aerial tissue formation	Galegoids
AGO10	Complementary sequence binding	Adaxial–abxaial polarity formation	Green plants
FT protein	Signaling	Floral morphogenesis	Angiosperms
LEAFY	Intercellular communication through gradient formation	Flower patterning	Land plants

We further establish the functional and biological significance for selecting these candidate genes in the developmental gene toolkit in plants with PLAZA 2.0 for comparative genomics in plants. This shows the phylogenetic evolution of all those genes consequently. Therefore a genetic toolkit for plant development can be prepared considering all the protein molecules mentioned above as a future project.

REFERENCES

1. Floyd SK, Bowman JL, The ancestral development toolkit of land plants, *Int. J. Plant Sci.* **168**(1):1–35 (2007).

2. Newman SA, The developmental genetic toolkit and the molecular homology–analogy paradox, *Biol. Theory* **1**(1):12–16 (2006).

3. Kenrick P, Crane PR, The origin and early evolution of plants on land, *Nature* **389**:33–39 (Sept. 2007).

4. Cronk Q, Plant evo-devo (evolution of plant development). *Sci. Topics*, Aug. 15, 2008 (available at http://www.scitopics.com/Plant_evo_devo_evolution_of_plant_development.html).

5. Graham LE, Cook ME, Busse JS, The origin of plants: Body plan changes contributing to a major evolutionary radiation, *Proc. Natl. Acad. Sci. USA* **97**(9):4535–4540 (April 2000).

6. Srivastava L, *Plant Growth and Development: Hormones and Environment*, Academic Press, New York, 2002.

7. Whang SS, Confocal microscopy study of *Arabidopsis* embryogenesis using GFP: mTn, *J. Plant Biol.* **52**(4):312–318 (Aug. 2009).

8. Proseus TE, Boyer SB, Turgor pressure moves polysaccharides into growing cell walls of Chara corallina, *Ann. Bot.* **95**(6):967–979 (2005).

9. Cosgrove DJ, Loosening of plant cell walls by expansins, *Nature* **407**(21):321–326 (Sept. 2000).

10. Fleming AJ, McQueen-Mason S, Mandel T, Kuhlemeier C, Induction of leaf primordia by the cell wall protein expansin, *Science* **276**:1415–1418 (1997).

11. Hall Q, Cannon MC, The cell wall hydroxyproline-rich glycoprotein RSH is essential for normal embryo development in *Arabidopsis*, *Plant Cell* **14**:1161–1172 (2002).

12. Shevell DE, Leu WM, Gillmor CS, Xia G, Feldman KA, Chua NH, EMB30 is essential for normal cell division, cell expansion, and cell adhesion in *Arabidopsis* and encodes a protein that has similarity to Sec7, *Cell* **77**:1051–1062 (1994).

13. Bonifacino JS, Jackson CL, Endosome-specific localization and function of the ARF activator GNOM, *Cell* **112**(2):141–142 (2003).

14. Geldner N, Cell polarity in plants: A PARspective on PINs, *Curr. Opin. Plant Biol.* **12**(1):42–48 (2009).

15. Friml J, Vieten A, Sauer M, Weijers D, Schwarz H, Hamann T, Offringa R, Jürgens G, Efflux-dependent auxin gradients establish the apical-basal axis of *Arabidopsis*, *Nature* **426**:147–153 (2003).

16. Gao X, Nagawa S, Wang G, Yang Z, Cell polarity signaling: Focus on polar auxin transport, *Mol. Plant* **1**(6):899–909 (2008).

17. Blilou I, Xu J, Wildwater M, Willemsen V, Paponov I, Friml J, Heidstra R, Aida M, Palme K, Scheres B, The PIN auxin efflux facilitator network controls growth and patterning in *Arabidopsis* roots, *Nature* **433**:39–44 (2005).

18. Feraru E. et al, PIN polar targeting, *Plant Physiol.* **147**:1553–1559 (2008).

19. Dhonukshe P. et al, Generation of cell polarity in plants links endocytosis, auxin distribution and cell fate decisions, *Nature* **456**:962–966 (2008).

20. Christensen SK, Dagenais N, Chory J, Weigel D, Regulation of auxin response by the protein kinase PINOID, *Cell* **100**(4):469–478 (2000).

21. Dhonukshe P, Kleine-Vehn J, Friml J, Cell polarity, auxin transport, and cytoskeleton-mediated division planes: Who comes first? *Protoplasma* **226**(1–2):67–73 (2005).

22. Geldner N, Friml J, Stierhof YD, Jurgens G, Palme K, Auxin transport inhibitors block PIN1 cycling and vesicle trafficking, *Nature* **413**:425–428 (2001).

23. Hou G, Kramer VL, Wang YS, Chen R, Perbal G, Gilroy S, Blancaflor EB, The promotion of gravitropism in *Arabidopsis* roots upon actin disruption is coupled with the extended alkalinization of the columella cytoplasm and a persistent lateral auxin gradient, *Plant J.* **39**:113–125 (2004).

24. Szymanski DB, Plant cells taking shape: New insights into cytoplasmic control, *Curr. Opinion Plant Biol.* **12**:735–744 (2009).

25. Nick P, Han M-J, An G, Auxin stimulates its own transport by shaping actin filaments, *Plant Physiol.* **151**:155–167 (2009).

26. Mathur J, Martin H, Microtubules and microfilaments in cell morphogenesis in higher plants, *Curr. Biol.* **12**:R669–R676 (2002).

27. Kandasamy MK, McKinney EC, Meagher RB, A single vegetative actin isovariant overexpressed under the control of multiple regulatory sequences is sufficient for normal *Arabidopsis* development, *Plant Cell* **21**(3):701–718 (2009).

28. Huang S, An YQ, McDowell JM, McKinney EC, Meagher RB, The *Arabidopsis* ACT11 actin gene is strongly expressed in tissues of the emerging inflorescence, pollen, and developing ovules, *Plant Mol. Biol.* **33**(1):125–139 (1997).

29. Griffith ME, Mayer U, Capron A, Ngo QA, Surendrarao A, McClinton R, Jürgens G, Sundaresan V, The TORMOZ gene encodes a nucleolar protein required for regulated division planes and embryo development in *Arabidopsis*, *Plant Cell* **19**(7):2246–2263 (2007).

30. Chen J-G, Gao Y, Jones AM, Differential roles of *Arabidopsis* heterotrimeric G-protein subunits in modulating cell division in roots, *Plant Physiol.* **141**(3):887–897 (2006).

31. Ullah H, Chen J-G, Temple B, Boyes DC, Alonso JM, Davis KR, Ecker JR, Jones AM, The β-subunit of the *Arabidopsis* G protein negatively regulates auxin-induced cell division and affects multiple developmental processes, *Plant Cell* **15**(2):393–409 (2003).

32. Harper RM, Stowe-Evans EL, Luesse DR, Muto H, Tatematsu K, Watahiki MK, Yamamoto K, Liscum E, The NPH4 locus encodes the auxin response factor ARF7, a conditional regulator of differential growth in aerial *Arabidopsis* tissue, *Plant Cell* **12**(5):757–770 (2000).

33. Tatematsu K, Kumagai S, Muto H, Sato A, Watahiki MK, Harper RM, Liscum E, Yamamoto KT, MASSUGU2 encodes Aux/IAA19, an auxin-regulated protein that functions together with the transcriptional activator NPH4/ARF7 to regulate differential growth responses of hypocotyl and formation of lateral roots in *Arabidopsis thaliana*, *Plant Cell* **16**(2):379–393 (Feb. 2004).

34. Esmon CA, Tinsley AG, Ljung K, Sandberg G, Hearne LB, Liscum E, A gradient of auxin and auxin-dependent transcription precedes tropic growth responses, *Proc. Natl. Acad. Sci.* **103**(1):236–241 (2006).

35. Hutvagner G, Simard MJ, Argonaute proteins: Key players in RNA silencing, Nat. *Rev. Mol. Cell. Biol.* **9**(1):22–32 (2008).

36. Liu Q, Yao X, Pi L, Wang H, Cui X, Huang H, The *ARGONAUTE10* gene modulates shoot apical meristem maintenance and establishment of leaf polarity by repressing miR165/166 in *Arabidopsis*, *Plant J.* **58**(1):27–40 (2009).

37. Teper-Bamnolker P, Samach A, The flowering integrator FT regulates SEPALLATA3 and FRUITFULL accumulation in *Arabidopsis* leaves, *Plant Cell* **17**(10):2661–2675 (2005).

38. Adrian J, Farrona S, Reimer JJ, Albani MC, Coupland G, Turck F, cis-Regulatory elements and chromatin state coordinately control temporal and spatial expression of flowering locus T in *Arabidopsis*, *Plant Cell* **22**(5):1425–1440 (May 2010).

39. Notaguchi M, Abe M, Kimura T, Daimon Y, Kobayashi T, Yamaguchi A, Tomita Y, Dohi K, Mori M, Araki T, Long-distance, graft-transmissible action of *Arabidopsis* flowering locus T protein to promote flowering, *Plant Cell Physiol.* **49**:1645–1658 (2008).

40. Wu X, Weigel D, Wigge PA, Signaling in plants by intercellular RNA and protein movement, *Genes Dev.* **16**:151–158 (2002).

41. Haywood V, Kragler F, Lucas WJ, Plasmodesmata pathways for protein and ribonucleoprotein signaling, *Plant Cell* **14**:S303–S325 (May 2002).

42. Winter CM, Austin RS, Reback MA, Wu M, Yamaguchi A, Li H, Wagner D, LEAFY target genes reveal a direct link between external stimulus response and flower development, *Proc. 21st Int. Conf. Arabidopsis Research*, Japan 2010.

43. Moyroud E, Kusters E, Monniaux M, Koes R, Parcy F, LEAFY blossoms, *Trends Plant Sci.* **15**(6):346–352 (June 2010).

44. Maizel A, Busch MA, Tanahashi T, Perkovic J, Kato M, Hasebe M, Weigel D, The floral regulator LEAFY evolves by substitutions in the DNA binding domain, *Science* **308**(5719):260 (2005).

45. Liu C, Thong Z, Yu H, Coming into bloom: the specification of floral meristems. *Development* **136**:3379–3391 (2009). doi:10.1242/dev.033076.

46. Kato T, Morita MT, Tasaka M, Defects in dynamics and functions of actin filament in *Arabidopsis* caused by the dominant-negative actin fiz1-induced fragmentation of actin filament, *Plant Cell Physiol.* **51**(2):333–338 (2010). doi:10.1093/pcp/pcp189.

47. Sessions A, Yanofsky MF, Weigel D, Cell-cell signaling and movement by the floral transcription factors LEAFY and APETALA1, *Science* **289**(5480):779 (2000). doi: 10.1126/science.289.5480.779.

48. Kenrick P, Crane P, *The Origin and Early Diversification of Land Plants: A Cladistic Study*. Smithsonian Institution Press, Washington, DC, 1997.

49. Hamilton A, Hamilton P, *Plant Conservation: An Ecosystem Approach*, Earthscan, London, 2006, p. 2.

50. Wang H-C, Moore MJ, Soltis PS, Bell CD, Brockington SF, Alexandre R, Davis CC, Latvis M, Manchester SR, Soltis DE, Rosid radiation and the rapid rise of angiosperm-dominated forests, *Proceedings of the National Academy of Sciences* **106**(10):3853–3858 (2009).

51. Scotland RW, Wortley AH, How many species of seed plants are there?, *Taxon* **52**(1):101–104 (2003).

52. Soltis DE, Soltis PS, Endress PK, Chase MW, *Phylogeny and Evolution of the Angiosperms*, Sinauer, Sunderland, MA, 2005.

53. Goodstein DM, Shu S, Howson R, Neupane R, Hayes RD, Fazo J, Mitros T, Dirks W, Hellsten U, Putnam N, Rokhsar DS, Phytozome: a comparative platform for green plant genomics, *Nucleic Acids Res.* **40**(D1):D1178–D1186 (2012).

54. Proost S, Van Bel M, Sterck L, Billiau K, Van Parys T, Van de Peer Y, Vandepoele K, PLAZA: a comparative genomics resource to study gene and genome evolution in plants, *Plant Cell* **21**:3718–3731 (2009).

BIBLIOGRAPHY

Cannon MC, Terneus K, Hall Q, Tan L, Wang Y, Wegenhart BL, Chen L, Lamport DT, Chen Y, Kieliszewski MJ, Self-assembly of the plant cell wall requires an extensin scaffold, *Proc. Natl. Acad. Sci. USA* **105**(6):2226–2231 (2008).

Corbesier L, Vincent C, Jang SH, Fornara F, Fan QZ, Searle I, Giakountis A, Farrona S, Gissot L, Turnbull C, Coupland G, FT protein movement contributes to long-distance signaling in floral induction of *Arabidopsis*, *Science* **316**:1030–1033 (2007).

Donaldson JG, Jackson CL, A cell-centered approach to developmental biology, *Curr. Opin. Cell Biol.* **12**:475–482 (2000).

Dupree P, Plant embryogenesis: Cell division forms a pattern, *Curr. Biol.* **6**(6):683–685 (June 1996).

Geldner N, The Arabidopsis GNOM ARF-GEF mediates endosomal recycling, auxin transport, and auxin-dependent plant growth, *Cell* **112**:219–230 (2003).

Jaeger KE, Wigge PA, FT protein acts as a long-range signal in *Arabidopsis*, *Curr. Biol.* **17**:1050–1054 (2007).

Jürgens G, Apical-basal pattern formation in the *Arabidopsis* embryo: Studies on the role of the *gnom* gene, *Development* **117**:149–162 (1993).

Jürgens G, Apical-basal pattern formation in *Arabidopsis* embryogenesis, *EMBO J.* **20**:3609–3616 (2001).

Kleine-Vehn J, Dhonukshe P, Swarup R, Bennett M, Friml J, Subcellular trafficking of the Arabidopsis auxin influx carrier AUX1 uses a novel pathway distinct from PIN1, *Plant Cell* **18**(11):3171–3181 (2006).

Kleine-Vehn J, Langowski L, Wisniewska J, Dhonukshe P, Brewer PB, Friml J, Cellular and molecular requirements for polar PIN targeting and transcytosis in plants, *Mol. Plant* **1**(6):1056–1066 (2008).

Kleine-Vehn J, Friml J, Polartargeting and endocytic recycling in auxin-dependent plant development, *Annu. Rev. Cell Dev. Biol.* **24**:447–473 (2008).

Kleine-Vehn J, Dhonukshe P, Sauer M, Brewer PB, Wisniewska J, Paciorek T, Benkova E, Friml J, ARF GEF-dependent transcytosis and polar delivery of PIN auxin carriers in *Arabidopsis*, *Curr. Biol.* **18**:526–531 (2008).

Lyndon RF, *Plant Development: The Cellular Basis*, Unwin Hyman, London, 1990.

Mayer U, Büttner G, Jürgens G, Apical-basal pattern formation in the *Arabidopsis* embryo: Studies on the role of the *gnom* gene, *Development* **117**:149–162 (1993).

Ma H, Plant G proteins: The different faces of GPA1, *Curr. Biol.* **11**:R869–R871 (2001).

Merks R, Glazier J, Statistical mechanics and its applications, *Phys A. Appl. Biol. Syst.* **352**(1):113–130 (July 2005).

Mathieu J, Warthmann N, Kuttner F, Schmid M, Export of FT protein from phloem companion cells is sufficient for floral induction in *Arabidopsis*, *Curr. Biol.* **17**:1055–1060 (2007).

Niklas KJ, Simulation of organic shape: The roles of phenomenology and mechanism, *J. Morphol.* **219**(3):243–246 (2005).

Niklas KJ, Spatz H-C, Vincent J, Plant biomechanics: An overview and prospectus, *Am. J. Bot.* **93**:1369–1378 (2006).

Perrot-Rechenmann C, Cellular responses to auxin: Division versus expansion, *Cold Spring Harbor Perspect. Biol.* **2**(5):a001446 (May 2010).

Salazar-Ciudad I, Looking at the origin of phenotypic variation from pattern formation gene networks, *J. Biosci.* **34**:573–587 (2009).

Schopfer P, Biomechanics of plant growth, *Am. J. Bot.* **93**:1415–1425 (2006).

Steinmann T, Geldner N, Grebe M, Mangold S, Jackson CL, Paris S, Galweiler L, Palme K, Jürgens G , Coordinated polar localization of auxin efflux carrier PIN1 by GNOM ARF GEF, *Science* **286**(5438):316–318 (1999).

Surpin M, Raikhel N, Traffic jams affect plant development and signal transduction, *Nature* **5**:100–109 (2004).

Zhang J, Nodzynski T, Pencik A, Rolcik J, Friml J, PIN phosphorylation is sufficient to mediate PIN polarity and direct auxin transport, *Proc. Natl. Acad. Sci.* **107**:918–922 (2010).

CHAPTER 2

PROTEIN SEQUENCE MOTIF INFORMATION DISCOVERY

BERNARD CHEN

2.1 INTRODUCTION

Proteins can be regarded as one of the most important elements in the process of life; they can be grouped into different families according to their sequential or structural similarities. Many biochemical tests suggest that a sequence determines conformation completely, because all the information that is necessary for specifying protein interaction sites with other molecules is embedded into the protein's amino acid sequence. The close relationship between protein sequence and structure plays an important role in current analysis and prediction technologies. Therefore, understanding the hidden relationships between protein structures and their sequences is an important task in modern bioinformatics research. The biological term *sequence motif* denotes a relatively small number of functionally or structurally conserved sequence patterns that occur repeatedly in a group of related proteins. These motif patterns may be able to predict the structural or functional area of other proteins, such as enzyme binding sites, DNA or RNA binding sites, prosthetic attachment sites, and protein–protein interaction sites.

PROSITE [1], PRINTS [2], and BLOCKS [3] are three of the most popular motif databases. PROSITE is a method for determining the function of uncharacterized proteins translated from genomic or cyclic DNA (cDNA) sequences. It consists of a database of biologically significant sites and patterns formulated in such a way that with appropriate computational tools, it can rapidly and reliably identify to which known family of protein (if any) the new sequence belongs [1]. Analysis of 3D structures of PROSITE patterns suggests that recurrent sequence motifs imply common structure and function. Fingerprints, a group of conserved motifs used to characterize a protein family, from PRINTS, contain several motifs from different regions of multiple sequence alignments, increasing the ability to

Algorithmic and Artificial Intelligence Methods for Protein Bioinformatics. First Edition.
Edited by Yi Pan, Jianxin Wang, Min Li.
© 2014 John Wiley & Sons, Inc. Published 2014 by John Wiley & Sons, Inc.

predict the existence of similar motifs because individual parts of the fingerprint are mutually conditional [2]. The blocks are multiply aligned ungapped segments corresponding to the most highly conserved regions of proteins. The *BLOCKS database* is constructed automatically by searching for the most highly conserved regions in groups of proteins documented in the PROSITE database [3]. Since sequence motifs from PROSITE, PRINTS, and BLOCKS are developed from multiple alignments, these sequence motifs search for conserved elements of sequence alignment only from the same protein family and carry little information about conserved sequence regions, which transcend protein families [4].

The commonly used tools for protein sequence motif discovering include MEME [5], Gibbs sampling [6], and BlockMaker [7]. Some newer algorithms include MITRA [8], ProfileBranching [9], and generic motif discovery algorithm for sequential data [10]. When using these tools, users are asked to give several protein sequences, normally presented in the FASTA format, as the input data. Again, sequence motifs discovered by the above mentioned methods may carry little information that crosses family boundaries because the size of the input dataset is limited.

Some researchers [4,11,28] have tried to obtain protein sequence motifs that are universally conserved across protein family boundaries. To achieve this goal, the input dataset has to be large enough to somehow represent all known protein sequences. Han and Baker [11] have used the K-means clustering algorithm to find recurring protein sequence motifs. They selected a set of initial points as the centroids at random. Zhong et al. [4] proposed an improved K-means clustering algorithm to obtain initial centroid locations more wisely. Because K-means clustering performance is very sensitive to initial point selection, the experiment by Zhong et al. [4] shows improved results. Those authors [4] used the K-means clustering algorithm instead of other more advanced clustering technology primarily because of the extremely large input dataset. Since K-means clustering is known for its efficiency, other clustering methods with higher spatiotemporal costs may not be suitable for this task.

2.2   GRANULE COMPUTING APPROACHES

Granular computing [16–26] represents information in the form of aggregates, also called *information granules*. For a huge and complicated problem, it applies the divide-and-conquer concept to split the original task into several smaller subtasks to save time and space complexity. Also, in the process of splitting the original task, it comprehends the problem without including meaningless information. As opposed to traditional data-oriented numeric computing, granular computing is knowledge-oriented [18].

2.2.1   *K*-Means Clustering Algorithm

The process of grouping a set of physical or abstract objects into classes of similar objects is called *clustering* [27]. A cluster is a collection of data objects that are similar to one another within the same cluster and are dissimilar to the objects in other clusters. In terms of machine learning, clustering is a typical example of unsupervised learning that indicates that the learning process does not rely on predefined classes. Therefore, clustering is a form of learning by observation, rather than by examples [27].

The K-means clustering algorithm proceeds as followings:

1. The K-means clustering algorithm randomly selects k objects from the dataset to represent the initial cluster centroids.
2. For each remaining object, according to the given distance calculation measurement, the object is assigned to the closest cluster.
3. After step 2, each cluster computes the new centroid of the cluster by averaging all members of the cluster.
4. Steps 2 and 3 iterate until all the centroids remain at the same position.

The pseudocode of the basic K-means clustering algorithm is presented in Figure 2.1.

Among all clustering algorithms, the K-means one has the advantages of easy interpretation and implementation, high scalability, and low computation complexity. K-means clustering takes the user input parameter k, and partitions a set of n objects into k clusters so that the resulting intracluster similarity is high but the intercluster similarity is low [27].

2.2.2   Fuzzy C-Means Clustering Algorithm

Fuzzy C-means (FCM) [29,30] is a clustering algorithm that allows one segment of data to belong to one or more clusters. Minimization of the following objective function is the main principle of FCM:

$$J_m = \sum_{i=1}^{N} \sum_{j=1}^{C} u_{ij}^m \| x_i - c_j \|^2, \qquad 1 \le m < \infty$$

```
(1)   arbitrarily choose K objects as the initial centroid;
(2)   repeat
(3)         (re)assign each remaining object to the cluster to
            which the object is the most Similar, based on the
            mean value of the object in the cluster;
(4)         update the cluster mean;
(5)   until no change;
```

Figure 2.1   The K-means clustering algorithm [27].

The fuzzification factor m is any real number greater than 1; U_{ij} is defined as the degree of membership for each data member x_i in the cluster j. The term x_i is the ith member of d-dimensional measured data, c_j is the d-dimensional center of the cluster, and $|| * ||$ is any norm expressing the similarity between any measured data and the center. Two major execution mathematical functions for FCM are the update of membership U_{ij} and cluster centers C_j defined as the follows:

$$u_{ij} = \frac{1}{\sum_{k=1}^{C} \left(\frac{\| x_i - c_j \|}{\| x_i - c_k \|} \right)^{2/(m-1)}}$$

$$c_j = \frac{\sum_{i=1}^{N} u_{ij}^{m} \cdot x_i}{\sum_{i=1}^{N} u_{ij}^{m}}$$

The Fuzzy C-means clustering algorithm proceeds in the following steps, which are very similar to those for the K-means clustering algorithm:

1. The FCM clustering algorithm randomly selects k objects from the dataset to represent the initial cluster centroids.
2. For each object, according to the given distance calculation measurement, calculate the degree of membership U_{ij} with all clusters.
3. After step 2, each cluster computes the new centroid of the cluster C_j.
4. Steps 2 and 3 iterate until all the centroids remain at the same position or a termination criterion.

The pseudocode for the basic fuzzy C-means clustering algorithm is presented in Figure 2.2.

```
(1)  initialize membership function matrix, U(0), and randomly
        select a set of initial centroids.;
(2)  repeat
(3)        at k-step: update U(k) to U(k+1) by the function
              of uij;
(4)        calculate the centroid information by cj function;
(5)  until |U(k+1) − U(k)| < ε [19];
```

Figure 2.2   The fuzzy C-means clustering algorithm.

2.2.3 The Fuzzy Greedy *K*-Means (FGK) Model

A granular computing model called *fuzzy–greedy-K-means model* (FGK model) has been proposed [28] to detect protein sequence motifs that transcend protein family boundaries. The FGK model works by using FCM to build a set of information granules and then apply the greedy *K*-means clustering algorithm to obtain the final information. Instead of randomly selecting initial seeds in each round of the original *K* means, the greedy *K*-means clustering algorithm collects five set of results generated by original *K* means and then select the initial centroids from centroids of the high-quality clusters in previous results. Because the centroids in higher-quality clusters have the potential to generate better clusters in the sixth round, the selection procedure into several steps: initially gathering centroid seeds belonging to clusters with the highest-quality measurement and then decreasing the quality measurement threshold gradually. For example, in the protein sequence motif discovery process, the sixth-round initial centroid selection procedure is divided into five steps: initially gathering centroid seeds belonging to clusters with structural similarity >80% and then proceeding with 75%, 70%, 65%, and 60%. For each new selected new centroid candidate, its distance is checked against all points that are already selected in the initialization array. If the minimum distance of a new point between all existing centroids is greater than the threshold distance, this point will be included in the initialization array as a new centroid (because this point is dissimilar to all other points); otherwise, the new point is too close with existing centroids and should be discarded. (because this point is similar to some points that already existed in the initial centroid pool). Experimental results with different threshold are given in the next section. The major advantages of the FGK model are reduced spatiotemporal complexity, filtered outliers, and higher-quality granular information results [28]. The basic concept of the FGK model is depicted in Figure 2.3.

2.3 EXPERIMENTAL SETUP

2.3.1 Experimental Dataset

Since the major purpose of this work is to obtain protein sequence motif information across protein family boundaries, the dataset of our work is intended to represent all known protein sequences. However, without a systematic approach, it is very difficult to extract useful knowledge from an extremely large volume of data. We apply the basic principle of selecting representative protein files from the whole PDB database and then using the profile in the Homology-derived Secondary Structure of Proteins (HSSP) database [13] to expand each file.

The dataset used in this work includes 2710 PDB protein sequences obtained from the Protein Sequence Culling Server (PISCES) [12]. Among these 2710

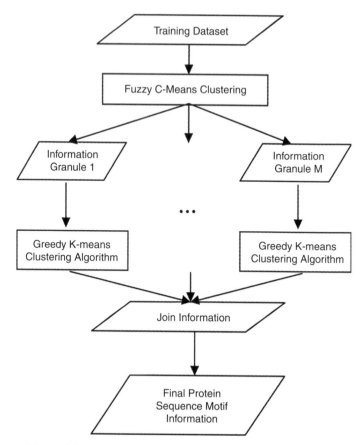

Figure 2.3   Sketch of the fuzzy greedy *K*-means (FGK) model.

protein sequences, no sequence in this database shares more than 25% sequence identity. HSSP is a derived database merging structural (3D) and sequence (1D) information. For each protein of known 3D structure from the Protein Data Bank (PDB), the database has a multiple sequence alignment of all available homologs and a sequence profile characteristic of the family [13]. At the end of each HSSP file, it calculates the occurrence percentage of every amino acid on each sequence position. An example of the 1b25 HSSP file is given in Figure 2.4.

The sliding-window technique with nine successive residues is generated from protein sequences. Each window represents one sequence segment of nine contiguous positions. More than 560,000 segments are generated by this method. Each window corresponds to a sequence segment, which is represented by a 9×20 matrix; 20 rows represent 20 amino acids and 9 columns represent each position of the sliding window. For the frequency profiles (HSSP) representation for sequence segments, each position of the matrix represents the frequency for a specified amino acid residue in a sequence position for the multisequence alignment.

```
## SEQUENCE PROFILE AND ENTROPY
 SeqNo PDBNo   V   L   I   M   F   W   Y   G   A   P   S   T   C   H   R   K   Q   E   N   D
     1    1 A   0  22   6  72   0   0   0   0   0   0   0   0   0   0   0   0   0   0   0   0
     2    2 A   3   0   0   3  14   0  22  22   6   3   0   3   0   0   3  14   0   3   0   6
     3    3 A   0   0   0   0   0   0   2  93   2   0   0   0   0   0   2   0   0   0   0   0
     4    4 A   0   0   2   0  13  26  50   0   2   0   0   2   0   0   2   0   0   0   2   0
     5    5 A   0   0   0   4   0  20   0   0  17   0   0  17   4  11   0   7   7   0  13   0
     6    6 A   0   0   0   0   0   0   0  72   0   0   2   0   2   4   2   0   0   2   9   7
     7    7 A   2   0   0   0   0   0   0   0   0   0   0   2   0   2  45  47   0   0   2   0
     8    8 A  27   3  55   5   2   0   0   2   0   0   3   3   0   0   0   0   0   0   0   0
     9    9 A   5  68   5   0   0   0   3   0  18   0   0   0   0   0   0   0   0   0   0   0
    10   10 A   5   2   0   0   7   3   8   0   0   0   0   0   0   3  58   2   0   3   3   5
    11   11 A  65   0  33   0   0   0   0   0   2   0   0   0   0   0   0   0   0   0   0   0
    12   12 A   0   0   0   0   0   0   0   0   0   0   0   0   0   0   0   0   0   0  35  65
    13   13 A   0  95   0   3   0   0   0   0   0   0   0   2   0   0   0   0   0   0   0   0
    14   14 A   0   0   0   0   0   0   0   7   3   0  38  37   0   0   2   3   0   3   3   3
    15   15 A   0   0   0   0   0   0   0   2   8   0  17  30   0   0   5   8   0  10  12   8
    16   16 A   0   3   0   2   0   0   2  45   2   0   2   0   0   0  18  10   2  12   3   0
```

Figure 2.4 Part of the 1b25 HSSP file. Columns 1 and 2 (on left) give the PDB protein sequence number and chain number, respectively. For each amino acid location, the tabulation gives 20 numbers representing the percentage of the occurrence of each amino acid.

We also obtained secondary structure from the Dictionary of Secondary Structure of Proteins (DSSP) [14], which is a database of secondary structure assignments for all protein entries in the Protein Data Bank (PDB), for each sequence segment. The main uses of secondary structure information are to evaluate sequence clusters. Originally, DSSP allocates the secondary structure to eight different classes. However, in this study, those eight classes are reclassified into three categories according to the following conversion model: assigning *H*, *G*, and *I* to *H* (helices), assigning *B* and *E* to *E* (sheets), and assigning all others to *C* (coils).

2.3.2   Distance Measure

Since the Manhattan distance is featured by every position of the frequency profile equally, this distance measure is the most suitable measurement for this research [4,11]. The following formulation is adopted to obtain the distance between two sequence segments [8,15].

$$\text{Dissimilarity} = \sum_{i=1}^{L}\sum_{j=1}^{N}|F_k(i,j) - F_c(i,j)|$$

where L is the window size, $N = 20$ representing 20 different amino acids; $F_k(i,j)$ is the value of the matrix at row i and column j, representing the sequence segment; and $F_c(i,j)$ is the value of the matrix at row i and column j, and representing the centroids of a given sequence cluster. The lower the dissimilarity value, the higher the similarity between the two segments.

2.3.3   Secondary Structural Similarity Measure

The cluster's average structure is calculated using the following formula:

$$\text{Secondary structural similarity} = \frac{\sum_{i=1}^{ws} \max(p_{i,H}, p_{i,E}, p_{i,C})}{ws}$$

where ws is the window size and $P_{i,H}$ denotes the frequency of occurrence of helix among the segments for the cluster in position i; $P_{i,E}$ and $P_{i,C}$ are defined in a similar way. If the structural homology for a cluster exceeds 70%, the cluster can be considered structurally identical [13]. If the structural homology for the cluster is between 60% and 70%, the cluster can be viewed as weakly structurally homologous [4].

2.3.4   HSSP-BLOSUM62 Measure

BLOSUM62 [15] is a scoring matrix based on known alignments of diverse sequences. By using this matrix, we may discern the consistency of the amino acids appearing in the same position of the motif information generated by our method. Because different amino acids appearing in the same position should be close to each other, the corresponding value in the BLOSUM62 matrix will give a positive value. Hence, the measure is defined as follows:

$$\text{If } k = \begin{cases} 0 \text{ or } 1 \quad \text{then } \text{HSSP} - \text{BLOSUM62 measure} = 0 \\ \text{else: HSSP--BLOSUM62 measure} = \dfrac{\sum_{i=1}^{k-1}\sum_{j=i+1}^{k}\text{HSSP}_i \cdot \text{HSSP}_j \cdot \text{BLOSUM62}_{ij}}{\sum_{i=1}^{k-1}\sum_{j=i+1}^{k}\text{HSSP}_i \cdot \text{HSSP}_j} \end{cases}$$

where k is the number of amino acids with frequency higher than a certain threshold in the same position (in this chapter, 8% is the threshold). HSSP_i indicates the percent of amino acid i to appear. BLOSUM62 denotes the value of BLOSUM62 on amino acids i and j. The higher HSSPBLOSUM62 value indicates more significant motif information.

2.3.5   Parameter Setup for Fuzzy C-Means Clustering

For fuzzy C-means clustering, the fuzzification factor is set to 1.05 and the number of clusters is equal to 10. These settings yielded the best results for the dataset specified in 2.1. To separate information granules from FCM results, the membership threshold is set to 13%; 800 is the number used for total number of clusters. The formula that determines how many clusters should be included in each information granule is:

$$C_k = \frac{n_k}{\sum_{i=1}^{m} n_i} \times \text{total number of clusters}$$

where C_k denotes the number of clusters assigned to information granule k, n_k is the number of members belonging to information granule k, and m is the number of clusters in FCM. Table 2.1 summarizes the results from FCM.

Although the total data size increased from 413 to 529 MB (megabytes) and the total number of members increased from 562,745 to 721,390, we deal with only one information granule at a time. Therefore, the goal of reduced space complexity is achieved.

2.4   PROTEIN SEQUENCE MOTIF INFORMATION DISCOVERED BY FGK MODEL

2.4.1   Execution Time

In Table 2.2, the average K-means execution time for all information granules and the original dataset is given on the left column. A graph that compares the

TABLE 2.1   Summary of Results Obtained by Fuzzy C Means

Dataset	Number of Members	Number of Clusters	Data Size (MB)
Granule 0	136,112	151	99.9
Granule 1	68,792	76	50.5
Granule 2	86,094	95	63.2
Granule 3	65,361	72	47.9
Granule 4	63,159	70	46.3
Granule 5	120,130	133	88.2
Granule 6	128,874	143	94.6
Granule 7	4,583	5	3.3
Granule 8	43,254	48	31.7
Granule 9	5,032	6	3.7
Total	721,390	799	529
Original dataset	562,745	800	413

TABLE 2.2   Execution Time Comparison Table

Dataset	Running Time (s)
Granule 0	60,546
Granule 1	15,198
Granule 2	23,603
Granule 3	13,680
Granule 4	12,771
Granule 5	46,230
Granule 6	53,430
Granule 7	83
Granule 8	6,072
Granule 9	107
Total	231,720
Original dataset	1,285,928

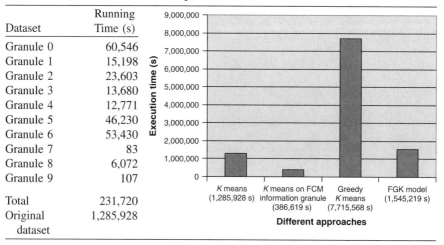

average execution time for all methods mentioned in this chapter is shown in the right column. From the graph, "K means" represents the average execution time for applying the original K-means algorithm on the intact dataset once. "K means on FCM separated data" gives the average runtime for executing the original K-means algorithm on the information granules obtained by fuzzy C-means clustering. The total execution time shown for "K means on FCM separated data" on the graph equals the sum of the execution time of all informational granules plus the time required by the fuzzy C-means clustering algorithm (154,899 s).

The third method, "greedy K means," requires the original K-means clustering algorithm to be executed 5 times and the sixth iteration to obtain the result. Without discussing the trivial details, their method requires six iterations of the K-means clustering algorithm on the original dataset. Therefore, the value shown on the graph equals the K-means value times 6. The last method, "FGK model," is the model presented in this chapter. The method to compute the total required time equals the sum of execution time on all information granules times 6 plus one iteration time required by FCM.

With comparison of the execution times, the FGK model requires only 20% of application the greedy K-means clustering algorithm on the whole dataset and almost equals the time needed for one round by original K-means clustering on the whole dataset. This result shows that the granular computing model really decreases the time complexity of this task.

2.4.2 Protein Sequence Motif Quality

The major difference (improvement) occurs on the evaluation measure of secondary structural similarity as we expected. In Table 2.3, we give the HSSP-BLOSUM62 measure (the last column) and average percentage of sequence segments belonging to clusters with high structural similarity (the second and third columns) for different methods. To fully compare these results, we include the result of applying the K-means clustering algorithm on original data, the result of using the K-means clustering algorithm on information granules, and the results of adapting the FGK model with different distance threshold setup for the greedy K-means clustering algorithm. "FGK model 200" indicates that the dataset is clustered by the FGK model with the new greedy initialization K-means clustering algorithm, and the distance threshold is set as 200. "FGK model 250," "FGK model 300," "FGK model 350," and "FGK model 400" are defined similarly.

The results of Table 2.3 reveal that the quality of clusters improved dramatically by applying granular computing techniques that utilize FCM to separate the

TABLE 2.3 Comparison of HSSP-BLOSUM62 Measure and Percentage of Sequence Segments Belonging to Clusters with High Structural Similarity

Method	>60% (%)	>70% (%)	H-B Measure
Traditional	25.82	10.44	0.2543
FCM K means	37.14	12.99	0.3589
FGK model 200	42.45	14.14	0.3393
FGK model 250	42.77	14.06	0.3443
FGK model 300	41.08	13.89	0.3311
FGK model 350	37.47	13.49	0.3489
FGK model 400	37.62	13.86	0.3676

whole dataset into several information granules. In the FCM *K*-means approach, the average percentage of clusters with structural similarity >60% increased by 11%, which translates to more than 90 meaningful sequence motifs that cannot be disclosed by traditional methods but are discovered by our approach. Also, the increase in HSSP-BLOSUM62 measurement from 0.254 to 0.358 proves that the motif information is more consistent and meaningful under the granular computing strategy.

For "FGK model 250," although the HSSP-BLOSUM62 measurement decreased slightly, the result achieves the highest percentage (42.77%) of clusters with high structural similarity among all methods. It indicates that the greedy initialization method can reveal some hidden motif information that the traditional one cannot. By comparing the result that was generated different approaches, we realized that the FGK model has the ability to improve the quality of clusters from the traditional *K*-means approach.

2.4.3 Protein Sequence Motif Presentation Format

After discovering more than 300 high-quality sequence motifs, how to present these useful recurring patterns is another research issue. The most important issue in this visualization work is that the protein sequence motifs discovered by computer scientists have to be easily understood by biologists. A motif information representation that utilizes graphical amino acid logos that is widely used by biologists is presented in this section. Figure 2.5 illustrates some sequence motifs generated from the FGK model. The following format is used for representation of each motif table:

- The upper box gives the number of members belonging to this motif, the secondary structural similarity, and the average HSSP-BLOSUM62 value.
- The graph demonstrates the type of amino acid frequently appearing in the given position by amino acid logo. It only shows the amino acid appearing with a frequency of >8%. The height of symbols within the stack indicates the relative frequency of each amino or nucleic acid at that position.
- The *x*-axis label indicates the representative secondary structure (S), the HSSP-BLOSUM62 measure (H-B), and the hydrophobicity value (Hyd.) of the position. The hydrophobicity value is calculated from summation of the frequencies of occurrence of Leu, Pro, Met, Trp, Ala, Val, Phe, and Ile.

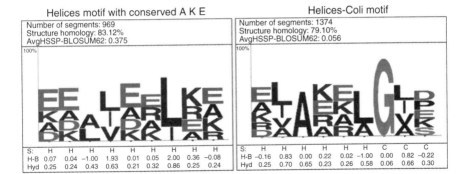

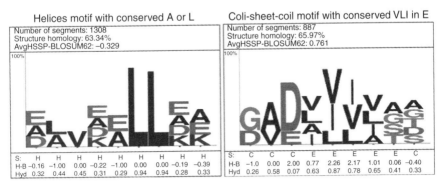

Figure 2.5   Sequence motif examples: (a) helix motif with conserved A K E; (b) helix coil motif; (c) helix motif with conserved A; (d) coil motif with conserved A G S; (e) helix motif with conserved A or L; (f) coil–sheet–coil motif with conserved VLI in E.

REFERENCES

1. Hulo N, Sigrist CJA, Le Saux V, Langendijk-Genevaux PS, Bordoli L, Gattiker A, De Castro E, Bucher P, Bairoch A, Recent improvements to the PROSITE database, *Nucleic Acids Res.* **32**:134–137 (2004).

2. Attwood TK, Blythe MJ, Flower DR, Gaulton A, Mabey JE, Maudling N, McGregor L, Mitchell AL, Moulton G, Paine K, PRINTS and PRINTS-S shed light on protein ancestry, *Nucleic Acids Res.* **30**:239–241 (2002).

3. Henikoff S, Blocks +: A non-redundant database of protein alignment blocks derived from multiple compilations, *Bioinformatics* **15**:471–479 (1999).

4. Zhong W, Altun G, Harrison R, Tai, PC, Pan Y, Improved K-means clustering algorithm for exploring local protein sequence motifs representing common structural property, *IEEE Trans. Nanobiosci.* **4**:255–265 (2005).

5. Bailey TL, Elkan C, *Fitting a Mixture Model by Expectation Maximization to Discover Motifs in Bipolymers*, Dept. Computer Science and Engineering, Univ. California, San Diego, 1994.

6. Lawrence CE, Altschul SF, Boguski MS, Liu JS, Neuwald AF, Wootton JC, Detecting subtle sequence signals: A Gibbs sampling strategy for multiple alignment, *Science* **262**:208–214 (1993).

7. Henikoff S, Henikoff JG, Alford WJ, Pietrokovski S, Automated construction and graphical presentation of protein blocks from unaligned sequences, *Gene.* **163**(2):GC17–26 (1995 Oct 3).

8. Eskin E, Pevzner PA, Finding composite regulatory patterns in DNA sequences, *Bioinformatics* **18**:354–363 (2002).

9. Price A, Ramabhadran S, Pevzner PA, Finding subtle motifs by branching from sample strings, *Bioinformatics* **19**:149–155 (2003).

10. Jensen KL, Styczynski MP, Rigoutsos I, Stephanopoulos GN, A generic motif discovery algorithm for sequential data, *Bioinformatics* **22**:21–28 (2006).

11. Han KF, Baker D, Recurring local sequence motifs in proteins, *J. Mol. Biol.* **251**:176–187 (1995).

12. Wang G, Dunbrack RL, PISCES: A protein sequence culling server, *Bioinformatics* **19**:1589–1591 (2003).

13. Sander C, Schneider R, Database of homology-derived protein structures and the structural meaning of sequence alignment, *Proteins: Struct. Funct. Genet.* **9**:56–68 (1991).

14. Kabsch W, Sander C, Dictionary of protein secondary structure: Pattern recognition of hydrogen-bonded and geometrical features, *Biopolymers* **22**:2577–2637 (1983).

15. Henikoff S, Henikoff JG, Amino acid substitution matrices from protein blocks, *Proc. Natl. Acad. Sci. USA* **89**:10915–10919 (1992).

16. Lin TY, Granular computing: Fuzzy logic and rough sets, in Zadeh LA, Kacprzyk J, ed., *Computing with Words in Information/Intelligent Systems*, Physica Verlag, Heidelberg 1999, pp. 183–200.

17. Lin TY, Granular computing on binary relations I: Data mining and neighborhood systems, *Rough Sets Knowl. Discov.* **1**:107–121 (1998).

18. Lin TY, Data mining and machine oriented modeling: A granular computing approach, *Appl. Intell.* **13**:113–124 (2000).

19. Yao YY, On modeling data mining with granular computing, *Proc. 25th Annual Int. Computer Software and Applications Conf.*, 2001, pp. 638–643.

20. Tang Y, Zhang YQ, Huang Z, Hu X, Granular SVM-RFE gene selection algorithm for reliable prostate cancer classification on microarray expression data, *Proc. 5th IEEE Symp. Bioinformatics and Bioengineering, (BIBE 2005)*, 2005, pp. 290–293.

21. Yao YY, Granular computing, *Comput. Sci. (Ji Suan Ji Ke Xue)* **31**:1–5 (2004).

22. Yao YY, A partition model of granular computing, *Lect. Notes Comput. Sci. Trans. Rough Sets* **1**:232–253 (2004).

23. Yao Y, Perspectives of granular computing, *Proc. 1st Int. IEEE Conf. Granular Computing*, 2005.

24. Yao YY, Zhong N, Granular computing using information tables, in *Data Mining, Rough Sets and Granular Computing*, 2002, pp. 102–124.

25. Yao YY, Yao JT, Granular computing as a basis for consistent classification problems, *Proc. PAKDD (Pacific Asia Knowledge Discovery and Data Mining)* **2**:101–106 (2002).

26. Lin TY, Data mining: Granular computing approach, in Zhong N, Zhou L. (ed.), *Methodologies for Knowledge Discovery and Data Mining, Lecture Notes in Artificial Intelligence Proc. PAKDD* **3**:24–33 (1999).

27. Han J, Kamber M, *Data Mining: Concepts and Techniques*, Morgan Kaufmann, 2006.

28. Chen B, Tai PC, Harrison R, Pan Y, FGK model: An efficient granular computing model for protein sequence motifs information discovery, *Proc. Int. Conf. Computational and Systems Biology* (CASB), Dallas, 2006.

29. Dunn JC, A fuzzy relative of the ISODATA process and its use in detecting compact well-separated clusters, *J. Cybernet.* **3**:32–57 (1973).

30. Bezdek JC, *Pattern Recognition with Fuzzy Objective Function Algorithms*, Plenum Press, New York, 1981.

CHAPTER 3

IDENTIFYING CALCIUM BINDING SITES IN PROTEINS

HUI LIU and HAI DENG

3.1 INTRODUCTION

The number of experimentally and computationally derived structural models available in databases has been steadily increasing with the emergence of structural genomics projects worldwide. One important problem in current biology and chemistry is to assign proteins with functions based on 3D structure. Calcium, one of the most important metals for life, is responsible for regulating many biological processes through its interactions with numerous calcium binding proteins in different biological environments [1,2]. Identifying the calcium binding sites is not only critical for the study of individual proteins but also helpful for revealing the general factors involved in such as the mechanisms governing calcium binding affinity, metal selectivity, and calcium-induced conformation change [3]. Sites are defined by a 3D location and a local neighborhood with a common structural or functional role. Non-calcium-binding sites are locations where the function does not occur or a different function is present. According to structural features, calcium binding sites can be classified as continuous or discontinuous [4,5]. Continuous calcium binding sites consist of amino acids adjacent in primary sequence, usually in a highly conserved loop flanked by the helix–loop–helix, whereas discontinuous calcium binding sites consist of residues that are spatially proximate in the folded structure but distant in the sequence, and do not have conserved calcium binding loops and flanked helices.

Identification of the calcium binding sites in proteins is one of the main barriers to understanding the role of calcium in biological systems. Numerous efforts have been devoted to predicting and visualizing calcium binding sites in proteins with high accuracy and speed. Yamashita and coworkers [6] reported that metal ions bind at centers of high hydrophobicity contrast, which was further

Algorithmic and Artificial Intelligence Methods for Protein Bioinformatics. First Edition.
Edited by Yi Pan, Jianxin Wang, Min Li.
© 2014 John Wiley & Sons, Inc. Published 2014 by John Wiley & Sons, Inc.

embedded within a shell of carbon-containing hydrophobic atom groups. They embedded the whole protein structure into a 3D grid and measured hydrophobicity contrast at each gridpoint in order to predict metal binding sites on the basis of this observation. Nayal and Di Cera [7] applied a similar approach to improve performance through replacing the contrast function with valence function with a clear cutoff between calcium binding and non-calcium-binding sites (nonsites). The computational calculations of both grid algorithms are intensive and thus not suitable for predicting calcium binding sites in proteins with required speed and accuracy. Several methods, such as FEATURE, protein seqFEATURE, or MetSite [8–15], used statistical approaches for recognizing calcium binding sites based on a variety of physical and chemical features in calcium binding sites and nonsites. Rychlewski et al. [15] illustrated the capability of predicting the precise locations of calcium binding sites with high coordination numbers based on the Fold-X empirical forcefield. However, the success rate of their results is low.

To overcome the disadvantages of the abovemeintioned approaches, we illustrate three methods based on the geometric and other key features of calcium binding sites in this chapter. The first method, called GG [16], applied a graph theory algorithm by taking advantage of its capability of extracting key features of the system [17,18]. GG has obtained high performance with >90% site sensitivity and 80% site selectivity, and more than 95% of the sites with four or more ligands have been accurately identified within 1 Å of the documented calcium ions. Their results have demonstrated that a cluster of four or more oxygen atoms has a high potential for calcium binding. The second method named as GG2.0 is an enhanced version of the GG method to predict calcium binding sites in proteins [19]. GG2.0 applies the maximal clique algorithm to find biggest local oxygen clusters and calculate the geometric filter related to the ratio between the size of the first shell and the second shell of calcium binding sites by using an optimization tool. Their results not only achieve the high performance of 98% site sensitivity and 86% site selectivity but also demonstrate that some oxygen clusters satisfying geometric criteria are not calcium binding sites with some fixed residue combinations. GSVM [20], a supervised classification model, is built by absorbing the advantages of statistical approaches and graph theory algorithm. On the basis of the maximal oxygen clusters, a putative calcium center (PCC) is located by minimizing the average distance between PCC and every oxygen atom for one maximal cluster. Spherical regions centered on PCC are chosen as putative calcium binding sites. GSVM distinguish between calcium binding sites and non-calcium-binding sites by taking spatial distribution of biophysical and biochemical properties as an input variable for a binary classification task. High performance with site sensitivity and site selectivity has been obtained through GSVM.

The rest of the chapter is organized as follows: Section 3.2 illustrates datasets, performance measurement, and detailed implementation of three methods: GG, GG2.0, and GSVM. Experimental results and discussion are presented in Section 3.3. Conclusions are included in Section 3.4.

3.2 METHODS

3.2.1 Datasets

To compare these three methods with previous finding, we select a total of 123 proteins and 231 calcium binding sites in three datasets, which are queried from the metalloprotein database and browser (MDB) with the conditions that every calcium binding protein structure from PDB has resolution of <2.0 Å from X-ray crystallography, each site has a coordination number of >3, excluding water oxygen, and the PDB entry must be in the PDBSELECT nonhomology list. Nayal-Di Cera's 7 dataset (dataset I) contains 32 proteins with 62 calcium binding sites. Dataset II from Pidcock and Moore 5 has 44 proteins and 94 calcium binding sites, which are obtained from 515 fully normalized crystal structures of calcium binding proteins deposited in PDB from 1994 to 1998 with a resolution ranging from 1.0 to 2.5 Å. Liang's dataset (dataset III) contains 91 calcium binding sites from 54 proteins, and 14 non-calcium-binding proteins. These datasets are summarized in Table 3.1.

3.2.2 Performance Measurement

A qualified clique is a true prediction (TP) if its putative of calcium ion location falls into the cutoff distance (3.5 Å in our studies) from a documented calcium ion in a crystal structure. A documented calcium binding site is a true prediction site (TPS) if there is any prediction within the cutoff distance from this site. The performance of our studies are evaluated by *site sensitivity* (SEN) and *site selectivity* (SEL), which represent the percentage of TPS in the total sites and the percentage of TP in the total predictions, respectively.

$$SEN = \frac{TPS}{total\ sites}$$

$$SEL = \frac{TP}{total\ predictions}$$

TABLE 3.1 Description of Three Datasets (Ca$-$O $\le$ 3.5 Å)

Dataset	Total Proteins	Total Sites	Number of Sites with >4 Oxygen Cliques	Number of Sites with 3 Oxygen Cliques	Number of Sites with ≤ 2 Oxygen Cliques
I	32	62	55 (88.71%)	7	0
II	44	94	81 (86.17%)	7	6
III	54	91	80 (87.91%)	8	3

3.2.3   GG Algorithm

3.2.3.1 Graph Algorithm   For a given protein structure as shown in Figure 3.1, the coordinates in the PDB file of oxygen atoms are extracted first. The distances between every two oxygen atoms are calculated. A graph $G(V,E)$ is constructed accordingly, in which V is the set of all oxygen atoms and each edge in E exists between a pair of oxygen atoms apart within an O—O cutoff distance (6.0 Å in GG algorithm 17). The graph construction uses $O(n^2)$, where $n = |V(G)|$ is the number of oxygen atoms. A clique Q is a subset of V such that every two vertices of Q are connected by an edge. The number of vertices in the clique is defined as the size of a clique.

Instead of exhaustive search in grid methods, we use a backtracking algorithm to find cliques of certain sizes in G. The time complexity of GG is linear because of the specificity of the graph G construction from a protein structure. Further more, the number of cliques is far less than the number of the gridpoints. Therefore, GG is more computational efficient compared with the previous methods. The pseudocode for finding cliques of four vertices in G is shown as Figure 3.2.

3.2.3.2 Geometry Algorithm   The point that has the same distance to the four vertices of a clique is defined as the circumcenter (CC). The distance between CC and vertices of a clique is called psdCa—O. In order to eliminate false positives, a clique is considered as a putative calcium binding site only if psdCa—O falls into the range (R_1, R_2), where R_1 and R_2 are the lower and upper limits, respectively. Since the space for calcium binding should not be occupied by other atoms, GG algorithm further applied a D-filter to eliminate any cliques that contain nonoxygen atoms within a short distance (D-filter) from the CC. The complexity of this step algorithm is $O(nm)$, where m is the number of all atoms other than oxygen. Dataset I was used to optimize the parameters such as psdCa—O range and D-filter in order to achieve high accuracy and speed. By using an O—O cutoff of 6.0 Å, a psdCa—O range of 1.8–3.0 Å and a D-filter equal to the psdCa—O, the best performance was obtained.

3.2.3.3 Removal of Redundant Predictions   A merging algorithm was adopted to remove redundant predictions in one location. All putative sites in a protein are input in a vector and sorted by psdCa—O. The putative sites within 3.5 Å (center–center distance) from it are deleted once the one with the shortest psdCa—O is determined. The merging procedure is repeated until the vector is empty. The computational complexity is not larger than $O(n^2)$ because it depends on the number of total comparisons.

3.2.3.4 Computational Complexity Analysis   The computational complexity of GG is $O(n + n^2 + nm)$ from the three steps of this algorithm, which can be simplified to $O(nm)$ because it is the dominant component.

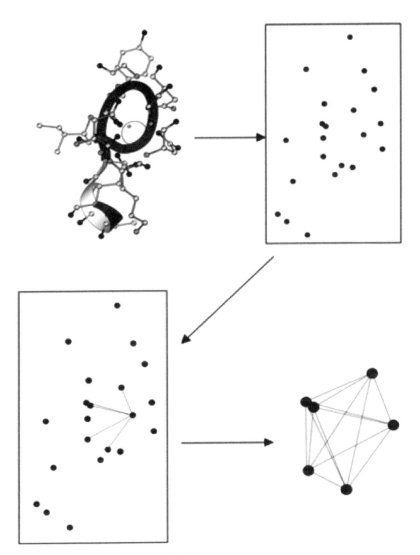

Figure 3.1 The schematic model of a GG program is shown. The oxygen atom positions (dark dots) are extracted from the protein structure, while the other atoms (light dots) are excluded. The distances between two oxygen atoms are calculated and an edge is assigned if the distance is below a cutoff distance (O—O cutoff). A potential calcium binding position is a clique (bottom right), which is a group in which every oxygen atom is linked to all other members of the group by edges.

```
1. Loop through all vertices a in V
2.   Loop through all vertices b in the adjacecy list of a
3.   output V:=V-{a} if no such b exists
4.     Loop through all vertices c adjacent to both a and b
5.     output V:=V-{a} if no such c exists
6.       Loop through all vertices d adjacent to both a, b, and c
7.         output clique {a,b,c,d}
8.       output V:=V-{a} if no such d exists
```

Figure 3.2 Pseudocode of the GG algorithm for finding all cliques of size 4.

3.2.4 GG2.0 Algorithm [19]

3.2.4.1 A Geometric Criterion After oxygen cliques are found by using a graph algorithm similar to GG17, a carbon cluster around every oxygen cluster is also obtained because each oxygen atom is connected to one carbon atom. The *least variance point* (LVP) is defined as the geometric point that has a smallest variance with respect to every other atom/vertex of the cluster/clique. There exists a corresponding carbon cluster surrounding every oxygen cluster. These two clusters are thus called *twin clusters*, and the LVP of the oxygen cluster is chosen as the center of the twin clusters. The optimization function of fminsearch in the Matlab software was used to obtain the coordinates of the LVP of a cluster. Then the radius of oxygen/carbon cluster (RO/RC) can be calculated as

$$RO = \frac{\sum_{i=1}^{k} \text{dist}(LVP,O)}{k}$$

$$RC = \frac{\sum_{i=1}^{k} \text{dist}(LVC,O)}{k}$$

where and are the distances between the LVP and each oxygen or carbon ligand, respectively, and k is the number of vertices of a cluster. The RO/RC ratio reflects the size of an oxygen/carbon shell to some extent; thus we defined the ratio between the RO and the RC for every twin cluster as r_RO_RC. To eliminate false positives, r_RO_RC was used as a filter within some range for a putative calcium binding site. Since the carbon shell will become smaller when a calcium binding site has a bidentate residue as ligand, we adjust r_RO_RC to ar_RO_RC as the filter. From the experiments, the results obtained by using ar_RO_RC are much better than those obtained by r_RO_RC. The r_RO_RC and ar_RO_RC are calculated as

$$r\_RO\_RC = \frac{RO}{RC}$$

$$ar\_RO\_RC = r\_RO\_RC - 0.05 * NB$$

where NB is the number of bidentate residues in a putative calcium binding site.

3.2.4.2 A Chemic Criterion Some oxygen clusters satisfying the geometric criteria are not around calcium binding sites from the experimental results. We observe some patterns of residue combination for non-calcium-binding sites in those clusters of size 4. The patterns are summarized as the chemic criteria, as follows:

1. If a cluster contains a backbone carbonyl oxygen atom, it is considered to consist of putative sites.
2. If a cluster contains two sidechain carboxylate atoms from different residues, the cluster is considered to consist of putative sites.

3.2.5 GSVM Algorithm

3.2.5.1 Graph Algorithm GSVM adopted a graph algorithm similar to that of GG17 to obtain all oxygen clusters, which were all maximal cliques of the graph constructed by the coordinates of oxygen atoms of a protein. A putative calcium center (PCC) was located to be the point that has the shortest distance to every oxygen atom in the oxygen cluster. A 7.0-Å spherical region centered on PCC is built. All the spherical regions are chosen as putative calcium binding sites. Hundreds of (sphere, PCC) pairs for every protein structure are obtained by in this way.

3.2.5.2 Classifying Calcium Binding Sites and Nonsites by Support Vector Machine (SVM) Distinguishing between calcium binding sites and nonsites is a binary classification problem. Given a training dataset `Dtrain` that includes pairs of measurements, each consisting of a feature vector $x(i)$ in a d-dimensional feature space R^d with a corresponding ("target") class label $y(i) \epsilon \{-1, 1\}, 1 \leq i \leq n$, the goal is to find a classifier (from the training dataset) with a mapping or a function $y = f(x, \theta)$ that can predict a value y given an input vector of measured values x and a set of unknown parameters θ.

The accuracy of an SVM model depends largely on the selection of the model parameters. To determine the parameters of C and Γ, GSVM [20] conducts a cross-validation process on the training dataset. Cross-validation is also used to estimate the generalization capability on new samples that are not in the training dataset. A k-fold cross-validation randomly splits the training dataset into k approximately equal-sized subsets, leaves out one subset, builds a classifier on the remaining samples, and then evaluates classification performance on the unused subset. This process is repeated k times for each subset to obtain cross-validation performance over the whole training datasets. GSVM adopts 5 as the k value.

3.2.5.3 Feature Data Encoding There is a significant meaning for the prediction performance to select an appropriate data encoding scheme to represent the microenvironments of calcium binding sites and nonsites because it largely determines the quality of feature extraction of SVM models. The spatial distributions of biophysical and biochemical properties surrounding calcium binding sites differ significantly from those surrounding the control nonsites [11]. For every putative calcium binding site, GSVM extract biophysical and biochemical properties from every spherical region into a feature vector. The feature descriptors of protein structure include four groups, atom-based features, chemical group–based features, residue-based features, and secondary structure–based features. The atom-based features consist of the number of carbons, number of nitrogens, number of oxygen atoms, sum of hydrophobicity values of all atoms within a putative calcium binding site, and sum of charge values of all atoms within a putative calcium binding site. Examples of chemical group–based feature include number of hydroxyls, number of amides, number of amines, number of carbonyls, number of ring structures, and number of peptides. Standard 20 amino acids can be classified into five groups: hydrophobic, charged, nonplolar, polar, and acidic. GSVM counted the number of amino acids within a putative calcium binding site for every group, then encoded into residue-based features. Secondary structure–based features include the number of ALPHA, the number of BETA, the number of COIL, and the number of HET within a putative calcium binding site. In one word, the spatial distributions of biophysical and biochemical properties for every (sphere, PCC) pair were encoded into a 20-dimensional feature vector. Figure 3.3c,d describes the construction of a feature vector.

3.2.5.4 *Data Preprocessing*   There are several hundreds of putative calcium binding sites found for every protein structure. The putative site is labeled as +1 if the PCC of a putative site is located within 3.5 Å of the documented calcium ion; otherwise it is labeled −1. Unfortunately, the class imbalance problem exists because the number of positive site samples is relatively rare as compared with that of negative site samples. For example, given 1AG9, there are 5 positive samples but 232 negative samples. Since only support vectors (SVs) are used for classification and many majority samples far from the decision boundary can be removed without affecting the classification [21], SVM is more accurate on

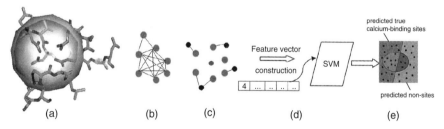

Figure 3.3   Schematic diagram of GSVM: (a) 7.0-Å spherical region around a calcium ion; (b) the extracted oxygen atom (red dots) and constructed graph *G*. (c) a maximal clique of size 6 in graph *G* with calcium center (blue dot) (the black dots represent carbon atoms located within the spherical region); (d) for the spherical region, construction of a feature vector (e.g., one feature is the number of atoms); (e) the feature vector is taken as the input variable for SVM that distinguishes sphere samples between calcium binding sites and non-calcium-binding sites.

TABLE 3.2   Example of Imbalanced Data in Dataset II

PDB ID	Number of Samples	Number of Positive Samples	Number of Negative Samples	Changed
1AG9	232	5 (2.15%)	145	5 (3.44%)
1B90	106	11 (10.38%)	61	11 (18.03%)
1CE5	105	4 (3.81%)	74	4 (5.40%)
1EG2	618	15 (2.43%)	380	15 (3.95%)
—	—	—	—	—
Total	13,520	444 (3.28%)	8654	444 (5.13%)

moderately imbalanced data compared with other standard classifiers. However, a SVM classifier can be sensitive to high class imbalance data, which results in a drop in the classification performance on the positive class. It is prone to generating a classifier that has a strong estimation bias toward the majority class, resulting in a large number of false negatives. The methods proposed to solve imbalanced classification can be categorized into the following three different types: cost-sensitive learning, oversampling the minority class, or undersampling the majority class [21].

There are 13,520 samples in dataset I where the positive:negative ratio is about 1:29 as shown in Table 3.2. If the PCC of a negative sample site falls within the cutoff distance (3.0 Å in our study) of its neighboring negative sample site, one of these two will be removed from the dataset. Thus, by removal of close negative spherical regions, majority negative samples are undersampled. The positive:negative ratio is reduced to 1:18 as shown in column, of Table 3.2; however, it is still highly imbalanced. The libsvm23 program implemented in RapidMiner [22] for binary classification was used with fivefold cross-validation. The cost matrix used for cost-sensitive learning was defined as [+1 − 1; 10 0], which means that the costs for the error of predicting +1 as −1 are 10 times higher than the other error type. The problem of imbalanced data is further alleviated through cost-sensitive learning.

3.3   RESULTS AND DISCUSSION

A SEN of 91% and a SEL of 77% have been achieved for the prediction of 91 calcium binding sites in dataset II when a true prediction is assumed if the predicted calcium is within 3.5 Å of the documented calcium ions by using an O—O cutoff of 6.0 Å a psdCa—O range of 1.8–3.0 Å and a D-filter equal to psdCa—O. Under the same condition, a SEN of 87% and a SEL of 74% have been achieved in dataset III as shown in Figure 3.4a. The SEN and SEL are 84% and 59% for dataset II and 80% and 55% for dataset III, respectively (Fig. 3.4b) if the standard of a true prediction is that the predicted calcium is within 1 Å of the documented calcium ions. As in dataset I, 6 of 11 sites with three or

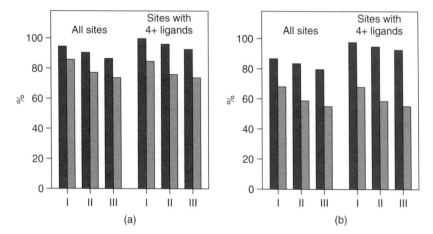

Figure 3.4 The sensitivity (black bars) and selectivity (gray bars) of the GG program with a O—O distance cutoff of 6.0 Å and the psdCa—O distance range cutoff of 1.8–3.0 Å. The standard of a true prediction is that the predicted calcium position is within 3.5 Å (a) or 1.0 Å (b) threshold distance to the documented calcium ions. The results of all sites are shown on the left, and the results considering only the sites with four or more ligands are shown on the right.

fewer ligands in dataset II and 4 of 13 in dataset III have been identified within 3.5 Å of the real calcium, but none of the predictions is within 1 Å of the real calcium. If we consider only the calcium binding sites with four or more ligands as real sites, the SENs for datasets I, II, and III increase to 98%, 95%, and 93%, respectively, with the true prediction standard of within 1.0 Å of the documented calcium ions (as shown in Fig 3.4). Although the performance of the prediction was lower by including these less popular calcium binding sites or non-calcium-binding proteins, it confirms the practicability of high site selectivity, sensitivity, and accuracy of GG algorithm.

GSVM classified all (sphere, PCC) pairs into two types: calcium binding sites and non-calcium-binding sites. To obtain maximum accuracy, 20 experiments with fivefold cross-validation were conducted for every dataset. The summary results of experiments are presented in Table 3.3. For dataset I, the total predictions made by GSVM was 379 (column 5 in Table 3.3) and the total number of TPs was 356 (column 6 in Table 3.3), while 59 of 62 documented sites were predicted. Thus, the sensitivity was $59/62 = 95\%$ (column 7 in Table 3.3), whereas the selectivity was $356/379 = 94\%$ (column 8 in Table 3.3).

GG2.0 queried from the metalloprotein database and browser (MDB) [23] with the conditions that every calcium-binding protein structure from PDB [24] have a resolution <2.0 Å from X-ray crystallography, each site have a coordination number >3 excluding water oxygen, and the PDB entry be in the PDBSELECT nonhomology list (Hobohm and Sander) in order to acquire a high-resolution and nonhomology dataset of proteins with calcium binding sites. The retrieved dataset

TABLE 3.3 Summary Performance of Datasets I, II, and III

Dataset	Total Proteins	Total Sites	TPS	Total Predictions	TP	SEN	SEL
I	32	62	59	379	356	95%	94%
II	44	94	85	478	411	90%	87%
III	54	91	85	495	436	93%	91%

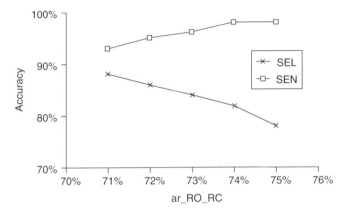

Figure 3.5 Effect of ar_RO_RC on prediction accuracy.

contains 163 proteins of 345 sites. After excluding the PDB entries containing a calcium binding site that does not conform to the same requirement as the Fold-X method, we find that the training dataset contains 121 protein structure files with all 240 calcium binding sites finally. Four calcium binding sites a have coordinated ligand number of <4 each and are not taken into account for calculating prediction accuracy in the testing dataset containing 20 proteins.

As seen from Figure 3.5, without using the chemical filter, GG2.0 can obtain the prediction accuracy of the SENs ranging from 92% to 98% with SELs ranging from 87% to 78%. There is a tradeoff between the SEN and the corresponding SEL. Since SEN with a higher value than SEL is preferred, 74% is taken as the empirical value of ar_RO_RC for the filter threshold. Using the chemical filter with an ar_RO_RC of 75%, the GG2.0 obtains the best site sensitivity of 98%, but the SEL increases from 82% to 86%. This means that the chemical filter is the absolute filter to exclude non calcium-binding oxygen clusters.

Several methods such as Feature and SeqFeature based on the statistic function of the physicochemical environment around functional sites have been developed for predicting calcium-binding sites [5,6,7,8,9]. These methods predict the calcium binding sites by a scoring system taking into account multiple properties such as secondary structures, chemical groups, and atom types for which high sensitivity and selectivity have been claimed. The same dataset investigated by

Altman et al. using Feature was analyzed by GG program [12]. The standard of true prediction of calcium binding sites is within 6.0 Å of the documented calcium for FEATURE in contrast to 1.0 Å for the prediction using GG. Even though the SEN from FEATURE is similar to that from the GG with the sacrifice of SEL for the sites with four or more oxygen ligand atoms, GG has achieved SEN of 95% within 1 Å of the structural resolution. The experimental results have shown that the GG program not only provided high prediction sensitivity without the use of vast statistical properties but also retained a greater site resolution to the documented calcium positions. This is very important for the application of testing the functions of the proteins with required resolution and accuracy. GG2.0 is an enhanced version of the GG method to predict calcium binding sites in proteins. it not only reduces the search space of the GG but also reveals certain geometric relation between the oxygen shell and carbon shell of calcium binding sites. Additionally, it indicates that some oxygen clusters from a group of residues with certain combination are formed possibly as a result of to hydrogen bonds instead of calcium ionic bonds. The two proposed filters in GG2.0 are useful for designing calcium binding sites in proteins. GSVM combines the advantages of GG and statistical methods. It is observed that GSVM has better site sensitivity and selectivity compared with GG. For two reasons: (1) the biophysical and biochemical properties of environments around sites are smoothly incorporated into feature vectors, so more features are used to select calcium binding sites; and (2) the SVM has superior generalization capability, and is a good tool for the binary classification problem. Moreover, GSVM actually builds a general model, which can be used to test numerous various features to identify significant ones related to forming calcium binding sites.

3.4   CONCLUSION

Identifying calcium binding sites is very important for the study of proteins. It is strongly needed to develop methodology for predicting calcium binding sites in proteins with high accuracy and high speed. Three methodologies are reviewed in this chapter, which are GG 17, GG2.0 20, and GSVM 21. GG using graph theory has revealed new features of calcium binding in proteins and the developed program may facilitate the understanding and prediction of functions of calcium roles in biological systems based on oxygen coordination, which can be provided by homology modeling based on the sequence information. GG can be a powerful tool for automated analysis of large structural genomic databases with sensitivity of >85% in addition to its capability of provided structural resolution (within 1 Å of the documented ions and with high speed). The GG2.0, as an enhanced version of the GG method, reduces the search space of GG, and further captures certain geometric relation between the oxygen shell and the carbon shell of calcium binding sites. GSVM adopts a statistical learning method to classify calcium binding sites and nosites based on constructed regions using a graph algorithm. Thus, GSVM absorbs advantages of both statistical learning and graph theory. Moreover, GSVM provides a means for building a general model that can be used to test and select significant features directly related to forming calcium binding sites.

REFERENCES

1. Silva JJRF, Williams RJP, *The Biological Chemistry of the Elements*, Oxford Univ. Press, 1991.

2. Linse S, Forsen S, Determinants that govern high-affinity calcium binding, *Adv. 2nd Messenger Phosphoprot. Res.* **30**:89–151 (1995).

3. Ikura M, Calcium binding and conformational response in ef-hand proteins, *Trends Biochem. Sci.* **21**(1): 14–17 (1996).

4. Yang W, Lee HW, Hellinga H, Yang JJ, Structure analysis, identification and design of calcium-binding sites in proteins, *Proteins* **47**:344–356 (2002).

5. Pidcock E, Moore GR, Structural characteristics of protein binding sites for calcium and lanthanide ions, *J. Biol. Inorg. Chem.* **6**:479–489 (2001).

6. Yamashita MM, Wesson L, Eisenman G, Eisenberg D, Where metal ions bind in proteins, *Proc. Natl. Acad. Sci. USA* **87**:5648–5652 (1990).

7. Nayal M, Di Cera E, Predicting Ca^{2+}-binding sites in proteins, *Proc. Natl. Acad. Sci. USA* **91**:817–821 (1994).

8. Wei L, Huang ES, Altman RB, Are predicted structures good enough to preserve functional sites? *Struct. Fold. Design* **7**:643–650 (1997).

9. Sodhi JS, Bryson K, McGuffin LJ, Ward JJ, Wernisch L, Jones DT, Predicting metal-binding site residues in low-resolution structural models, *J. Mol. Biol.* **342**:307–332 (2004).

10. Kuntz ID, Blaney JM, Oatley SJ, Langridge R, Ferrin TE, A geometric approach to macromolecule-ligand interactions, *J. Mol. Biol.* **161**:269–288 (1982).

11. Bagley SC, Altman RB, Characterizing the microenvironment surrounding protein sites. *Protein Sci.* **4**:622–635 (1995).

12. Liang MP, Banatao DR, Klein TE, Brutlag DL, Altman RB, webFEATURE: An interactive web tool for identifying and visualizing functional sites on macromolecular structures, *Nucleic Acids Res.* **31**:3324–3327 (2003).

13. Liang MP, Brutlag DL, Altman RB, Automated construction of structual motifs for predicting functional sites on protein structures, *Proc. Pacific Symp. Biocomputing*, pp. 2003, 204–215.

14. Katchalski-Katzir E, Shariv I, Eisenstein M, Friesem AA, Aflalo C, Vakser IA, Molecular surface recognition: determination of geometric fit between proteins and their ligands by correlation techniques, *Proc. Natl. Acad. Sci. USA* **89**:2195–2199 (1992).

15. Rychlewski L, Fischer D, Elofsson A, LiveBench-6: Large-scale automated evaluation of protein structure prediction servers, *Proteins* **53**(Suppl. 6): 542–547 (2003).

16. Deng H, Chen G, Yang W, Yang JJ, Predicting calcium-binding sites in proteins—a graph theory and geometry approach, *Proteins* **64**:34–42 (2006).

17. Samudrala R, Moult J, A graph-theoretic algorithm for comparative modeling of protein structure, *J. Mol. Biol.* **279**:287–302 (1998).

18. Canutescu AA, Shelenkov AA, Dunbrack RL Jr, A graph-theory algorithm for rapid protein side-chain prediction, *Protein Sci.* **12**:2001–2014 (2003).

19. Liu H, Deng H, Identifying calcium-binding sites with oxygen-carbon shell geometric and chemic criteria: A graph-based approach, *Proc. 2008 IEEE Int. Conf. Bioinform. Biomedi. (BIBM 2008)*, Philadelphia, PA, pp. 2008, 407–410.

20. Liu H, Metts N, Identifying calcium-binding sites in proteins by analyzing the microenvironment surrouding protein sites via SVMs, *Proc. 2009 World Congress in Computer Science, Computer Engineering, and Applied Computing*, Las Vegas, Nevada, pp. 834–839, 2009.

21. Akbani R, Kwek S, Japkowicz N, Applying support vector machines to imbalanced data sets, *Proc. 15th Eur. Conf. Machine Learning*, Pisa, Italy, pp. 39–50, 2004.

22. See http://rapid-i.com/.

23. Castagnetto J, Hennessy S, Roberts V, Getzoff E, Tainer J, Pique M, MDB: The metalloprotein database and browser at the scripps research institute, *Nucleic Acids Res,* **30**(1): 379–382 (2002).

24. Berman HM, Westbrook J, Feng Z, Gilliland G, Bhat TN, Weissig H, Shindyalov IN, Bourne PE, The protein data bank, *Nucleic Acids Res.* **28**(1): 235–242 (2000).

CHAPTER 4

REVIEW OF IMBALANCED DATA LEARNING FOR PROTEIN METHYLATION PREDICTION

ZEJIN DING and YAN-QING ZHANG

4.1 INTRODUCTION

Protein posttranslational modifications (PTMs) bring many diversified modifications to the polypeptide of a protein and play very important roles in many biological processes, such as influencing structural and functional diversity, determining cellular plasticity and dynamics, and impacting transcription activity, [1,2]. Protein methylation is one important type of posttranslational modification; it is a reversible modification and takes place dominantly on arginine and lysine residue [3]. Since the discovery of methylation in the mid-1960s [4], researchers have found its significant contributions in various biological processes, such as transcriptional regulation, RNA processing, signal transduction, DNA repair, genome stability, and heterochromatin compaction.

However, the molecular mechanism underlying methylation is still poorly understood. A genomewide search of methylated substrates is highly needed to unravel many unknown functions of protein arginine methyltransferases (PRMTs) in biological processes and cellular components. But performing actual laboratorial experiments to verify all residues in human proteins is too costly and time-consuming, and hence infeasible. Therefore, effective computational learning methods to predict methylation sites will greatly help researchers expedite the process of finding potentially methylated residues in new protein sequences. Several computational methods for methylation prediction have been developed in the literature, where most of them use support vector machines (SVMs) [5] as the learning algorithm and focus on extracting effective features from peptide sequences. However, the number of methylated residues is far less than unmethylated ones, causing the dataset for SVM modeling to be highly imbalanced.

Algorithmic and Artificial Intelligence Methods for Protein Bioinformatics. First Edition.
Edited by Yi Pan, Jianxin Wang, Min Li.
© 2014 John Wiley & Sons, Inc. Published 2014 by John Wiley & Sons, Inc.

Directly using SVM to train the data may lead to significantly biased classifiers with highly skewed hyperplanes, which always classify any new sequences as unmethylated examples. Therefore, solving the imbalanced data learning problem should be considered as one important step in accurate methylation prediction.

In this chapter, we focus on the study of computational predictions on this particular PTM—protein arginine methylation. We aim to provide a comprehensive review of the study of arginine methylation prediction. We extensively investigate all existing methylation prediction methods and servers; thoroughly review all feature extracting schemes used for sequence encoding; and carefully summarize and compare all processing steps in their methodologies, including data collection, feature extraction and selection, classifier training and evaluation, and result discussion. Finally, we suggest several future directions that are worthy of continuous research on methylation predictions. We hope that readers will be inspired to solve other PTM prediction or bioinformatics problems after reading this chapter.

4.2 PROTEIN AND METHYLATION

Proteins consist of one or more polypeptides and fold to particular 3D structures. A polypeptide is a linear polymer chain consisting of many amino acids and chained by the peptide bonds between the carboxyl and amino groups of neighboring amino acid. Amino acids, also called *residues*, are encoded genetically, and there are only 20 kinds of amino acids in total. However, a sequence of these amino acids can produce a countless number of combinations, resulting in millions of functional proteins, as well as largely diversified life forms. A typical protein contains hundreds or thousands of amino acid residues. In essence, the primary amino acid sequence determines the 3D structure and functionality of a protein.

The genetic material present in the nucleus of eukaryotic cells is tightly packaged into chromatin, which functions as a structural and dynamic scaffold in the regulation of various nuclear processes, including transcription, DNA replication and repair, mitosis, and apoptosis [6,7]. Among different chromatin modifications, the histone arginine methylation is catalyzed by protein arginine methyltransferases (PRMTs) that transfer the methyl group from S-adenosyl-L-methionine (AdoMet, SAM) to the guanidino group of arginines in histone or nonhistone protein substrates, resulting in mono and di-methylarginine residues in substrate proteins (Fig. 4.1).

The η-nitrogens of an arginine residue in a protein can be monomethylated or dimethylated, with either both methyl groups on single terminal nitrogen (asymmetric dimethylated arginine) or on either nitrogens (symmetric dimethylated arginine) by protein arginine methyltransferases (PRMTs) [3]. Currently, protein methylation has been intensely studied in the histones—the main protein components of chromatin because of its important role in epigenetic regulation of gene function.

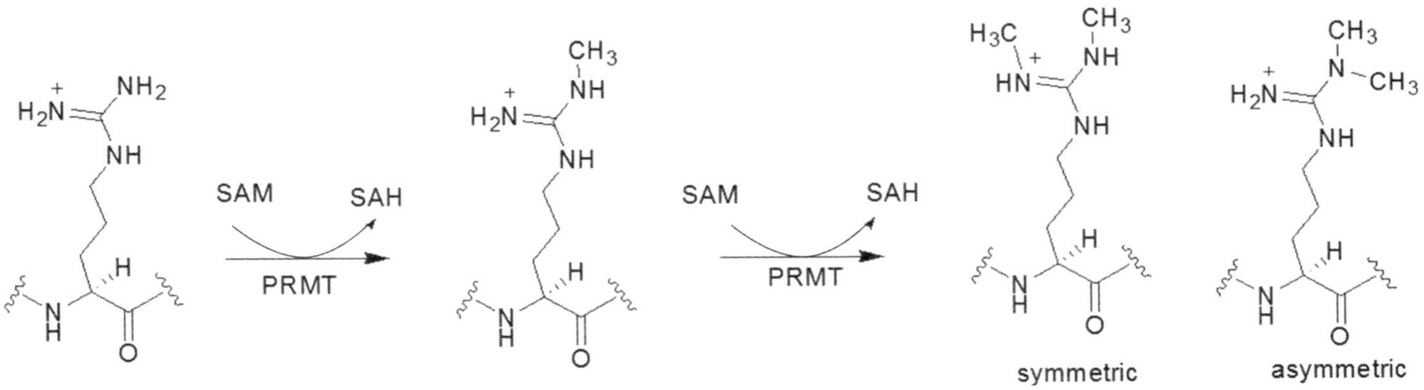

Figure 4.1 Protein arginine methylation catalyzed by PRMTs.

Eleven PRMT family members have been identified at the protein and genomic levels in human tissues or cells and categorized into two major types: types 1 and 2, according to substrate and product specificity [3,8]. Type 1 enzymes (PRMT1,3,4,6,8) catalyze the transfer of the methyl group from S-adenosyl-L-methionine (SAM, AdoMet) to the guanidinonitrogen atoms of arginine residue to produce ω-NG monomethylarginines (MMA, L-NMMA) and ω-NG,NG-asymmetric dimethylarginines (ADMA) (for a review see Ref. 3). Type 2 enzymes (PRMT5,7,9) catalyze the formation of MMA and ω-NG,N′G-symmetric dimethylarginines (SDMA). Of note, the enzymatic activity of PRMT2,10,11 remains uncharacterized. PRMT-catalyzed arginine methylation has been shown to be involved in many biological processes, including signal transduction, gene transcriptional regulation, RNA transport, RNA splicing, and embryonic development [3].

Clearly, arginine methylation has a strong impact on the ability of the PRMT substrates to perform their biological functions. A challenging problem in the study of protein arginine methylation is to understand and explore the substrate specificity of PRMTs. Thus far, only limited numbers of substrates of PRMTs (∼50–70 confirmed reports in total for all the PRMT members) have been identified and experimentally verified. Improved computer-aided analysis of the existing PRMT substrates will yield new insight into the diversity of PRMT substrates, and identify new PRMT targets and related biological pathways.

4.3 RELATED WORKS ON METHYLATION PREDICTION

The first protein methylation predictor is the AutoMotif server designed by Plewczynski et al. [9], which aims to predict all single-residue PTMs; methylation prediction is only a small focus of their service. At the same time, Daily et al. [10] focused on the relation between intrinsic disorder and protein modification, and built a particular server called MethylationPredictor based on SVM learning. Later, Chen et al. presented another robust prediction web server, MeMo [11], which has thus far continuously provided predicting services and returned results immediately. Since then, a few other research groups also joined the parade to study the prediction of methylation modifications in proteins and publish their predictors. To date, all the computational methylation prediction methods described in the literature are AutoMotif [9], MethylationPredictor [10], MeMo [11], MASA [12], BPB-PPMS [13], FS-GSVM [14], and NNA-MF [15].

As each of these methods has its own special method for solving this prediction problem, we provide a comprehensive and in depth review in the following sections by comparing every step in the process, including data collection, feature extraction and selection, classifier training and evaluation, and finally discussion of results.

Before moving forward to the comparisons, we point out a fundamental assumption used in all aforementioned predicting methods—the possibility that an arginine residue might be methylated is determined largely by the physicochemical properties of its neighboring residues and the overall biological characteristics presented from these flanking residues. This assumption is popularly and implicitly used in predicting other kinds of PTMs or protein biological properties, such as the prediction of protein secondary structure [16,17] and solvent accessible area [18].

4.3.1 Data Collection

To build a computational prediction model, first an initial training dataset needs to be collected for an algorithm to learn from. In this case, the training dataset includes methylated sequences (the positive class) and unmethylated sequences (the negative class).

The main strategy for collecting methylated sequences in those prediction methods is to search through the Swiss-Prot database [19]. As Swiss-Prot has high-quality manually annotated protein sequence databases, it is easy to write scripts to collect all the "experimentally verified" methylated residues. For example, MethylationPredictor uses a Perl script called BioPerl to search specific terms related to methylated proteins [10]. A positive (methylated) set is created by checking the MOD_RES field, which contains methylarginine or methyllysine in the annotations of proteins; MOD_RES values marked as "probable," "possible," or "potential," "by similarity" are excluded, and the negative set consists of all nonmethylated arginine or lysine in the same protein sequences in MethylationPredictor.

Besides searching Swiss-Prot to find methylated sequences, some researchers searched the PubMed literature to manually check experimentally verified methylation residues. For example, MeMo authors searched the PubMed with keywords *methylation lysine* and *methylation arginine* and found about 1700 scientific articles, containing 264 arginine methylarginines [11]. They combined the manually curated data and Swiss-Prot data together to form the positive training set, resulting in total 273 positive methylated arginines.

To further refine the quality of collected protein sequences, a homology reducing process is often used to remove extra similar sequences or fragments. For example, MeMo authors first use BLASTCLUST [20] to cluster all protein sequences. Sequences sharing 30% similarity will be realigned through BL2SEQ [20], in order to check whether the methylated sites from two or more different sequences are at the same location. If this is so, then only one methylated residue is retained in the final positive set, while the other is removed. Methylation-Predictor, MASA, and BPB-PPMS also employed similar homology removing strategy.

After the homology reduction process, every methylated or nonmethylated arginine is considered as a training example for later modeling. According to the assumption mentioned previously, the flanking sequences are important in determining the status of methylation in the middle residue. Hence, a sequence fragment containing neighboring residues with the center residue is considered as one example. The length of such fragment is normally chosen between 7 and 25 in many computational experiments, as this range is shown to be effective in prediction. From a biological perspective, a neighboring residue too far away from a target residue should not have a favorable impact on its methylation status. The length of sequence fragments is also called *window size* in the literature.

The negative datasets are created from the unmethylated arginines within the same methylated protein sequences. In other words, all the arginines that are not marked as "experimentally verified" methylation belong to the negative class. However, as un-methylated residues are significantly more numerous than methylated ones, the resulting dataset is highly imbalanced. Table 4.1 summarizes all the data information collected in the seven methylation prediction methods according to data collection stage.

4.3.2 Feature Extraction and Selection

Biological information underlying methylation-related sequences needs to be extracted into meaningful computational vectors in order to build accurate prediction models. This is the encoding or feature extraction step, which is the main procedure that differentiates the aforementioned seven methylation predictors.

Domain knowledge and statistical analysis are the primary strategies used to explore the underlying biological information within those methylated protein sequences. Based on mathematical analysis and biological characteristics, several effective encoding schemes for protein sequences have already been developed in literature, such as physicochemical properties, BLOSUM Matrix[21], PSSM

TABLE 4.1 Summary of the Seven Arginine Prediction Methods in Data Collecting Step

Predictor	Year	Data Source	Raw Data Size	Reduced Data Size	Fragment Size	Web Service
AutoMotif	2005	Swiss-Prot version 42	NA[a]	NA	9 aa	Yes (NA)
Methylation Predictor	2005	Swiss-Prot version 45 + Ong et al. [44]	116 + 1315 −	84 + 757 −	25 aa	Yes (NA)
MeMo	2006	Swiss-Prot version 48 + ~1700 articles	273 + 1395 −	247 + 1211 −	15 aa	Yes
MASA	2009	Swiss-Prot version 55 + MeMo data	303 + 1216 −	246 +	13 aa	Yes
BPB-PPMS	2009	Swiss-Prot version 56	434 +	216 + 1980 −	11 aa	Yes
FS-GSVM	2009	MeMo data	—	247 + 1211 −	15 aa	No
NNA-MF	2011	Swiss-Prot version 57.9	190 + 2377 −	(no reduce)	11 aa	No

[a]NA means data or service not available; fragment size is the best size when used for training or prediction.

Matrix[20], etc. Other schemes combine a few basic encoding methods together to build longer and more informative vectors. In this section, we will introduce several basic feature extraction methods as well as some advanced encoding schemes used in the seven methylation prediction algorithms.

4.3.2.1 Feature Extraction

4.3.2.1.1 Orthogonal Code   Orthogonal encoding treats the limited number of amino acids as values for a nominal feature. Hence, a 20-bit binary value is sufficient to represent each amino acid. First, it ranks all amino acids according to their one-letter name alphabetically. For example, alanine is first, arginine is the second, and so on. Then, the 20-bit representation will have a one in its *i*th position, where *i* is its ranking number. All other positions will have zeros. For example, alanine is converted to 10000 00000 00000 00000, arginine is 01000 00000 00000 00000, and so on. Each bit is considered as on feature, so the total features for a training example is expressed as $20*N$, where N is the size of each sequence fragment.

4.3.2.1.2 BLOSUM Matrix   To include the evolutionary divergent information among protein sequences, a block of an amino acid substitution matrix (BLOSUM) was developed by Henikoff and Henikoff [21]. They scanned the BLOCKS protein database for conserved subsequences of different protein families and then counted the relative frequencies of amino acids and their substitution probabilities. A log-odds score is used to measure each of the 210 possible substitutions among the 20 amino acids. Several sets of BLOSUM matrices have been generated using different alignment databases, while BOLSUM62 is the most popular one used in computational predictions for protein properties. The values in the BLOSUM62 matrix are substitution scores that represent the chance of one amino acid being substituted by all other amino acids. Hence, each amino acid is also represented by 20 log-odds scores. The total feature dimension for a protein sequence of size N is still $20*N$ features. This encoding scheme is better than orthogonal code in the prediction perspective, as protein evolutionary characteristics are embedded.

4.3.2.1.3 Physicochemical Properties   The 20 amino acids have very different physical and chemical properties. Encoding these properties into the feature representation makes more sense in building better predicting models. Such amino acids properties include the status of being polar, charged, aromatic, small, tiny, hydrophilic/hydrophobic, and aliphatic. These physicochemical features can be represented by 8 binary bits in total. The detailed feature values of 20 amino acids can be found at http://prowl.rockefeller.edu/aainfo/pchem.htm.   Physicochemical features have shown to be very effective in predicting many protein properties, such as secondary structures [22], peptide binding [23], and protein subcellular localization [24].

4.3.2.1.4 PSSM Matrix   So far, the preceding representations for each amino acid are constant vectors, that is, position-independent matrices. In other words, regardless of where a particular kind of residue is in a fragment, it always receives the same encoding vector everywhere when it occurs. However, from a biological perspective, the same residue may carry different information during the history of evolution. A residue in a conversed region normally shows stronger functional relevance than one in a nonconversed area.

The position-specific scoring matrix (PSSM) created by position-specific iterated BLAST (PSI-BLAST) [20] is a popular matrix for measuring the conversation information for protein sequences. PSI-BLAST is a powerful sequence searching method, which performs multiple sequence alignments to find similar protein sequences to a query sequence from a protein database. PSI-BLAST constructs a PSSM from the resulting multiple alignment. The conservation for each amino acid is measured by the likelihood that this amino acid will mutate to all 20 amino acids in that position in the multialignment results. Hence, amino acid in every position of a protein sequence will receive a special vector (in most cases unique) of 20 values, depicting its evolutionary conversation characteristics in that position. In PSI-BLAST searching, the whole sequence is required in order to find the best matches during alignments. Hence, the input will be the whole protein sequences from the previous step, not just the sliced fragment. After the whole PSSM matrix is constructed, the PSSMs for a particular fragment can be sliced as PSSM features. The total feature size for a length N sequence is also $20*N$.

4.3.2.1.5 Secondary Structure   Structure information of protein sequences normally has certain preference around modified residues in many kinds of PTMs. Hence, extracting protein structure features may better facilitate the prediction of methylated residues. There are four levels of protein structure: primary sequence, secondary structure, tertiary structure, and quaternary structure. Primary sequences have been used in previous encoding schemes, while the other three levels are normally difficult to collect or unavailable in most cases. In particular, the tertiary and quaternary structures of proteins require sophisticated technologies such as X-ray crystallography [25] or nuclear magnetic resonance spectroscopy (NMR) [26] to reconstruct. Hence, the only possible structure level for fast and efficient prediction is the protein's secondary structure. Another reason is that there are already many available prediction tools for protein secondary structure, which can provide highly accurate predictions. For example, PSIPRED [16] is one simple and reliable method for SS prediction, using two feedforward neural networks as learning algorithms. PSIPRED 2.0 can achieve a mean Q_3 score of 80.6% across 40 submitted target domains without obvious sequence similarity to structures presented in the Protein Data Bank (PDB). There are only three types of secondary structure: helix (H), sheet (E), and coil (C). As each residue receives a prediction on its SS property, it can be easily converted into a 3-bit number vector. For example, helix is encoded as 100, sheet is encoded as 010, and coil is encoded as 001.

4.3.2.1.6 Solvent-Accessible Surface Area The relationships between PTMs and solvent ASA have been suggested in several publications. For example, Pang et al. [27] showed that protein methylation has preference in regions that are intrinsically disordered and easily accessible. Hence, Shien et al. first used solvent ASA properties in the feature extraction step for methylation prediction [12]. As few protein sequences have known tertiary structures in PDB for computing solvent ASA, predicted values based on primary sequences are normally used. The RVP-net [18] is an effective ASA prediction tool, and it outputs a real value—the percentage of solvent ASA area of each amino acid on protein sequence. RVP-net uses neighboring residue information to build a predicting classifier based on a neural network, resulting in a mean absolute error of 18.0–19.5% between the predicted and experimental values of ASA per residue. Similarly, the full sequence needs to input RVP-net, and then the resulting value sequences are sliced accordingly to match methylated and nonmethylated fragments. Obviously, each residue has only one float feature for its ASA property.

4.3.2.1.7 Intrinsic Disorder Many studies have shown that intrinsically disordered regions are conversed in several different PTMs such as methylation and acetylation. Hence, the structural disorder is considered as another new biological feature. MethylationPredictor [10] is the first method to emphasizes the correlation between intrinsically disordered regions and methylation, and uses them as one main predicting feature. Later, MF-NNA also embedded this feature during encoding. However, MethylationPredictor uses several predictors of structural disorder, including VL2 [28], VL3 [29], and a *B*-factor predictor [30], while MF-NNA only uses one: VSL2 [31]. Each residue will receive one value for each predictor, and the full sequence needs to be used as input for these predictors.

4.3.2.1.8 Statistical Profile Statistical analysis on biological data has shown to be effective in solving many complicated problems, such as in feature selection for microarray expression data [32] and sampling for multiple sequence alignments [33]. As methylated and unmethylated peptide fragments have both been created from the data collection step, performing simple statistical analysis on both sequence sets can detect discriminative features. One example is biprofile Bayes feature extraction proposed in Shao et al. [13]. Their underlying motivation is that each protein sequence should theoretically exhibit different characteristics in positive and negative feature spaces, respectively. Their proposed position-specific profiles combine the posterior probability of every residue in a fragment in both positive and negative datasets. The posterior probability can be estimated by the occurrence of each amino acid at each position in the positive and negative datasets. Hence, each position will receive two real values as the biprofile feature. The total size of biprofile features is $2*N$.

4.3.2.2 Feature Combination As each feature extraction is independent, one can combine several feature sets together to cover more information to enhance prediction accuracy. Several methylation prediction servers mentioned earlier have applied this concept to aggregate a few extraction methods together to create robust representing vectors for protein peptides. For example, MASA mixes orthogonal encoding, PSSM, secondary structure, and solvent ASA together and performs extensive experiments to find the best combinations in terms of better prediction accuracy; FS-GSVM [14] also combines several feature sets in their methods together, including physicochemical property, secondary structure, PSSM, and solvent ASA. Each amino acid is represented in 32 features in FS-GSVM.

4.3.2.3 Feature Selection However, too many combined features may introduce redundant or correlated features that are not helpful in the later classification modeling step. Hence, feature selection methods can be used to choose relevant features to the methylated statuses of residues. For example, MethylationPredictor first applies a t test to each individual feature to rank its importance, and then uses principal-component analysis (PCA) to reduce dimensionality. The NNA-MF and FE-GSVM both use the mRMR [34] (minimum redundancy and maximum relevance) algorithm to perform an explicit feature selection step before building the classifier.

In Table 4.2 we summarize the feature extraction and feature selection steps that are used in the seven methylation methods.

4.3.3 Classification Method and Evaluation

Given the assumption that methylated residue is determined by the biological or mathematical characteristics of its neighboring residues, protein methylation prediction is a classic binary classification task. The training data can be generated from previous data collection and feature extraction steps, and now the goal in

TABLE 4.2 Summary of Feature Extraction Strategies Used in the Seven Prediction Methods

Predictor	Bin	BLO62	PhCh	PSSM	SS	SASA	ID	Bi-P	Feature Selection
AutoMotif	✓	✓		✓					
Methylation Predictor			✓	✓			✓		t test and PCA
MeMo	✓								
MASA	✓			✓	✓	✓			
BPB-PPMS								✓	
FS-GSVM			✓	✓	✓	✓			mRMR
NNA-MF			✓	✓				✓	mRMR

Notation: BLO62—BLOSUM62; PhCh—physicochemical; SS—secondary structure; SASA—solvent ASA; Bi-P—Bi-Profile; ID—intrinsic disorder this step is to choose an appropriate classification algorithm and build an accurate prediction model.

Of many classification or supervised machine learning algorithms, most existing methylation predictors chose support vector machines (SVMs) to build the classifier. A particular reason is that SVM has shown its higher prediction accuracy in many classification tasks in different domains, such as text mining, image segmentation, and bioinformatics. SVM have also been used in solving many other protein sequence related problems, such as secondary structure prediction [35], protein fold recognition [36], and protein–protein interaction [37].

4.3.3.1 SVM Modeling

As a supervised machine learning method, SVM applier the *structural risk minimization* (SRM) principle in statistical learning theory to minimize the boundary of the expected risk [5]. For binary classification problems, the SVM algorithm creates a hyperplane to separate the data into two classes with the maximum margin. If a clear separation hyperplane does not exist, a kernel strategy can be used to project the original feature space to a high-dimensional feature space. In the transformed space, the separating hyperplane is built with maximum margin and minimum error, which corresponds to a nonlinear function in the original space.

4.3.3.2 Imbalanced Data Learning

The first challenging issue when building accurate classifiers for methylation is the highly imbalanced training data. Methylated residues such as arginine and lysine are significantly fewer in number than those unmethylated ones, meaning that the positive examples are much less than negative examples in the collected training data. Many traditional learning algorithms suffer from this imbalanced data distribution, and generate drastically biased predicting models such that these models classify any new examples into negative classes. Obviously, these biased models are useless if they are used in methylation prediction servers.

Imbalanced data learning is one of the challenging topics in the machine learning community, and it has been studied for more than a decade. Hundreds of imbalance learning algorithms have been published and applied in solving real-world problems. Generally, as summarized by Ahmad et al. [38], there are two different approaches to solving this problem; one is from a data perspective, and the other is from an algorithm perspective. The first type mainly uses undersampling or oversampling strategies to create balanced data and then apply traditional learning algorithms; the latter type tries to design advanced learning algorithms, to internally impose more learning impact on the minority class.

So far, most of the existing SVM-based methylation predictors have used random undersampling strategies to tackle the data imbalance issue. For example, MeMo applied random sampling on the unmethylated training set to maintain same number of examples of positives and negatives before building classifiers. MASA tried different ratios when performing the undersampling on negative data, and they found that the optimal ratio between the size of positive class and negative class to be around 1 : 5. The most recent predictor, BPB-PPMS, revealed a ratio of $1:3$ between size of methylated and un-methylated set as the best ratio to maintain as many negative data and as high an accuracy as possible.

The only predictor that attempted to solve this imbalance problem from the algorithm perspective is the FE-GSVM, which employed an effective granular SVM repetitive undersampling (GSVM-RU [39]) method to build an accurate classifier on both positive and negative classes. The main idea behind GSVM-RU is that, although a single round of SVM learning cannot create a "good" hyperplane for classification, multiple times of SVM learning and discarding previous support vectors from the majority class may push the hyperplane away from the minority class. By this procedure, the hyperplane will be more evenly located in the middle of two feature spaces. All examples from the minority class will be retained during all SVM learning iterations, while the support vectors from majority class will be excluded during learning process. Gradually, the samples in the majority class will be fewer in number, and then the classification hyperplane will be adjusted into an appropriate position. Clearly, compared to undersampling, the benefit of GSVM-RU is no information loss; every example has to be used at least once for training, and some vectors are evaluated before removal. FS-GSVM has shown that using GSVM-RU on this imbalance problem can be effective, on the basis of their experimental results. We believe that this direction should be further investigated because of its better learning ability and robustness.

4.3.3.3 *Other Classification Modeling*   Out of the seven predictors mentioned above, the NNA-MF [15] is the only one that used a different classification model: the *nearest-neighbor algorithm* (NNA). NNA is a simple but widely used machine learning method, and it predicts a new example as the same category of its nearest neighbor. A distance function needs to be defined in order to determine which example is the closest. In NNA-MF, such distance is defined as

$$\text{Dist}\,(v_i, v_j) = 1 - * \frac{v_i * v_j}{\|v_i\| * \|v_j\|},$$

where v_i and v_j are the feature vectors of two sequence fragments. To address the imbalanced training data issue, NNA-MF used a different method instead of random undersampling. They split the majority negative class into small chunks such that each is of relatively the same size as those in the positive class. Then, each chunk is combined with the positive class to form a new training subset and to build a new NNA model. In total, they built 11 NNA predictors on the collected methylated arginine data. The final prediction of a new example from those predictors is integrated with a simple majority voting system.

4.3.3.4 *Classification Evaluation*   To fairly evaluate the classification performance of those learned models, two other issues need to be addressed: finding appropriate testing datasets and good prediction metrics.

For the first issue, cross-validation is a standard method for creating several groups of training data and testing data, in order to collect an unbiased classification performance. The procedure is as follows. Given a whole training dataset D, split it into k same-sized data folds $D_1, D_2, \ldots, D_k$; then, for each fold D_i, use $D - D_i$ as a new training set to build a classifier, and use D_i as the testing set to make predictions. The overall performance is the average result of those predictions on every fold. k is normally chosen from 3,5,7,10, or larger. If k is selected as n—the size of whole dataset D, meaning that every example will be used as a single testing set—then the procedure is called *leave-one-out cross-validation* (LOOCV). Another way to find testing data is to intentionally create independent new examples that are never shown in the whole training dataset. For example, in NNA-MF, the authors collected 84 methylarginine proteins, and randomly selected 10 of them as the independent testing sets, in order to evaluate several other predictors, including MeMo and BPB-PPMS.

For the second issue, an effective performance metric is needed to measure the accuracy for both negative class and positive class. Traditional accuracy on the whole dataset is no longer appropriate because it will be biased toward the majority class. For example, if a dataset contains only 5% positive examples, then a classifier predicting everything as negative will still have an accuracy of 95%. Several statistical measurements can be used to solve this problem, such as sensitivity and specificity, Matthews correlation coefficient (MCC), and area under the curve receiver operating characteristic (AUC-ROC). For example, predictor MeMo reports four measures in their results: accuracy, sensitivity, specificity, and MCC; BPB-PPMS shows AUC in their results, in addition to four other metrics; meanwhile, FS-GSVM reports accuracy, sensitivity, specificity, g-means, and AUC.

Table 4.3 summarizes the main strategies used in this classification modeling and evaluation step for the seven existing predictors.

4.3.4   Result Discussion

The results of the seven methylation prediction methods are summarized in three directions: computational performance, biological findings, and prediction servers.

TABLE 4.3   Classification and Evaluation Settings for Seven Methylation Predictors

Predictor	Learning Models	Imbalance Processing	Validation Method	Independent Testing
AutoMotif	SVM	NA	NA	NA
MethylationPredictor	SVM	Undersampling	LOOCV	No
MeMo	SVM	Undersampling	7-fold CV	No
MASA	SVM	Undersampling	10-fold jackknife	Yes
BPB-PPMS	SVM	Undersampling	5-fold CV	Yes
FS-GSVM	GSVM	GSVM-RU	7-fold CV	No
NNA-MF	NNA	Data splitting	Jackknife CV	Yes

4.3.4.1 Computational Performance As each method uses its special feature extracting or model building step, we collected their cross-validation performance ratings together in a single table and compared (Table 4.4). Differences between these classification performances may suggest the variations in effectiveness of these methods. However, as the training data and testing data were quite different when the authors built those predicting models, such comparisons may not be accurate. An obvious trend is that new predictors are generally better than older ones. This is because new methylated proteins are continuously being identified in the literature, and hence the volume of training data is growing and the prediction model is improving in terms of accuracy.

Some of the seven predictors used an independent testing dataset to compare the prediction performance. For example, MASA created a balanced dataset with 30 methylated arginines and 30 unmethylated arginines, to verify that MASA is better than MeMo in terms of precision, sensitivity, specificity, and accuracy. BPB-PPMS also randomly generates an independent test set with 15 methylated arginines in 11 proteins in the rat lumbar spinal cord and p53 [13]. The results showed the sensitivity of BPB-PPMS to be much higher when an appropriate threshold was chosen. NNA-MF intentionally left 10 proteins as the independent testing set, and compared with both MeMo and BPB-PPMS. The sensitivity of NNA-MF far exceeded that of both MeMo and BPB-PPMS. However, their performance is only better than that of MeMo and worse than BPB-PPMS in terms of specificity, accuracy, and MCC.

4.3.4.2 Biological Findings The biological findings behind those features and values are valuable computational results. We discuss several findings here to understand the biological mechanism under protein arginine methylation. First, the MethylationPredictor authors performed statistical analysis on flanking residues around methylated arginines, and they found that a distinctive indication

TABLE 4.4 Optimal Cross-Validation Results in the Seven Methylation Predictors

Predictor	Best Sequence Size	Kernel	Accuracy (%)	SN (%)	SP (%)	PPV (%)	MCC	AUC (%)
AutoMotif	9 aa	NA	NA	36.28	—	78.00	—	—
Methylation Predictor	NA	Poly	77.9	73.6	82.2	—	—	85.0
MeMo	15 aa	RBF	86.70	69.60	89.20	—	0.54	—
MASA	13 aa	—	84.8	82.1	87.4	86.6	0.796	—
BPB-PPMS	11 aa	RBF	87.98	74.71	94.32	—	0.7729	92.54
FS-GSVM	15 aa	RBF	86.69	72.55	88.04	—	—	84.47
NNA-MF	11 aa	NA	74.25	74.39	74.11	—	0.4852	—

Notation: SN—sensitivity/recall; SP—specificity; PPV—positive prediction value/precision; MCC—Matthews correlation coefficient; AUC—area under the curve (ROC)

for arginine methylation region is glycine–arginine-rich (GAR). This is actually a well-known property for arginine methylation; arginines located GAR motifs are preferred sites of methylation of several PRMTs [40]. The association between methylation and intrinsic disorder had been computationally verified in MethylationPredictor; accuracies of methylated arginine residues predicted to be in disordered regions are much higher than those unmethylated arginines.

MeMo only used the orthogonal representation and simple SVM for classification; hence they did not provide much analysis on the feature side. But they suggested designing more powerful methyltransferase family–specific predictors, and to use other machine learning techniques. MASA authors checked the effectiveness of different groups' extracted features, and found that the combination of PSSM and solvent ASA is the best in terms of computational performance. They double-checked their method by training models from predicted values and testing them on methylated proteins with available 3D structures; the result is very confident: 80.5% of positive test data have been identified. BPB-PPMS employed the statistical biprofiles only as extracted features; hence, their discussion of feature impact to methylation mechanism is not presented. However, they provide a case study to verify their methodology; a more recent study on experimentally verified methylation sites in Tat protein [41] has confirmed high prediction accuracy for BPB-PPMS.

Noticeably, NNA-MF performed quite in-depth biological feature analysis on their results. NNA-MF incorporated three groups of features and employed an incremental strategy and mRMR for feature selection. In addition, they built 11 prediction models from the methylation training data. Hence, they can easily collect the frequency of each feature on these 11 models, and measure the impacts of each feature, as well as each group of features. From sequence conversation (PSSM matrix) aspects, position AA1, AA4, AA6, AA8, and AA11 have a greater influence on the prediction of methylarginine than do other positions. As to amino acid's physicochemical property, the closest preceding residue and two subsequent residues of a center residue are most important in determining the methylation status, and electrostatic charge and secondary structure properties contribute more than do other properties. Interestingly, the structural disorder features on the right side of a methylarginine structure show much greater influence than do those on the left side; the disorder feature on AA9 is important for the identification of methylarginine. Finally, in the optimal feature set, 75.5% are PSSM features, meaning that PSSM features are most important to methylation; 22.5% are amino acid factors, meaning that characteristics of neighboring amino acids also play an important role; and 2% are disorder features, which means that disorder features are not relevant to methylation status in comparison to other features.

4.3.4.3 Prediction Servers The last important contributions from these methylation predictors are the five public available web-based prediction servers: AutoMotif, MethylationPredictor, MeMo, MASA, and BPB-PPMS. So far, only MeMo, MASA, and BPB-PPMS are currently available. Researchers can submit valid protein sequences (in FASTA format) to these servers, and choose interested methylated types, such as arginine or lysine. The prediction results are normally immediately returned to the user, with detailed methylated residues and their probabilities. Both MASA and BPB-PPMS provide a threshold option for users who are interested in higher sensitivity. Prediction results from MASA have more predicted information than others; in addition to residue type, position, and probability of methylation, it outputs the predicted ASA real values as well. In order to quickly return the prediction scores, some slow feature extracting process has been removed from constructing such web service. For example, computing PSSM matrix for a whole protein sequence normally takes several minutes; hence none of the current web services have embedded PSSM encoding. It is used only when conducting experimental analysis.

With these fast methylation prediction services, researchers no longer need to perform biological experiments to verify every arginine or lysine in a sequence; they can submit the interested sequences to these servers and verify only those residues that are highly possible. Hence, these efficient prediction services can greatly enhance the productivity of researchers in identifying new methylated proteins, in order to further understand the fundamental biological process.

4.4 CONCLUSION

In this chapter, we introduced the protein methylation prediction problem and reviewed all the current computational approaches to solve this problem. As one kind of PTM, methylation is relatively less studied than other PTMs, for instance, in comparison to phosphorylation. More recent studies on this prediction topic are also inadequate, as we found only about 7 methylation prediction methods published in the literature.

The challenges for solving this particular prediction task are twofold: (1) extracting abundant and relevant features from protein sequences and (2) building effective classification models on highly imbalanced data. We summarized all the feature extraction strategies that are popularly used in methylation prediction (some are also popular in other PTM predictions), and hope that readers can be motivated to create new feature categories on protein sequence. Computational results in some of these methods have suggested strong correlations between certain types of features and methylation.

As methylated residues are significantly fewer in number than unmethylated ones, the known training dataset is highly imbalanced. Most existing methylation predictors simply use random sampling to create balanced datasets for training, suffering from information loss. However, one interesting method—the FS-GSVM—uses GSVM-RU to tackle this imbalance data issue. Additionally, Ding proposed a new highly imbalanced data learning framework to solve this challenging data issue [38]. We believe that utilizing these new imbalance data learning techniques will be a practical direction for new methylation predictors.

Another direction of future computational methylation study is to identify the specific PRMT substrates for possible methylation residues. So far, the existing predictors have been able to predict the position and probability of methylation only for a related amino acid. However, when verifying these positions in real biological experiments, a particular PRMT substrate needs to be used. Although there does exist some simple rules about the characteristics of PRMT substrates [e.g., PRMT1 (like PRMT3) mediates methylation typically within the archetypal Arg–Gly or Arg–Gly–Gly sequence [42]], such an over simplified rule cannot account for all the existing PRMT substrates. More recent studies have shown that the substrate specificity of PRMT1 is far broader than the typical RGG paradigm and suggest that many of the cellular functions of PRMT1 may not yet have been explored [43]. A better computer-aided analysis of the existing PRMT substrates should yield new insight into the diversity of PRMT substrates, and identify new PRMT targets and related biological pathways.

ACKNOWLEDGMENTS

This work is partially supported by the Molecular Basis of Disease Program at Georgia State University, Atlanta.

REFERENCES

1. Seo J, Lee K-L, Post-translational modifications and their biological functions: Proteomic analysis and systematic approaches, *J. Biochem. Mol. Biol.* **37**(1):35–44 (2004).

2. Walsh CT, Garneau-Tsodikova S, Gatto GJ Jr, Protein posttranslational modifications: The chemistry of proteome diversifications, *Angew. Chem. Int. Ed.* **44**:7342–7372 (2005).

3. Bedford MT, Richard S, Arginine methylation: An emerging regulator of protein function, *Mol. Cell* **18**:263–272 (2005).

4. Paik WK, Kim S, Enzymatic methylation of protein pabp1 identified as an arginine fractions from calf thymus nuclei, *Biochem. Biophys. Res. Commun.* **29**:14–20 (1967).

5. Vapnik V, Cortes C, Support vector networks, *Machine Learn.* **20**(3):273–293 (1995).

6. Holbert MA, Marmorstein R, Structure and activity of enzymes that remove histone modifications, Curr. *Opin. Struct. Biol.* **15**(6):673–680 (2005).

7. Tchurikov NA, Molecular mechanisms of epigenetics, *Biochemistry* **70**(4):406–423 (2005).

8. Lee DY, Teyssier C, Strahl BD, Stallcup MR, Role of protein methylation in regulation of transcription, *Endocr. Rev.* **26**(2):147–170 (2005).

9. Plewczynski D, Tkacz A, Wyrwicz LS, Rychlewski L, AutoMotif server: Prediction of single residue post-translational modifications in proteins, *Bioinformatics* **21**(10):2525–2527 (2005).

10. Daily K, Radivojac P, Dunker A, Intrinsic disorder and protein modifications: Building an SVM predictor for methylation, *Proc. IEEE Symp. Computational Intelligence in Bioinformatics and Computational Biology*, San Diego, CA, 2005, pp. 475–481.

11. Chen H, Xue Y, Huang N, Yao X, Sun Z, MeMo: A web tool for prediction of protein methylation modifications, *Nucleic Acids Res.* **34**:249–253 (2006).

12. Shien DM, Lee TY, Chang WC, Hsu JB, Horng JT, Hsu PC, Wang TY, Huang HD, Incorporating structural characteristics for identification of protein methylation sites, *J. Comput. Chem.* **30**(9):1532–1543 (2009).

13. Shao J, Xu D, Tsai SN, Wang Y, Ngai SM, Computational identification of protein methylation sites through bi-profile Bayes feature extraction, *PLoS One* **4**(3):e4920 (2009).

14. Ding ZJ, Zhang Y-Q, Xie N, Zheng YG, Identifying new methylation arginine via granular decision fusion with SVM modeling, *Proc. 2009 Int. Joint Conf. Bioinformatics, Systems Biology and Intelligent Computing*, Shanghai, 2009, pp. 237–241.

15. Hu LL, Li Z, Wang K, Niu S, Shi XH, Cai YD, Li HP, Prediction and analysis of protein methylarginine and methyllysine base on multisequence features, *Biopolymers* **95**(11):763–771 (2011).

16. Jones DT, Protein secondary structure prediction based on position-specific scoring matrices, *J. Mol. Biol.* **292**:195–202 (1999).

17. Pirovano W, Heringa J, Protein secondary structure prediction, *Methods Mol. Biol.* **609**:327–348 (2010).

18. Ahmad S, Gromiha MM, Sarai A, RVP-net: Online prediction of real valued accessible surface area of proteins from single sequences, *Bioinformatics* **19**(14):1849–1851 (2003).

19. Boeckmann B, Bairoch A, Apweiler R, Blatter MC, Estreicher A, Gasteiger E, Martin MJ, Michoud K, O'Donovan C, Phan I, Pilbout S, Schneider M, The SWISS-PROT protein knowledgebase and its supplement TrEMBL in 2003, *Nucleic Acids Res.* **31**:365–370 (2003).

20. Altschul SF, Madden TL, Schaffer AA, Zhang J, Zhang Z, Miller W, Lipman DJ, Gapped BLAST and PSI-BLAST: A new generation of protein database search programs, *Nucleic Acids Res.* **25**:3389–3402 (1997).

21. Henikoff S, Henikoff JG, Amino acid substitution matrices from protein blocks, *Proc. Nat. Acad. Sci. USA* **89**(22):10915–10919 (1992).

22. Wang LH, Liu J, Li YF, Zhou HB, Predicting protein secondary structure by a support vector machine based on a new coding scheme, *Genome Inform.* **15**(2):181–190 (2004).

23. Ray S, Kepler TB, Amino acid biophysical properties in the statistical prediction of peptide-MHC class I binding, *Immunome Res.* **3**:9 (2007).

24. Sarda D, Chua GH, Li KB, Krishnan A, pSLIP: SVM based protein subcellular localization prediction using multiple physicochemical properties, *BMC Bioinform.* **6**:152 (2005).

25. Jan D, *Principles of Protein X-Ray Crystallography*, Springer, Berlin, 2006.

26. Wüthrich K, The way to NMR structures of proteins, *Nat. Struct. Biol.* **8**:923–925 (2001).

27. Pang CN, Hayen A, Wilkins MR, Surface accessibility of protein post-translational modifications, *J. Proteome Res.* **6**:1833–1845 (2007).

28. Vucetic S, Brown CJ, Dunker AK, Obradovic Z, Flavors of protein disorder, *Proteins* **52**:573–584 (2003).

29. Obradovic Z, Peng K, Vucetic S, Radivojac P, Brown CJ, Dunker AK, Predicting intrinsic disorder from amino acid sequence, *Proteins* **53**(S6):566–572 (2003).

30. Radivojac P, Obradovic Z, Smith DK, Zhu G, Vucetic S, Brown CJ, Lawson JD, Dunker AK, Protein flexibility and intrinsic disorder, *Protein Sci.* **13**(1):71–80 (2004).

31. Peng K, Radivojac P, Vucetic S, Dunker AK, Obradovic Z, Length-dependent prediction of protein intrinsic disorder, *BMC Bioinform.* **7**:208 (2006).

32. Ding ZJ, Zhang Y-Q, Zhao Y, Data shuffling and statistical analysis on microarray data for gene selection—a comparative study on filtering methods, *Int. J. Funct. Informatics Personal. Med.* **3**(3):183–203 (2011).

33. Lawrence CE, Altschul SF, Boguski MS, Liu JS, Neuwald AF, Wootton JC, Detecting subtle sequence signals: A Gibbs sampling strategy for multiple alignment, *Science* **262**(5131):208–214 (1993).

34. Peng H, Long F, Ding C, Feature selection based on mutual information: Criteria of max-dependency, max-relevance, and min-redundancy, IEEE Trans. *Pattern Anal. Machine Intell.* **27**(8):1226–1238 (2005).

35. Hua S, Sun Z, A novel method of protein secondary structure prediction with high segment overlap measure: Support vector machine approach, *J. Mol. Biol.* **308**(2):397–407 (2001).

36. Ding C, Dubchak I, Multi-class protein fold recognition using support vector machines and neural networks, *Bioinformatics* **17**:349–358 (2001).

37. Rashid M, Ramasamy S, Raghava GP, A simple approach for predicting protein-protein interactions, Curr. *Protein Peptide Sci.* **11**(7):589–600 (2010).

38. Ding Z, *Diversified Ensemble Classifiers for Highly Imbalanced Data Learning and Their Application in Bioinformatics*, Computer Science Dissertations, Georgia State Univ. Paper 60, 2011.

39. Tang Y, Zhang Y-Q, Chawla NV, Krasser S, SVMs modeling for highly imbalanced classification, *IEEE Trans. Syst. Man Cybernet*. (Pt. B) **39**(1):281–288 (2009).

40. Bedford MT, Arginine methylation at a glance, *J. Cell Sci.* **120**(Pt. 24):4243–4246 (2007).

41. Xie B, Invernizzi CF, Richard S, Wainberg MA, Arginine methylation of the human immunodeficiency virus type 1 Tat protein by PRMT6 negatively affects Tat Interactions with both cyclin T1 and the Tat transactivation region, *J. Virol.* **81**:4226–4234 (2007).

42. Blanchet F, Schurter BT, Acuto O, Protein arginine methylation in lymphocyte signaling, *Curr. Opin. Immunol.* **18**:321–328 (2006).

43. Wooderchak WL, Zang T, Zhou ZS, Acuña M, Tahara SM, Hevel JM, Substrate profiling of PRMT1 reveals amino acid sequences that extend beyond the "RGG" paradigm, *Biochemistry* **47**:9456–9466 (2008).

44. Ong S-E, Mittler G, Mann M, Identifying and quantifying in vivo methylation sites by heavy methyl silac, *Nat. Methods* **1**:119–126 (2004).

CHAPTER 5

ANALYSIS AND PREDICTION OF PROTEIN POSTTRANSLATIONAL MODIFICATION SITES

JIANJIONG GAO, QIUMING YAO, CURTIS HARRISON BOLLINGER, and DONG XU

5.1 INTRODUCTION

Protein has a wide range of essential functions in living cells, including building and repair of body tissues (structural or storage proteins), catalysis of biochemical reactions (enzymes), regulation of growth and metabolism (hormones), water balancing (membrane proteins), and nutrient transport (transporters or carriers). A protein synthesized immediately after translation from mRNA is typically called an *immature protein*, which is often not fully functional. In order to carry out specific functions in cells, new proteins usually undergo a process called *posttranslational modification* (PTM). PTM plays key roles in many cellular processes such as signaling, cellular differentiation, protein degradation, protein stability, gene expression regulation, protein function regulation, and protein interactions [1]. Irregular PTM activity is often a cause or consequence of many diseases such as cancer [2].

It has been estimated that there are more than 200 types of PTMs mediated by enzymes consisting of 5% of the proteome [3]. Many of these enzymes, such as transferases (e.g., kinases and phosphatases) and ligases, add or remove various types of chemical groups such as phosphate, acyl group, lipid, glycans, or even peptides covalently at amino acid sidechains. Many of these processes are reversible and can thereby change the protein confirmation back and forth or transduce the signal molecules. Other enzymes, such as proteases, perform proteolytic cleavage at specific points on protein backbones, which are involved in the posttranslational processes including terminal methionine removal, signal

Algorithmic and Artificial Intelligence Methods for Protein Bioinformatics. First Edition.
Edited by Yi Pan, Jianxin Wang, Min Li.
© 2014 John Wiley & Sons, Inc. Published 2014 by John Wiley & Sons, Inc.

TABLE 5.1   PTMs Studied in This Chapter

PTM Type	Modified Amino Acid	Function
Phosphorylation	Phosphoserine Phosphothreonine Phosphotyrosine	Signaling pathway, protein degradation, cell cycle, growth, apoptosis
Glycosylation	O-GlcNAc-serine O-GlcNac-threonine	Protein folding, protein stability, protein activity
Methylation	N6-methyllysine Omega-N-methylarginine	Regulation of gene expression, protein stability
Acetylation	N6-acytyl-lysine	Regulation of gene expression, cellular localization
Palmitoylation	S-palmitoylcysteine	Cellular localization
SUMOylation	SUMOylatedlysine	Cellular localization, apoptosis
Sulfation	Sulfotyrosine	Protein–protein interaction

peptide cleavage, or zymogen activation. In this chapter, we focus on a few common covalent PTMs, listed in Table 5.1.

More recently, proteomics data of various PTM sites are accumulating rapidly, thanks to high-throughput mass spectrometry studies [4–13] and associated web resources (Table 5.2). In particular, protein phosphorylation has been extensively characterized and annotated, especially in humans. Nevertheless, our knowledge of protein PTM is still limited. As a result, computational prediction of PTM sites is also becoming an increasingly active research area. Table 5.3 lists PTM site prediction tools.

We developed a standalone bioinformatics tool, Musite, specifically designed for large-scale prediction of PTM sites. PTM site prediction was modeled as an unbalanced binary classification problem. High-quality proteomics data in multiple organisms were collected from several sources, listed in Table 5.2. Three sets of features [k-nearest-neighbor (KNN) scores, disorder scores, and amino acid frequencies] were extracted from the collected data. The extracted features were then combined using a support vector machine (SVM) to train prediction models for the PTMs in Table 5.1 by a comprehensive machine learning method called *bootstrap aggregation*. Cross-validation tests showed that our bootstrap aggregating method performed well. Besides the standalone version of Musite (http://musite.sourceforge.net/), a web server version named Musite.net was also implemented (http://musite.net).

5.2 MUSITE: A MACHINE LEARNING APPROACH

Posttranslational modification site prediction is a binary classification problem. For example, considering phosphoserine prediction, serine residues can be classified into two categories: phosphoserines or positive data and non-phosphoserines (serines that cannot be phosphorylated) or negative data. Note that our aim is to predict whether a residue can be modified by a specific PTM regardless of cell state or biological condition. Musite framework was designed for PTM site prediction in three processes: (1) data collection and preparation, (2) feature extraction, and (3) classifier/prediction model training and evaluation.

5.2.1 Data Collection

We collected high-quality experimentally verified data from several resources in Table 5.2. The numbers of sites for each PTM that we collected are listed in Table 5.4.

5.2.2 Feature Extraction

Feature selection and extraction is an important step in identifing patterns that characterize the commonalities within each class and differences between classes.

TABLE 5.2 Summary of PTM Databases

Database	Website	Species	PTM
UniProt/Swiss-Prot [14]	`http://uniprot.org/`	All species	All
HPRD [15]	`http://www.hprd.org/`	Human	All
dbPTM [16]	`http://dbptm.mbc.nctu.edu.tw/`	All species	All
PhosphoSitePlus	`http://www.phosphosite.org/`	Mainly human and mouse	Multiple
PHOSIDA [17,18]	`http://www.phosida.com/`	Multiple species	Multiple
Phospho.ELM [19–21]	`http://phospho.elm.eu.org/`	Mainly human and mouse	Phosphorylation
PhsophoPep [22,23]	`http://www.phosphopep.org/`	Yeast, worm, fly, human	Phosphorylation
P3DB [24]	`http://p3db.org/`	Plants	Phosphorylation
PhosPhAt [25,26]	`http://phosphat.mpimp-golm.mpg.de/`	*Arabidopsis thaliana*	Phosphorylation
Phosphomouse [13]	`https://gygi.med.harvard.edu/phosphomouse/`	Mouse	Phosphorylation
O-GlycBase	`http://www.cbs.dtu.dk/databases/OGLYCBASE/`	All species	Glycosylation

TABLE 5.3   Summary of PTM Site Prediction Tools

Tool Name	Website	PTM Type
AutoMotif [27,28]	http://ams2.bioinfo.pl/	Multiple
ELM [29]	http://elm.eu.org/	Multiple
Minimotif Miner [30–32]	http://mnm.engr.uconn.edu/	Multiple
Musite [33,34]	http://musite.sf.net and http://musite.net	Multiple
PROSITE [35,36]	http://ca.expasy.org/prosite/	Multiple
ScanSite [37]	http://scansite.mit.edu/	Multiple
Scan-x [38]	http://scan-x.med.harvard.edu/	Multiple
DISPHOS [39]	http://www.dabi.temple.edu/disphos/	Phosphorylation
GPS [40]	http://gps.biocuckoo.org/	Phosphorylation
NetPhos [41,42]	http://www.cbs.dtu.dk/services/NetPhos/	Phosphorylation
NetPhorest [43]	http://netphorest.info/	Phosphorylation
KinasePhos [44]	http://kinasephos2.mbc.nctu.edu.tw/	Phosphorylation
DictyOGlyc [45]	http://www.cbs.dtu.dk/services/DictyOGlyc/	GlcNac
EnsembleGly [46]	http://turing.cs.iastate.edu/EnsembleGly/	*O/N/C*-glycosylation
GPP [47]	http://comp.chem.nottingham.ac.uk/glyco/	*N/O*-glycosylation
NetCGlyc [48]	http://www.cbs.dtu.dk/services/NetCGlyc/	*C*-mannosylation
NetGlycate [49]	http://www.cbs.dtu.dk/services/NetGlycate/	Lysine glycation
NetOGlyc [50]	http://www.cbs.dtu.dk/services/NetOGlyc/	GalNAc
Oglyc [51]	http://www.biosino.org/Oglyc/	*O*-glycosylation
YingOYang [52]	http://www.cbs.dtu.dk/services/YinOYang/	Ying–yang sites
Big-PI Predictor [53]	http://mendel.imp.ac.at/sat/gpi/gpi_server.html	GPI
PredGPI [54]	http://gpcr.biocomp.unibo.it/predgpi/	GPI
Myristoylator [55]	http://ca.expasy.org/tools/myristoylator/	*N*-Terminal myristoylation
PrePS [56]	http://mendel.imp.ac.at/sat/PrePS/	Prenylation
SUMOsp [57,58]	http://sumosp.biocuckoo.org/	SUMOylation
CSS-Palm [59,60]	http://csspalm.biocuckoo.org/	Palmitoylation
NBA-Palm [61]	http://www.bioinfo.tsinghua.edu.cn/NBA-Palm/	Palmitoylation

TABLE 5.3   (*Continued*)

Tool Name	Website	PTM Type
BPB-PPMS [62]	`http://www.bioinfo.bio.cuhk` `.edu.hk/bpbppms/`	Methylation
MASA [63]	`http://masa.mbc.nctu.edu.tw/`	Methylation
NetAcet [64]	`http://www.cbs.dtu.dk/services` `/NetAcet/`	Acetylation
PredMod [65]	`http://ds9.rockefeller.edu/basu` `/predmod.html`	Acetylation
UbiPred [66]	`http://iclab.life.nctu` `.edu.tw/ubipred/`	Ubiquitination
Sulfinator [67]	`http://ca.expasy` `.org/tools/sulfinator/`	Sulfation
SulfoSite [68]	`http://sulfosite.mbc.nctu.edu.tw/`	Sulfation

TABLE 5.4   **Numbers of PTM Sites Collected**

PTM	Modified Residue Type	Number of Modified Residues
Phosphorylation	Phosphoserine	65,822
	Phosphothreonine	14,478
	Phosphotyrosine	5,725
Acetylation	N6-acetyllysine	4,121
Methylation	N6-methyllysine	230
	Omega-*N*- methylarginine	60
Sulfation	Sulfotyrosine	193
SUMOylation	SUMOylated lysine	299
Palmitoylation	*S*-palmitoylcysteine	212
GlcNAcation	*O*-GlcNAc-serine	137
	O-GlcNAc-threonine	91

Musite extracts three sets of features: *k*-nearest-neighbor (KNN) scores, protein disorder scores, and amino acid frequencies.

5.2.2.1   *K-Nearest-Neighbor (KNN) Scores*

KNN scores were extracted as follows to measure the local sequence similarity between query sites and known PTM sites:

1. For a query site (possible PTM site), find its *k* nearest neighbors in positive and negative sets, respectively, according to local sequence similarity. The similarity metric was derived from the BLOSUM62 matrix.
2. Calculate the average distances from the query sequence to all neighbors in the positive and negative sets.

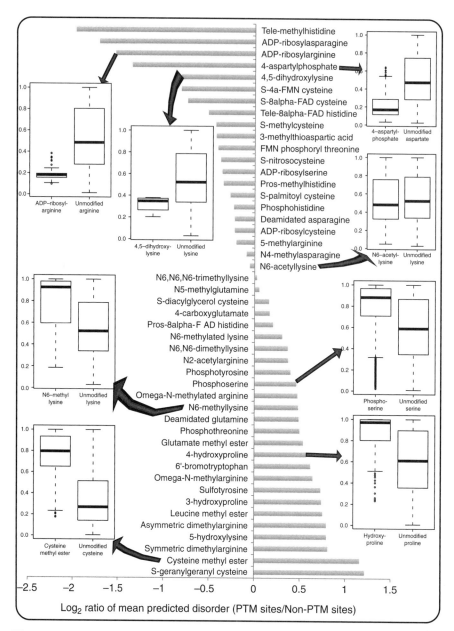

Figure 5.1   Correlation between PTM and protein disorder. The horizontal axis (abscissa) represents the log ratio of mean predicted disorder score of PTM sites versus that of non-PTM sites. A value below 0 means that the corresponding PTM is enriched in structure regions; otherwise, it is enriched in disordered regions. The vertical axis (ordinate) from top to bottom represents PTMs sorted from being most significantly enriched in structure regions to being most significantly enriched in disordered regions. Boxplots of predicted disorder scores of a few representative types of PTM sites and their non-PTM counterparts are also shown.

3. Sort the neighbors by the distances and pick the k nearest neighbors.
4. Calculate KNN score as the percentage of positive neighbors (PTM sites) in its k nearest neighbors.
5. Repeat steps 1–4 at different neighbor sizes (k) values to obtain multiple KNN scores as features that reflect different properties of neighbors with various ranges of similarities.

5.2.2.2 Predicted Protein Disorder Scores Protein disorder has been shown to be correlated with PTMs [39,69]. The correlations between various PTMs and protein disorders are summarized in Figure 5.1 according to results that we previously reported [69]. Predicted protein disorder scores were extracted as features by the following procedure:

1. Predicting disordered regions in the query protein sequence using a disorder prediction tool VSL2B [70].
2. Extracting predicted disorder scores for the residues around each candidate site.
3. Taking the average scores surrounding each site with different window sizes as features for the PTM predictor.

5.2.2.3 Local Amino Acid Frequency It has been observed that amino acids around PTM sites have different compositions. For example, around phosphorylation sites, rigid, buried, neutral amino acids (W, C, F, I, Y, V, L) were significantly depleted, while flexible, surface-exposed amino acids (S, P, E, K) were significantly enriched [39]. We extracted amino acid frequencies around candidate sites with window size of 13 (6 residues from each side of a candidate site) as features.

5.2.3 Classifier Training

Using the extracted features, we trained classifies by a machine learning ensemble meta-algorithm called *bootstrap aggregating* or *bagging* [71] as follows:

1. Extract a training set from a training set by sampling with replacement from positive dataset and negative dataset, respectively, with the same number of data points (say, 2000) in each dataset.
2. Train an SVM classifier using the training set. SVMlight V6.02 [72] is used.
3. Repeat steps 1 and 2 multiple times to obtain several trained classifiers.
4. Submit features extracted for a query to all trained classifiers from step 3, and take the averaged output as the prediction score for the query site.

5.2.4   Evaluation

To evaluate Musite, cross-validation tests were performed. Receiver operating characteristic (ROC) curves were calculated and plotted based on specificities [Eq. (5.1)] and sensitivities [Eq. (5.2)] by taking different thresholds:

$$\text{Specificity} = \frac{\text{true negative}}{(\text{true negative}) + (\text{false positive})} \qquad (5.1)$$

$$\text{Sensitivity} = \frac{\text{true positive}}{(\text{true positive}) + (\text{false negative})} \qquad (5.2)$$

The results of cross-validation tests for phosphorylation site prediction were reported earlier [33]. For each of the other PTMs, we performed fivefold cross-validation tests according to the following procedure. The positive data were first divided into five groups. Each group was then combined with the same number of randomly selected negative data points, forming a sub-dataset. Each time, one of the five sub-datasets was retained as the validation data. All the remaining positive and negative data were used to train a prediction model. The validation data were then submitted to the trained model for prediction. The cross-validation process was repeated 5 times with each sub-dataset used exactly once as the validation data. Sensitivities at different specificity levels in each cross-validation run were calculated according to Equations (5.1) and (5.2). Figure 5.2 shows the receiver operating characteristic (ROC) curve by averaging the sensitivities at different specificities over five cross-validations.

5.3   MUSITE IMPLEMENTATION

5.3.1   Core Modules of Musite Open-Source Framework

With its GNU GPL open-source license and extensible API, Musite provides an open framework for PTM site prediction applications. The Musite framework contains six core modules (more details on these modules are described in an earlier work [34]):

1. The data module defines core data structures representing protein information, PTMs, prediction models, prediction results, and other parameters.
2. The input/output (IO) module supports reading from or writing to files of various formats, including FASTA, Musite XML, and UniProt XML.
3. The feature extraction module defines different types of features extracted from data.
4. The classifier module provides a set of binary classifiers and aggregated classifier.
5. The training/prediction module implements the machine learning procedure for model training and prediction.

6. The user interface (UI) module provides friendly graphical user interface (GUI) to functionalities such as PTM site prediction, prediction result analysis, and customized prediction model training.

5.3.2 Musite.net: A Web Server

Musite.net is a web implementation and extension of Musite standalone application. Musite.net provides a uniform interface for submitting query sequences and analyzing prediction results for different PTMs in various species. Besides phosphorylation, it currently supports prediction of acetylation, methylation, sulfation, SUMOylation, palmitoylation, and GlcNAcation. As PTM data are accumulating rapidly, we will continue to update the prediction models and build new models for more PTMs and species.

On Musite.net, a prediction request can be submitted using a web form. One can select a prediction model according to PTM types, organisms, or kinase types (for phosphorylation site prediction), and submit either sequences or accession

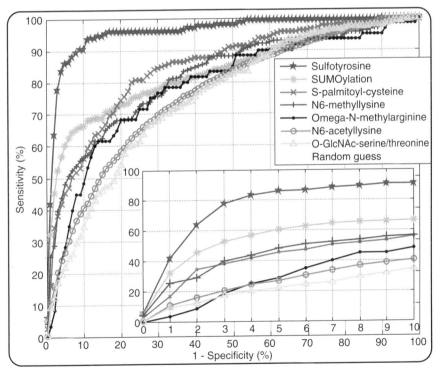

Figure 5.2 ROC curves of Musite predictions of PTM sites. A curve for each PTM represents the average sensitivities and specificities for difference thresholds over five cross-validation runs. The bottom right figure is the zoomed-in region with high prediction specificities (0.9−1).

numbers of the query proteins for prediction. The prediction result is presented in an interactive output page as illustrated in Figure 5.3. One can turn on or off different representations of the prediction result: the protein sequence with highlighted predicted sites, a plot of specificity levels against residue positions, and a table listing predicted sites. Using a slider, one can adjust the significance threshold to any specificity level. If multiple sequences are submitted, the prediction result for each individual sequence can be expanded or shrunk to help the user focus on predictions of interest. The prediction result can be exported to a tab-delimited text file for further analysis.

Musite.net can also be accessed by direct URLs (e.g., `http://musite.net/ ?acc=uniprot:P04637&model=Phosphorylation.H.sapiens.general .tyr`). Similar to the web form submission, one should select the model and provide either the accession number or sequence of the query protein. Direct URLs enable other websites to hyperlink to Musite. For instance, P3DB [24] has linked to Musite in its phosphoprotein pages, to enable users who are interested in predicted phosphorylation sites to easily navigate from experimental phosphorylation data in P3DB to predicted results at Musite.net.

Musite.net also provides a RESTful web service (`http://musite.net/ service`) that can be accessed programmatically. Bioinformatics developers can utilize this web service to integrate the PTM site prediction capacity of Musite.net into their own bioinformatics applications.

5.4 SUMMARY

By taking advantage of the large magnitude of experimentally verified PTM sites and utilizing a comprehensive machine learning method, Musite provides a useful bioinformatics software system for PTM site prediction. Musite has a few unique functionalities, including customized model training from users' own data and continuous adjustment of stringency levels of prediction results. Musite was also the first open-source project intended for PTM site prediction, making it very easy to add new features or explore new machine learning methods for PTM prediction. We provided standalone and web server versions of Musite, both with intuitive graphical user interface (GUI) to access the prediction models that we trained. The standalone version can be used for up to proteome-wide PTM site prediction in an automated fashion, while the web server is meant to provide quick access of PTM site prediction for light jobs. With the Musite project, we determined to build a platform for community use that enables both computational and experimental biologists to obtain a better prediction and understanding of protein PTMs.

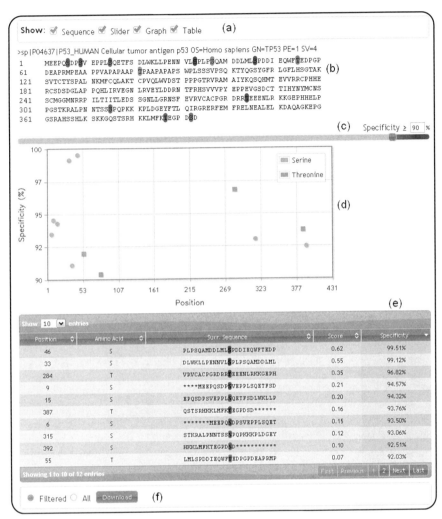

Figure 5.3 Example of a prediction result page; as an example, the query protein with UniProt accession P04637 was submitted for prediction of general phosphoserines/threonines. (a) different presentations of the prediction result can be selected (by default, sequence and slider are selected); (b) the query sequences with predicted PTM sites are highlighted in different colors on the basis of prediction confidence; (c) A slider is provided to control the stringency threshold (any threshold of specificity between 0% and 100% can be set); (d) a plot of specificities against residue positions is made available; (e) a table of predicted PTM sites is presented; (f) the prediction result can be downloaded as a tab-delimited text file.

ACKNOWLEDGMENTS

We would like to thank Dr. Jay J. Thelen and Dr. A. Keith Dunker for helpful discussions. This work was supported by funding from the National Institute of Health (Grants R21/R33 GM078601 and R01 GM100701) and National Science Foundation (Grant DBI-0604439)

REFERENCES

1. Seo J, Lee KJ, Post-translational modifications and their biological functions: Proteomic analysis and systematic approaches, *J. Biochem. Mol. Biol.* **37**(1):35–44 (2004).

2. Krueger KE, Srivastava S, Posttranslational protein modifications: Current implications for cancer detection, prevention, and therapeutics, *Mol. Cell. Proteomics* **5**(10):1799–1810 (2006).

3. Walsh C, *Posttranslational Modification of Proteins: Expanding Nature's Inventory*, Roberts Publishers, 2006.

4. Beausoleil SA, Jedrychowski M, Schwartz D, Elias JE, Villen J, Li J, Cohn MA, Cantley LC, Gygi SP, Large-scale characterization of HeLa cell nuclear phosphoproteins, *Proc. Natl. Acad. Sci. USA* **101**(33):12130–12135 (2004).

5. Olsen JV, Blagoev B, Gnad F, Macek B, Kumar C, Mortensen P, Mann M, Global, *in vivo*, and site-specific phosphorylation dynamics in signaling networks, *Cell* **127**(3):635–648 (2006).

6. Villen J, Beausoleil SA, Gerber SA, Gygi SP, Large-scale phosphorylation analysis of mouse liver, *Proc. Natl. Acad. Sci. USA* **104**(5):1488–1493 (2007).

7. Chi A, Huttenhower C, Geer LY, Coon JJ, Syka JE, Bai DL, Shabanowitz J, Burke DJ, Troyanskaya OG, Hunt DF, Analysis of phosphorylation sites on proteins from *Saccharomyces cerevisiae* by electron transfer dissociation (ETD) mass spectrometry, *Proc. Natl. Acad. Sci. USA* **104**(7):2193–2198 (2007).

8. Munton RP, Tweedie-Cullen R, Livingstone-Zatchej M, Weinandy F, Waidelich M, Longo D, Gehrig P, Potthast F, Rutishauser D, Gerrits B, Panse C, Schlapbach R, Mansuy IM, Qualitative and quantitative analyses of protein phosphorylation in naive and stimulated mouse synaptosomal preparations, *Mol. Cell. Proteomics* **6**(2):283–293 (2007).

9. Sugiyama N, Nakagami H, Mochida K, Daudi A, Tomita M, Shirasu K, Ishihama Y, Large-scale phosphorylation mapping reveals the extent of tyrosine phosphorylation in *Arabidopsis*, *Mol. Syst. Biol.* **4**:193 (2008).

10. Zhai B, Villen J, Beausoleil SA, Mintseris J, Gygi SP, Phosphoproteome analysis of *Drosophila melanogaster* embryos, *J. Proteome Res.* **7**(4):1675–1682 (2008).

11. Boersema PJ, Foong LY, Ding VM, Lemeer S, van Breukelen B, Philp R, Boekhorst J, Snel B, den Hertog J, Choo AB, Heck AJ, In depth qualitative and quantitative profiling of tyrosine phosphorylation using a combination of phosphopeptide immuno-affinity purification and stable isotope dimethyl labeling, *Mol. Cell. Proteomics*: **9**(1):84–89 (2010).

12. Choudhary C, Kumar C, Gnad F, Nielsen ML, Rehman M, Walther TC, Olsen JV, Mann M, Lysine acetylation targets protein complexes and co-regulates major cellular functions, *Science* **325**(5942):834–840 (2009).

13. Huttlin EL, Jedrychowski MP, Elias JE, Goswami T, Rad R, Beausoleil SA, Villen J, Haas W, Sowa ME, Gygi SP, A tissue-specific atlas of mouse protein phosphorylation and expression, *Cell* **143**(7):1174–1189 (2010).

14. Farriol-Mathis N, Garavelli JS, Boeckmann B, Duvaud S, Gasteiger E, Gateau A, Veuthey AL, Bairoch A, Annotation of post-translational modifications in the Swiss-Prot knowledge base, *Proteomics* **4**(6):1537–1550 (2004).

15. Prasad TS, Kandasamy K, Pandey A, Human protein reference database and human proteinpedia as discovery tools for systems biology, *Methods Mol. Biol.* **577**:67–79 (2009).

16. Lee TY, Huang HD, Hung JH, Huang HY, Yang YS, Wang TH, dbPTM: an information repository of protein post-translational modification, *Nucleic Acids Res.* **34**(database issue):D622–D627 (2006).

17. Gnad F, Gunawardena J, Mann M, *PHOSIDA* 2011: The posttranslational modification database, *Nucleic Acids Res.* **39**(database issue):D253–D260 (2011).

18. Gnad F, Ren S, Cox J, Olsen JV, Macek B, Oroshi M, Mann M, PHOSIDA (phosphorylation site database): Management, structural and evolutionary investigation, and prediction of phosphosites, *Genome Biol.* **8**(11):R250 (2007).

19. Diella F, Cameron S, Gemund C, Linding R, Via A, Kuster B, Sicheritz-Ponten T, Blom N, Gibson TJ, Phospho.ELM: A database of experimentally verified phosphorylation sites in eukaryotic proteins, *BMC Bioinformatics* **5**:79 (2004).

20. Diella F, Gould CM, Chica C, Via A, Gibson TJ, Phospho.ELM: A database of phosphorylation sites—update 2008, *Nucleic Acids Res.* **36**(database issue):D240–D244 (2008).

21. Dinkel H, Chica C, Via A, Gould CM, Jensen LJ, Gibson TJ, Diella F, Phospho.ELM: A database of phosphorylation sites—update 2011, *Nucleic Acids Res.* **39**(database issue):D261–D267 (2011).

22. Bodenmiller B, Campbell D, Gerrits B, Lam H, Jovanovic M, Picotti P, Schlapbach R, Aebersold R, PhosphoPep—a database of protein phosphorylation sites in model organisms, *Nat. Biotechnol.* **26**(12):1339–1340 (2008).

23. Bodenmiller B, Malmstrom J, Gerrits B, Campbell D, Lam H, Schmidt A, Rinner O, Mueller LN, Shannon PT, Pedrioli PG, Panse C, Lee HK, Schlapbach R, Aebersold R, PhosphoPep—a phosphoproteome resource for systems biology research in *Drosophila* Kc167 cells, *Mol. Syst. Biol.* **3**:139 (2007).

24. Gao J, Agrawal GK, Thelen JJ, Xu D, P3DB: A plant protein phosphorylation database, *Nucleic Acids Res.* **37**(database issue):D960–D962 (2009).

25. Durek P, Schmidt R, Heazlewood JL, Jones A, MacLean D, Nagel A, Kersten B, Schulze WX, PhosPhAt: The *Arabidopsis thaliana* phosphorylation site database. An update, *Nucleic Acids Res.* **38**(database issue):D828–D834 (2010).

26. Heazlewood JL, Durek P, Hummel J, Selbig J, Weckwerth W, Walther D, Schulze WX, PhosPhAt: A database of phosphorylation sites in *Arabidopsis thaliana* and a plant-specific phosphorylation site predictor, *Nucleic Acids Res.* **36**(database issue):D1015–D1021 (2008).

27. Plewczynski D, Tkacz A, Wyrwicz LS, Rychlewski L, AutoMotif server: Prediction of single residue post-translational modifications in proteins, *Bioinformatics* **21**(10):2525–2527 (2005).

28. Plewczynski D, Tkacz A, Wyrwicz LS, Rychlewski L, Ginalski K, AutoMotif server for prediction of phosphorylation sites in proteins using support vector machine: 2007 update, *J. Mol. Model.* **14**(1):69–76 (2008).

29. Puntervoll P, Linding R, Gemund C, Chabanis-Davidson S, Mattingsdal M, Cameron S, Martin DM, Ausiello G, Brannetti B, Costantini A, Ferre F, Maselli V, Via A, Cesareni G, Diella F, Superti-Furga G, Wyrwicz L, et al, ELM server: A new resource for investigating short functional sites in modular eukaryotic proteins, *Nucleic Acids Res.* **31**(13):3625–3630 (2003).

30. Balla S, Thapar V, Verma S, Luong T, Faghri T, Huang CH, Rajasekaran S, del Campo JJ, Shinn JH, Mohler WA, Maciejewski MW, Gryk MR, Piccirillo B, Schiller SR, Schiller MR, Minimotif Miner: A tool for investigating protein function, *Nat. Methods* **3**(3):175–177 (2006).

31. Rajasekaran S, Balla S, Gradie P, Gryk MR, Kadaveru K, Kundeti V, Maciejewski MW, Mi T, Rubino N, Vyas J, Schiller MR, Minimotif miner 2nd release: A database and web system for motif search, *Nucleic Acids Res.* **37**(database issue):D185–D190 (2009).

32. Schiller MR, Minimotif miner: A computational tool to investigate protein function, disease, and genetic diversity, *Current Protocols in Protein Science*, 2007, Unit 2.12, Chap. 2.

33. Gao J, Thelen JJ, Dunker AK, Xu D, Musite, a tool for global prediction of general and kinase-specific phosphorylation sites, *Mol. Cell. Proteomics* **9**(12):2586–2600 2010.

34. Gao J, Xu D, *The* Musite open-source framework for phosphorylation-site prediction, *BMC Bioinformatics* **11**(Suppl 12):S9 2010.

35. de Castro E, Sigrist CJ, Gattiker A, Bulliard V, Langendijk-Genevaux PS, Gasteiger E, Bairoch A, Hulo N, ScanProsite: Detection of PROSITE signature matches and ProRule-associated functional and structural residues in proteins, *Nucleic Acids Res.* **34**(web server issue):W362–W365 (2006).

36. Gattiker A, Gasteiger E, Bairoch A, ScanProsite: A reference implementation of a PROSITE scanning tool, *Appl. Bioinformatics* **1**(2):107–108 (2002).

37. Obenauer JC, Cantley LC, Yaffe MB, Scansite 2.0: Proteome-wide prediction of cell signaling interactions using short sequence motifs, *Nucleic Acids Res.* **31**(13):3635–3641 (2003).

38. Schwartz D, Chou MF, Church GM, Predicting protein post-translational modifications using meta-analysis of proteome scale data sets, *Mol. Cell. Proteomics* **8**(2):365–379 (2009).

39. Iakoucheva LM, Radivojac P, Brown CJ, O'Connor TR, Sikes JG, Obradovic Z, Dunker AK, The importance of intrinsic disorder for protein phosphorylation, *Nucleic Acids Res.* **32**(3):1037–1049 (2004).

40. Xue Y, Ren J, Gao X, Jin C, Wen L, Yao X, GPS 2.0, a tool to predict kinase-specific phosphorylation sites in hierarchy, *Mol. Cell. Proteomics* **7**(9):1598–1608 (2008).

41. Blom N, Gammeltoft S, Brunak S, Sequence and structure-based prediction of eukaryotic protein phosphorylation sites, *J. Mol. Biol.* **294**(5):1351–1362 (1999).

42. Blom N, Sicheritz-Ponten T, Gupta R, Gammeltoft S, Brunak S, Prediction of post-translational glycosylation and phosphorylation of proteins from the amino acid sequence, *Proteomics* **4**(6):1633–1649 (2004).

43. Miller ML, Jensen LJ, Diella F, Jorgensen C, Tinti M, Li L, Hsiung M, Parker SA, Bordeaux J, Sicheritz-Ponten T, Olhovsky M, Pasculescu A, Alexander J, Knapp S, Blom N, Bork P, Li, S, Cesareni G, Pawson T, et al, Linear motif atlas for phosphorylation-dependent signaling, *Sci. Signal.* **1**(35):ra2 (2008).

44. Wong YH, Lee TY, Liang HK, Huang CM, Wang TY, Yang YH, Chu CH, Huang HD, Ko MT, Hwang JK, KinasePhos 2.0: A web server for identifying protein kinase-specific phosphorylation sites based on sequences and coupling patterns, *Nucleic Acids Res.* **35**(web server issue):W588–W594 (2007).

45. Gupta R, Jung E, Gooley AA, Williams KL, Brunak S, Hansen J, Scanning the available *Dictyostelium discoideum* proteome for *O*-linked GlcNAc glycosylation sites using neural networks, *Glycobiology* **9**(10):1009–1022 (1999).

46. Caragea C, Sinapov J, Silvescu A, Dobbs D, Honavar V, Glycosylation site prediction using ensembles of support vector machine classifiers, *BMC Bioinformatics* **8**:438 (2007).

47. Hamby SE, Hirst JD, Prediction of glycosylation sites using random forests, *BMC Bioinformatics* **9**:500 (2008).

48. Julenius K, NetCGlyc 1.0: Prediction of mammalian *C*-mannosylation sites, *Glycobiology* **17**(8):868–876 (2007).

49. Johansen MB, Kiemer L, Brunak S, Analysis and prediction of mammalian protein glycation, *Glycobiology* **16**(9):844–853 (2006).

50. Julenius K, Molgaard A, Gupta R, Brunak S, Prediction, conservation analysis, and structural characterization of mammalian mucin-type *O*-glycosylation sites, *Glycobiology* **15**(2):153–164 (2005).

51. Li S, Liu B, Zeng R, Cai Y, Li Y, Predicting *O*-glycosylation sites in mammalian proteins by using SVMs, *Comput. Biol. Chem.* **30**(3):203–208 (2006).

52. Gupta R, Brunak S, Prediction of glycosylation across the human proteome and the correlation to protein function, *Proc. Pacific Symp. Biocomputing* 2002, pp. 310–322.

53. Eisenhaber B, Bork P, Eisenhaber F, Prediction of potential GPI-modification sites in proprotein sequences, *J. Mol. Biol.* **292**(3):741–758 (1999).

54. Pierleoni A, Martelli PL, Casadio R, PredGPI: A GPI-anchor predictor, *BMC Bioinformatics* **9**:392 (2008).

55. Bologna G, Yvon C, Duvaud S, Veuthey AL, *N*-Terminal myristoylation predictions by ensembles of neural networks, *Proteomics* **4**(6):1626–1632 (2004).

56. Maurer-Stroh S, Koranda M, Benetka W, Schneider G, Sirota FL, Eisenhaber F, Towards complete sets of farnesylated and geranylgeranylated proteins, *PLoS Comput. Biol.* **3**(4):e66 (2007).

57. Ren J, Gao X, Jin C, Zhu M, Wang X, Shaw A, Wen L, Yao X, Xue Y, Systematic study of protein sumoylation: Development of a site-specific predictor of SUMOsp 2.0, *Proteomics* **9**(12):3409–3412 (2009).

58. Xue Y, Zhou F, Fu C, Xu Y, Yao X, SUMOsp: A web server for sumoylation site prediction, *Nucleic Acids Res.* **34**(web server issue):W254–W257 (2006).

59. Ren J, Wen L, Gao X, Jin C, Xue Y, Yao X, CSS-Palm 2.0: An updated software for palmitoylation sites prediction, *Protein Eng. Design Select.* **21**(11):639–644 (2008).

60. Zhou F, Xue Y, Yao X, Xu Y, CSS-Palm: Palmitoylation site prediction with a clustering and scoring strategy (CSS), *Bioinformatics* **22**(7):894–896 (2006).

61. Xue Y, Chen H, Jin C, Sun Z, Yao X, NBA-Palm: Prediction of palmitoylation site implemented in Naive Bayes algorithm, *BMC Bioinformatics* **7**:458 (2006).

62. Shao J, Xu D, Tsai SN, Wang Y, Ngai SM, Computational identification of protein methylation sites through bi-profile Bayes feature extraction, *PLoS One* **4**(3):e4920 (2009).

63. Shien DM, Lee TY, Chang WC, Hsu JB, Horng JT, Hsu PC, Wang TY, and Huang HD, Incorporating structural characteristics for identification of protein methylation sites, *J. Comput. Chem.* **30**(9):1532–1543 (2009).

64. Kiemer L, Bendtsen JD, Blom N, NetAcet: prediction of *N*-terminal acetylation sites, *Bioinformatics* **21**(7):1269–1270 (2005).

65. Basu A, Rose KL, Zhang J, Beavis RC, Ueberheide B, Garcia BA, Chait B, Zhao Y, Hunt DF, Segal E, Allis CD, Hake SB, Proteome-wide prediction of acetylation substrates, *Proc. Natl. Acad. Sci. USA* **106**(33):13785–13790 (2009).

66. Tung CW, Ho SY, Computational identification of ubiquitylation sites from protein sequences, *BMC Bioinformatics* **9**:310 (2008).

67. Monigatti F, Gasteiger E, Bairoch A, Jung E, The Sulfinator: predicting tyrosine sulfation sites in protein sequences, *Bioinformatics* **18**(5):769–770 (2002).

68. Chang WC, Lee TY, Shien DM, Hsu JB, Horng JT, Hsu PC, Wang TY, Huang HD, Pan RL, Incorporating support vector machine for identifying protein tyrosine sulfation sites, *J. Comput. Chem.* **30**(15):2526–2537 (2009).

69. Gao J, Xu D, Correlation between posttranslational modification and intrinsic disorder in protein, *Proc. Pacific Symp. Biocomputing* 2012, Big Island, Hawaii, pp. 94–103.

70. Obradovic Z, Peng K, Vucetic S, Radivojac P, Dunker AK, Exploiting heterogeneous sequence properties improves prediction of protein disorder, *Proteins* **61**(Suppl 7):176–182 (2005).

71. Breiman L, Bagging predictors. *Machine Learn.* **24**(2):123–140 (1996).

72. Thorsten J, *Learning to Classify Text Using Support Vector Machines: Methods, Theory and Algorithms*, Kluwer Academic Publishers, 2002, p. 224.

PART II

PROTEIN ANALYSIS AND PREDICTION

CHAPTER 6

PROTEIN LOCAL STRUCTURE PREDICTION

WEI ZHONG, JIEYUE HE, ROBERT W. HARRISON,
PHANG C. TAI, and YI PAN

6.1 INTRODUCTION

Studying the protein sequence–structure relationship is one of the most active bioinformatics research areas. A better understanding of the protein sequence–structure correlation can improve effectiveness and efficiency of local protein structure prediction [1]. Many biochemical tests indicate that a protein's sequence can determine that protein's structure completely because all the information that is necessary to specify protein interactions with other molecules is embedded in the protein's sequence [2]. These studies provide experimental support for exploring the protein sequence–structure relationship using data mining techniques. The structure-cluster-based approach, the sequence-cluster-based approach, and the clustering support vector machine (SVM) are used to explore the sequence–structure relationship for local protein structure prediction.

6.2 STRUCTURAL CLUSTER APPROACH

For the structural–cluster approach, protein structural segments are grouped into different structural clusters using multiple structural alignments [3] and unsupervised clustering algorithms [4–6]. Each cluster is associated with a representative local structural prototype. Yang and Wang utilized multiple structural alignments to produce a large set of structure-based sequence profiles [3]. In this multiple structural alignment, sequence segments that have structure similar to that of seed sequence segments are used to construct local structure-based sequence

Algorithmic and Artificial Intelligence Methods for Protein Bioinformatics. First Edition.
Edited by Yi Pan, Jianxin Wang, Min Li.
© 2014 John Wiley & Sons, Inc. Published 2014 by John Wiley & Sons, Inc.

profiles, which are stored in the LSBSP1 data library. On the basis of these local structure-based sequence profiles, the consensus approach is adopted to predict the structure of a query sequence segment. The second approach used the unsupervised clustering algorithm to generate 3D protein fragments represented by a structural alphabet of 16 protein blocks [4–6]. The library of 120 overlapping prototypes is constructed with high 3D local approximation based on these protein fragments. A system of experts developed from the 120 prototypes optimize the discrimination from sequences of a given prototype from the others, using logistic regression. For a sequence segment whose structure is to be predicted, all experts calculate probabilities of sequence–structure correlation for the prototypes and propose the top scorers for the structural candidates based on the ranking. This system achieved a prediction rate of 51.2% per the sequence window.

6.3   SEQUENCE CLUSTER APPROACH

For the sequence cluster approach, sequence segments are clustered into high-quality sequence clusters with the K-means clustering algorithm [7,8] and multiple sequence alignment [9] to explore the protein sequence–structure correlations. In 2000, the hidden Markov model (HMM) was established on the basis of high-quality sequence clusters in order to predict the backbone torsion angles for local protein structure [10–11]. The clustering algorithm is critical to exploring how protein sequences correspond to local 3D protein structure in these approaches. The conventional clustering algorithm, such as the K-means and K-nearest-neighbor algorithms, assumes that the distance between samples can be calculated with exact precision [12]. When the distance function for these clustering algorithms is not well defined, the clustering algorithm may not be effective in discovering the complex sequence–structure relationship. Consequently, the majority of sequence segments in some sequence clusters are weakly mapped to the representative structure of their assigned clusters.

6.4   SUPPORT VECTOR MACHINES FOR LOCAL PROTEIN STRUCTURE PREDICTION

The support vector machine (SVM) has shown superior classification performance in various bioinformatics applications because of its strong generalization capability [13]. It can deal with the nonlinear relationship by implicitly mapping input samples from the input feature space into another high-dimensional feature space with the nonlinear kernel function. Consequently, SVM is preferred over the conventional clustering algorithm for exploring the nonlinear protein sequence–structure relationship. Since its training time complexity is at least quadratic to the number of samples, SVM trainings for very large datasets are slow processes [13]. The task of learning the sequence–structure correlation using an SVM becomes more challenging when each subspace of the whole protein sample space corresponds to different local 3D structures [14].

Many SVM training algorithms have been proposed to enhance the efficiency of SVM trainings for large datasets while maintaining reasonable performance. These algorithms can be divided into three major classes:

1. *Decomposition Algorithms.* Decomposition algorithms [13,15,16] partition a large quadratic programming (QP) problem into a series of smaller QP subproblems, that can be easily and efficiently tackled. Although the decomposition algorithm can expedite the training process, they do not scale well with the size of datasets since the kernel matrix may grow beyond the available memory during the optimization process.

2. *Selective Sampling Techniques.* These algorithms handle large datasets by selecting a small number of high-quality training samples intelligently from the whole dataset in order to improve the learning capacity of SVM [17,18]. The selective sampling techniques may reduce the classification perfor- mance of SVM when a single effective decision boundary is difficult to form for the protein datasets that have multiple sequence–structure distri- bution patterns in different sample subspaces.

3. *Multiple SVM Systems.* These include the Bayesian committee machine (BCM) [19], SVM ensembles [20], clustering support vector machines (CSVMs) [12], and supergranule support vector machines (GSVMs) [21]. Experimental results show that the performance of BCM and SVM ensem- bles is worse than that of a single SVM, especially when the dataset expands and becomes more complicated [19,20,21].

6.5 CLUSTERING SUPPORT VECTOR MACHINES FOR LOCAL PROTEIN STRUCTURE PREDICTION

In order to overcome disadvantages of building one SVM over the whole sample space, the clustering support vector machine (CSVM) was proposed to predict distance matrices, torsion angles, and secondary structures for backbone α-carbon atoms of protein sequence segments [12]. During the CSVM construction phase, the K-means clustering algorithm partitions sequence segments into multiple clus- ters. Then, each SVM in the CSVM model is built for one sequence cluster produced by the clustering algorithm in order to clarify the unique nonlinear sequence–structure relationship in each cluster. During the testing phase, the clustering algorithm provides the initial cluster assignment for the given sequence segment. If the SVM modeled for the assigned cluster predicts the sequence seg- ment as positive, this sequence segment has the potential to be closely mapped to the representative structure of this cluster. Consequently, the representative 3D structure for this cluster can be safely assigned to this sequence segment. If the SVM modeled for the assigned cluster predicts the sequence segment as negative, the frequency profiles of this sequence segment are not closely related to the representative local 3D structure of this cluster. As a result, initial cluster assignment by the clustering algorithm is not reliable. The greedy algorithm is utilized to select the next closest cluster based on the distance function. The previous procedure is repeated until one SVM trained for the selected cluster predicts the sequence segment as positive. Compared with the K-means clustering algorithm, CSVM can estimate how closely protein sequences correspond with local 3D structures using the nonlinear kernel. Consequently, CSVM can provide the additional dependable information for cluster membership assignment. The experimental results show that CSVM can improve accuracy of local protein structure prediction significantly compared to the K-means clustering algorithm [12].

6.5.1 *K*-Means Clustering Algorithm

The K-means clustering algorithm is selected to partition the whole sample space into multiple clusters. In each cluster, sequence segments with similar characteristics are grouped together. Consequently, a complex data mining project is divided into a series of computationally tractable simpler tasks. After several experiments, 800 clusters that are deemed relatively suitable for this application are selected [14].

Sequence segments with 11 continuous positions are generated, using the sliding-window method. In total 500,000 sequence segments are produced in the training dataset. These sequence segments of 11 continuous positions represented by the HSSP frequency profiles [23] are clustered into different groups with the K-means algorithm.

The distance score of the given sequence segment for each cluster is calculated after comparing the HSSP frequency profile for this sequence segment with the centroid of each cluster. A lower distance score indicates that the sequence segment is closer to the centroid for the given cluster, which is the average frequency profile of sequence segments for the given cluster.

The following formula calculates the distance score of a given sequence segment for a specified cluster [25].

$$\text{Distance score} = \sum_{i=1}^{L} \sum_{j=1}^{N} |F_k(i,j) - F_c(i,j)| \tag{6.1}$$

Here, L is the window size and N is 20; $F_k(i,j)$ is the value of frequency profile at row i and column j for the sequence segment k, while $F_c(i,j)$ is the value of the matrix at row i and column j for the centroid of the cluster.

An average frequency profile reveals how often amino acids occur in each position of a given cluster. The following formula calculates the frequency of the amino acid of type R at the specified position of the average frequency profile for a sequence cluster:

$$f_R = \frac{\text{Num}_R}{\text{total\_number}} \tag{6.2}$$

Here, Num_R is the number of amino acid of R in the specified position of the sequence cluster and *total number* is the total number of amino acids in the specified position of the sequence cluster.

The reliability score of a given sequence segment for a cluster assesses how often the amino acids of the given sequence segments match more frequently occurring amino acids in the corresponding position of a cluster. A higher reliability score indicates that the sequence segment can be assigned to the given cluster more reliably, as

$$\text{Reliability score} = \sum_{i=1}^{L} F_c(i,j) \qquad (6.3)$$

where $F_c(i,j)$ is the value of the matrix at row i and column j for the average frequency profile of the cluster. The value of j is determined by the type of amino acid in the specified position of the sequence segment.

Five clusters with the top five smallest distance scores for the sequence segment are selected in order to exclude some less significant clusters for cluster assignment purposes. The sequence segment is assigned to the cluster with the highest reliability score among these top five clusters. If there is a tie, the cluster with the smaller distance score is selected.

The distance scores efficiently reduce the number of candidate clusters based on similarity between the frequency profile of the given sequence segment and the centroid of each cluster. The reliability score evaluates how well amino acids of the sequence segment match very frequently occurring amino acids in the conversed positions of the average cluster frequency profiles. Combined information from the distance score and the reliability score can improve effectiveness of cluster assignment noticeably since the distance score and the reliability score each convey independent biological information.

6.5.2 Training CSVMs for Each Cluster

Since the distribution patterns for frequency profiles belonging to different clusters are quite different, training of CSVMs is customized for each cluster belonging to different cluster groups. The CSVMs for clusters in the bad cluster group are trained to select sequence segments whose structure can be reliably predicted. The CSVMs for clusters in the good cluster group are designed to filter out sequence segments whose structure may not be reliably predicted.

The RBF kernel function is chosen for training each SVM. The RBF kernel parameters, including j, γ, and C, are optimized through the grid search process [13]. In each cluster, the structure deviation of positive sequence segments from the representative structure of this cluster is within a given threshold. The negative sample is similarly defined. Frequency profiles of positive sequence segments may be closely correlated with the given 3D representative structure of specified clusters. Frequency profiles of negative sequence segments are not closely mapped to the representative 3D structure. Labeling sequence segments as positive or negative offers important training patterns for CSVMs to learn the underlying sequence–structure relationship for each cluster.

6.5.3   Local Protein Structure Prediction by CSVMs

The clustering algorithm first assigns sequence segments whose structures are to be predicted to the specific cluster. Then CSVM trained for this cluster is utilized to assess how close this sequence segment is nonlinearly related to the 3D representative local structure of this cluster. If the sequence segment is identified as positive by CSVM, this segment has the strong potential to be closely mapped to the representative 3D local structure for this cluster. As a result, the representative 3D local structure of this cluster can be safely assigned to the sequence segment. If the sequence segment is predicted as negative, this segment may not closely correspond to the 3D local structure for this cluster. Consequently, the structure of this segment cannot be reliably predicted by this cluster. This cluster is deleted from the cluster candidate group. The next cluster from the cluster candidate group is selected by the cluster membership function. This process is repeated until one CSVM trained for the selected candidate cluster identifies the sequence segment as positive. The whole CSVM algorithm is displayed in Figure 6.1. Basically, the sequence segments that are incorrectly assigned by the conventional clustering algorithm are reclassified by the CSVMs model.

6.6   EXPERIMENTAL RESULTS

6.6.1   Training Set and Independent Test Set

The training set obtained from the Protein Sequence Culling Server (PISCES) [25] includes 2000 protein sequences. The training dataset is used to produce sequence clusters and the CSVM model. The independent test set consists of 200 protein sequences from the recent release of PISCES. The 3D structure of protein sequences is obtained from the Protein Data Bank (PDB) [26]. Any two protein sequences in the dataset share less than 25% similarity.

6.6.2   Prediction Accuracy Metrics

In order to assess the performance of different models, structure prediction accuracy of sequence segments in terms of secondary structure accuracy, the distance matrix root mean square deviation (dmRMSD) and torsion angle RMSD (taRMSD) are calculated.

The term Q_3 is a popular performance measure in protein secondary structure prediction. It refers to the three-state overall percentage of correctly predicted

---

Clustering Support Vector Machine Model

1. Granulating the whole sequence feature space into clusters
   by the K-means algorithm
   WHILE (the training error is bigger than the threshold
   values)
   {
     Converting sequences into segments by the sliding window
        method
     Assigning each segment to the specific cluster by
        membership functions
     Updating the centroid and the frequency profile for each
        cluster
   }

2. Training CSVM for each granule
   Classifying clusters into different groups based on the
        training accuracy
   FOR each cluster
   {
     Labeling each training sample as positive or negative
        respectively for different cluster groups
     Modeling each CSVM for each cluster by optimizing RBF
        kernel parameters (j, y, and C) with the grid search
        algorithm
   }

3. Predicting protein structure by the CSVMs algorithm
   While (there are clusters in the cluster group)
     {
       Allocating a given sequence segment to a cluster
          in the cluster group by membership functions
       Predicting the property of the given sequence
          segment by CSVM modeled for the selected
          cluster
       If (the given sequence segment is predicted as
          positive)
          {
             Assigning the corresponding structure of
                the selected cluster to this sequence
                segment leave the loop
          }
       remove the selected cluster from the cluster
          group
     }
   randomly assigning a structure to the sequence segment

Figure 6.1 The CSVM model [12].

residues. The following formula is used to calculate secondary structure accuracy [27]:

$$Q_3 = \frac{\sum_{i \in \{H,E,C\}} \text{number of residues correctly predicted}_i}{\sum_{i \in \{H,E,C\}} \text{number of residues in class } i}. \tag{6.4}$$

The following formula is used to calculate dmRMSD [28]:

$$\text{dmRMSD} = \sqrt{\frac{\sum_{i=1}^{L}\sum_{j=i+1}^{L}(\alpha_{i \to j}^{s1} - \alpha_{i \to j}^{\text{ADM}})^2}{M}}. \tag{6.5}$$

$$M = \frac{(L \times L - L)}{2}. \tag{6.6}$$

where $\alpha_{i \to j}^{\text{ADM}}$ is the distance between α-carbon atom i and α-carbon atom j in the average distance matrix of a cluster; M is the number of distances in the distance matrix in this formula.

The following formula is used to calculate taRMSD:

$$\text{taRMSD} = \sqrt{\frac{\sum_{k=1}^{L}\left\{\left(\varphi_{ki} - \varphi_{kj}\right)^2 + \left(\psi_{ki} - \psi_{kj}\right)^2\right\}}{2L}} \tag{6.7}$$

Here, φ_{kj} is φ in position k of the representative angle for a cluster and ψ_{kj} is ψ in position k of the representative angle for a cluster; terms φ and ψ are defined by Karp [2].

6.6.3 Classification of Clusters into Different Groups

Clusters with high training accuracy are given priority in predicting structures of sequence segments. If structures of sequence segments cannot be predicted by high-quality clusters, clusters with lower training accuracy are selected for structure prediction.

Training secondary structure accuracy for a given cluster is the average training accuracy of sequence segments in the training set predicated by this cluster. Training dmRMSD of a given cluster is the average training dmRMSD of sequence segments in the training set predicated by this cluster. Training taRMSD of a given cluster is defined similarly. Test secondary structure accuracy, test dmRMSD, and test taRMSD are defined similarly for each cluster in the independent test set.

Table 6.1 displays the criteria used to categorize clusters into different groups according to training accuracy. Clusters in the good cluster group have training

TABLE 6.1   Standard for Classification of Clusters into Different Groups

Cluster Group	Secondary Structure Accuracy (%)	dmRMSD (Å)	taRMSD
Bad	60–70	>1.5	>30°
Average	70–80	1–1.5	25–30°
Good	>80	<1	<25°

TABLE 6.2   Threshold for Evaluating Accuracy Criteria 1 and 2 for Each Cluster

Accuracy Criterion	Secondary Structure Accuracy (%)	dmRMSD (Å)	taRMSD
1	>70	<1.5	<30°
2	>80	<1	<25°

secondary structure accuracy of >80%, training dmRMSD of <1 Å, and training taRMSD of <25°. The bad cluster group and the average cluster group are defined similarly. In this work, 30 clusters are randomly selected from each cluster group to test the effectiveness of the prediction model.

6.6.4 Structure Prediction Accuracy Criteria

Only joint information on secondary structure, torsion angle, and distance matrix can represent protein structure precisely. To thoroughly compare the prediction performance of these algorithms, two sets of accuracy criteria, termed accuracy criteria 1 and accuracy criteria 2 are defined. Accuracy criteria 1 and 2 consider secondary structure accuracy, dmRMSD, and taRMSD simultaneously. Table 6.2 provides the threshold for evaluating accuracy criteria 1 and 2 for each cluster. Accuracy criteria 2 for one cluster consist of is the percentage of sequence segments with secondary structure accuracy of >80%, dmRMSD of <1 Å, and taRMSD of <25° in the test set for this cluster. Accuracy criteria 2 reflect the percentage of sequence segments with the most reliable structure prediction for this particular cluster. Accuracy criteria 1 are defined similarly. Accuracy criteria 1 calculate the percentage of sequence segments with are acceptable level of structure prediction for one cluster.

6.6.5 Experimental Results and Analysis

Figure 6.2 shows average accuracy, precision, and recall of CSVMs for different cluster groups. Besides accuracy, precision and recall are also the important indicators for the generalization power of SVM. Only if accuracy, precision, and recall are balanced, can SVM can accomplish strong learning capability.

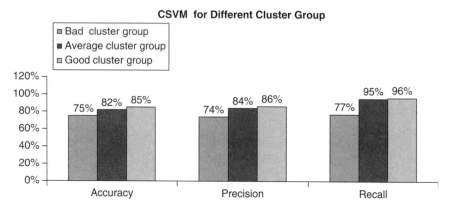

Figure 6.2   Average accuracy, precision, and recall of CSVMs for different cluster groups.

Equations (6.8) and (6.9) show how to calculate precision and recall. Figure 6.2 indicates that CSVM trained for different cluster groups is effective in discriminating between positive and negative samples. CSVMs trained for the bad cluster group are able to choose sequence segments whose structure can be predicted reliably. The high recall value for CSVMs belonging to the good cluster group shows that CSVMs did not misclassify sequence segments whose structure can be accurately predicted. The high-precision value for CSVMs belonging to the good cluster group demonstrates that CSVMs belonging to the good cluster group can effectively filter out sequence segments whose structure cannot be reliably predicted.

$$\text{precision} = \frac{TP}{TP + FP} \tag{6.8}$$

$$\text{recall} = \frac{TP}{TP + FN} \tag{6.9}$$

Figure 6.3 compares the secondary structure accuracy between the conventional clustering algorithm and the CSVM model. Secondary structure accuracy for the bad cluster group increases by 8.32% when the CSVM model is applied. Secondary structure accuracy for the average cluster group increases by 3.22% when the CSVM model is applied.

Figure 6.4 compares dmRMSD values between the conventional clustering algorithm and the CSVMs model. The dmRMSD error for the bad cluster group reduces by 10.82% when the CSVM model is applied. The dmRMSD error for the average cluster group reduces by 6.90%. The dmRMSD error for the good cluster group reduces by 2.91% when the CSVM model is applied.

Figure 6.5 compares the taRMSD between the conventional clustering algorithm and the CSVM model. The taRMSD error for the bad cluster group reduces

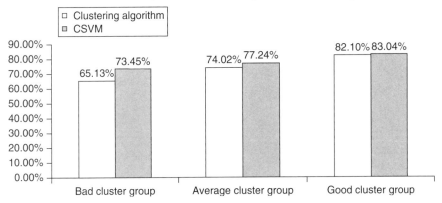

Figure 6.3 Comparison of secondary structure accuracy between the clustering algorithm and CSVM model.

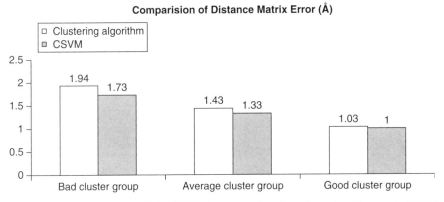

Figure 6.4 Comparison of dmRMSD between the clustering algorithm and CSVM model.

by 13.75% when the CSVM model is applied. The taRMSD error for the average cluster group reduces by 5.20% when the CSVM model is applied. The taRMSD error for the good cluster group reduces by 1.51% when the CSVM model is applied.

Accuracy criteria 1 and 2 measure three performance metrics at the same time. Since three metrics evaluate the prediction performance in different perspectives, including all three metrics can provide rigorous assessment of effectiveness for structure prediction. Figure 6.6 compares accuracy criteria 1 between the conventional clustering algorithm and the CSVMs model. Figure 6.7 compares accuracy criteria 2 between the conventional clustering algorithm and the CSVM model for different cluster groups.

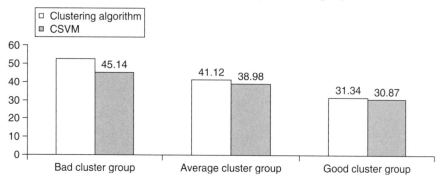

Figure 6.5 Comparison of taRMSD between the clustering algorithm and CSVM model

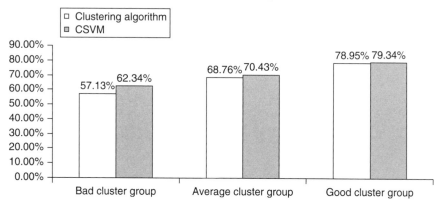

Figure 6.6 Comparison of accuracy criterion 1 between the clustering algorithm and the CSVMs model for different cluster groups.

Figures 6.6 and 6.7 demonstrate that the CSVMs model can improve the prediction performance under the most rigorous evaluation standards. Experimental results indicate that CSVMs are effective in recognizing the complex patterns of frequency profiles for each cluster. Compared with the traditional clustering algorithm, CSVMs can improve local structure prediction accuracy noticeably.

The distribution patterns of frequency profiles vary for different cluster groups. For example, the distribution pattern of frequency profiles for the bad cluster group is diverse while the distribution pattern of frequency profiles for the good cluster group is compact. The customized learning process for different cluster groups can clarify the sequence–structure relationship more effectively. SVM

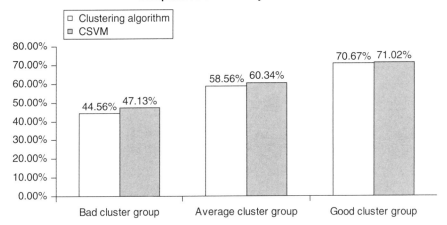

Figure 6.7 Comparison of accuracy criterion 2 between the clustering algorithm and the CSVM model for different cluster groups.

training for very large datasets is the slow process, due to the high training time complexity. The special features of CSVMs enable the training tasks for each CSVM to be parallelized. Parallel training processes can increase the speed for the data mining task for very large datasets.

REFERENCES

1. Rahman A, Zomaya AY, An overview of protein-folding techniques: Issues and perspectives, *Int. J. Bioinformatics Res. Appl.* **1**:121–143 (2005).

2. Karp G, *Cell and Molecular Biology (Concepts and Experiments)*, 3rd ed., Wiley, 2002, pp. 52–65.

3. Yang AS, Wang LY, Local structure prediction with local structure-based sequence profiles, *Bioinformatics* **19**(10):1267–1274 (2003).

4. De Brevern1 AG, Benros1 C, Gautier R, Valadié H, Hazout1 S, Etchebest C, Local backbone structure prediction of proteins, *Silico Biol.* **4**(3):381–386 (2004).

5. Etchebest C, Benros C, Hazout S, de Brevern AG, A structural alphabet for local protein structures: Improved prediction methods, *Proteins: Struct. Funct. Bioinformatics* **59**:810–827 (2005).

6. Benros C, de Brevern AG, Etchebest C, Hazout S, Assessing a novel approach for predicting local 3D protein structures from sequence, *Proteins: Struct. Funct. Bioinformatics* **62**:865–880 (2006).

7. Han KF, Baker D, Recurring local sequence motifs in proteins, *J. Mol. Biol.* **251**(1):176–187 (1995).

8. Han KF, Baker D, Global properties of the mapping between local amino acid sequence and local structure in proteins, *Proc. Natl. Acad. Sci. USA* **93**(12):5814–5818 (1996).

9. Hunter CG, Subramaniam S, Protein local structure prediction from sequence, *Proteins: Struct. Funct. Genet.* **50**:572–579 (2003).

10. Bystroff C, Thorsson V, Baker D, HMMSTR: A hidden markov model for local sequence-structure correlations in proteins, *J. Mol. Biol.* **301**:173–190 (2000).

11. Bystroff C , Baker D, Prediction of local structure in proteins using a library of sequence-structure motifs, *J. Mol. Biol.* **281**:565–577 (1998).

12. Zhong W, He J, Harrison R, Tai PC, Pan Y, Clustering support vector machines for protein local structure prediction, *Expert Syst. Appl.* **32**(2):518–526 (2007).

13. Vapnik V, *Statistical Learning Theory*, Wiley, New York, 1998.

14. Zhong W, Altun G, Harrison R, Tai PC, Pan Y, Improved *K*-means clustering algorithm for exploring local protein sequence motifs representing common structural property, *IEEE Trans. Nanobiosci.* **4**(3):255–265 (2005).

15. Platt J, Fast training of support vector machines using sequential minimal optimization, *Advances in Kernel Methods: Support Vector Learning*, MIT Press, 1999, pp. 185–208.

16. Joachims T, Making large-scale support vector machine learning practical, *Advances in Kernel Methods: Support Vector Machines*, MIT Press, 1999, pp. 169–184.

17. Khan L, Awad M, Thuraisingham B, A new intrusion detection system using support vector machines and hierarchical clustering, *Int. J. Very Large Data Bases* **16**(4):507–521 (2007).

18. Li XO, Cervante J, Yu W, Support vector classification for large data sets by reducing training data with change of classes, *Proc. 2008 IEEE Int. Conf. Systems, Man and Cybernetics*, 2008, pp. 2609–2614.

19. Tresp V, A bayesian committee machine, *Neural Comput.* **12**(11):2719–2741 (2000).

20. Valentini G, An experimental bias-variance analysis of SVM ensembles based on resampling techniques, *IEEE Trans. Systems, Man and Cybernetics, Pt. B: Cybernetics* **35**(6):1252–1271 (2005).

21. Chen B, Johnson M, Protein local 3D structure prediction by super granule support vector machines (Super GSVM), *BMC Bioinformatics* **10**(11):S15 (2009).

22. Gupta SK, Rao KS, Bhatnagar V, *K*-means clustering algorithm for categorical attributes, *Proc. Data Warehousing and Knowledge Discovery (DaWaK-99)*, Florence, Italy, 1999, pp. 203–208.

23. Sander C, Schneider R, Database of homology-derived protein structures and the structural meaning of sequence alignment, *Proteins: Struct., Funct., Genet.* **9**(1):56–68 (1991).

24. Han JW, Kamber M, *Data Mining: Concepts and Techniques*, 2nd ed., Morgan Kaufmann, 2006.

25. Wang G, Dunbrack RL Jr, PISCES: A protein sequence-culling server, *Bioinformatics* **19**(12):1589–1591 (2003).

26. Berman HM, Westbrook J, Bourne PE, The protein data bank, *Nucleic Acids Res.* **28**:235–242 (2000).

27. Hu H, Pan Y, Harrsion R, Tai PC, Improved protein secondary structure prediction using support vector machine with a new encoding scheme and advanced tertiary classifier, *IEEE Trans. Nanobiosci.* **2**(4):265–271 (2004).

28. Kolodny R, Linial N, Approximate protein structural alignment in polynomial time, *Proc. Natl. Acad. Sci. USA* **101**:12201–12206 (2004).

CHAPTER 7

PROTEIN STRUCTURAL BOUNDARY PREDICTION

GULSAH ALTUN

7.1 INTRODUCTION

At the present state of the art in protein bioinformatics, it is not yet possible to predict protein structure [43]. Proteins are among the major components of living organisms and are considered to be the working and structural molecules of cells. They are composed of building block units called *amino acids* [25,34]. These amino acids dictate the structure of a protein [49].

Many machine learning approaches and new algorithms have been proposed to solve the protein structure prediction problem [5,7,13,15,31,41]. Among the machine learning approaches, support vector machines (SVMs) have attracted a lot of attention because of their high prediction accuracy [1]. Since protein data consist of sequence and structural information, another widely used approach for modeling these structured data is to analyze them as graphs. In computer science, graph theory has been widely studied; however, more recently it has been applied to bioinformatics. In out research, we introduced new algorithms based on statistical methods, graph theory concepts, and machine learning for the protein structure prediction problem.

In this chapter, we describe a novel encoding scheme and a computational method using machine learning for prediction starting and ending points of secondary structure elements. Most computational methods have been developed with the goal to predict the secondary structure of every residue in a given protein sequence. However, instead of predicting the structure of each and every residue, a method that can correctly predict where each secondary structure segment (e.g., α helices, β sheets, or coils) in a protein starts and ends could be much more reliable since fewer predictions would be required. Our system makes only one prediction to determine whether a given sequence segment is the start

Algorithmic and Artificial Intelligence Methods for Protein Bioinformatics. First Edition.
Edited by Yi Pan, Jianxin Wang, Min Li.
© 2014 John Wiley & Sons, Inc. Published 2014 by John Wiley & Sons, Inc.

or end of any secondary structure H, E, or C, whereas the traditional methods must be able to predict each and every residue's structure correctly in the segment in order to make that decision. We compared the traditional existing binary classifiers to the new binary classifiers proposed in this chapter and achieved an accuracy much higher than that of the traditional approach.

In summary, we propose methods for predicting protein secondary structure and detecting transition boundaries of secondary structures of helices (H), coils (C), and sheets (E). Detecting transition boundaries instead of the structure of individual residues in the whole sequence is much easier. Thus, our problem is reduced to the problem of finding these transition boundaries.

7.2 BACKGROUND

In this chapter, we present problem definitions and discuss our motivation for research, and related work. This section gives a general background for the methods that we propose.

7.2.1 Prediction of Protein Structure

Proteins are polymers of amino acids containing a constant mainchain (linear polymer of amino acids) or backbone of repeating units with a variable sidechain (sets of atoms attached to each α carbon of the mainchain) attached to each [33]. Proteins play a variety of roles that define particular functions of a cell [33]. They are a critical component of all cells and are involved in almost every function performed by them. Proteins are building blocks of the body controls; they facilitate communication with cells and transport substances. Biochemical reactions among enzymes also contain protein. The transcription factors that turn genes on and off are proteins as well.

A protein consists primarily of amino acids, which determine its structure. There are 20 amino acids that can produce countless combinations of proteins [25,36]. There are four levels of structure in a protein:

Level 1 is the primary structure of the protein, which is its amino acid sequence. A typical protein contains 200–300 amino acids.

Level 2 is the secondary structure, which is formed of recurring shapes called helices, strands, and coils as shown in Figure 7.1. Many proteins contain helices and strands.

Level 3 is the tertiary structure of a protein, which is the spatial assembly of helices and sheets and the pattern of interactions between them. This is also called the *folding pattern* of a protein.

Many proteins contain more than one polypeptide chain; the combinations two or more polypeptide chains in a protein make up its quaternary structure [9,18].

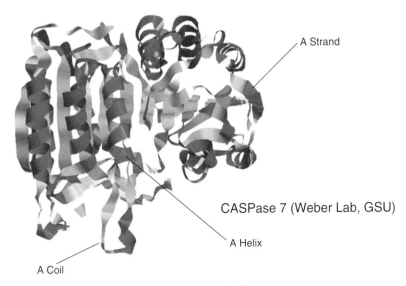

A Strand

CASPase 7 (Weber Lab, GSU)

A Helix

A Coil

Figure 7.1   CASPASE 7 protein.

The protein in Figure 7.1 is a CASPase 7 protein borrowed from the Weber lab in the Georgia State University (GSU) Biology Department.

Proteins interact with DNA (deoxyribonucleic acid), RNA (ribonucleic acid), and other proteins in their tertiary and quaternary states. Therefore, knowing the structure of a protein is crucial for understanding its function.

Large volumes of genes have been sequenced more recently. Therefore, the gap between known protein sequences and protein structures that have been experimentally determined is growing exponentially. The Protein Data Bank (PDB) [10] contains many proteins whose amino acid sequences are known; however, only a small fraction of these protein structures are known [7,10] because nuclear magnetic resonance (NMR) and X-ray crystallographic techniques take years to determine the structure of one protein. Therefore, access to computational tools to predict the structure of a protein is very important and necessary. Although only a few of the computational methods proposed for protein structure prediction yield 100% accurate results, even an approximate model can help experimental biologists guide their experiments. The ability to predict the secondary and tertiary structures of a protein from its amino acid sequence is still a major challenge in bioinformatics. With the methods available today, protein tertiary structure prediction is a very difficult task even when starting from exact knowledge of protein backbone torsion angles [11]. It has also been suggested that protein secondary structure delimits the overall topology of the proteins [35]. It is believed that predicting the protein secondary structure provides insight into, and an important starting point for, prediction of the tertiary structure of the protein, which leads to understanding the function of the protein. There have been many approaches toward revealing the protein secondary structure from the primary sequence information [17,22,37–40,50,51].

7.2.2   Protein Secondary Structure Prediction Problem Formulation

In this work, we adopted the most generally used Dictionary of Secondary Structure of Proteins (DSSP) secondary structure assignment scheme [29]. The DSSP classifies the secondary structure into eight different classes: H (α helix), G (3_{10} helix), I (π helix), E (β strand), B (isolated β bridge), T (turn), S (bend), and—(rest). These eight classes were reduced for the purposes of this work into three regular classes based on the following method: H, G, and I, to H; E, to E; and all others, to C. In this work, H represents helices; E represents sheets and C represents coils.

The formulation in stated is Problem 7.1.

Problem 7.1   Given a protein sequence $a_1 a_2 \ldots a_N$, predict the secondary structure. To do this, find the state of each amino acid a_i as being either H (helix), E (β strand), or C (coil).

The quality of secondary structure prediction is measured with a *three-state accuracy* score denoted as Q_3. The Q_3 formula is the percent of residues that match reality as follows:

$$Q_3 = \frac{\sum_{i \in \{H,E,C\}} \text{ number of residues correctly predicted}_i}{\sum_{i \in \{H,E,C\}} \text{ number of residues in class}_i} \tag{7.1}$$

The Q_3 index is one of the most commonly used performance measures in protein secondary structure prediction. It refers to the three-state overall percentage of correctly predicted residues.

7.2.3   Previous Work on Protein Secondary Structure Prediction

The protein secondary structure prediction problem has been studied widely for almost 25 years. Many methods have been developed for the prediction of secondary structure of proteins. In the initial approaches, secondary structure predictions were performed on single sequences rather than families of homologous sequences [21]. The methods were shown to be ~65% accurate. Later, with the availability of large families of homologous sequences, it was found that when these methods were applied to a family of proteins rather than a single sequence, the accuracy increased well above 70%. Today, many proposed methods utilize evolutionary information such as multiple alignments and PSI-BLAST profiles [2]. Many of those methods that are based on neural networks, SVM, and hidden Markov models have been very successful [5,7,13,15,31,41]. The accuracy of these methods reaches ~80%. An excellent review of the methods for protein secondary structure prediction has been published by Rost et al. [41].

7.2.4 Support Vector Machines

The support vector machines (SVM) algorithm is a modern learning system designed by Vapnik and Cortes [46]. Based on statistical learning theory, which explains the learning process from a statistical perspective, the SVM algorithm creates a hyperplane that separates the data into two classes with the maximum margin. Originally, it was a linear classifier based on the optimal hyperplane algorithm. However, by applying the kernel method to the maximum-margin hyperplane, Vapnik and his colleagues proposed a method for building a non-linear classifier. In 1995, Cortes and Vapnik suggested a soft-margin classifier, which is a modified maximum-margin classifier that allows for misclassified data. If there is no hyperplane that can separate the data into two classes, the soft-margin classifier selects a hyperplane that separates the data as cleanly as possible with a maximum margin [16].

Support vector machine learning is related to recognizing patterns from the training data [1,19]. The SVM software program SVM^{light} is an implementation of SVMs in C [26]. In this chapter, we adopt this SVM^{light} software, which is an implementation of Vapnik's SVMs [45]. This software also provides methods for assessing the generalization performance efficiently.

SVM^{light} consists of a learning module (svm_learn) and a classification module (svm_classify). The classification module can be used to apply the learned model to new examples.

The format for training data and test data input file is as follows:

```
<line> .=. <target> <feature>:<value> <feature>:<value> …
<target> .=. +1 | -1 | 0 | <float>
<feature> .=. <integer> | ''qid''
<value> .=. <float>
```

For classification, the target value denotes the class of the example; $+1$ and -1, as the target values, denote positive and negative examples, respectively.

7.3 NEW BINARY CLASSIFIERS FOR PROTEIN STRUCTURAL BOUNDARY PREDICTION

Proteins consist primarily of amino acids, which determine the structure of a protein. Protein structure has three states: primary structure, secondary structure, and tertiary structure. The *primary structure* of the protein is its amino acid sequence; the *secondary structure* is formed from recurring shapes: α helix, β sheet, and coil. The *tertiary structure* of the protein is the spatial assembly of helices and sheets and the pattern of interactions between them. Predicting the secondary and tertiary structures of proteins from their amino acid sequences is an important problem; knowing the structure of a protein aids in understanding how the functions of proteins in metabolic pathways map for whole genomes, in deducing evolutionary relationships, and in facilitating drug design.

It is strongly believed that protein secondary structure delimits the overall topology of the proteins [21] Therefore, since the mid-1980s, many researchers have tried to understand how to predict the secondary structure of a protein from its amino acid sequence. Many algorithms and machine learning methods have been proposed for this problem [2,30,32]. The algorithms for predicting secondary structure of proteins have reached a plateau of roughly 90%. Much more success has occurred with motifs and profiles [15].

The common approach to solve the secondary structure prediction problem has been to develop tools that predict the secondary structure for each and every amino acid (residue) of a given protein sequence. Here, we propose new binary classifiers that do not require the correct prediction of each and every residue in a given protein segment. The new binary classifiers predict only the start or end of a helix, sheet or coil. We illustrated this concept in Figure 7.2, which is a schematic representation of the tertiary structure of a protein with its secondary structure regions colored in different shades. The point where one secondary structure element ends and another one begins is called a *structural transition* throughout this chapter.

Protein sequences may have specific residue preferences at the end or start of secondary structure segments. For example, it has been shown that specific residue preferences exist at the end of helices, which is called *helix capping*. More recent research has suggested that it is possible to detect helix capping motifs [6]. However, these results reflect a linear decision function based on amino acid frequencies. It is well known that nonlinear decision functions, for example, those implemented with support vector machines (SVMs), dramatically outperform linear decision functions when the underlying data are nonlinear [46]. In this work, we use a machine learning approach based on SVM to predict the helix capping regions of a given protein sequence. These helix capping regions indicate where a helix ends. The same method is also used for predicting the start

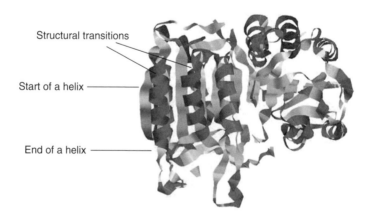

Figure 7.2 Structural transitions of a protein.

points of helices and to predict the endpoints and startpoints of coils and sheets. The ending and starting points of secondary structures are also called *structural transition boundaries*.

7.3.1 Problem Formulation

In this study, we adopted the most generally used DSSP secondary structure assignment scheme [29]. As mentioned in Section 7.2.2, the eight classes were reduced into three regular classes based on the following method: H, G, and I were reduced to H; E, to E; and all others, to C.

7.3.1.1 Traditional Problem Formulation for Secondary Structure Prediction   The traditional problem formulation is stated as exactly the same as Problem 7.1.

Given a protein sequence $a_1 a_2 \ldots a_N$, find the state of each amino acid a_i as being either H (helix), E (strand), or C (coil).

As mentioned earlier, the metric Q_3 is used to measure the quality of the secondary structure prediction. The Q_3 score, which is termed *three-state accuracy*, represents the percent of residues that match reality. Most of the previous research adopted Q_3 as an accuracy measurement.

7.3.1.2 New Problem Formulation for Transition Boundary Prediction
The new problem formulation is stated as follows.

Problem 7.2   Given a protein sequence profile, find the state of each amino acid a_i as being either (1) the start of a H (helix), E (β strand), or C (coil); (2) the end of a H (helix), E (β strand), or C; or (3) neither of the above (denoted as X: doesn't matter).

Here, we used a new scoring scheme that we call Q_T (where T denotes transition), which is similar to Q_3; however, Q_T is the percent of residues that match reality. We had to change the scoring scheme to Q_T because the Q_3 scoring scheme takes into account all the residues whereas Q_T factors in only the residues that are necessary for prediction.

$$Q_T = \frac{\sum_{i \in \{H,E,C\}} \text{ number of correctly predicted transition residues}_i}{\sum_{i \in \{H,E,C\}} \text{ number of transition residues}_i} \qquad (7.2)$$

In the Q_T scoring scheme, the number of correctly predicted transition residues of class H, E, or C is divided by the number of all transition residues of class H, E, or C.

7.3.2 Method

7.3.2.1 Motivation   Given a protein sequence of a 9-mer, let the middle element of this 9-mer be the starting position of a helix as shown in Figure 7.3. Our goal is to determine whether the middle residue is the start or end of a helix. If we use the traditional binary classifiers (such as $H/\sim H$), first we must correctly identify all the residues in the whole segment. We need to correctly predict three consecutive residues as H (at least four residues are needed for a helix), and the remaining residues should be $\sim H$. In this case, we have to make nine predictions, and ideally we should be correct all 9 times. However, the probability that we can predict all nine residues correctly in the protein segment is at maximum 0.35 if we assume that our chance of making each prediction correctly is 0.9 and that this probability of success is independent of the other predictions.

In the next section, we explore how to overcome the problem of making nine predictions for a given 9-mer and how to reduce it to a problem of making only one prediction per 9-mer.

7.3.2.2 A New Encoding Scheme for Prediction of Starts of H, E, and C   The goal of our new encoding scheme is shown in Figure 7.4, where a

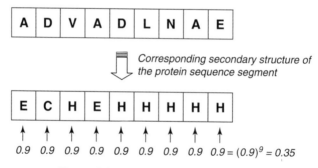

Figure 7.3   A 9-mer with helix junction.

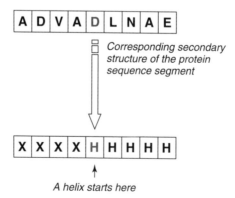

Figure 7.4   New encoding scheme for the helix startpoint.

new binary classifier has to make only one guess instead of nine guesses. Here, the new encoding scheme for representing the starting points of helices is shown as an example. The same encoding is applied to both sheets and coils.

Figure 7.4 illustrates the new encoding scheme.

For the middle residue to be classified as the start of a helix, the rules of the new encoding scheme are as follows:

1. The residues corresponding to X values can be C, H, or E, but no two consecutive H values are allowed.
2. The secondary structure of the middle residue must be H.
3. All residues after the middle residue must be H.

If all three rules are satisfied, the protein segment is represented by the new encoding scheme as the start of a helix (H_{start}). If not, the protein segment is represented as $\sim H_{start}$ (not the start of a helix).

7.3.2.3 A New Encoding Scheme for Prediction of Ends of H, E, and C

Similar to the the the method described in Section 7.3.2.2, the new encoding scheme for representing the ends of helices is shown as an example is in Figure 7.5. The same encoding is applied to sheets and coils.

In the new encoding scheme, the protein sequences are classified as shown in Figure 7.6.

The rules of the new encoding scheme are listed below. These are similar to the rules listed in Section 7.3.2.2, but are used to predict the ends of secondary structures. For the middle residue to be classified as a helix end, the conditions are as follows:

1. The residues corresponding to X values can be C, H, or E, but no two consecutive H values are allowed.
2. The secondary structure of the middle residue must be H.
3. All residues before the middle residue must be H.

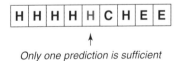

Only one prediction is sufficient

Figure 7.5   A 9-mer with helix end.

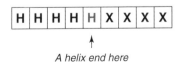

A helix end here

Figure 7.6   New encoding scheme for helix start.

If all three rules are satisfied, the protein segment is represented by the new encoding as the end of a helix (H_{end}). If not, the protein segment is represented as $\sim H_{end}$ (not the end of an helix).

7.3.3 New Binary Classifiers

In the traditional secondary structure prediction approach, usually six binary classifiers, such as three "1 versus rest" classifiers ($H/\sim H$, $E/\sim E$, and $C/\sim C$) and three "1 versus 1" classifiers (H/E, E/C, and C/H) are used. Here, the numeral 1 in the "1 versus rest" classifier refers to a positive class and the term *rest* indicates a negative class. Likewise, the expression "1's in 1 versus 1" classifier refers to positive class and negative class, respectively. For example, the classifier $H/\sim H$ classifies the testing sample as helix or not helix, and the classifier E/C classifies the testing sample as sheet or coil.

The following six new binary classifiers are proposed:

Binary Classifier 1: $H_{start}/\sim H_{start}$. This binary classifier classifies the positive samples as the start of a helix and negative samples as not being the start of a helix.

Binary Classifier 2: $E_{start}/\sim E_{start}$. This binary classifier classifies the positive samples as the start of a sheet and negative samples as not being the start of a sheet.

Binary Classifier 3: $C_{start}/\sim C_{start}$. This binary classifier classifies the positive samples as the start of a coil and negative samples as not being the start of a coil.

Binary Classifier 4: $H_{end}/\sim H_{end}$. This binary classifier classifies the positive samples as the end of a helix and negative samples as not being the end of a helix.

Binary Classifier 5: $E_{end}/\sim E_{end}$. This binary classifier classifies the positive samples as the end of a sheet and negative samples as not being the end of a sheet.

Binary Classifier 6: $C_{end}/\sim C_{end}$. This binary classifier classifies the positive samples as the end of a coil and negative samples as not being the end of a coil.

7.3.4 SVM Kernel

We used a radial basis function (RBF) kernel because it was optimal when used for secondary structure prediction:

$$K(x,y) = e^{-\gamma \|x-y\|^2} \tag{7.3}$$

Here, x and y are two input vectors containing different feature values and γ is the radial basis kernel parameter. Radial basis kernels depend on a numerical representation of the input data.

7.3.5 Selection of Window Size

In order to choose an optimal window size for the proposed encoding scheme for a given protein segment, we tried different window sizes on the smaller dataset RS126. We used the position-specific scoring matrix (PSSM) profiles of the dataset RS126 during the tests. As a prediction method, we used the SVM RBF kernel. Using the sliding-window scheme, we extract first each k-mer from a protein sequence. Each k-mer is classified as a positive or negative sample. If the middle residue satisfies the encoding scheme as described in Section 7.3.2, it is marked as a positive sample: H_{start}, E_{start}, or C_{start}. Otherwise it is marked as a negative sample: $\sim H_{start}$, $\sim E_{start}$, or $\sim C_{start}$,

Figure 7.7 shows the Q_T prediction accuracy results of all the six new binary classifiers used with the SVM RBF kernel and the RS126 dataset. The prediction accuracy of SVM varied for different window sizes. The best overall prediction accuracy was achieved with window size 9.

Figure 7.8 shows the Q_T prediction accuracy results of all the six new binary classifiers used with the SVM RBF kernel and the CB513 dataset. The prediction

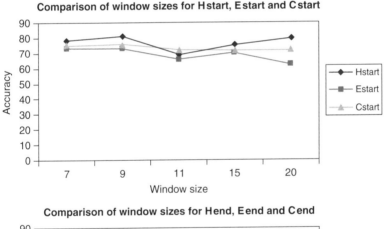

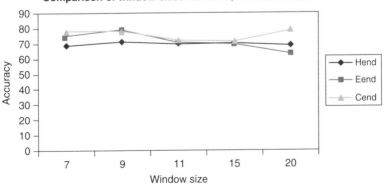

Figure 7.7   Accuracy of H_{end}, E_{end}, and C_{end} binary classifiers for the RS126 dataset.

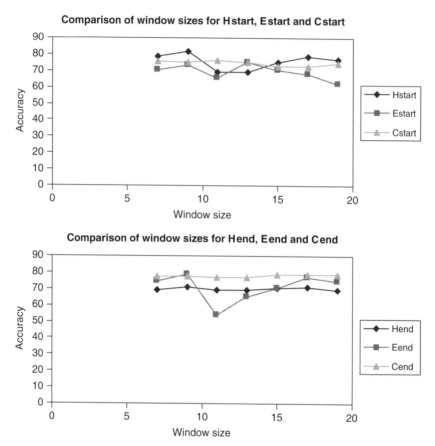

Figure 7.8 Accuracy of H_{end}, E_{end}, and C_{end} binary classifiers for CB513 dataset.

accuracy of SVM varied for different window sizes. The best overall prediction accuracy was achieved when the window size was 9 for CB513 data, which is similar to the results of RS126 data shown in Figure 7.7.

For the latter experiments and for the larger CB513 dataset, a window size of 9 was used to test the new binary classifiers.

7.3.6   Test Results of Binary Classifiers

Table 7.1 shows the Q_T prediction accuracy results of all six binary classifiers $H_{start}/\sim H_{start}$, $E_{start}/\sim E_{start}$, $C_{start}/\sim C_{start}$ and $H_{end}/\sim H_{end}$, $E_{end}/\sim E_{end}$ and $C_{end}/\sim C_{end}$ used with the SVM RBF kernel with a window size of 9. We used the PSSM profiles of the dataset CB513 during these tests. Since there were many negative samples, we balanced the negative and positive samples in the dataset by randomly choosing from the negative samples for training the SVM. The results are given in Table 7.1. The probability of SVM correctly predicting the

TABLE 7.1   Prediction Accuracies of the New Binary Classifiers

Binary Classifier	Accuracy (TP+TN)/ (TP+TN+FN+FP)	Recall (TP/TP+FN)	Specificity (TN/TN+FP)	Precision (TP/(TP+FP)
$H_{start}/{\sim}H_{start}$	81.5	78.5	84.16	83.33
$E_{start}/{\sim}E_{start}$	73.16	73.33	73.16	73.16
$C_{start}/{\sim}C_{start}$	75.33	78.33	72	74.33
$H_{end}/{\sim}H_{end}$	71.33	86.16	66.66	69.5
$E_{end}/{\sim}E_{end}$	78.66	82	75.33	77.66
$C_{end}/{\sim}C_{end}$	77.66	79	76	77.5

Notation: TP—true positive; TN—true negative; FP—false positive; FN—false negative.

start of helices is 81.5%, which is much higher than the 35% theoretical bound for per-residue prediction. The probability of successfully predicting the end of a helix is also high—approximately 71.33%. This shows that there is more of a signal in the data indicating the start of helices than there is a stop signal. The start and end positions of strands and coils are predicted with approximately 75% accuracy.

These results show that, by training a classifier such as SVM to predict the secondary structure transition boundaries, one can detect where helices, strands, and coils begin and end with high accuracy. Furthermore, these secondary structure transition boundaries are detected in an attempt to perform only one prediction at a time rather than trying to predict correctly all the residues in a given sequence segment, the probability of which would theoretically be only roughly 35%.

7.3.7   Accuracy as a Function of Helix Size

Figure 7.9 compares the prediction accuracy levels of helix starting and ending points as a function of the number of turns in the helix. One can see that the

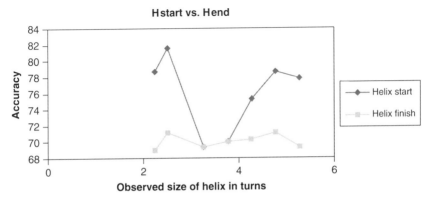

Figure 7.9   Accuracy levels of H_{start} and H_{end}.

prediction accuracies of the binary classifiers $H_{start}/{\sim}H_{start}$ and $H_{end}/{\sim}H_{end}$ reach a maximum value when the helix has 2.25 turns. Since a helix has about 4 residues per turn, this corresponds to a window size of 9 residues. At different number of turns of a helix, the accuracies are lower. This also proves that choosing a window size of 9 residues is optimal for the transition boundary prediction problem.

7.3.8 Comparison between Traditional Binary Classifiers and New Binary Classifiers

Several studies focus on determining where the structural segments start and end. Aydin et al. have shown that new dependence models and training methods bring further improvements to single-sequence protein secondary structure prediction [7]. Their results improve most Q_3 accuracy results by 2%, which shows that considering amino acid patterns at segment borders increases the prediction accuracy. Some other approaches focus on finding the end of helices. The reason for this is that the helices (α-helices) are the most abundant regular secondary structure and that a certain residue preference exists at the ends of helices [48]. However, current secondary structure prediction programs cannot identify the ends of helices correctly in most cases. The same rule applies to strands, although the residue preferences for strand termini are not as strong as in helices. Wilson et al. used cumulative pseudo-free-energy calculations to predict helix start positions and achieved 38% prediction accuracy. We achieved ${\sim}80\%$ Q_T accuracy using SVM, which is, of course, significantly higher.

One could question what our Q_3 overall prediction accuracy is. Most of the current secondary structure prediction methods attempt to solve the problem at a perresidue level, whereas we try to solve the prediction at a persegment level. In this work, we proposed binary classifiers that target prediction of the start and end positions of helices, strands, and coils. Therefore, to compare our prediction accuracy to the current prediction methods, we derived a method that converts our Q_T accuracy results to the standard Q_3 and vice versa.

7.3.8.1 *Estimates of Q_3 from Q_T and Q_T from Q_3* When traditional binary classifiers such as "1 versus rest" classifiers ($H/{\sim}H$, $E/{\sim}E$, and $C/{\sim}C$), and "1 versus 1" classifiers (H/E, E/C, and C/H) are used, their prediction accuracies are measured using a Q_3 metric. In the Q_3 measurement, predictions for each and every residue of a protein sequence are performed. To determine whether a given protein sequence is the start or end of a secondary structure with the traditional binary classifiers, each residue's secondary structure must be predicted first. However, it is clear that, even with the 90% accuracy per residue, the probability of independently predicting k residues correctly is 0.9 to the kth order. In order to calculate a Q_3 measurement of a given protein sequence window (of size k), a prediction for each and every residue in that window must be made using the traditional binary classifiers. However, with the proposed new binary

classifiers, only one prediction per window is suffices to indicate whether that window represents the end or start of a helix, sheet, or coil. Besides, the overall prediction probability is slightly pessimistic because the estimates may not be fully independent.

In light of this reasoning, to compare our results to those of the traditional binary classifiers that calculate the prediction accuracy per residue, we derived a method using the following assumption. Given a protein segment of window size k, we assumed that the prediction of each residue in that window is truly independent of the other residues in that window. Then, we converted the traditional Q_3 accuracy measurement to our accuracy measurement Q_T, using the following equation:

$$Q_T = Q_3^{(\text{window size})} \tag{7.4}$$

This formula basically states that the fewer the number of predictions made for a given protein window, the higher the chances are that the prediction is correct. Using the traditional binary classifiers, given a protein window of size k, we must make k predictions to see what that protein sequence segment is. Using the binary classifiers proposed in this work, only one prediction is enough. The inverse of Equation (7.3) is

$$Q_3 = e^{\ln(Q_T)/k} \tag{7.5}$$

The inverse of this formula gives us the corresponding Q_3 accuracy as a function of Q_T.

7.3.8.2 Traditional Versus New Binary Classifiers

In order to make a fair comparison, we took Q_3 measurements for the $H/{\sim}H$, $E/{\sim}E$, and $C/{\sim}C$ binary classifiers from References 23 and 24, which provide one of the highest Q_3 measurements for these binary classifiers, and estimated their Q_T measurements. We also converted the Q_T results in Table 7.1 to Q_3 measurements and listed the results in Tables 7.2 and 7.3.

Table 7.2 shows our Q_T accuracy calculations converted to the corresponding Q_3 accuracies. When Q_3 accuracies are converted to Q_T measurements as shown in Table 7.3, the accuracies are low. (*Note:* These estimates are based on the assumption that each residue prediction is independent of all the others.) These results show that using the new binary classifiers gives prediction accuracy higher

TABLE 7.2 Estimated Q_3 Results

Binary Classifiers	Q_T Converted to Q_3	
	Q_T	Q_3
$H/{\sim}H$	83.17	96.31
$E/{\sim}E$	80.5	95.67
$C/{\sim}C$	76.5	94.65

TABLE 7.3 Estimated Q_T Results

Binary Classifiers	Q_3 Converted to Q_T	
	Q_3	Q_T
$H/{\sim}H$	87.18	50.35
$E/{\sim}E$	86.02	47.09
$C/{\sim}C$	77.47	36.01

Sources: $Q3$ measurements from Hu et al. [23] and Hua and Sun [24].

TABLE 7.4 Protein ID: CBG

Binary Classifier	Accuracy	Recall	Specificity	Precision
$H_{start}/{\sim}H_{start}$	0.77	0.62	0.77	0.13
$E_{start}/{\sim}E_{start}$	0.80	0.53	0.81	0.9
$C_{start}/{\sim}C_{start}$	0.71	0.59	0.72	0.17
$H_{end}/{\sim}H_{end}$	0.79	0.54	0.80	0.13
$E_{end}/{\sim}E_{end}$	0.81	0.59	0.82	0.11
$C_{end}/{\sim}C_{end}$	0.72	0.57	0.73	0.17

TABLE 7.5 Protein ID: CELB

Binary Classifier	Accuracy	Recall	Specificity	Precision
$H_{start}/{\sim}H_{start}$	0.89	0.2	0.99	0.03
$E_{start}/{\sim}E_{start}$	0.75	0.39	0.78	0.13
$C_{start}/{\sim}C_{start}$	0.58	0.27	0.62	0.07
$H_{end}/{\sim}H_{end}$	0.91	0.70	0.92	0.17
$E_{end}/{\sim}E_{end}$	0.79	0.42	0.82	0.17
$C_{end}/{\sim}C_{end}$	0.63	0.51	0.64	0.13

than that obtained using the traditional binary classifiers. These results also prove that it is better to make predictions using a per segment window rather than per residue. In other words, we should split the data into large chunks (segments) and make predictions using these segments instead of attempting to predict each and every piece of data (residues).

7.3.9 Test Results on Individual Proteins Outside the Dataset

In order to prove that the new proposed encoding scheme works, we have run double-blind tests on individual proteins. The test results are given in Table 7.4. In all test cases, the accuracy, recall and specificity values are high as expected; however, the precision values are low (see also Tables 7.5–7.8). This is due to the unbalanced nature of the dataset. In our training datasets, we have many negative samples whereas the positive samples constitute roughly 1% of the number of

TABLE 7.6   Protein ID: BAM

Binary Classifier	Accuracy	Recall	Specificity	Precision
$H_{start}/\sim H_{start}$	0.79	0.57	0.79	0.09
$E_{start}/\sim E_{start}$	0.69	0.50	0.69	0.06
$C_{start}/\sim C_{start}$	0.66	0.75	0.65	0.16
$H_{end}/\sim H_{end}$	0.76	0.86	0.76	0.11
$E_{end}/\sim E_{end}$	0.78	0.62	0.78	0.11
$C_{end}/\sim C_{end}$	0.72	0.56	0.73	0.16

TABLE 7.7   Protein ID: AMP1

Binary Classifier	Accuracy	Recall	Specificity	Precision
$H_{start}/\sim H_{start}$	0.70	0.64	0.70	0.08
$E_{start}/\sim E_{start}$	0.79	0.11	0.82	0.02
$C_{start}/\sim C_{start}$	0.73	0.65	0.73	0.15
$H_{end}/\sim H_{end}$	0.84	0.55	0.85	0.12
$E_{end}/\sim E_{end}$	0.83	0.67	0.83	0.11
$C_{end}/\sim C_{end}$	0.72	0.67	0.72	0.16

TABLE 7.8   Protein ID: ADD1

Binary Classifier	Accuracy	Recall	Specificity	Precision
$H_{start}/\sim H_{start}$	0.86	0.77	0.87	0.28
$E_{start}/\sim E_{start}$	0.84	0.88	0.84	0.11
$C_{start}/\sim C_{start}$	0.65	0.66	0.65	0.16
$H_{end}/\sim H_{end}$	0.74	0.59	0.75	0.14
$E_{end}/\sim E_{end}$	0.86	0.88	0.86	0.13
$C_{end}/\sim C_{end}$	0.80	0.37	0.84	0.18

the negative sets. This is a major problem with these kinds of datasets. The false positives (FPs) are high because we are dealing with 100 times more examples of negative cases than positive cases. These results imply that it is very difficult to obtain a high precision, because of the unbalanced nature of the datasets. The false positives overwhelm the correct matches. This is the truly difficult aspect of using minority classes. The good accuracy shows that there is a signal in the data that we can extract. However, because there are so many more negative matches, we obtain a large number of FPs. What we discover by this analysis is that there is a signal that SVM selects because we have high accuracy; however, we cannot obtain high precision values because there are very few examples of the minority classes. Therefore, we give the results for both balanced data and unbalanced data.

TABLE 7.9   Test 1, Random Subset 1

Binary Classifier	Accuracy	Recall	Specificity	Precision
$H_{start}/{\sim}H_{start}$	80	80	80	80
$E_{start}/{\sim}E_{start}$	73	77	68	71
$C_{start}/{\sim}C_{start}$	73	72	73	73
$H_{end}/{\sim}H_{end}$	70	77	64	68
$E_{end}/{\sim}E_{end}$	81	84	78	80
$C_{end}/{\sim}C_{end}$	76	80	72	76

TABLE 7.10   Test 2, Random Subset 2

Binary Classifier	Accuracy	Recall	Specificity	Precision
$H_{start}/{\sim}H_{start}$	81	79	83	83
$E_{start}/{\sim}E_{start}$	72	78	67	70
$C_{start}/{\sim}C_{start}$	70	73	68	69
$H_{end}/{\sim}H_{end}$	73	76	70	72
$E_{end}/{\sim}E_{end}$	78	82	74	77
$C_{end}/{\sim}C_{end}$	75	79	71	75

TABLE 7.11   Test 3, Random Subset 3

Binary Classifier	Accuracy	Recall	Specificity	Precision
$H_{start}/{\sim}H_{start}$	87	84	91	90
$E_{start}/{\sim}E_{start}$	75	74	77	76
$C_{start}/{\sim}C_{start}$	72	73	71	72
$H_{end}/{\sim}H_{end}$	74	84	64	70
$E_{end}/{\sim}E_{end}$	80	83	77	79
$C_{end}/{\sim}C_{end}$	81	84	77	79

7.3.10   Test Results on Randomly Selected Data Subsets

In order to ensure that we did not simply select a subset of the negative data for balancing the dataset that optimized our method's prediction probabilities, we tested our method using 10 different randomly chosen different subsets of the data. These test results show that our proposed method works and that it is possible to train an SVM algorithm to learn where the helices, strands, and coils begin and end. (See Tables 7.9–7.18.)

7.3.11   Additional Test Results on Randomly Selected Data Subsets

To ensure that we did not simply select a subset of the data that optimized our method's prediction probabilities when we balanced the dataset, we tested our method using 10 different randomly chosen different subsets of the data.

TABLE 7.12 Test 4, Random Subset 4

Binary Classifier	Accuracy	Recall	Specificity	Precision
$H_{start}/\sim H_{start}$	84	83	84	84
$E_{start}/\sim E_{start}$	73	71	75	74
$C_{start}/\sim C_{start}$	73	79	68	71
$H_{end}/\sim H_{end}$	76	80	73	75
$E_{end}/\sim E_{end}$	78	84	71	75
$C_{end}/\sim C_{end}$	78	79	77	79

TABLE 7.13 Test 5, Random Subset 5

Binary Classifier	Accuracy	Recall	Specificity	Precision
$H_{start}/\sim H_{start}$	80	80	81	81
$E_{start}/\sim E_{start}$	74	74	74	74
$C_{start}/\sim C_{start}$	78	79	77	77
$H_{end}/\sim H_{end}$	76	78	72	81
$E_{end}/\sim E_{end}$	79	82	75	77
$C_{end}/\sim C_{end}$	81	83	79	81

TABLE 7.14 Test 6, Random Subset 6

Binary Classifier	Accuracy	Recall	Specificity	Precision
$H_{start}/\sim H_{start}$	82	79	85	84
$E_{start}/\sim E_{start}$	72	70	73	72
$C_{start}/\sim C_{start}$	75	76	74	74
$H_{end}/\sim H_{end}$	79	87	71	75
$E_{end}/\sim E_{end}$	78	81	75	77
$C_{end}/\sim C_{end}$	78	81	74	77

TABLE 7.15 Test 7, Random Subset 7

Binary Classifier	Accuracy	Recall	Specificity	Precision
$H_{start}/\sim H_{start}$	83	83	82	81
$E_{start}/\sim E_{start}$	79	86	71	77
$C_{start}/\sim C_{start}$	71	72	70	71
$H_{end}/\sim H_{end}$	73	75	71	72
$E_{end}/\sim E_{end}$	82	82	82	82
$C_{end}/\sim C_{end}$	76	78	73	76

TABLE 7.16   Test 8, Random Subset 8

Binary Classifier	Accuracy	Recall	Specificity	Precision
$H_{start}/\sim H_{start}$	84	82	85	85
$E_{start}/\sim E_{start}$	81	84	77	81
$C_{start}/\sim C_{start}$	72	78	66	70
$H_{end}/\sim H_{end}$	74	79	70	72
$E_{end}/\sim E_{end}$	81	85	77	79
$C_{end}/\sim C_{end}$	80	83	76	79

TABLE 7.17   Test 9, Random Subset 9

Binary Classifier	Accuracy	Recall	Specificity	Precision
$H_{start}/\sim H_{start}$	85	83	88	87
$E_{start}/\sim E_{start}$	79	84	74	78
$C_{start}/\sim C_{start}$	74	78	69	72
$H_{end}/\sim H_{end}$	74	82	71	66
$E_{end}/\sim E_{end}$	80	84	76	79
$C_{end}/\sim C_{end}$	78	85	71	76

TABLE 7.18   Test 10, Random Subset 10

Binary Classifier	Accuracy	Recall	Specificity	Precision
$H_{start}/\sim H_{start}$	83	80	86	85
$E_{start}/\sim E_{start}$	73	73	73	73
$C_{start}/\sim C_{start}$	75	78	73	74
$H_{end}/\sim H_{end}$	73	80	67	70
$E_{end}/\sim E_{end}$	80	84	75	78
$C_{end}/\sim C_{end}$	79	83	75	79

These test results show that our proposed method works and that it is possible to train an SVM algorithm to learn where the helices, strands, and coils begin and end when features are reduced according to the clique algorithm. (See Tables 7.19–7.28.)

7.3.12   Conclusion

In this section, we proposed a new way to look at the protein secondary prediction problem. Most of the current methods use the traditional binary classifiers such as $H/\sim H$ and require the correct prediction of every residue's secondary structure. This approach gives an overview of the secondary structure of a sequence. However, to determine whether a sequence segment is a helix, sheet, or coil using the traditional binary classifier, most of the residues in the sequence segment must be classified correctly. Even with a 90% probability that each residue

TABLE 7.19   Test 1, Random Subset 1

Binary Classifier	Accuracy	Recall	Specificity	Precision
$H_{start}/\sim H_{start}$	82	80	83	83
$E_{start}/\sim E_{start}$	81	86	74	80
$C_{start}/\sim C_{start}$	73	78	71	68
$H_{end}/\sim H_{end}$	80	85	75	79
$E_{end}/\sim E_{end}$	80	82	77	79
$C_{end}/\sim C_{end}$	77	82	72	76

TABLE 7.20   Test 2, Random Subset 2

Binary Classifier	Accuracy	Recall	Specificity	Precision
$H_{start}/\sim H_{start}$	83	80	85	84
$E_{start}/\sim E_{start}$	79	85	72	77
$C_{start}/\sim C_{start}$	73	80	73	70
$H_{end}/\sim H_{end}$	79	86	71	77
$E_{end}/\sim E_{end}$	80	85	74	77
$C_{end}/\sim C_{end}$	81	84	76	80

TABLE 7.21   Test 3, Random Subset 3

Binary Classifier	Accuracy	Recall	Specificity	Precision
$H_{start}/\sim H_{start}$	84	82	85	85
$E_{start}/\sim E_{start}$	82	88	75	80
$C_{start}/\sim C_{start}$	76	77	75	75
$H_{end}/\sim H_{end}$	78	86	70	76
$E_{end}/\sim E_{end}$	80	84	75	78
$C_{end}/\sim C_{end}$	77	82	72	76

TABLE 7.22   Test 4, Random Subset 4

Binary Classifier	Accuracy	Recall	Specificity	Precision
$H_{start}/\sim H_{start}$	83	80	86	85
$E_{start}/\sim E_{start}$	83	86	79	83
$C_{start}/\sim C_{start}$	76	73	79	78
$H_{end}/\sim H_{end}$	81	88	72	80
$E_{end}/\sim E_{end}$	81	82	80	81
$C_{end}/\sim C_{end}$	79	78	79	80

TABLE 7.23   Test 5, Random Subset 5

Binary Classifier	Accuracy	Recall	Specificity	Precision
$H_{start}/\sim H_{start}$	85	82	87	86
$E_{start}/\sim E_{start}$	78	82	74	78
$C_{start}/\sim C_{start}$	72	76	68	71
$H_{end}/\sim H_{end}$	77	81	72	77
$E_{end}/\sim E_{end}$	83	84	81	82
$C_{end}/\sim C_{end}$	80	82	77	79

TABLE 7.24   Test 6, Random Subset 6

Binary Classifier	Accuracy	Recall	Specificity	Precision
$H_{start}/\sim H_{start}$	83	80	86	85
$E_{start}/\sim E_{start}$	81	83	78	81
$C_{start}/\sim C_{start}$	74	76	72	73
$H_{end}/\sim H_{end}$	85	89	80	84
$E_{end}/\sim E_{end}$	82	87	78	80
$C_{end}/\sim C_{end}$	78	83	72	77

TABLE 7.25   Test 7, Random Subset 7

Binary Classifier	Accuracy	Recall	Specificity	Precision
$H_{start}/\sim H_{start}$	82	79	84	84
$E_{start}/\sim E_{start}$	80	85	74	79
$C_{start}/\sim C_{start}$	71	78	65	69
$H_{end}/\sim H_{end}$	79	85	73	78
$E_{end}/\sim E_{end}$	81	83	79	80
$C_{end}/\sim C_{end}$	77	82	71	76

TABLE 7.26   Test 8, Random Subset 8

Binary Classifier	Accuracy	Recall	Specificity	Precision
$H_{start}/\sim H_{start}$	83	83	84	84
$E_{start}/\sim E_{start}$	80	85	75	79
$C_{start}/\sim C_{start}$	77	78	75	76
$H_{end}/\sim H_{end}$	79	85	72	76
$E_{end}/\sim E_{end}$	79	83	75	77
$C_{end}/\sim C_{end}$	80	82	76	80

TABLE 7.27   Test 9, Random Subset 9

Binary Classifier	Accuracy	Recall	Specificity	Precision
$H_{start}/{\sim}H_{start}$	81	81	82	82
$E_{start}/{\sim}E_{start}$	79	88	70	76
$C_{start}/{\sim}C_{start}$	74	71	77	76
$H_{end}/{\sim}H_{end}$	81	88	74	80
$E_{end}/{\sim}E_{end}$	82	84	81	82
$C_{end}/{\sim}C_{end}$	80	83	76	79

TABLE 7.28   Test 10, Random Subset 10

Binary Classifier	Accuracy	Recall	Specificity	Precision
$H_{start}/{\sim}H_{start}$	85	83	87	86
$E_{start}/{\sim}E_{start}$	81	84	77	81
$C_{start}/{\sim}C_{start}$	74	76	72	73
$H_{end}/{\sim}H_{end}$	82	85	78	81
$E_{end}/{\sim}E_{end}$	79	83	76	78
$C_{end}/{\sim}C_{end}$	79	85	73	77

is correctly predicted independently, the cumulative probability of being correct for all the residues in the sequence segment is low (~35%). We propose six new binary classifiers that could be used to classify all the residues in a given protein sequence segment when attempting to determine whether the sequence segment is a helix, strand, or coil. In our binary classifiers, only one classification is made per segment. To apply these binary classifiers, we proposed a new encoding scheme for data representation. Our results show that it is possible to train an SVM to learn where the helices, strands, and coils begin and end.

We proposed six new binary classifiers that are used to predict the starts and end of secondary structures of protein. For these binary classifiers, we also proposed a new encoding scheme. Our current encoding scheme takes into account only the information as to whether a protein window is the end or start of a secondary structure. It does not factor in where in the protein that sequence window belongs. Depending on whether it occurs at the beginning or end of a sequence, the occurrence of a transition boundary could be changed drastically. The new binary classifiers currently do not use the information that stipulates that a sequence window be at the start or end of protein; however, these classifiers can be improved in the future to represent this information.

Another future improvement could be to find common amino acid patterns that make up the transition boundaries. If there are common amino acid patterns (motifs), this information could be added to the encoding scheme and an SVM could be additionally trained with these patterns to ensure a more accurate prediction. These common patterns could lead to rules stipulating, for instance, order in which amino acids represent transition boundaries. These rules can later be embedded into the encoding scheme or put into a new kernel function of SVM.

The correct detection of transition boundaries could be used to predict the tertiary structure of a protein. For instance, each transition boundary could also be a possible domain boundary. Proteins usually contain several domains or independent functional units that have their own shape and function. All these remain as promising topics for future research.

7.4 CONCLUSION

We propose six new binary classifiers that are used for predicting the start and end of secondary structures of protein. With these binary classifiers, it is easier to train an SVM since only one prediction per protein segment is necessary for concluding whether it is a helix, strand, or coil. In order to use these binary classifiers, we also proposed a new encoding scheme for data representation. Our results show that it is possible to train an SVM to learn where the helices, strands, and coils begin and end. We have achieved close to 90% accuracy, whereas traditional binary classifiers can attain a maximum only accuracy of only 35% for a window size of 9.

Detecting transition boundaries instead of the structure of individual residues in the whole sequence is much easier. Thus, our problem is reduced to the task of finding these transition boundaries. Our work provides new insights on accurately prediction of protein secondary structure and may help determine tertiary structure as well; this could be used by biologists to help solve the critically important problem of how proteins fold. A protein's tertiary structure is critical to its ability to perform its biological functions correctly and efficiently.

REFERENCES

1. Abe S, *Support Vector Machines for Pattern Classification*, Springer-Verlag, 2005.
2. Altschul SF, Madden TL, Schaffer AA, Zhang J, Zhang Z, Miller W, Lipman DJ, Gapped BLAST and PSI-BLAST: A new generation of protein database search programs, *Nucleic Acids Res.* **25**(17):3389–3402 (1997).
3. Altschul SF, Gish W, Miller W, Myers EW, Lipman DJ, Basic local alignment search tool, *J. Mol. Biol.* **215**(3):403–410 (1990).
4. Altun G, Zhong W, Pan Y, Tai PC, Harrison RW, A new seed selection algorithm that maximizes local structural similarity in proteins, *Proc. Int. IEEE Conf. Engineering in Medicine and Biology (EMBC'06)*, Aug. 2006, pp. 5822–5825.
5. Altun G, Hu H-J, Brinza D, Harrison RW, Zelikovsky A, Pan Y, Hybrid SVM kernels for protein secondary structure prediction, *Proc. Int. IEEE Conf. Granular Computing (GRC 2006)*, May 2006, pp. 762–765.
6. Aurora R, Rose G, Helix capping, *Protein Sci.* **7**:21–38 (1998).

7. Aydin Z, Altunbasak Y, Borodovsky M, Protein secondary structure prediction for a single-sequence using hidden semi-Markov model, *BMC Bioinformatics.* **7**(1):178 (2006).

8. Baxevanis AD, Ouellette BF. *Bioinformatics: A Practical Guide to the Analysis of Genes and Proteins*, Wiley, 2005.

9. Berg JM, Tymoczko JL, Stryer L, *Biochemistry*, 5th ed., Freeman WH, New York, 2002.

10. Berman H, Henrick K, Nakamura H, Markley JL, The worldwide Protein Data Bank (wwPDB): Ensuring a single, uniform archive of PDB data, *Nucleic Acids Res.* **35**: (Jan. 2007).

11. Birzele F, Kramer S, A new representation for protein secondary structure prediction based on frequent patterns, *Bioinformatics*, **22**(21):2628–2634 (2006).

12. Butenko S, Wilhelm W, Clique-detection models in computational biochemistry and genomics, *Eur. J. Oper. Res.* **17**(1):1–17 (2006).

13. Breiman L, Random forests, *Machine Learn.* **45**(1):5–32 (2001).

14. Breiman L, Cutler A, Random forest (available at `http://www.stat.berkeley.edu/~breiman/RandomForests/cc_software.htm`).

15. Bystroff C, Thorsson V, Baker D, HMMSTR: A hidden Markov model for local sequence structure correlations in proteins, *J. Mol. Biol.* **301**:173–190 (2000).

16. Burges C, A tutorial on support vector machines for pattern recognition, *Data Mining Knowl. Discov.* **2**(2):121–167 (1998).

17. Casbon J, *Protein Secondary Structure Prediction with Support Vector Machines*, MSc thesis, Univ. Sussex, Brighton, UK, 2002.

18. Chou PY, Fasman GD, Prediction of protein conformation, *Biochemistry* **13**(2):222–245 (1974).

19. Cristianini N, Shawe-Taylor J, *An Introduction to Support Vector Machines*, Cambridge Univ. Press, 2000.

20. Efron B, Tibshirani R, *An Introduction to the Bootstrap*, Chapman & Hall, New York, 1993.

21. Fleming PJ, Gong H, Rose GD, Secondary structure determines protein topology, *Protein Sci.* **15**:1829–1834, (2006).

22. Garnier J, Osguthorpe DJ, Robson B, Analysis of the accuracy and implications of simple methods for predicting the secondary structure of globular proteins, *J. Mol. Biol.* **120**:97–120 (1978).

23. Hu H, Pan Y, Harrison R, Tai PC, Improved protein secondary structure prediction using support vector machine with a new encoding scheme and an advanced tertiary classifier, *IEEE Trans. Nanobiosci.* **3**(4):265–271 (2004).

24. Hua S, Sun Z, A novel method of protein secondary structure prediction with high segment overlap measure: Support vector machine approach, *J. Mol. Biol.* **308**:397–407 (2001).

25. Ignacimuthu S, *Basic Bioinformatics*, Narosa Publishing House, 2005.

26. Joachims T, Making large-scale SVM learning practical. *Advances in Kernel Methods—Support Vector Learning*, Schölkopf B, Burges C, Smola A. (ed.), MIT Press, Cambridge, MA, 1999.

27. Jones D, Protein secondary structure prediction based on position-specific scoring matrices, *J. Mol. Biol.* **292**:195–202 (1999).

28. Jones NC, Pevzner PA, *An Introduction to Bioinformatics Algorithms*, MIT Press, Cambridge, MA.

29. Kabsch W, Sander C, Dictionary of protein secondary structure: Pattern recognition of hydrogen-bonded and geometrical features, *Biopolymers* **22**(12):2577–2637 (1983).

30. Karypis G, YASSPP: Better kernels and coding schemes lead to improvements in protein secondary structure prediction, *Proteins* **64**(3):575–586 (2006).

31. Kim H, Park H, Protein secondary structure prediction based on an improved support vector machines approach, *Protein Eng.* **16**(8):553–560 (2003).

32. Kloczkowski A, Ting KL, Jernigan RL, Garnier J, Combining the GOR V algorithm with evolutionary information for protein secondary structure prediction from amino acid sequence, *Proteins*, **49**:154–166, (2002).

33. Kurgan L, Homaeian L, Prediction of secondary protein structure content from primary sequence alone—a feature selection based approach, *Machine Learn. Data Mining Pattern Recogn.* **3587**:334–345 (2005).

34. Lesk AM, *Introduction to Protein Science—Architecture, Function and Genomics*, Oxford Univ. Press, 2004.

35. Ostergard PRJ, A fast algorithm for the maximum clique problem, *Discrete Appl. Math.* **120**(1–3):197–207 (2002).

36. Przytycka T, Aurora R, Rose GD, A protein taxonomy based on secondary structure, *Nat. Struct. Biol.* **6**:672–682 (1999).

37. Przytycka T, Srinivasan R, Rose GD, Recursive domains in proteins, *J. Biol. Chem.* **276**(27):25372–25377 (2001).

38. Qian N, Sejnowski TJ, Predicting the secondary structure of globular proteins using neural network models, *J. Mol. Biol.* **202**:865–884 (1988).

39. Riis SK, Krogh A, Improving prediction of protein secondary structure using structured neural networks and multiple sequence alignments, *J. Comput. Biol.* **3**(1):163–184 (1996).

40. Rost B, Sander C, Prediction of secondary structure at better than 70% accuracy, *J. Mol. Biol.* **232**:584–599 (1993).

41. Rost B, Sander C, Schneider R, Evolution and neural networks—protein secondary structure prediction above 71% accuracy, *Proc. 27th Hawaii Int. Conf. System Sciences*, Wailea, HI, 1994, vol. 5, pp. 385–394.

42. Rost B, Rising accuracy of protein secondary structure prediction, in: Chasman D, ed., *Protein Structure Determination, Analysis, and Modeling for Drug Discovery*, Marcel Dekker, New York, 2003, pp. 207–249.

43. Tramontano A, *The Ten Most Wanted Solutions in Protein Bioinformatics*, Chapman & Hall/CRC Mathematical Biology and Medicine Series.

44. Vanschoenwinkel B, Manderick B, Substitution matrix based kernel functions for protein secondary structure prediction, *Proc. Int. Conf. Machine Learning and Applications*, 2004.

45. Vishveshwara S, Brinda KV, Kannan N, Protein structure: Insights from graph theory, *J. Theor. Comput. Chem.* **1**:187–211 (2002).

46. Vapnik V, Cortes C, Support vector networks, *Machine Learn.* **20**(3):273–293 (1995).

47. West DB, *Introduction to Graph Theory*, 2nd ed., Prentice-Hall, 2001.

48. Wilson CL, Boardman PE, Doig AJ, Hubbard SJ, Improved prediction for *N*-termini of a-helices using empirical information, *Proteins: Struct., Funct., Bioinformatics* **57**(2):322–330 (2004).

49. Xiong J, *Essential Bioinformatics*. Cambridge Univ. Press, 2006.

50. Zhong W, Altun G, Harrison R, Tai PC, Pan Y, Improved *K*-means clustering algorithm for exploring local protein sequence motifs representing common structural property, *IEEE Trans. Nanobiosci.* **4**(3):255–265 (2005).

51. Zhong W, Altun G, Tian X, Harrison R, Tai PC, Pan Y, Parallel protein secondary structure prediction schemes using Pthread and OpenMP over hyper-threading technology, *J. Supercomput.* **41**(1):1–16 (July 2007).

CHAPTER 8

PREDICTION OF RNA BINDING SITES IN PROTEINS

ZHI-PING LIU and LUONAN CHEN

8.1 INTRODUCTION

Protein–RNA interactions play a key role in a number of biological processes in DNA packaging and replication, mRNA processing, protein synthesis, assembly, and function of ribosomes and eukaryotic spliceosomes. A reliable identification of RNA binding sites in proteins is important for functional annotation and site-directed mutagenesis. However, it is time-consuming and labor-intensive to detect the interaction sites in proteins by traditional experimental methods. There are some computational methods that have been proposed to address this challenge. Generally, prediction of RNA binding sites is based on the sequence and structure features identified from protein and its RNA partner. The residue properties as well as various element features are detected and combined together into description vectors to represent the interacting events. For the encoding scheme, numerous methods have been proposed to describe the interacting preferences of protein residue and its RNA partners. In this chapter, we provide an introduction for the prediction of RNA binding sites in proteins by machine learning algorithms, such as neural network, naive Bayes, support vector machines, and random forest. On the basis of these classification methods, we can identify the RNA binding sites of proteins by various features underlying the interaction.

8.2 BACKGROUND

It is crucial to decipher the mechanism of how proteins interact with other molecules in the understanding of cellular processes [2,12,38]. RNA undergoes diverse posttranscriptional regulation of gene expression, including regulation of its transportation, localization, and decay [10]. In many cases, this process

Algorithmic and Artificial Intelligence Methods for Protein Bioinformatics. First Edition.
Edited by Yi Pan, Jianxin Wang, Min Li.
© 2014 John Wiley & Sons, Inc. Published 2014 by John Wiley & Sons, Inc.

occurs through elements on the mRNA molecule that interact with the hundreds of RNA binding proteins existing in the cell [12,24]. Interactions between proteins and RNA molecules play an essential role in a variety of biological activities, such as posttranscriptional gene regulation, alternative splicing, translation, and infections by RNA viruses [31]. Therefore, it is important to understand the principle of protein–RNA interactions and identify their interaction sites when selecting activators and inhibitors in rational drug design. RNA recognition by proteins is mediated primarily by certain classes of RNA binding domains and motifs [25,28]. The correlated patterns of sequence and structure in RNA binding proteins can then be recognized to bind to specific RNA sequences and folds. In recognition of RNA functional importance in living molecules and close association with protein in its activities, experimental and computational studies of protein–RNA complexes have been substantially increased [8,15]. Various approaches have been proposed to study protein–RNA interactions [24], but precise mechanisms of interaction are far from for fully understood. Therefore, to clearly elucidate protein–RNA interacting patterns, it is necessary to develop a reliable method for predicting protein–RNA interacting sites, in particular by exploiting the increasingly accumulated data of protein–RNA complexes.

Many studies indicate that there is a strong relationship between interaction residues and their compositions in protein–RNA complexes [7,8,18]. In building a machine learning method for predicting protein–RNA binding sites, two factors play crucial roles in the predictor:

1. *Features Encoded to Represent and Characterize Protein–RNA Binding Sites.* Obviously, the sequence and structure features of binding residues are the contributors of how the RNA binding events in proteins [11,25]. Various interaction features discovered by analyzing the property of interacting sites will give us useful information to understand how protein interacts with RNA with specificity. The message transforming between protein residues and their interacting nucleotides of RNA molecule is also a descriptor of the interaction propensity. It will improve the identification process by considering the interaction features underlying the partnership between protein residues and RNA nucleotides. These physicochemical features, sequence conservation score, evolutionary information, and interaction propensity could be identified and integrated together as the descriptors of the interacting patterns between protein residues and RNA nucleotides.

2. *Computational Algorithms of the Classifier.* These include neural network (NN), naive Bayes (NB), and support vector machine (SVM). Random forest (RF) is also an alternative algorithm with potential improvements [5]. So far, a number of feature-based machine learning techniques have been developed to predict RNA binding residues in proteins. For instance, Jeong et al. [13] proposed a NN method for predicting RNA binding sites by using weighted evolutionary profiles. BindN [35] was used with a SVM-based classifier to predict potential RNA or DNA binding residues in proteins by sequence

features. RNABindR [32] generated a NB classifier to predict RNA binding amino acid residues in proteins. We considerably improved the prediction performance of protein RNA binding sites using integrated properties by a RF classifier [23].

In this chapter, we mainly describe the protocols of predicting RNA binding sites in proteins by feature based machine learning methods. The available protein–RNA complexes from the Protein Data Bank (PDB) [4] are selected to build the data source and define the binding sites in proteins. Various features of sequence and structure are derived comprehensively to represent protein residues for characterizing the protein–RNA binding events. The features are collected and combined together by encoding feature vectors. Machine learning methods (e.g., NN, NB, SVM, RF) are implemented to ascertain the features underlying the RNA binding residues as well as those of non-RNA-binding residues. To check the prediction performance of these predictors, cross-validation processes are used to show the efficiency and effectiveness of these pipelines. Furthermore, the trained predictors are used to predict novel RNA binding sites in proteins. In this chapter, we also compare these features and those of the existing methods. In particular, we identify the importance of each feature in determining the specificity of protein–RNA interaction, as well as the contribution of various hybrid features in the prediction.

8.3 FRAMEWORK OF PREDICTION

Figure 8.1 is a flowchart showing steps involved in the prediction of RNA binding sites in proteins. The framework of these steps can be summarized as follows. Given a protein [sequence or structure shown in diagram (a)], the task involved in this prediction is to annotate where the RNA binding events take place [shown in structure (c)] by a predictor [shown in diagram (b)]. The predictor is often built by a classifier trained on available protein–RNA binding information. Given protein–RNA complexes, we first define the RNA binding residues from their three-dimensional (3D) structures [diagram (d)]. In these feature-based machine learning approaches, a crucial step is to identify the features of these binding residues, such as sequence-based features of physicochemical atoms and structure-based features of solvent accessible surface areas. Often, we also identify some defined features that are considered to be closely related to the interaction between protein and RNA. Each protein residue is then represented by a derived feature vector [diagram (e)]. In the training dataset, we implement a machine learning algorithm to learn the distinctive features underlying these RNA binding residues as well as non-RNA-binding residues. The predictor is trained to distinguish the features of RNA binding residues and those of non-RNA-binding residues simultaneously [graph (f)]. The prediction performance of the classifier is often evaluated by a cross-validation process [graph (g)]. After we achieve acceptable training results, we can use the predictor to predict

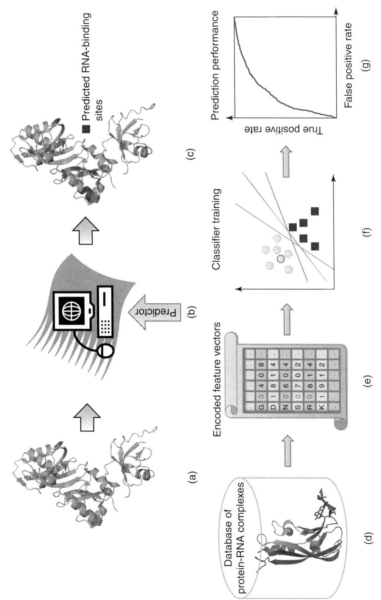

Figure 8.1 Framework for predicting RNA binding sites in proteins.

RNA binding sites in a novel protein after the target protein is encoded with the same feature vectors as described in the training data.

The overall prediction performance for a predictor is first evaluated by the statistical measurements in the cross-validation, such as fivefold cross-validation; that is, the whole dataset is randomly partitioned into five groups of equal size. To ensure that the training process is completely independent from the test data, the classifier is trained on the four groups and tested on the control group, and each of them is chosen for the assessment one by one. The predictive results are evaluated by different measures, including sensitivity (SN), specificity (SP), accuracy (ACC), F measure, and Matthews correlation coefficient (MCC). Mathematically, they are defined by the following equations:

$$SN = \frac{TP}{TP + FN}$$

$$SP = \frac{TN}{TN + FP}$$

$$ACC = \frac{TP + TN}{TP + FP + TN + FN}$$

$$F\,measure = \frac{2 \times SN \times SP}{SN + SP}$$

$$MCC = \frac{TP \times TN - FP \times FN}{\sqrt{(TP + FN)(TP + FP)(TN + FP)(TN + FN)}}$$

where TP, FN, FP, and TN are the numbers of true positive, false negative, false positive, and true negative residues in the prediction, respectively. To present the interrelationship of specificity and sensitivity of the identification, the receiver operating characteristic (ROC) curve is often used, and the area under the ROC curve (AUC) is also calculated. The F measure is the harmonic mean of sensitivity and specificity. Usually the maximum F measure point is chosen as the cutoff for sensitivity and specificity in ROC curves of the prediction performance. The MCC value ranges between 1 (all predictions are correct) and -1 (none are correct).

The purpose of cross-validation is to evaluate the efficiency and effectiveness of the proposed prediction method on available protein–RNA complexes. When we intend to identify the RNA binding sites in a novel protein, the former built classifier can be trained in the whole dataset. After the corresponding features of the predicting protein are encoded, the RNA binding residues can be predicted by the trained predictor. The generalization and extension ability of prediction plays a crucial role in the applications. The flexibility and scale of application are highly related to the required features in the proposed predictor. For instance, some structure-based features in a protein are not available when there is no 3D structure. In these cases, we can train the predictor by sequence-based features, and then the RNA binding sites can be predicted only by sequence information.

8.4 DESCRIPTION FEATURES OF PROTEIN RNA BINDING SITES

For predicting RNA binding sites in proteins by machine learning methods, we need to encode the residues by various descriptors mined from available protein sequences and structures. Compared to some energy-based methods for defining features of the protein–RNA interaction sites, sequence-derived and structure-derived features focus mainly on the physicochemical patterns, evolutionary information, solution accessible surfaces, and sidechain environment of residues. Roughly, these features can be categorized into sequence-derived and structure-derived classes. Some of them, such as interaction propensity, are also defined by this available information.

8.4.1 Definition of RNA Binding Sites

RNA binding events often take place at the pockets or cavities on protein surfaces [1,22,26]. When we train the predictor, we need to define positive samples as well as negative samples, that is, true RNA binding residues and true non-RNA-binding residues in the proteins. When the 3D structure of protein–RNA complex is available, the closest distance between the atoms of protein residue and that of its partner RNA nucleotide residue can be easily calculated. When the distance is shorter than that of a given threshold, the amino acid residue is defined as RNA binding residue [32]. Furthermore, some energy-based methods are proposed to define the RNA binding residues in proteins. For instance, a residue is defined as an RNA binding residue if any of its nonhydrogen atoms is within van der Waals contact or hydrogen binding distance to any RNA nonhydrogen atom directly or indirectly by a bridging water molecule [1,39]. Several methods, such as ENTANGLE, can be used to detect the interacting residues by searching appropriate hydrogen bonding and stacking, electrostatic, hydrophobic, and van der Waals interactions between protein and RNA residues [1]. The structure information can also be implemented to define RNA binding sites. For instance, on comparison of solvent accessible surface area of the protein structure with and without RNA, the degree of difference of residues can be used to distinguish RNA binding residues with non-RNA-binding residues [18].

8.4.2 Sequence-Based Features

It is relatively easy to obtain the sequence information of interacting protein and RNA. Hence, the sequence-derived features are wildly implemented in building the feature vectors. Strong biases of different types of amino acid residues in RNA binding sites have been reported, such as the abundancy of arginine-rich motifs [1]. This motivates the inclusion of residue information in the prediction. Often,

20 types of amino acids and their physicochemical characteristics are identified and represented as the feature descriptors. The physicochemical characteristics of an amino acid residue can be described by three values: number of atoms, number of electrostatic charge, and number of potential hydrogen bonds [21,23,29]. The hydrophobic effect is also shown to be important in protein–RNA binding. The hydrophobicity of an amino acid residue can be described by the hydrophobic index designed by Sweet and Eisenberg [30].

Evolutionary information is often used to locate the functional sites of RNA binding. The position-specific scoring matrix (PSSM) is a commonly used representation of evolutionary patterns in biological sequences. For a PSSM profile, a residue a_i at position i in a protein sequence is presented by an evolutionary information vector consisting of loglikelihoods for 20 different amino acids [6]. The sequence conservation status is given by the weighted positions of RNA binding events. The values of sequence conservation for amino acids are often obtained by PSI-BLAST [3] search of the protein chain sequence in a nonredundant sequence database [34]. The round of iteration can be set to be 3, and the result of the PSI-BLAST search well be a PSSM. Specifically, the conservation score of each residue is referred to the corresponding diagonal value of the matrix [23].

8.4.3 Structure-Based Features

These former values are related only to protein sequence and do not contain any structural information. When the 3D structure of the protein–RNA complex is available, some important structure features can be derived to characterize these amino acid residues. Secondary structure information has been shown to be correlated with protein–RNA interaction [1,31]. Two types of secondary structures are RNA binding type. (1) binding between α-helix or loop and a groove of the RNA pockets and (2) binding between β-sheet surface and unpaired RNA bases [11,39]. It is expected to improve the prediction accuracy of RNA binding residues after inclusion of such features. The secondary structure of an amino acid residue can be calculated by DSSP algorithm [16]. It would be divided into three states: helix, sheet, and coil. DSSP secondary structure types I, G, and H are considered as helix; types E and B are considered as sheet; types T, S, and blank are considered as coil. We can use (1,0,0), (0,1,0), and (0,0,1) to represent the three types, respectively [23,37].

The area accessible to a solvent on a protein surface is important in the protein function of binding RNA. The relative accessible surface area delineates the local solvent environment of protein–RNA interaction [23]. This should improve the prediction of RNA binding residues in proteins. The accessible surface area of an amino acid can generally be calculated by DSSP [16]. Then we calculate the relative property by dividing the accessible surface area by the accessible surface area of fully exposed amino acids. The accessible surface areas of the fully exposed amino acids are available according to Rost and Sander [27].

The pK_a value of an amino acid sidechain defines the pH-dependent characteristic of a protein. The descriptor represents the pH-dependence of activity and protein stability. This is an important factor in determining environmental characteristics of a protein [9]. It is widely used in the prediction of protein–RNA binding sites for its important effect on the protein environment [23,35]. The normal pK_a values of amino acids in calculating protein sidechain environment properties [9] can be implemented in the descriptors of characterizing the protein residues.

To distinguish the RNA binding sites of protein, various descriptors are derived from available information. They are usually combined together as feature vectors to encode the residues. We often define some new descriptors to represent the residue specificity to distinguish the RNA binding events. For instance, some statistical information of binding or interaction propensity between protein and RNA residues can be derived [23,31].

8.4.4   Derived Features of Interaction Propensity

To improve the state of the art in machine learning methods for predicting protein–RNA binding residues, some methods have been developed to define various measurements of binding propensity between protein and its RNA partners [31]. We also introduced a new interaction propensity for binding residues that highlights residue pairs on protein–RNA interface [23]. Protein–RNA interactions are reported to involve a number of nonpolar weak interactions. Also, the interactions often occur in a patch on the surface [15,18]. Therefore, a statistical measure of binding residue pairs in the protein–RNA interface definitely sheds new light on the binding characteristics and features. These derived features are expected to improve the accuracy of predicting RNA binding residues in proteins.

In several previous studies, strong biases have been reported in the types of amino acids, presenting in protein–RNA interfaces such as the abundant occurrence of arginine-rich motifs [15,17,18,31]. Terribilini et al. [31], defined the interface propensity for each amino acid type χ as

$$P(\chi) = \log_2 \frac{\text{percentage of residues of one type } \chi \text{ in interfaces}}{\text{percentage of residues of one type } \chi \text{ in entire dataset}}$$

Apparently, an interface propensity value greater than 0 indicates that an amino acid is overrepresented in RNA–protein interfaces relative to the protein sequence as a whole.

Kim et al. [17] defined an interaction propensity for each of the 20 amino acids binding each of the four nucleotides, respectively. Amino acids on the protein surface were determined if the relative accessibility was >5% [20]. The interaction propensity P_{ab} between amino acid a and nucleotide b was then defined by [17]

$$P_{ab} = \frac{\dfrac{N_{ab}}{\sum_{i,j} N_{ij}}}{\dfrac{N_a}{\sum_i N_i} \dfrac{N_b}{\sum_j N_j}}$$

where

N_{ab} = number of amino acid residues a interacting with nucleotide residue b

$\sum_{i,j} N_{ij}$ = total number of interacting pairs of any amino acid and nucleotide

N_a = number of amino acids a

$\sum_i N_i$ = total number of amino acids

N_b = number of nucleotides b

$\sum_j N_j$ = total number of nucleotides

$N_{ab}/(\sum_{i,j} N_{ij})$ = ratio of occurrence of amino acid a and nucleotide b to total number of all amino acids binding to any nucleotide on protein surface.

$N_b/(\sum_j N_j)$ = ratio of frequency of nucleotide b to that of all nucleotides on surface.

In 2006, another interaction propensity was defined by amino acid residue singlet interface propensity and residue doublet propensity in protein–RNA interfaces [18]. The residue singlet interface propensity (P_i) was calculated for each amino acid type i as a fraction of the frequency that i contributes to a protein–RNA interface compared to the frequency that i contributes to a protein surface:

$$P_i = \frac{f_i}{\overline{f}_i}$$

$$f_i = \frac{n_i}{\sum_{i=1}^{20} n_i}, \qquad \overline{f}_i = \frac{\overline{n}_i}{\sum_{i=1}^{20} \overline{n}_i}$$

Here, n_i is the number of amino acid type i on the protein surface and $\overline{n}_i$ is that in the RNA interface. The number n_i was obtained from the population of nonhomologous proteins in the PDB and $\overline{n}_i$ was determined from the data for protein–RNA complexes [18]. Similarly, the residue doublet interface propensity P_{ij} was calculated as follows. The frequency f_{ij} of doublet amino acid type ij on the protein surface and that in the protein–RNA interface $\overline{f}_{ij}$ were calculated from the number of residue doublets as

$$f_{ij} = \frac{n_{ij}}{\sum_{i=1}^{20} \sum_{j=1}^{20} n_{ij}} = f_i \times f_j \times C_{ij}$$

$$\overline{f}_{ij} = \frac{\overline{n}_{ij}}{\sum_{i=1}^{20} \sum_{j=1}^{20} \overline{n}_{ij}} = \overline{f}_i \times \overline{f}_j \times \overline{D}_{ij}$$

where n_{ij} is the number of doublet type ij on the protein surface and $\overline{n}_{ij}$ is that in the RNA interface. Terms $f_i, f_j, \overline{f}_i, \overline{f}_j$ are given in the single interface propensity, and C_{ij} and D_{ij} are the surface and interface residue doublet coefficient, respectively. If amino acid types i and j have no correlation on the protein surface, then $C_{ij} = 1.0$ and in the RNA interface, $D_{ij} = 1.0$. Then, the residue doublet preference in the RNA interface was determined to be

$$Q_{ij} = \frac{\bar{f}_{ij}}{f_{ij}} = P_i \times P_j \times \frac{D_{ij}}{C_{ij}}$$

where P_i and P_j are the residue singlet interface propensities. The residue doublet interface propensity was defined as

$$P_{ij} = \frac{D_{ij}}{C_{ij}}$$

The mutual interaction propensity between protein residues and its binding RNA partners will discriminatively characterize the RNA binding residues in protein sequences, and the derived features from the structure information will benefit the prediction accuracy of a classifier that considers the mutual relationship between interacting residues and nucleotides. With this in mind, we identified and quantified the mutual dependence between protein residues and RNA nucleotide by calculating a new measure: mutual interaction propensity [23]. We highlighted the important role of the neighbor residues in determining the specificity of biochemical features and the preference for interaction with nucleotides for an amino acid residue [31,36]. Hence, we defined the mutual interaction propensity of a residue triplet and a nucleotide. A triplet is regarded as interacting with a nucleotide when its central residue interacts with the nucleotide. The mutual interaction propensity was defined as

$$S(x,y) = \sum_{p,r} f_{p,r}(x,y) \log_2 \frac{f_{p,r}(x,y)}{f_p(x) f_r(y)}$$

where x represents a residue triplet, y represents a nucleotide (i.e., $y \in \{A, G, C, U\}$); $f_{p,r}(x,y) = N_{p,r}(x,y)/\sum_{x,y} N_{p,r}(x,y)$ represents the frequency of x interacting y in the protein–RNA pair (p,r), where $N_{p,r}(x,y)$ is the number of residue triplet x binding to nucleotide y and $\sum_{x,y} N_{p,r}(x,y)$ is the total number of residue triplet and nucleotide pairs in the protein–RNA pair (p,r); and $f_p(x) = N_p(x)/\sum_x N_p(x)$ represents the frequency of the residue triplet x in protein p, where $N_p(x)$ is the number of residue triplet x and $\sum_x N_p(x)$ is the total number of all residue triplets in the protein p. Similarly, $f_r(y) = N_r(y)/\sum_y N_r(y)$ represents the frequency of a nucleotide y, where $N_r(y)$ is the number of nucleotide y and $\sum_y N_r(y)$ is the total number of nucleotides in the RNA r. The interaction propensity of a triplet x and a nucleotide y is calculated on all interacting protein–RNA pairs in the dataset. We identify the binding specificity of mutual interaction propensity between the existing triplets and four RNA nucleotides. A protein sequence of length l residues corresponds to $l - 2$ triplets, and every triplet will get its corresponding values of mutual propensity with four types of nucleotides individually. The derived feature of mutual interaction propensity of each residue ($l - 2$ centers in the triplets) was described by the four values [23].

8.4.5 Encoding Scheme

We determine the properties and various features of binding residue from sequence and structure profiles. The combination of information from different sources would enable us to encode protein residues into feature vectors after deriving the features of RNA binding residues as well as those of non-RNA-binding residues. They are encoded into a vector to represent the elements of residue characterization. The information of neighbor residues is usually contained when we formulate the feature vectors. A sliding-window technique is often implemented to encode the amino acid residues. From instance, we can use the windows of odd number s size of residues in the encoding scheme. Whether a residue binds RNA is determined by the middle residue (itself) and its neighbor $s - 1$ residue profile. The feature vectors representing the residue in the window were then encoded by properties of the s residues. Individual residues were then represented in feature vectors with the same-length elements. The number of elements in the feature vector would be determined by the chosen feature descriptors.

8.5 EXISTING METHODS

Methods NN, NB, SVM, and RF are the classic machine learning methods. So far, some methods based on these classifiers have respectively been proposed to predict RNA binding sites in proteins by various features. Table 8.1 lists some methods and their corresponding features used to train the predictors. Jeong et al. [13] proposed a NN-based method for predicting RNA binding sites by using amino acid types (AA) and secondary structure elements (SS). Then, Jeong and Miyano [14] improved the prediction performance of NN classifier by using

TABLE 8.1 Some Available Methods for Predicting RNA Binding Sites in Proteins

Software	Classifier	Feature(s)	Reference
—	NN	AA, SS, PSSM	14
BindN	SVM	SSI, pK_a, HP, MM	35
RNAbindR	NB	IP, RSA, SE, HP, SS, EP	32
RISP	SVM	PSSM	33
RNAProB	SVM	PSSM	6
PPRint	SVM	PSSM	19
PRINTR	SVM	PSSM, SSI, RSA, SS	37
PiRaNhA	SVM	PSSM, IP, RSA, HP	29
PRNA	RF	MIP, PC, HP, pK_a, PSSM, SS, RSA	23
RBRpred	SVM	SSI, PSSM, RSA, SS	39

the weighted profiles of PSSM. Wang and Brown [35] proposed a SVM-based classifier to predict RNA binding residues in proteins by using single-sequence information (SSI) plus three biochemical sequence features, including side chain pK_a value (pK_a), hydrophobicity index (HP), and molecular mass of amino acid (MM). RNABindR [32] implemented a NB classifier to predict RNA binding amino acid residues in proteins by features of interface propensity (IP), relative accessible surface area (RSA), sequence entropy (SE), hydrophobicity (HP), secondary structure (SS), and electrostatic potential (EP). PPRint [19] implemented a SVM-based method in the identification using PSSM. RNAProB [6] is also a SVM-based method by using the evolutionary information of smoothed PSSM. Tong et al. [33] also proposed a RNA interaction site prediction (RISP) method using SVM in conjunction with evolutionary information of amino acid sequences in terms of their PSSMs. PRINTR [37] developed a method for the prediction of protein residues that interact with RNA using SVM by single-sequence information (SSI), PSSM, predicted secondary structure (SS), relative solvent-exposed surface area (RSA). Spriggs et al. [29] improved the prediction performance by a SVM-based classifier using four properties of PSSM, interface propensity (IP), relative solvent accessibility (RSA), and hydrophobicity (HP). We proposed a RF method for combining various features of interacting protein and RNA [23]. Mutual interaction propensity (MIP) and sequence-derived features, such as physicochemical characteristics (PC), hydrophobicity (HP) and sidechain pK_a value (pK_a), as well as structure-derived features, including PSSM conservation value, relatively accessible surface (RAS), and secondary structure (SS), are integrated together to train the predictor. Zhang et al. [39] proposed a sequence-based model for the prediction of RNA binding residues. They implemented five feature sets (12 features) based on the single-sequence information (SSI), evolutionary conservation (PSSM), the predicted secondary structure (SS), and the predicted relative solvent accessibility (RSA). A SVM classifier was built on these features after processing by feature selection.

8.6   FEATURE ANALYSIS AND COMPARISON STUDY

We represented protein residues as feature vectors individually by identifying sequence and structure information potentially contributing to the RNA binding events. These features of binding residues and nonbinding residues are implemented to train a classifier to learn the underlying residue patterns of protein–RNA interaction. Some of the descriptors in the feature vector, such as *relative accessible surface* and *secondary structure*, can be calculated only after 3D protein structure is available. The defined feature of interaction propensity can also be implemented when structure information is known. Apparently, it is valuable to determine and compare the importance of these different descriptors about their contributions to the prediction. Moreover, the comparisons of machine learning methods will provide valuable information on the discriminative classifiers for predicting RNA binding sites in proteins.

In our published paper on predicting RNA binding residues in proteins [23], we investigated comparisons between various methods and numerous features. The effectiveness and efficiency provided evidence for substantial feasibility of the prediction for protein–RNA binding residues by feature-based machine learning methods. We generally categorized our residue features into sequence-based and structure-based descriptors. We composed a dataset of 205 protein–RNA interaction pairs from RsiteDB [28]. As shown in Table 8.1, we identified MIP, PC, HP, SS, and PSSM conservation values and pK_a values of these residues to encode the feature vectors. We trained and tested our RF-based predictors and achieved high performance of prediction by combining various features [23]. To evaluate the contribution of each feature for the prediction accuracy, we tested the performance of some selected features in these descriptors. Table 8.2 presents the results of prediction performance of the fivefold cross validation by subtracting one of the descriptors individually in the scoring scheme. After subtracting each descriptor individually while describing these residues, we found decreased accuracy of prediction in comparison to the accuracy obtained when we used all the descriptors. For instance, when we omitted the defined MIP, ACC, and F measure, the AUC became 75.8%, 0.751, and 0.828, respectively, in comparison to 84.5%, 0.859, and 0.923 that we obtained individually using all descriptors.

We also investigated the prediction performance by combining different sequence-derived features and structure-derived features [23]. The details of prediction results are shown in Table 8.3. Table 8.3 also shows the results of the prediction based on the combined sequence features and those of structure features, respectively. When we employed the scheme of combining these features based only on sequence (without Structure features), our RF-based method achieved a prediction accuracy of 81.4%, 0.832 F measure and 0.905 AUC value. Our method can obtain 82.6% ACC, 0.847 F measure, and 0.917 AUC without sequence features. The results indicate that with the combination of all these descriptors, the predictor can identify more information for better classifying protein–RNA binding residues from nonbinding ones. Here, MIP represents mutual interaction propensity, PC represents physicochemical characteristics, HP represents hydrophobicity, PSSM represents PSSM conversation value, ACC represents accessible surface, SS represents secondary structure, and

TABLE 8.2 Prediction Results Obtained by Subtracting Descriptor

Without Feature	SN (%)	SP (%)	ACC (%)	F Measure	AUC
MIP	75.9	74.3	75.8	0.751	0.828
PC	82.9	87.1	83.3	0.849	0.920
HP	83.7	86.4	84.0	0.850	0.920
PSSM	82.2	85.9	82.6	0.840	0.912
RSA	82.9	83.2	82.9	0.840	0.905
SS	83.5	86.9	83.9	0.851	0.920
pK_a	83.4	86.7	83.8	0.850	0.920

TABLE 8.3   **Predictive Results Obtained by Combinations of Different Descriptors**

Without Composition (With Composition) of Features	SN (%)	SP (%)	ACC (%)	F Measure	AUC
HP, ACC, SS (MIP + PC + PSSM + pk_a)	81.5	85.7	81.9	0.836	0.908
PC, ACC, SS, pKa (MIP + HP + PSSM)	81.9	85.7	82.3	0.838	0.911
PC, HP, PSSM (MIP + ACC + SS + pK_a)	83.0	86.5	83.3	0.847	0.917
PC, HP, pK_a (MIP + PSSM + ACC + SS)	83.7	86.7	84.0	0.852	0.922
MIP, ACC, SS (PC + HP + PSSM + pK_a)	72.7	68.5	72.3	0.705	0.774
MIP, PC, HP, PSSM, pK_a (ACC + SS)	62.0	67.5	62.5	0.646	0.709
MIP, PC, pK_a (HP + PSSM + ACC + SS)	74.1	74.6	74.2	0.744	0.824
MIP, PSSM, SS (PC + HP + ACC + pK_a)	69.6	73.3	70.0	0.714	0.795
Structure features (MIP + PC + HP + PSSM + pK_a)	80.9	85.6	81.4	0.832	0.905
Sequence features (MIP + ACC + SS)	82.0	87.5	82.6	0.847	0.917

pK_a represents sidechain pK_a value, respectively. The comparison study results have shown the importance of residue properties in the identification of binding specificity. These features can be used to construct the structural markers and motifs for discriminating RNA binding sites as well as nonbinding ones [22,23].

For available machine learning methods of NN, NB, SVM, and RF, we also compared the prediction results of these predictors on the benchmark dataset. We explored these algorithms using the same process of performing training and test steps [23]. In the 205 protein chains, we randomly conducted a training set of 105 protein chains as well as a test set of the remaining 100 chains. We trained these classifiers and then implemented the prediction and validation in the test set to evaluate the performance of the machine learning methods. Figure 8.2 shows the ROC curves of prediction by different classifiers in the test set. The performance details are given in Table 8.4. In Figure 8.2, AUC values of RF-based, SVM-based, NN-based, and NB-based predictors are 0.912, 0.801, 0.782, and 0.713, respectively. The RF-based method performs better than other classifiers in our dataset. As to the prediction results of the other known methods listed in Table 8.1, such as RNABindR, BindN, and PPRint, they are also available in our published paper [23].

TABLE 8.4 Comparison of Results for Different Machine Learning Methods

Method	SN (%)	SP (%)	ACC (%)	F Measure	AUC	MCC
RF	81.9	86.8	82.4	0.843	0.912	0.488
SVM	75.7	73.7	75.5	0.747	0.801	0.335
NN	70.6	72.2	70.7	0.714	0.782	0.280
NB	65.3	68.1	65.6	0.667	0.713	0.211

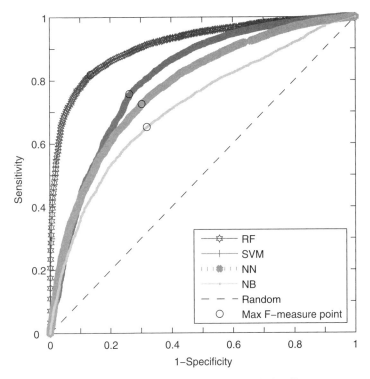

Figure 8.2 ROC performance of several classifiers.

8.7 CONCLUSION

In this chapter, we provided an overview for predicting RNA binding sites in proteins on the basis of various features by machine learning methods. The physicochemical features, sequence-derived features, and structure-derived features were identified in various protein–RNA complexes. The interacting sites of protein and RNA were encoded into features, and the interaction events between these residues were signed with labels to distinguish the binding residues and nonbinding residues. Various features representing the interaction of an amino acid and its partner nucleotides were encoded into feature vectors. The features were then used to train a machine learning classifier. To assess the prediction performance of these predictors, currently the cross-validation technique is widely implemented. The statistical assessments were analyzed and compared by various strategies of encoding features and selecting machine learning algorithms. The comparisons in these existing methods show their advantages and characteristics. In the training set, the residues were encoded into feature vectors representing the RNA binding specificities in proteins. The learning and validation processes in protein–RNA complexes will provide evidence for the effectiveness of predictors. After training of those computational methods, the predictors can directly be used to predict the RNA binding residues in a protein. The sequence information and structure information, if available, of the targeted protein will be identified as the input features. The methods based only on sequence would provide broader coverage of prediction. Clearly, the accuracy and coverage of prediction are closely related to the available information, encoded mechanisms, and the classifiers.

ACKNOWLEDGMENTS

We thank Professor Xiang-Sun Zhang, Dr. Ling-Yun Wu, and Dr. Yong Wang of the Chinese Academy of Sciences (CAS) for helpful discussions and comments. This work was supported by the National Natural Science Foundation of China (NSFC) under Grants 31100949, 61134013, 91029301, and 61072119; by Shanghai NSF under Grant 11ZR1443100; and by the Knowledge Innovation Program of Shanghai Institutes for Biological Sciences (SIBS) of CAS with Grant 2011KIP203; by the Chief Scientist Program of SIBS, CAS with Grant 2009CSP002; and by the SA-SIBS Scholarship Program; This research was also partially supported by the National Center for Mathematics and Interdisciplinary Sciences, CAS.

REFERENCES

1. Allers J, Shamoo Y, Structure-based analysis of protein-RNA interactions using the program ENTANGLE, *J. Mol. Biol.* **311**:75–86 (2001).
2. Chen L, Wang RS, Zhang XS, *Biomolecular Network: Methods and Applications in Systems Biology*, John Wiley & Sons. 2009.
3. Altschul SF, Madden TL, Schaffer AA, Zhang J, Zhang Z, Miller W, Lipman DJ, Gapped BLAST and PSI-BLAST: A new generation of protein database search programs, *Nucleic Acids Res.* **25**:3389–3402 (1997).
4. Berman HM, Westbrook J, Feng Z, Gilliland G, Bhat T, Weissig H, Shindyalov I, Bourne P, The Protein Data Bank, *Nucleic Acids Res.* **28**:235–242 (2000).
5. Breiman L, Random forests, *Machine Learn.* **45**:5–32 (2001).
6. Cheng CW, Su EC, Hwang JK, Sung TY, Hsu WL, Predicting RNA-binding sites of proteins using support vector machines and evolutionary information. *BMC Bioinformatics* **9**(Suppl 12):S6 (2008).

7. Doherty EA, Batey RT, Masquida B, Doudna JA, A universal mode of helix packing in RNA, *Nat. Struct. Biol.* **8**(4):339–343 (2001).

8. Ellis JJ, Broom M, Jones S, Protein-RNA interactions: Structural analysis and functional classes, *Proteins* **66**:903–911 (2007).

9. Gibas CJ, Subramaniam S, Explicit solvent models in protein pKa calculations, *Biophys. J.* **71**:138–147 (1996).

10. Glisovic T, Bachorik JL, Yong J, Dreyfuss G, RNA-binding proteins and post-transcriptional gene regulation, *FEBS Lett.* **582**:1977–1986 (2008).

11. Hall KB, RNA-protein interactions, *Curr. Opin. Struct. Biol.* **12**:283–288 (2002).

12. Han LY, Cai CZ, Lo SL, Chung MC, Chen YZ, Prediction of RNA-binding proteins from primary sequence by a support vector machine approach, *RNA* **10**:355–368 (2004).

13. Jeong E, Chung IF, Miyano S, A neural network method for identification of RNA-interacting residues in protein, *Genome Inform.* **15**:105–116 (2004).

14. Jeong E, Miyano S, *A Weighted Profile Based Method for Protein-RNA Interacting Residue Prediction*, LNCS Series, vol. 3939, 2006, pp. 123–139.

15. Jones S, Daley DT, Luscombe NM, Berman HM, Thornton JM, Protein-RNA interactions: A structural analysis, *Nucleic Acids Res.* **29**:943–954 (2001).

16. Kabsch W, Sander C, Dictionary of protein secondary structure: Pattern recognition of hydrogen-bonded and geometrical features, *Biopolymers* **22**:2577–2637 (1983).

17. Kim H, Jeong E, Lee SW, Han K, Computational analysis of hydrogen bonds in protein-RNA complexes for interaction patterns, *FEBS Lett.* **552**:231–239 (2003).

18. Kim OT, Yura K, Go N, Amino acid residue doublet propensity in the protein-RNA interface and its application to RNA interface prediction, *Nucleic Acids Res.* **34**:6450–6460 (2006).

19. Kumar M, Gromiha MM, Raghava GP, Prediction of RNA binding sites in a protein using SVM and PSSM profile, *Proteins* **71**:189–194 (2008).

20. Lee B, Richards FM, The interpretation of protein structures: Estimation of static accessibility, *J. Mol. Biol.* **55**:379–400 (1971).

21. Li N, Sun Z, Jiang F, Prediction of protein-protein binding site by using core interface residue and support vector machine, *BMC Bioinformatics* **9**:553 (2008).

22. Liu ZP, Wu LY, Wang Y, Zhang XS, Chen L, Bridging protein local structures and protein functions, *Amino Acids* **35**:627–650 (2008).

23. Liu ZP, Wu LY, Wang Y, Zhang XS, Chen L, Prediction of protein-RNA binding sites by a random forest method with combined features, *Bioinformatics* **26**:1616–1622 (2010).

24. Lunde BM, Moore C, Varani G, RNA-binding proteins: Modular design for efficient function, *Nat. Rev. Mol. Cell. Biol.* **8**:479–490 (2007).

25. Morozova N, Allers J, Myers J, Shamoo Y, Protein-RNA interactions: Exploring binding patterns with a three-dimensional superposition analysis of high resolution structures, *Bioinformatics* **22**:2746–2752 (2006).

26. Perez-Cano L, Solernou A, Pons C, Fernandez-Recio J, Structural prediction of protein-RNA interaction by computational docking with propensity-based statistical potentials, *Proc. Pacific Symp. Biocomputing*, Kamuela, Hawaii, 2010, vol. **15**, pp. 293–301.

27. Rost B, Sander C, Conservation and prediction of solvent accessibility in protein families, *Proteins* **20**:216–226 (1994).

28. Shulman-Peleg A, Shatsky M, Nussinov R, Wolfson HJ, Prediction of interacting single-stranded RNA bases by protein-binding patterns, *J. Mol. Biol.* **379**:299–316 (2008).

29. Spriggs RV, Murakami Y, Nakamura H, Jones S, Protein function annotation from sequence: Prediction of residues interacting with RNA, *Bioinformatics* **25**:1492–1497 (2009).

30. Sweet RM, Eisenberg D, Correlation of sequence hydrophobicities measures similarity in three dimensional protein structure, *J. Mol. Biol.* **171**:479–488 (1983).

31. Terribilini M, Lee JH, Yan C, Jernigan RL, Honavar V, Dobbs D, Prediction of RNA binding sites in proteins from amino acid sequence, *RNA* **12**:1450–1462 (2006).

32. Terribilini M, Sander JD, Lee JH, Zaback P, Jernigan RL, Honavar V, Dobbs D, RNABindR: A server for analyzing and predicting RNA-binding sites in proteins, *Nucleic Acids Res.* **35**:W578–W584 (2007).

33. Tong J, Jiang P, Lu Z, RISP: A web-based server for prediction of RNA-binding sites in proteins, *Comput. Methods Programs Biomed.* **90**:148–153 (2008).

34. The UniProt Consortium: The Universal Protein Resource (Uniprot), *Nucleic Acids Res.* **36**:D190–D195 (2008).

35. Wang L, Brown SJ, BindN: A web-based tool for efficient prediction of DNA and RNA binding sites in amino acid sequences, *Nucleic Acids Res.* **34**:W243–W248 (2006).

36. Wang L, Eghbalnia HR, Markley JL, Nearest-neighbor effects on backbone alpha and beta carbon chemical shifts in proteins, *J. Biomol. NMR* **39**(3): 247–257 (2007).

37. Wang Y, Xue Z, Shen G, Xu J, PRINTR: Prediction of RNA binding sites in proteins using SVM and profiles, *Amino Acids* **35**:295–302 (2008).

38. Weigt M, White RA, Szurmant H, Hoch JA, Hwa T, Identification of direct residue contacts in protein-protein interaction by message passing, *Proc. Natl. Acad. Sci. USA* **106**:67–72 (2009).

39. Zhang T, Zhang H, Chen K, Ruan J, Shen S, Kurgan L, Analysis and prediction of RNA-binding residues using sequence, evolutionary conservation, and predicted secondary structure and solvent accessibility, *Curr. Protein Pept. Sci.* **11**(7): 609–628 (2010).

CHAPTER 9

ALGORITHMIC FRAMEWORKS FOR PROTEIN DISULFIDE CONNECTIVITY DETERMINATION

RAHUL SINGH, WILLIAM MURAD, and TIMOTHY LEE

9.1 INTRODUCTION

Cysteine residues have a property unique among the amino acids, in that they can pair to form a covalent bond, known as a *disulfide bond* (S—S bond). These bonds are so named because they occur when each cysteine's sulfhydryl group becomes oxidized following this the reaction:

$$S—H + S—H \rightarrow S—S + 2H \tag{9.1}$$

Because disulfide bonds impose length and angle constraints on the backbone of a protein, knowledge of the location of these bonds can significantly help in understanding the space of possible stable tertiary structures into which the protein folds. The disulfide bond pattern of a protein also can have an important effect on its function. For example, Angata et al. [1] showed that the sterical structure formed by intramolecular disulfide bonds in the polysialyltransferase ST8Sia IV is critical for catalyzing the polysialylation of the neural cell adhesion molecule (NCAM). NCAM has an important role in neuronal development and regeneration. Figure 9.1 is a schematic representation of ST8Sia IV and the sialyltransferase of another gene family, ST6Gal I, showing how this contrast in disulfide bond structure impacts function. We define the *disulfide connectivity determination problem* as follows. Given the primary structure of a protein (i.e., the sequence of amino acid residues that constitute the protein), determine all

Algorithmic and Artificial Intelligence Methods for Protein Bioinformatics. First Edition.
Edited by Yi Pan, Jianxin Wang, Min Li.
© 2014 John Wiley & Sons, Inc. Published 2014 by John Wiley & Sons, Inc.

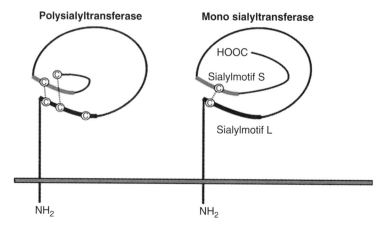

Figure 9.1   Schematic representation of ST8Sia IV and ST6Gal I, showing the functional importance of disulfide bonds. ST8Sia IV is a polysialyltransferase and contains two disulfide bonds (shown using thin lines with cysteines labeled ©). These two disulfide bonds bring the *C* terminus of the protein and the sialylmotifs L and S close together in space. In contrast, ST6Gal I lacks the cysteine at the COOH-terminal end; therefore, the COOH terminal is not close to sialylmotifs L or S. ST6Gal I does not catalyze polysialylation, but rather it transfers single sialic acid residue (monosialyltransferase) to the carbohydrate acceptor substrate. (Adapted from Angata et al. [1].)

the cysteine pairs that are connected by disulfide bonds. The reader may note that these cysteine pairs completely define the disulfide connectivity pattern of the protein. For example, the disulfide connectivity pattern for ST8Sia IV is C142—C292, C156—C356, and the cysteines C11 and C169 are not engaged in a disulfide bond (such cysteines are termed *free*.) The number following each C, in this example, refers to the cysteine residue's position in the primary sequence, which by convention begins at the unbounded *N* terminus of the protein.

Potentially, three classes of techniques can be used for determining the disulfide connectivity of a protein [26], includeing (1) crystallographic techniques producing high-resolution 3D structures of proteins, (2) techniques that detect disulfide bonds by analyzing the spectra obtained from the targeted digestion of an intact protein using mass spectrometry, and (3) algorithmic techniques that *predict* (or infer) the disulfide connectivity from sequence-based characteristics. Each of these classes of techniques comes with its advantages and disadvantages. For instance, determination of disulfide bonds can be achieved with high accuracy using X-ray crystallography or NMR. However, such methods require relatively large amounts (10–100 mg) of pure protein in a particular solution or crystalline state and are fundamentally low-throughput in nature. On the other hand, mass spectrometric methods can offer accurate bond identification and, in principle, can scale to any number of bonds with much less stringent sample purity requirements when compared to NMR or X-ray crystallography. However, the actual task of analyzing and identifying the MS/MS spectra corresponding to disulfide linkages is nontrivial and requires sophisticated algorithms. Furthermore, the search space that has to be analyzed increases rapidly as a function of the number of cysteines, peptides, and ion types being considered. Finally, techniques for algorithmic prediction of disulfide connectivity are based on utilizing local and global sequence characteristics. Consequently, these methods do not require significant data preparation and can be run in high-throughput settings. However, it may not always be possible to obtain a functional relationship (or mapping) between local or global sequence characteristics in the presence of specific disulfide bonds. Consequently, sequence-based methods can lead to higher false positive or false negative predictions, when compared to crystallographic or mass spectrometric techniques. Regardless, sequence-based predictors are relatively straightforward to use and often may be the only recourse, if access to crystallography or MS data is limited.

In the following sections, we first describe the algorithmic frameworks underlying sequence-based approaches to disulfide bond detection. Next, we introduce the fundamentals of mass spectrometry (MS) and finally present the algorithmic frameworks that can be used for determining disulfide bonds from MS data.

9.2 DETERMINING DISULFIDE BONDS FROM SEQUENCE INFORMATION: FORMULATIONS, FEATURES, AND ALGORITHMIC FRAMEWORKS

The basic idea underlying the determination of disulfide bonds from sequence information involves two main steps: (1) identifying global or local features that can be derived from sequence-level data and (2) inferring the relationship between these features and the disulfide connectivity. The inference process can be (1) unsupervised and based on similarity in some feature space, (2) supervised and involve a machine learning algorithm and a "training set," and (3) based on modeling the physics of the molecule. The gamut of different methods that have been proposed in the literature in this context can be understood by analyzing them from three correlated but different perspectives: (1) the specific problem that is being solved (*problem formulation*), (2) the global and/or local features that are extracted from the sequence-based information (*feature descriptors*), and (3) the algorithmic strategy that is used (*algorithmic solution frameworks*). In the following text, we discuss these perspectives in detail and analyze the prior research results obtained in each of these three contexts. For a more detailed review, we refer the reader to a paper by Singh [26].

9.2.1 Problem Formulations

The goal of computationally finding disulfide bonds can be attempted in terms of the following problem formulations:

- *Residue classification*—classify cysteine residues into those that are bonded and those not bonded.

- *Chain classification*—distinguish protein chains that contain disulfide bonds from those that do not.
- *Connectivity prediction*—determine all pairs of cysteine residues that are connected to each other by disulfide bonds.
- *Bridge classification*—determine whether a specific pair of cysteine residues are joined by a disulfide link.

The reader may note that the chain classification problem is subsumed by the residue classification formulation, since the identification of bonded cysteine residues can be used trivially to identify which chains contain disulfide bonds. Similarly, the connectivity prediction problem subsumes the question of bridge classification. At this point, a note on the computational complexity of this problem is due. If $C = \{c_1, c_2, \ldots, c_n\}$ are the cysteines in a protein, then the number of possible disulfide connectivity patterns (denoted as DMS hereafter) is [7,26]

$$\left|\text{DMS}\right| = (n-1)!! = \prod_{i=1}^{n/2}(2i-1) \qquad (9.2)$$

9.2.2 Feature Descriptors

9.2.2.1 *Global Feature Descriptors*   Since cysteines can occur in either oxidized or thiol forms, a number of global and local sequence-based descriptors have been designed for the residue classification and connectivity prediction problems. The global descriptors are typically based on capturing the statistical frequency of amino acid residues (also called the *amino acid composition*) in the protein. A variation of this idea lies in computing the statistical frequencies of oxidized and reduced cysteines on the surface and in the interior of the proteins. Another variation involves determining physicochemical properties such as hydrophobicity, positive, negative, polar, charged, small, tiny, aliphatic, aromatic, and proline and their negation at a position in the sequence, with the goal of comparing sequences by determining how well these properties are conserved [10,11]. A different type of global feature-based encoding was proposed by Mucchielli-Giorgi et al. [21]. In this encoding, the global features were encoded by a 23-element vector. In this vector, the first 20 elements described the relative abundance of each amino acid residue. Element 21 corresponded to the normalized size of the protein. For a given protein, elements 22 and 23 contained the number and frequency of occurrences of cysteines in the protein, respectively. The cysteine state sequence constitutes yet another global descriptor. The reader may note that for n cysteines, there are $2^n - 1$ possible state sequences (when interchain bonds are excluded). This descriptor has been used by Chen et al. [4].

All the aforementioned global descriptors have been used primarily in residue or chain classification problems. The problem of connectivity determination has given rise to a different set of global descriptors. Arguably, the most prominent of these is the contact potential graph [7]. For m cysteines, this descriptor consists of a completely connected graph G with m vertices. Each edge in this graph had nonzero weights corresponding to one of four formulations of contact potentials, representing the propensity for bond formation between the corresponding cysteine residues. The formulations used to derive the contact potentials by Fariselli and Casadio [7] included (1) the contact potential of Mirny and Shakhnovich [20], which is designed for protein folding and threading; (2) a contact potential derived by constrained optimization that maximized the difference between scores for correct cysteine pairing and incorrect pairings; (3) an odds ratio contact potential; and (4) a contact potential obtained using Monte -Carlo annealing.

9.2.2.2 *Local Feature Descriptors*   In contrast to the global descriptors, local descriptors focus on encoding the characteristics of the sequence environment around the cysteines. In one of the early works in this area, Muskal et al. [22], proposed a novel local descriptor scheme, modifications of which have been extensively used in later studies. In this scheme, each cysteine constituted the center of a window. Each residue inside the window was encoded by a 21-element vector. In this vector, each of the 20 elements corresponded to one of the 20 amino acids. The final element was used as an indicator in case the window overlapped a break in the chain or one of the termini. Within the window, a specific amino acid was encoded by assigning a value of 1 to its corresponding element and the value of 0 to all the other elements (except the indicator node). Muskal's goup experimented with different window sizes corresponding to different sizes of the flanking sequences and obtained best results with 14 flanking amino acid positions [22]. In Figure 9.2, an example illustrates a commonly employed variation of this descriptor, where a 20-element vector is used to encode the presence or absence of each amino acid residue in the neighborhood of a cysteine. The encoding framework proposed by Muskal et al. [22] was extended by Fariselli et al. [6] by considering eight different encodings of the input sequences. The basic encoding framework (employed in context of a single sequence input) was identical to that proposed by Muskal et al., [22]. The other seven encodings involved different features captured from multiple sequence profiles. In the case

---

Amino Acid Residue positions in the vector ={A,R,N,D,C,E,Q,G,H,I,L,K,M,F,P,S,T,W,Y,V}
Sample peptide sequence = DCAY

V_D={0,0,0,1,0,0,0,0,0,0,0,0,0,0,0,0,0,0,0,0}
V_C={0,0,0,0,1,0,0,0,0,0,0,0,0,0,0,0,0,0,0,0}
V_A={1,0,0,0,0,0,0,0,0,0,0,0,0,0,0,0,0,0,0,0}
V_Y={0,0,0,0,0,0,0,0,0,0,0,0,0,0,0,0,0,0,1,0}

Figure 9.2   Example illustrating the encoding of the local environment around a cysteine. The 20-element descriptor is a variation of the encoding approach proposed by Muskal et al. [22]. Each residue in the neighborhood of a cysteine is represented by a 20-element vector. Each position of this vector represents the presence (denoted by a 1) or absence (denoted by a 0) of a specific amino acid.

of multiple sequences, the sequence profile of the cysteine-containing segments taken from the HSSP files of the proteins were used [25]. A 21-element vector was used to encode each residue as in Muskal et al. [22]. However, the key distinction was that the first 20 elements in the vector represented the frequency of occurrence of the 20 amino acid residues in the multiple alignment. Furthermore, in computing the frequency, the central cysteine was also taken into account. In addition to the frequency of occurrence, other features that were considered by Fariselli et al. [6] included *charge, hydrophobicity, conservation weight, and relative entropy*, and their combinations. Frasconi et al. [13] proposed another variation of Muskal's encoding framework that consisted of a 24-element vector. The first 20 elements of the vector represented the relative abundance of specific amino acid residues in the sequence. Element 21 represented the ratio of the length of the sequence to the average length of sequences in the dataset. The ratio of the number of cysteines in the sequence to the maximum number of cysteines observed in the training set constituted element 22. Element 23 represented the ratio of the number of cysteines in the current sequence to the size of the sequence. The final element of the vector acted as a flag in case the sequence had an odd number of cysteines.

9.2.2.3 *Combinations of Local and Global Feature Descriptors*   The study by Vullo and Frasconi [29], presents an example of a descriptor that combines both global and local information. In this work, an undirected graph was used to represent connectivity pattern. Each vertex in the graph contained a description of the local environment of the bonded cysteine. The local environment was captured using a 20-element vector corresponding to a multiple-alignment profile in a local window around each cysteine. In another example, the notion of utilizing the specificities in the sequence neighborhood was extended to take advantage of cysteine distributions in secondary structure elements [8,9]. The cysteine separation profile is another commonly used descriptor that captures local-to-global characteristics. The idea of CSP is based on the observation that proteins with similar disulfide bonding patters share similar folds. Consequently, the separation between oxidized cysteine residues, called the *cysteine separation profile* (CSP), is used for determining disulfide connectivity. Approaches based on this idea encode the separation amongst cysteine residues as a vector. Given a protein P with $2n$ cysteine residues $C_1, C_2, ..., C_{2n}$, we can define its cysteine separation profile as follows:

$$CSP(P) = (C_2 - C_1, C_3 - C_2, ..., C_{2n} - C_{2n-1}) = (P_1, P_2, ..., P_{2n-1}) \qquad (9.3)$$

9.2.3 Algorithmic Solution Frameworks

Given the problem formulations described earlier and a choice of descriptors, the fundamental challenge lies in determining which cysteines participate in a disulfide bond. According to the class of algorithms used, the classical approaches to these problems can be grouped broadly into the following classes:

- *Determination of Classification Function Using Nearest-Neighbor Inference.* These techniques identify disulfide bonds according to the closest training sample(s) in the feature space. From a machine learning perspective, this class of methods constitutes examples of instance-based learning. Neighborhood-based inference has been employed primarily for the residue and chain classification problems.
- *Determination of Classification Function Using Machine Learning Algorithms.* Methods in this class have employed approaches such as neural networks, support vector machines, and logical regression in supervised settings to determine the classification function.
- *Methods Based On Modeling the Physics of Molecules.* This class of methods has been based primarily on modeling the problem as a graph, where cysteines constitute the vertices and the edges are weighted using some measure that is indicative of physicochemical interactions, such as contact potential or evolutionary information. Determining the disulfide connectivity is then cast as a graph-theoretic optimization problem.

9.2.3.1 *Techniques Based on Nearest-Neighbor Inference*

Fiser and Simon [11] observed that oxidized and reduced forms of cysteines rarely occurred simultaneously, except in cases when the cysteine was covalently bonded to heteroatoms, prosthetic groups, or other amino acids in active sites. A residue classification strategy was proposed on the basis of this observation. In this strategy, if the majority of the predicted cysteines in a molecule belonged to one oxidation state and had a high conservation score with respect to the group of oxidized cysteines and lower conservation scores with respect to the group of reduced cysteines, then the other cysteines in the other molecules were assigned to the same oxidation state. If the predicted number of reduced and oxidized cysteines was found to be equal, then the logarithms of the averages of the relative conservation scores for the predicted bonded cysteines and predicted free cysteines were compared. The cysteines in the molecule were predicted to be oxidized or reduced according to whichever relative conservation score was larger.

In the context of connectivity determination, Zhao et al. [33] used a neighborhood distance–based approach defined on the cysteine separation profiles to determine disulfide connectivity. The fundamental hypothesis underlying this method was that molecules having similar separation profiles have similar connectivity patterns. Given two proteins P^1 and P^2, the divergence between the corresponding cysteine separation profiles CSP(P^1) and CSP(P^2) was defined as in Equation (9.4), where i indexes the elements of the CSPs:

$$\mathrm{CSP}(P^1) - \mathrm{CSP}(P^2) = \sum_i |P^1_{\ i} - P^2_{\ i}| \tag{9.4}$$

For a given protein, its disulfide connectivity was predicted to be same as that of a database protein having the most similar cysteine separation profile. Despite its conceptual simplicity, this idea has been found to perform well in practice. Other approaches for predicting connectivity patters based on nearest-neighbor inference include comparisons with an annotated database, as done in the CysView server [18].

9.2.3.2 *Techniques Using Machine Learning Algorithm*

In an early approach Muskal et al. [22], proposed solving the problem of residue classification based on the use of a neural network to learn the influence of the local sequence environment according to whether a cysteine participated in a disulfide bond. A feedforward network with no hidden layers was employed and the network weights were learned using backpropagation. In the training cycle, each example from the training set was presented to the network and the network weights were updated. Once the total error over all samples in the training set converged to a minimum, the network weights were fixed and evaluations were conducted on the remaining data. A cysteine residue was classified as forming a disulfide bond or free, depending on the relative values of the two output neurons.

Mucchielli-Giorgi [21] used logistic regression for residue classification using a combination of global and local descriptors. The overall amino acid composition of the protein constituted the global descriptor, while the local descriptors consisted of two alternate encodings of residues in the local neighborhood. In the first encoding, the environment around each residue was described by a 20-dimensional binary vector, identical to the encoding scheme in Muskal et al. [22]. The second encoding captured the over(under)representation of an amino acid at a specific position in the neighborhood of the cysteine. The descriptors, either individually or in combination, were passed to the logistic function. If the output exceeded a threshold, the cysteine was predicted to be oxidized; otherwise, it was predicted to be free. The threshold itself was defined by minimizing the prediction error rate.

A hybrid approach for predicting the state of a cysteine was proposed by Martelli et al. [19] by accounting for the possible presence of other cysteines in the sequence and their respective states. A hidden Markov model (HMM) consisting of four states and specific interstate transitions was used to enforce this global constraint. The HMM probability parameters were estimated through outputs of state-specific neural networks, which were used to learn the local environment conductive to the bonding or nonbonding state of the cysteine residue on which the window was centered. The output of the neural network was then used as emission probabilities of the four-state HMM. Frasconi et al. [13] used another type of a hybrid classifier that consisted of two stages. In the first stage, global sequence descriptors were used to classify the sequence as having all, some, or none of its constituent cysteines participating in disulfide bonds. For sequences that were predicted to have a combination of free and disulfide-bonded residues, in the second stage, a classifier was trained to predict the bonding state. The classification framework was implemented as a probabilistic combination of support vector machines (SVMs).

In the context of connectivity determination, Vullo and Frasconi [29] used a recursive neural network (RNN) for scoring undirected graphs that represented connectivity patterns by their similarity to the correct graph. Each vertex in the connectivity graph contained 20-element vectors corresponding to a multiple-alignment profile in a local window around each cysteine. During the prediction stage, the score computed by the RNN was used to exhaustively search the space of all possible candidate graphs. Chen and Hwang [3] used multiple SVMs to predict the disulfide patterns using three descriptors: the CSP, the overall amino acid content, and the coupling between local sequence environments. In this formulation, each distinct disulfide pattern was considered as a separate class. The reader may note that this design implies that the increase in the number of classes with increase in the number of cysteines would be combinatorial. Interestingly, the authors were able to show that, given the learning strategy of the three descriptors, the cysteine separation profile provided the best overall results in terms of sensitivity and the fraction of proteins for which the entire disulfide connectivity was correctly predicted. Ceroni et al. [2] predicted the bonding state of cysteines using an SVM classifier based on both local and global features. Next, a bidirectional recurrent network was used to predict a globally correct sequence of bonding state assignments. The number of bonding states was enforced to be even, and the most likely set of bonding states was computed using the Viterbi algorithm. Prediction was carried out by running a trained neural network on all possible connectivity patterns and by selecting the one having the highest score.

9.2.3.3 *Methods Based on Modeling the Physics of Molecules*   One of the seminal works in the area of connectivity prediction, not based on machine learning, was proposed by Fariselli and Casadio [7]. In this method, first a completely connected graph G on m vertices, corresponding to the m cysteines was constructed. Next, edges in this graph were weighted using four different formulations of contact potential to reflect the propensity of bond formation between the corresponding cysteine residues. The specific contact potential formulations included (1) the contact potential due to Mirny and Shakhnovich [20], which was designed for protein folding and threading; (2) a contact potential derived by constrained optimization that maximized the difference between scores for correct cysteine pairing and incorrect ones; (3) an odds ratio contact potential; and (4) a contact potential obtained using Monte Carlo simulated annealing. Finally, the disulfide connectivity was determined by solving the maximum-weight perfect matching problem on G. Recall that the perfect matching of a graph is defined as a subset of its edges, such that each vertex in G has only one edge from the subset incident to it. The maximum-weight perfect matching finds a perfect matching that has the largest total weight of the edges. This problem can be formulated as a linear programming problem and can be solved in $O(m^3)$ time by using the Edmonds–Gabow algorithm [14]. Ferre and Clote [8] also determined disulfide connectivity by solving the maximum-weight matching problem on a graph where the edge weights were determined using the following schemes:

(1) monoresidue and diresidue weight matrices and (2) neural networks using local and evolutionary information obtained using PSI-BLAST.

9.3 ALGORITHMIC METHODS FOR DETERMINING DISULFIDE BONDS USING MASS SPECTROMETRY

We begin with a short description to mass spectrometry based experiment design and refer the interested reader for further details to Forner et al. [12], Nesvizhskii et al. [24], and Vitek [28]. Briefly, the mass spectrometric (MS) method consists of the following major steps:

1. A protease is used to digest a protein into peptides under nonreducing conditions. For example, trypsin cleaves a protein after each lysine and arginine residue. This step is necessary because the sensitivity of the mass spectrometer is higher for peptides than for proteins.

2. The peptides are injected into a liquid chromatography column (LC). The peptides elute sequentially from the LC column.

3. Each peptide is ionized by the addition of one or more protons and separated by the mass spectrometer based on the mass-to-charge ratio (m/z). The collection of mass spectra across elution time forms an LC-MS run, where peaks correspond to peptide ions. Since disulfide bonds present in the protein are not cleaved, structures with one or more peptides linked by disulfide bonds also appear with the other ionized peptides.

4. Finally, for identification, each ionized peptide, called a *precursor ion* henceforth, is isolated and undergoes collision-induced disociation (CID). The CID process results in fragment ions that constitute a secondary spectrum called MS/MS (or tandem MS or MS2) spectrum. Peak intensity in a spectrum is related to the abundance of peptides. Furthermore, distances between peaks in a MS/MS spectrum can be used to determine the peptide sequence of the corresponding LC-MS peak. If the precursor ion contains a disulfide bond, the fragmentation process typically keeps this bond intact. Thus, a disulfide bond can occur within cysteine residues of a single peptide (an intra-peptide bond) or between cysteine residues of different peptides (an interpeptide bond). The intrapeptide and interpeptide bonds can also occur simultaneously, yielding complex bonding topologies as illustrated in Figure 9.3.

The MS/MS spectrum can be regarded as a set of ordered number pairs. The sorted component of the pair is the charge-to-mass ratio, or m/z, of the peptide fragment. The other component is the intensity, which reflects the number of peptide fragments with the same m/z value. Figure 9.4 displays a small part of a tandem mass spectrum, where each m/z-versus-intensity value, or *mass peak*, could potentially correspond to the mass of a fragment of the protein that contains a disulfide bond. While a typical spectrum has several hundred such peaks,

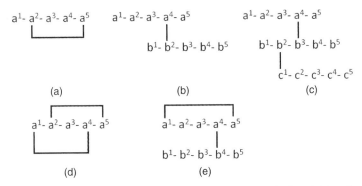

Figure 9.3 Examples of different kinds of disulfide bond topologies: (a) intrabond, with a disulfide bond between two cysteine residues, a^2 and a^5, in one peptide; (b) interbond, with a disulfide bond between two cysteine residues a^4 in one peptide and b^2 in the other; (c) tripeptide structure, with two interpeptide disulfide bonds; (d) multiple intrapeptide bonds; and (e) combination of interpeptide and intrapeptide bonds.

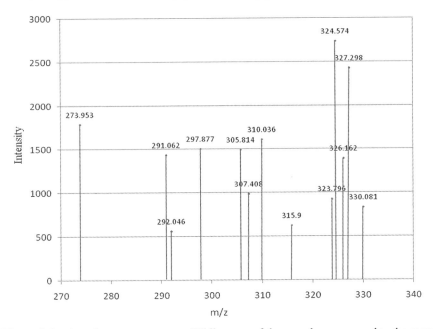

Figure 9.4 A tandem mass spectrum. While some of these peaks correspond to the mass of a subsequence of the amino acid sequence of the input protein sample, other peaks may result from noise, isotopic variation, neutral loss, and charge state uncertainty.

only a few of these peaks actually correspond to relevant information (for the given problem context). Other factors contribute to the information present in the MS/MS spectrum and need to be appropriately addressed to ensure correct analysis. We briefly outline some of these issues below and refer the reader to Lee et al. [15] for details on how these issues can be addressed:

- *Experimental noise* may occur as a result of chemical impurities in the protein sample, which generally result in mass peaks of low intensity, such as the peak at $m/z = 315.9$ in Figure 9.4.

- *Isotopic variation*, indicating that the constituent elements of a molecule have isotopes of differing mass, may occur. As a result, the same peptide fragment may appear as multiple peaks in the MS/MS spectrum. In Figure 9.6, the peaks at $m/z = 291.062$ and $m/z = 292.046$ may be due to isotopic variation.

- *Neutral loss*, refering to a peptide fragment's loss of an uncharged molecule, (usually water or ammonia) may also occur. For example, the peaks at $m/z = 305$ and $m/z = 326$ may both be measurements of the same peptide fragment.

- *Charge state uncertainty* occurs when peaks blend into each other because of lack of resolution during mass resolution. This is important because peptides may be ionized by the addition of more than one proton during mass spectrometric analysis.

9.3.1   Key Definitions and Concepts

A *disulfide bonded peptide structure* consists of one or more cysteine-containing peptides that contain one or more disulfide bonds. The *disulfide bond mass space* DMS = $\{Dm_i\}$ is defined as the set of mass values corresponding to every possible disulfide bonded peptide structure for a protein. Thus, the DMS corresponds to the *theoretical spectrum* of the peptides in a protein. During the ionization stage of mass spectrometric analysis, precursor ions are generated. A *precursor ion* is a peptide or disulfide bonded peptide structure that has been ionized, so that a charge to mass ratio associated with it appears as part of the mass spectrum of a protein. A *precursor ion mass space* PMS = $\{Pm_j\}$ is defined as the set of mass values of the precursor ions. The PMS is generated from the mass spectra after processing to account for noise, and constitutes the experimentally derived spectrum of the peptides. A *precursor match* (also called an *initial match*) between DMS and PMS occurs between elements Dm_i and Pm_j, which are sufficiently close in terms of mass. Mathematically, such a match can be declared if $|Dm_i - Pm_j| < T_{IM}$, where T_{IM} is defined as the *initial identification mass tolerance* (*threshold*), and denotes the amount of experimental variability that Pm_j is allowed to have in determining the match. In the following text, we denote the set of precursor matches as the *initial match* (*IM*) set between the PMS and the DMS.

To illustrate these definitions, let the amino acid sequence of a protein be EC^{2}GRNVNC^{8}TKAIQC^{14}LDEH, where the numbered superscripts represent the relative position in the amino acid sequence of each cysteine residue. Next, we simulate the action of the protease trypsin by dividing this protein into the peptides p_1=EC^{2}GR, p_2=NVNC^{8}TK, and p_3=AIQC^{14}LDEH. Since each of these peptides contains a single cysteine, the disulfide bond mass space

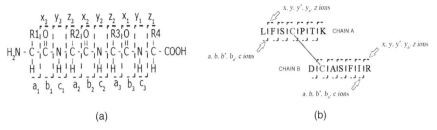

(a)   (b)

Figure 9.5 (a) Representation of some of the most common fragment ion types. Not included in the figure are b and y ions that have lost either a water molecule ($b°$, $y°$) or an ammonia molecule (b^*, y^*). (b) Fragment ions generated for a small pair of S–S-bonded peptides. Each possible fragmentation site (depicted by dashed lines) in both chains A and B, may generate 10 different ion types.

DMS $= \{m(p_1 + p_2), m(p_1 + p_3), m(p_2 + p_3)\}$, where $m(\cdot)$ denotes the total mass of the peptides enclosed in parentheses. If, for instance, an element of the precursor ion mass list is 1389 Da, and the initial identification mass tolerance $\varepsilon = 3$ Da, then the peptide structure $p_1 + p_3$ is added to the initial match because $m(p_1 + p_3) = 1388.59$ Da.

To produce the tandem mass spectrum data, peptides undergo collision-induced dissociation (CID), generating peptide fragments that are reintroduced into the mass spectrometer. The fragments produced are mostly either b ions containing the peptide's N terminus or y ions containing its C terminus. Other possible ion types include a, $b°$, b^*, c, x, $y°$, y^*, and z (see Fig. 9.5). A *cysteine-containing peptide fragment* is a peptide fragment that contains at least one amino acid identified as a cysteine residue. A *disulfide bonded peptide fragment structure* consists of one or more cysteine-containing peptide fragments that contain one or more disulfide bonds. The *disulfide-bonded fragment mass space* (FMS) $= \{Fm_i\}$ is defined as the set of the mass values of every disulfide-bonded fragment structure that can be obtained from fragment ions, which can be of types a, b, $b°$, b^*, c, x, y, $y°$, y^*, or z. The *tandem mass space* (TMS) $= \{Tm_j\}$ is the set mass values of the product ions obtained after the MS/MS step. A *validated match* (VM) between TMS and FMS is said to occur when $|Fm_i - Tm_j| < T_{VM}$, where T_{VM} is defined as the *validation mass tolerance* (*threshold*), the amount of experimental variability that Tm_j is allowed in determining the match.

As an illustration, let us suppose that there was an initial identification made for a simple interbonded structure, where the first peptide $p_1 =$ NVNCTK, and the second peptide $p_2 =$ AIQCLDEH. Table 9.1 shows all possible y and b ions that contain a cysteine, as well as the mass of each ion. Note that for y ions, an additional 18 Da is added to the sum of the residue mass values to account for the carboxylic acid group at the C terminus. Thus, each element of the FMS for this disulfide bond structure can now be generated by adding the mass of a fragment of peptide 1 with the mass of a fragment of peptide 2, and subtracting 2 Da, per formula (9.1). If an element of the MS/MS mass list TML is 1388 Da, and the

TABLE 9.1 Example of a Mass Table[a]

Number of Amino Acids	CLDEH (5)	QCLDEH (6)	IQCLDEH (7)	AIQCLDEH (8)
NVNC (4)	9	10	11	12
NVNCT (5)	10	11	12	13
NVNCTK (6)	11	12	13	14

[a]The numbers represent the masses of peptides–peptide combinations in daltons. The shaded elements of the table indicate peptide combinations that consist of 12 amino acids.

MS/MS mass tolerance $\tau = 1$ Da, then an element is added to the confirmed match, because an element of the FMS is m(NVNCT+QCLDEH) = 1388.59 Da.

On the basis of these observations, the key steps in determining the disulfide connectivity include:

1. Utilizing experimental data to obtain the precursor ion mass space PMS and the MS/MS mass space TMS.
2. Determining the initial match IM between the PMS and the disulfide bond mass space DMS
3. For each initial match, determining the confirmed match between the disulfide-bonded fragment mass space FMS and the TMS
4. Aggregating the confirmed matches into a weighted graph and determining the overall disulfide bond pattern

Before moving to specific methods that deal with this problem, we note that the sizes of both FMS and DMS grow exponentially. We have described the growth characteristics of the DMS in Equation (9.2). Here, we analyze how the FMS grows. For a disulfide-bonded peptide structure consisting of k peptides, considering that there are f different fragment ion types possible, up to f^k different fragment arrangements may occur in the FMS. If the ith fragment ion consists of p_i amino acid residues, then the size of the FMS for a disulfide-bonded peptide structure is formulated as follows:

$$|FMS| = f^k \times \prod_{i=1}^{n} p_i \qquad (9.5)$$

Part of the idea enumerated in steps 1–4 above is used in the MassMatrix system [31], which constitutes one of the established methods in this area. In the exploratory mode of MassMatrix, which coincides with our problem formulation, all cysteine residues are considered to be candidates for forming disulfide bonds. The algorithm therefore generates all possible combinations of disulfide bonds. The hypothetical peptides are fragmented using appropriate fragmentation models and scored against the experimental MS/MS spectra. The approach can analyze peptides with no more than two disulfide bonds, although it is possible to extend the methods to more bonds. In the following subsections, we study the anatomy of algorithmic methods for disulfide bond determination using MS/MS data using two methods designed by us, which extend the algorithmic approach taken in MassMatrix.

In the first method, called MS2DB [15–17], the theoretical spectra are exhaustively generated in an offline step and an indexing strategy is used to support efficient online search. However, the method, like MassMatrix, is restricted to bonding topologies involving a relatively small number of peptides. The second approach, called MS2DB+ [23], makes two fundamental departures from methods at the state of the art:

1. It uses a fragmentation model that allows for the consideration of not only b/y ions but also a, b°, b^{*}, c, x, y°, y^{*}, and z ions.
2. In order to deal with the ensuing growth in the FMS (see Fig. 5b for an illustration), MS2DB+ selectively generates the theoretical spectra using an approximation algorithm-based search formulation with data-driven parameter estimation.

This formulation considers only those regions of the search space where the correct solution resides with a high likelihood. In another departure from existing MS/MS-based methods, in both MS2DB and MS2DB+, the putative disulfide bonds are combined in a globally consistent pattern to yield the overall disulfide bonding topology of the molecule.

9.3.2 Matching by Offline Generation of Theoretical Spectrum and Efficient Search (MS2DB)

9.3.2.1 Finding the Initial Match In order to explain the strategy used by MS2DB to find the initial match, we first examine how to construct the DMS for each disulfide bond topology presented in Figure 9.3a–c. Then we will show how MS2DB generalizes this method to construct the disulfide bond mass space DMS for a topology consisting of an arbitrary number of peptides.

Let k denote the number of sites where an arbitrary protein A can be cleaved with a certain protease. As a result, A is divided into $k+1$ peptides. For the intrabonded case of Figure 9.3a, the time needed to construct the DMS equals the time required to search each peptide to determine which peptides contain two or more cysteine residues. Because there are $k+1$ peptides, the overall complexity involved in constructing the DMS for an intrabonded topology is $O(k)$. For the interbonded case of Figure 9.3b, if all $k+1$ peptides contain a cysteine residue, there will be $\frac{1}{2} k(k+1)$ unique pairs of consequences. Construction of the DMS then requires $O(k^2)$ time. For the tripeptide topology shown in Figure 9.3c, at most $\frac{1}{2} k(k+1)(k-1)$ unique triplets of subsequences can be formed, and so the DMS is constructed in $O(k^3)$ time. This condition is met in only the relatively unlikely condition that every peptide contains two or more cysteines. It is now straightforward to extrapolate to the n-peptide case, whose mass space requires

$O(k^n)$ time to compute. Because the DMS is searched for matches against the PMS, the next step is to arrange the DMS in such a way that they are approximately sorted by mass. This can be done without computing the mass of each peptide combination by noting that the number of amino acids in a peptide is directly proportional to its mass. For example, if the element contains a peptide combination that has a total of 12 amino acids, its mass will likely be larger than the mass of a peptide combination that has a total of 11 amino acids. Of course, it is also likely that multiple elements will have peptide combinations that have the same total number of amino acids. Because of these two characteristics, we now explore the use of a hash table to construct and search the DMS.

The hash table is a well-known data structure for efficient searching of a data space [5]. If the hash function satisfies the assumption of simple uniform hashing, then the expected time needed to search for an element is $O(1)$. Simple uniform hashing means that, given a hash table T, with $|T|$ buckets, any data element d_i is equally likely to hash into any bucket, independently of where any other element has hashed to. We store the DMS in a hash table. The number of amino acids in each peptide combination acts as the set of keys used for indexing into this table. Now the PMS elements must be converted to an equivalent number of amino acids in order to index into the DMS for matches. This can be done by use of the *expected match index*, as defined below.

Definition 9.1   The *expected match index* i_e is defined as the number used to index into a sorted or approximately sorted data structure to arrive at the region where a match is likely to be found. The expected match index is defined as $i_e = m_j/m_e$, where m_j is a value from a mass list and m_e is the *expected amino acid mass*. The expected amino acid mass is computed as the weighted mean of all 20 amino acids, specifically, $m_e = \sum_i w_i m(a_i)$, where w_i denotes the relative abundance of each amino acid and $m(a_i)$ is the mass of an amino acid residue. Using published values for mass values and relative abundances of each amino acid from the Swiss-Prot database (http://www.ebi.ac.uk/uniprot/), we obtain $m_e = 111.17\,\text{Da}$, with a weighted standard deviation of $\sigma_e = 28.86\,\text{Da}$.

Use of the expected match index is key to the algorithm used for this subproblem, which we call HashID. The pseudocode for this algorithm is presented in Figure 9.4. This algorithm uses a simple hashing function $h(d_i) = ||d_i||$, where d_i represents a peptide or peptide combination and the $|| \cdot ||$ denotes the number of amino acid residues in d_i. To illustrate how HashID works, consider a protein containing three cysteine-containing peptides, where $||p_1|| = 4$, $||p_2|| = 6$, and $||p_3|| = 8$. The combination $p_1 + p_2$ is hashed into bucket 10, $p_1 + p_3$ is hashed into bucket 12 and $p_2 + p_3$ is hashed into bucket 14. To illustrate how an initial match is obtained, let the precursor mass of a peptide have the value $m_j = 1387\,\text{Da}$. This results in $i_e = 12$. Accessing bucket 12 in the hash table, we compute the mass of the peptide combination in that bucket to be 1388.59. If the initial identification mass tolerance $T_{\text{IM}} = 3\,\text{Da}$, then an element is added to the initial match. All of the mass values in an accessed bucket must

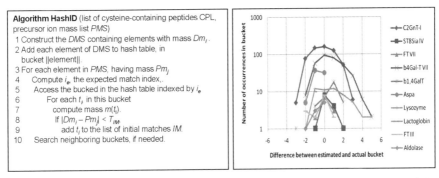

Figure 9.6 Pseudocode for the *HashID* algorithm (a) of MS2DB and analysis of the hashing-based indexing (b).

be computed and compared with m_j to determine whether there is a match. In addition, neighboring buckets are also searched in case they contain a peptide combination that has a matching mass. Clearly, for the procedure to be efficient, the number of neighboring buckets that have to be searched needs to be small. We next present an empirical study that demonstrates that this is indeed the case. In this study, the PMS for 10 proteins that underwent tandem mass spectrometric analysis was determined and for each element of the PMS, the expected match index i_e was calculated. Next, all the peptides that comprised the DMS were stored in the buckets based on the number of amino acids contained. As one can see from Figure 9.6b, nearly all combinations were placed within four buckets of the estimated bucket, thereby ensuring the locality of the search and therefore its efficiency.

To analyze the complexity of *HashID*, we consider each step in the *HashID* algorithm (Fig. 9.6) in turn. As discussed earlier, step 1 requires $O(k^n)$ time, where k is the number of cysteine-containing peptides following proteolytic digestion, and n is the maximum number of peptides in a disulfide-bonded peptide structure. Step 2 has a time complexity of $O(|DMS|)$, where $|DMS|$ denotes the size of the DMS. Step 3 has an overall complexity of $O(|PML|)$, where $|PML|$ denotes the size of the precursor ion mass list. Step 5 is $O(1)$, and steps 6–10 can all be considered to have a constant additive time complexity. Thus the overall time complexity of this algorithm is $O(k^n+(|DMS|+(|PML|))$. In practice, values of $p > 3$ are rarely observed, and values of $p > 5$ have not been reported to our knowledge. Consequently the effective complexity of this step is cubic.

9.3.2.2 *Finding the Confirmed Match*

In this section, we examine how to construct the disulfide bonded fragment mass space FMS in such a way that the expected match index can be used to identify the region where matches with the tandem mass space TMS are most likely to be found. We do this for a variety of disulfide bond topologies such as those presented in Figure 9.3. Because the initial match provides the sequence information for the disulfide-bonded peptide structure, the FMS elements that correspond to an expected match index can be generated without storing them in a precomputed state. To illustrate how this works, let us consider the topology of an interbonded pair of peptides (Fig. 9.3b). Let p_1 denote a peptide with its set of possible y ions denoted y_1 and the b ions denoted b_1. Similarly, let y_2 and b_2 denote the y ions and b ions for peptide p_2. Since p_1 and p_2 are disulfide-bonded, four types of fragment may occur: $y_1 + y_2$, $y_1 + b_2$, $b_1 + y_2$, and $b_1 + b_2$. A simple way to compute and display the FMS is to generate four tables based on these four types of fragment combinations. For example, in Table 9.1, each row represents the mass of a b ion of the peptide NVNCTK and each column represents the mass of a y ion of the peptide AIQCLDEH. If the ions used to form the mass tables are arranged in order of increasing number of amino acids, the set of elements in each table that represent a peptide pair whose sum total of amino acids equals the expected match index can be located in a straightforward manner. Visually, these elements correspond to a right-to-left diagonal region in a mass table. For example, the shaded diagonal region in Table 9.1 corresponds to a pair of peptides with a total amino acid count of 12. Thus, to determine a confirmed match, the masses of the elements in this region are computed using the sequence information, and these values are compared with an element of the TMS. A similar procedure is used for other bonding topologies.

The complexity involved in searching for a match for the interbonded topology corresponds to generating the elements of the diagonal: $O(\sqrt{(\|p_1\|)\|p_2\|})$, or $O(\|p\|)$, if $\|p_1\| \approx \|p_2\|$. The extension of this analysis to determine the time complexity involved in searching for a match for an n-peptide disulfide–bonded structure is now straightforward. The FMS for an n-peptide structure consists of 2^n n-dimensional sorted tables. Given an expected match index value, the region where matches are likely to be found has $n-1$ dimensions. Thus, the time complexity involved in determining a match with an element of the TML is $O(2^n \|p\|^{n-1})$. By contrast, an exhaustive search of the FMS requires a time complexity of $O(2^n \|p\|^n)$. The reduction achieved using indexing is significant for small values of n. On the basis of the previous discussion on the number of fragments that have been observed in the disulfide bonded peptide structure, the effective complexity reduces to cubic.

9.3.2.3 Determining the Global Bonding Pattern

The output of the previous step is a collection of validated matches between pairs of cysteines. Let the *validated match* $VM_{a,b}$ denote a match obtained from a disulfide bonded peptide structure with cysteines at locations a and b. To convert each $VM_{a,b}$ into a single number, we use as the edge weight the *match ratio r*, which is defined as the number of matches divided by the size of the tandem mass spectrum: $r = |VM|/|TMS|$. Next, we aggregate the collection of match ratios in a globally consistent manner to compute the overall disulfide bond pattern. For this we construct a weighted graph $G = \{V, E\}$ where each vertex v_i represents a cysteine residue in the protein and each edge $e_{a,b}$ represents a potential bond between

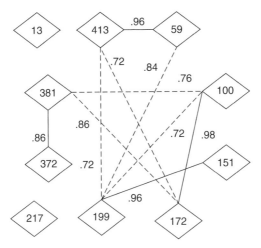

Figure 9.7 The weighted graph for C2GnT-I. Each edge weight corresponds to a match ratio. The solid edges represent the solution to the maximum-weight matching for this graph.

cysteines at locations a and b. If there is a match ratio $r_{a,b}$ that is greater than 50%, this number is assigned to the weight of the edge $e_{a,b}$. Thus G represents the set of all possible disulfide bond patterns for the protein. Figure 9.7 shows the resulting graph G for the protein C2GnT-I. The vertex labels represent the position of each cysteine residue in C2GnT-I's primary sequence, and numbers next to the edges come from the match ratio assignment.

Although G might represent the identified disulfide bond pattern, this is not the case in general. The solution sets of edges are constrained because an even number of bonded cysteine residues is required and a cysteine residue can be bonded to only one other cysteine residue. Thus, the number of vertices $|V| = 2B$, the number of edges $|E| = B$, and the number of incident edges to any vertex of degree$(v_i) = 1$ for any vertex where B denotes the number of disulfide bonds in a chain. As a result, the edge weighting function is found to be equivalent to the problem of computing the maximum-weight matching [7]. Finding the maximum-weight matching in a graph is a well-understood problem in graph theory. At present, the best performing algorithm that solves this problem for a fully connected graph was designed by Gabow [14]. This algorithm has a worst-case bound of $O(|C|^3)$. Since the other steps of this subproblem have runtimes that can be approximated by a constant, the overall time complexity for this subproblem, which we denote *GlobalMatch*, is $O(|C|^3)$. In Figure 9.7, the solid edges represent the solution to the maximum-weight matching for this graph.

9.3.2.4 *Computational Complexity and Limitations*   In the initial match step, the construction of the mass space requires $O(k^p)$ time, where k is the number of cysteine-containing peptides following proteolytic digestion, and p is the maximum number of peptides in a disulfide bonded peptide structure. Thus the

overall time complexity of this step is $O(k^p + |DMS| + |PML|)$. In nature, $p > 3$ are rarely observed, and $p > 5$ has not been reported to our knowledge. Consequently the effective complexity of this step is cubic. To analyze the complexity of the confirmation step, we note that the FMS for an n-peptide structure consists of 2^n n-dimensional sorted tables. Given an expected match index value, the region where matches are likely to be found has $n-1$ dimensions. Thus, the time complexity involved in determining a match with an element of the TML is $O(2^n ||p||^{n-1})$. The previous discussion of the number of fragments that have been observed in the disulfide bonded peptide structure indicates that the effective complexity reduces to cubic. Finally, the complexity of GlobalMatch is $O(c^3)$, where c is the number of cysteines in the protein. Thus, the overall complexity of this method is cubic, under the assumption that the DMS and FMS are precomputed. In the following text we present a method where these limitations are removed.

9.3.3 MS2DB+: A Fully Polynomial Time Method

In this section, we introduce and discuss the method that we proposed [23], which uses an approximation algorithm to generate the DMS and FMS. At a high level, this approach can be regarded as a two-stage database-based matching technique, where, in the first stage, the mass values of the theoretically possible disulfide-bonded peptide structures are compared with precursor ion mass values derived from the MS spectra. In the following, confirmatory stage, the theoretical spectra from the disulfide-bonded peptide structures are compared with MS/MS experimental spectra. An important characteristic of this method is that it considers multiple ion types: b, y, a, $b°$, b^*, c, x, $y°$, y^*, z. We remind the reader here that most methods consider only b/y ions to avoid an exponential increase in the search space. While few non-b/y ions are encountered in collision-induced dissociation (CID), some of these ions can be present with greater likelihood in dissociation methods such as electron capture dissociation (ECD), electron transfer dissociation (ETD), and electron detachment dissociation (EDD). We observed [23] that even in the case of CID, multiple instances of combinations between b/y ions and other ion types occurred. The chapter also showed how consideration of multiple ion types (other than b/y ions) led to improved accuracy in determining disulfide bonds, which were missed when only b/y ions were considered.

9.3.3.1 The Subset–Sum Problem and Polynomial Time Construction of DMS and FMS
Unlike MassMatrix or MS2DB, where the theoretical spectrum was generated prior to matching the experimental spectrum, the approach in MS2DB+ is based on the fact that since the experimental spectrum is available, it is unnecessary to generate the entire theoretical spectra for DMS and FMS. In other words, one can only generate the few disulfide bonded peptides whose mass is close to the (given) experimental spectra. This insight forms the basis of the polynomial time algorithm proposed by Murad et al. [23], who cast the generation of the select regions of the theoretical spectra in terms of the subset–sum problem. Recall that given the pair (S, t), where S is a set of positive integers and

$t \in \mathbf{Z}^+$, the subset–sum problem asks whether there exists a subset of S that adds up to t. While the subset–sum problem is itself NP-complete, it can be solved using approximation strategies to obtain near-optimal solutions, in polynomial time [5]. In the following, text we describe this strategy for reconstructing the DMS and FMS.

The central idea lies in obtaining an approximate solution to the subset–sum problem by trimming as many elements from *DMS* as possible based on a trimming parameter ε. The trimming is done in a manner such that if DMS* is the resultant trimmed set, then, for every element DMS$_i$ removed from DMS, there remains an element DMS$_i^*$ in DMS* that can be considered "sufficiently" close in terms of its mass to the deleted element DMS$_i$, as stipulated by the following equation:

$$\frac{\text{DMS}_i}{1 + \varepsilon} \leq \text{DMS}_i^* \leq \text{DMS}_i \tag{9.6}$$

The approximation algorithm for creating the partial DMS is described by the APPROX-DMS and TRIM routines, which are presented in Figure 9.8. The input to APPROX-DMS are (1) a sorted list of cysteine-containing peptides mass values (CCP); (2) a target mass value from the PMS list (PMS$_{\text{val}}$), (3) the trimming parameter ε, and (4) the initial match threshold (T_{IM}); which is set to ± 1.0 Da. In lines 2–8 of Figure 9.8, all the variables and data structures are initialized. In the following text we describe the APPROX-DMS routine. In lines 9–11 of Figure 9.8, the theoretical disulfide-bonded peptide structures are formed and stored in a data structure designated as TempSet. Line 10 excludes values greater than the PMS$_{\text{val}}$ plus an Initial Match threshold. Line 12 increments the DMS by invoking the routine MERGE, which returns a sorted set formed by merging the two sorted input sets DMS and TempSet, with duplicated values removed. In line 13, the TRIM routine is called to shorten the DMS set. Lines 14 and 15 examine whether the largest mass value in the constructed DMS set is sufficiently close

```
01. APPROX-DMS (CCP, PMSval, ε , TIM )
02.     DMS0 ← {0}
03.     IM ← { }
04.     TrimSet ← { }
05.     for i ← 0 to (|| CCP || – 1)
06.         PM ← CCPi
07.         TempSet ← { }
08.         DMSsize ← || DMS ||
09.         for j ← 0 to (DMSsize – 1)
10.             if ((PM + DMSj) ≤ (PMSval + TIM))
11.                 TempSetj ← PM + DMSj
12.         DMS ← MERGE (DMS, TempSet)
13.         DMS, Trimset ← TRIM (DMS, TrimSet, ε )
14.     if ((DMSmax) ≥ (PMSval - TIM))
15.         IM ← DMSmax
16.     return {IM, DMS, TrimSet}
```

```
17. TRIM (DMS, TrimSet, ε )
18.     n ← | DMS |
19.     max_value ← DMSn-1
20.     last ← max_value
21.     for i ← n-2 down to 0
22.         if last > (( 1+ ε ) × DMSi )
23.             DMS* ← DMSi
24.             last ← DMSi
25.         else
26.             TrimSet ← DMSi
27.     DMS* ← max_value
28.     return {DMS*, TrimSet }
```

```
01. APPROX-FMS (peptides, TMSval, δ , TIM )
02.     FMS0 ← {0}
03.     VM ← { }
04.     for i ← 0 to (|| peptides || - 1)
05.         TempSet ← { }
06.         Pepsequences ← peptidesi
07.         FragSet ← GENFRAGS (Pepsequences)
08.         for j ← 0 to (|| FMS || - 1)
09.             for k ← 0 to (||FragSet|| - 1)
10.                 if ((FragSetk + FMSj) ≤ (TMSval + TIM))
11.                     TempSet[ ] ← FragSetk + FMSj
12.         FMS ← MERGE (FMS, TempSet)
13.         FMS ← TRIM (FMS, δ )
14.     if ((FMSmax) ≥ (TMSval - TIM))
15.         VM ← FMSmax
16.     return { FMS, VM }
```

(a)   (b)

Figure 9.8 Pseudocode of the fully polynomial time approximation strategy. The APPROX-DMS and TRIM routines (a) are used to generate the DMS, while the APPROX-FMS routine (b) is combined with TRIM to generate the FMS.

to the targeted mass PMS_{val}. If so, an initial match occurs. In this approach, the trimming parameter ε is especially important; a large value of ε would cause meaningful fragments to be omitted from the DMS, while too small a value would lead to few data points being trimmed. We [23] estimated that this parameter used multiple-variable regression on a dataset consisting of nine proteins. The complexity of MERGE and TRIM routines is $O(|DMS|+|TempSet|)$ and $O(|DMS|)$, respectively. Further, for any fixed $\varepsilon > 0$, this algorithm is a $(1 + \varepsilon)$ approximation scheme. In other words, for any fixed ε, the algorithm runs in polynomial time. We [23] provided a formal proof of this property. In Table 9.2, we present an example illustrating the action of APPROX-DMS on the β-LG protein. The table presents snapshots of the DMS, TrimSet, and initial match (IM) sets for each CCP_i (cysteine-containing peptide) mass value during iterations of the trimming process.

In creating the FMS, we use a strategy similar to that used to generate the DMS. This involves again using an approximation algorithm to generate the theoretical spectra for all the IMs found during the first-stage matching. A parameter δ is next estimated and used to trim the FMS mass list in a manner identical to that used with the parameter ε for trimming the DMS as described above. The pseudocode of the APPROX-FMS procedure used for generating the *FMS* is shown in Figure 9.8b. In this pseudocode, the function GENFRAGS(.), in line 7, generates multiple fragment ions $(a, b, b^\circ, b^*, c, x, y, y^\circ, y^*, z)$ for peptide sequences in $Pep_{sequences}$, which contains the disulfide-bonded peptides involved in the IM that is being analyzed. Next, for each element in the FMS and for each fragment in FragSet (lines 8–11), new disulfide-bonded peptide fragment structures are formed. Line 10 rejects values greater than the TMS_{val}, considering the validation match threshold. In line 12, the current FMS set is combined with the disulfide-bonded peptide fragments set TempSet using MERGE. In line 13, the FMS is trimmed using the TRIM routine. Finally, a validation match (VM) is obtained (lines 14–15) in the cases where a correspondence can be established between the mass of the largest value in FMS and an experimentally determined mass value TMS_{val}, modulo the matching threshold.

9.3.3.2 Obtaining Globally Consistent Bond Topology

Once all the *validation matches* (VMs) are obtained, we have a "local" (bond-level) picture of the disulfide connectivity. This local information needs to be integrated to obtain a globally consistent view. The approach in MS2DB+ is similar to the one used in MS2DB. Specifically, we model the location of the putative disulfide bonds by edges in an undirected graph $G(V,E)$, where the set of vertices V corresponds to the set of cysteines. To each edge, we assign a match score. This score represents the combined importance of each single peak match within two spectra. Each specific peak match is weighted according to its intensity. The match score is given by

$$V_s = \frac{\sum_{j=1}^{n}(VM_i \times I_N)}{\sum_{j=1}^{n}(TMS_i \times I_N) \times 100} \tag{9.7}$$

TABLE 9.2 DMS, TrimSet, and IM Mass Sets for Each Cysteine Containing Peptide CCP_i Mass Value Generated from Tryptic Digestion of Protein β-Lactoglobulin (β-LG)[a]

i	CCP_i	DMS	TrimSet	IM
0	1064	{0, 1064}	{}	{}
1	1192	{0, 1064, 1192, 2254}	{}	{}
2	1658	{0, 1064, 1192, 1658, 2254, 2720, 2849}	{}	{}
3	1746	{0, 1064, 1192, 1658, 1746, 2254, 2720, 2849, 2937}	{2809}	{}
4	2275	{0, 1064, 1192, 1658, 1746, 2275, 2720, 2849, 2937}	{2254, 2809}	{}
5	2477	{0, 1064, 1192, 1658, 1746, 2275, 2477, 2720, 2849, 2937}	{2254, 2809}	{}
6	2535	{0, 1064, 1192, 1658, 1746, 2275, 2535, 2720, 2849, 2937}	{2254, 2477, 2809}	{}
7	2648	{0, 1064, 1192, 1658, 1746, 2275, 2535, 2648, 2720, 2849, 2937}	{2254, 2477, 2809}	{}
8	2776	{0, 1064, 1192, 1658, 1746, 2275, 2535, 2648, 2776, 2849, 2937}	{2254, 2477, 2720, 2809}	{}
9	2790	{0, 1064, 1192, 1658, 1746, 2275, 2535, 2648, 2776, 2849, 2937}	{2254, 2477, 2720, 2790, 2809}	{}
10	2930	{0, 1064, 1192, 1658, 1746, 2275, 2535, 2648, 2776, 2849, 2937}	{2254, 2477, 2720, 2790, 2809, 2930}	{}
11	3189	{0, 1064, 1192, 1658, 1746, 2275, 2535, 2648, 2776, 2849, 2937, 3189}	{2254, 2477, 2720, 2790, 2809, 2930}	{3189}

[a]The values presented here are retrieved at the end of each loop cycle (lines 5–17) in Figure 9.8.

where the numerator corresponds to the sum of each validation match for a disulfide bond multiplied by the matched MS/MS fragment normalized intensity value (I_N). Here, VM_i is a binary value that is set to 1 if a confirmatory match is found for fragment i. The denominator contains the sum of each experimental MS/MS fragment ion from TMS multiplied by I_N. Here, TMS_i is a binary variable that indicates the presence of a fragment i in the MS/MS spectrum. Finally, the globally optimal and consistent disulfide topology is found by computing the maximum-weight matching, as described earlier in an undirected graph $G(V,E)$, where the set of vertices V corresponds to the set of cysteines and the set of edges E contains all the putative S–S bonds found after the confirmatory match stage and weighted by the match score in Equation (9.7).

In addition to the empirical match score [Eq. (9.7)] calculated for each S–S bond determined by the MS-based framework, a probability-based scoring model proposed by Xu and Freitas [30] was also implemented. This model provided two scores, denoted pp and pp_2 scores. The pp score helps us evaluate whether the number of VMs could be a random number. The pp_2 score evaluates whether the total abundance (intensity) of VMs could be a random number. The formula used for calculating the pp value is presented in Equation (9.8), where n_{match} represents each confirmatory match found between a product ion and a theoretical fragment ion. Further, p_2 denotes the probability that a product ion randomly matches any of the fragment ions in the theoretical spectrum. In the equation used to calculate p_2, the term m is the product ion mass value, T_{VM} is the confirmatory match threshold, and r is the spectrum (mass) detection range.

$$pp = -\log \left(\sum_{x=n_{match}}^{n} \frac{n!}{x!\,(n-x)!} p_2^x (1-p_2)^{n-x} \right) \qquad (9.8)$$

where

$$p_2 = \frac{2m \times T_{VM}}{r} \qquad (9.9)$$

The formula for calculating the pp_2 value is shown in Equation (9.10), where I_{match} denotes the abundance (intensity) of an experimental product ion matched to a theoretical fragment ion, σ_y represents the variance for the distribution of the abundance of the ith product ion, and μ_y represents the mean for the distribution of the abundance of ith product ion:

$$pp_2 = -\log \left(\int_{I_{match}}^{\infty} \frac{e^{-(x-\mu_y)^2 / 2\sigma_y^2}}{\sqrt{2\pi}\,\sigma_y} dx \right) \qquad (9.10)$$

As an aside, the reader may note that MS2DB+ had better pp and pp_2 scores when compared to MassMatrix (higher pp and pp_2 scores are better, indicating smaller p values). In the next section, we present results that directly compare MassMatrix and MS2DB+ on a panel of disulfide bond–containing molecules.

9.4   EXPERIMENTAL RESULTS

In this section, we present results from the two methods MS2DB and MS2DB+. The underlying MS/MS data were obtained using a capillary liquid chromatography system coupled with a Thermo-Fisher LCQ ion trap mass spectrometer LC/ESI-MS/MS system, using the protocols described by Thomas et al. [27] and Yen and Macher [32]. These data represent the following nine eukaryotic glycosyltransferases (listed with their Swiss-Prot IDs): ST8Sia IV [Q92187], β-lactoglobulin [P02754], FucT VII [Q11130], C2GnT-I [Q09324], lysozyme [P00698], FT III [P21217], β1-4GalT [P08037], aldolase [P00883], and aspa [Q9R1T5]. For the method based on offline generation of theoretical spectra and online hashing-based search, an additional protein (human β1,4-galactosyltransferase VII) was also used. The disulfide bonding pattern for this protein is unknown.

9.4.1   Metrics

Given a set of molecules, if the true set of disulfide bonds are denoted by P and the set of cysteines not forming disulfide bonds by N, then the performance of a method can be assessed according to the following quantitative indicators:

- *True positive* (TP) *determination*, which occurs when disulfide bonds that are known to exist are correctly found by a method
- *False negative* (FN) *determination*, which occurs when bonds that are known to exist are not found by a method
- *True negative* (TN) *determination*, occurs when a method correctly identifies cysteine pairs that do not form a disulfide bond
- *False positive* (FP) *determination*, occurs when a method incorrectly assigns a disulfide link to a pair of cysteines, which are not actually bonded.

Instead of using these basic measures directly, it is common to combine them into the following measures [26]:

$$\text{Sensitivity } (Q_c) = \frac{TP}{P} \tag{9.11}$$

$$\text{Specificity } (Q_{nc}) = \frac{TN}{N} \tag{9.12}$$

$$\text{Accuracy } (Q_2) = \frac{TP + TN}{P + N} \tag{9.13}$$

$$\text{Matthew's correlation coefficient } (c) = \frac{TP \times TN - FP \times FN}{\sqrt{(TP + FN)(TP + FP)(TN + FP)(TN + FN)}} \tag{9.14}$$

9.4.2 Experimental Evaluation of MS2DB

The disulfide bond pattern for each of the 10 eukaryotic glycosyltransferases analyzed using this method is presented in Table 9.3. For this set, we make the following observations: (1) of the nine proteins for which the bonding topology is known, two have intrapeptide bonds, five are interbonded, and one consists of a combination of inter- and intrabonded cysteines; (2) two proteins have no disulfide bonds—these are used to test the method's ability to correctly analyze structures that do not contain any disulfide bonds; (3) the data for FT III contain a tripeptide structure with more than three peptides connected by two disulfide bonds; and (4) laboratory analysis of β4Gal-T determined that of the five cysteines present, two were free thiols (C214 and C307). Thus, only the remaining three cysteines were considered as possible sites for a disulfide bond. In addition, β4Gal-T functions as a homodimer, so disulfide bonds may form between cysteines across the dimer at the same cysteine location.

We compared the accuracy of our method with five predictive methods: DiANNA (http://clavius.bc.edu/~clotelab/DiANNA/), DISULFIND (http://disulfind.dsi.unifi.it/), PreCys (http://bioinfo.csie. ntu.edu.tw:5433/Disulfide/), DiPro (http://contact.ics.uci.edu/ bridge.html), and CysView (http://antigen.i2r.a-star.edu.sg/ CysV2/). These results are also presented in Table 9.3. Each method implements a specific machine learning technique. In DiANNA, the training phase of the neural network uses a prediction of the protein's secondary structure using PSIPRED as well as the profile arising from PSIBLAST-generated multiple alignment. In the DISULFIND system, the disulfide bonding state of each cysteine is first predicted by a binary classifier. Next, cysteines that are known to participate in the formation of bridges are paired to obtain a connectivity pattern. The PreCys system employs a two-level SVM. First, the bonding probability corresponding to each cysteine pair is estimated by the first SVM. Following this, each candidate connectivity pattern is scored by the second SVM with the confidence score, CSP search result, and the global information of the protein as inputs. The DiPro system also processes the protein's sequence in two steps. In the first step, a SVM is used to determine whether the sequence has disulfide bonds. Subsequently, neural networks and graph algorithms are used to predict the number of bonds, bonding states, and bonding patterns. Finally, the CysView system uses a dataset of annotated protein sequences and identifies and classifies them according to their disulfide connectivity patterns.

Next, we present our results in the form of a connectivity matrix as proposed by Martelli et al. [19] in Tables 9.4 and 9.5. In a connectivity matrix, each row and column is labeled with a cysteine location, and each element not on the diagonal corresponds to a possible disulfide bond. We present the connectivity matrices for four of the proteins from the dataset that we used in Tables 9.4 and 9.5. To conserve space, these tables display the results for two proteins each, one protein above the diagonal and the other below it. The diagonal region is shaded to indicate that disulfide bonds form between two cysteines that have

TABLE 9.3 Comparison of MS2DB with Prediction-Based Methods[a]

Protein (Abbreviation)	Disulfide Bond Structure	Peptide Bonding topology	DiANNA 1.1	DISULFIND	PreCys	DiPro 2.0	CysView	MS2DB
Mouse core 2 β1, 6-N-acetylglucosaminyltransferase I (C2GnT-I) Q09324	C59—C413, c090—C172, C151—C199, C372—C381, C13, C217, C234 free	Interbonded	C13—C172, C59—C217, C151—C234, C199—C372, C381—C413	> 10 cysteines	C59—C381, c090—C372, C151—C172, C199—C413	C372—C381, C13—C59, c090—C151, C172—C199	C13—C234, C59—C172, c090—C199, C217—C234	C59—C413, c090—C172, C151—C199, C372—C381
ST8Sia IV polysialyltransferase (ST8Sia IV) Q92187	C142—C292, C156—C356, C11, C169 free	Interbonded	C11—C156, C142—C292, C169—C356	All free	C142—C356, C156—C292	C292—C356, C142—C156	C11—C156, C142—C169	C142—C292, C156—C356
Human fucosyltransferase VII (FT VII) Q11130	C68—C76, C211—C214, C318—C321	Interbonded	C68—C321, C76—C211, C214—C318	C76—C318	C68—C76, C211—C214, C318—C321	C68—C76, C211—C214, C318—C321	C68—C76, C211—C214, C318—C321	C68—C76, C211—C214, C318—C321
Lysozyme P00698	C24—C145, C48—C133, C82—C98, C94—C112, c09 free	Two interbonded and two inter/intrabonded	C24—C145, C48—C133, C82—C98, C94—C112	C24—C145, C48—C133, C82—C98, C94—C112	C82—C145	C82—C98, C94—C112, c09—C24, C48—C145	c09—C143, C24—C112, C48—C94, C82—C98	C24—C145, C48—C133
Lactoglobulin P02754	C82—C126, C3, C12, C135, C137, C176 free	Interbonded	C12—C137, C82—C176, C126—C135	All free	All free	C3—C12, C122—C135	C3—C135, C12—C82	C82—C126
Human fucosyltransferase III (FT III) P21217	C81—C338, C91—C341, C16, C129, C143 free	Tripeptide	C16—C91, C81—C143, C129—C338	All free	C81—C91	C81—C91, C16—C29, C338—C341	All free	C81—C338, C91—C341
β -1, 4-galactosyltransferase (β1, 4-GalT) P08037	C134—C176, C247—C266, C23, C30, C342 free	Intrabonded	C23—C176, C30—C144, C266—C341	All free	C134—C247, C176—C266	C247—C266, C23—C30, C134—C176	C23—C30, C134—C176	C134—C176, C247—C266
Aldolase P00883	C73, C135, C115, C178, C202, C240, C290, C339 free	N/A	C73—C339, C135—C290, C115—C240, C178—C202	All free	All free	C290—C339, C135—C150, C178—C202	All free	All free
Aspartoacylase (Aspa) Q9R1T5	C4, C60, C66, C123, C145, C151, C217, C275 free	N/A	C4—C275, C60—C217, C66—C151, C123—C145	All free	All free	C60—C66, C217—C275, C145—C151	All free	C145—C349
Human β1, 4-galactosyltransferase VII (β4Gal-T VII) Q9UBV7	Unknown	N/A	C29—C214, C38—C75, C53—C324, C307—C316	All free	C29—C38, C59—C75	C316—C324, C29—C38, C53—C75	All free	C75—C75, C316—C374

[a]Included in the comparison are DiANNA, DISULFIND, PreCys, DiPro, and CysView. Note that DISULFIND does not support the prediction of proteins that contain more than 10 cysteines. C2GnT-I results were derived from combining data obtained from tryptic and tryptic–chymotryptic digestion.

TABLE 9.4 Below Diagonal, C2GnT-I Validation Testing Results; Above Diagonal, Lysozyme Validation Testing Results.

		10	24	48	82	94	98	112	133	145	Cysteine Location
13			TN	TN	TN	TN	TN	TN	TN	TN	10
59		TN		TN	TN	TN	TN	TN	TN	TP	24
100		TN	TN		TN	TN	TN	TN	TP	TN	48
151		TN	TN	TN		TN	FN	TN	TN	TN	82
172		TN	TN	TP	TN		TN	FN	TN	TN	94
199		TN	FP	FP	TP	TN		TN	TN	TN	98
235		TN	TN	TN	TN	TN	TN		TN	TN	112
372		TN	TN	TN	TN	TN	TN	TN		TN	133
381		TN	TN	FP	TN	FP	TN	TN	TP		145
413		TN	TP	TN	TN	FP	FP	TN	TN	TN	
Cysteine location		13	59	100	151	172	199	235	372	381	413

TABLE 9.5 Below Diagonal, FT III Validation Testing Results; Above Diagonal, Results for FucT VII

		68	76	211	214	318	321	Cysteine Location
16			TP	TN	TN	TN	TN	68
29		TN		TN	TN	TN	TN	76
81		TN	TN		TP	TN	TN	211
91		TN	TN	TN		TN	TN	214
143		TN	TN	TN	TN		TP	318
338		TN	TN	TP[a]	TP[a]	TN		321
341		FP	TN	TP[a]	TP[a]	TN	TN	
Cysteine location		16	29	81	91	143	338	341

[a]These cells are characterized by the identification of two disulfide bonds in a three-peptide disulfide bond structure; thus, the disulfide bonds occur at either C81—C338 and C91—C341 or C81—C341 and C91—C338.

differing locations. In this matrix, the "known" linkage patterns are indicated by a gray shaded matrix element. In addition, one of the classifications TP, FP, FN, or TN (defined above) is assigned to each matrix element.

9.4.3 Experimental Evaluation of MS2DB+

We present results from two experiments. The first experiment involves a direct comparison between MassMatrix and MS2DB+ and is presented in Table 9.6. The reader may note that every bond correctly determined by MassMatrix was also found by MS2DB+. However, some disulfide bonds were found by MS2DB+, that were not found by MassMatrix. Next, in Table 9.7, we present

TABLE 9.6 Comparison with MassMatrix[a]

Protein	Known Pattern	Proposed Method	MassMatrix
ST8Sia IV	$C^{142}C^{292}$, $C^{156}C^{356}$	$C^{142}C^{292}$ [V_s:131;pp:109;pp2:41], $C^{156}C^{356}$ [V_s:100;pp:97;pp2:6]	$C^{142}C^{292}$ [V_s^*:54;pp:15;pp2:13], $C^{156}C^{356}$ [V_s^*:77;pp:23;pp2:15]
β-LG	$C^{82}C^{176}$, $C^{122}C^{135}$	$C^{82}C^{176}$ [V_s:100;pp:49;pp2:16]	$C^{82}C^{176}$ [V_s^*:68;pp:14;pp2:14]
FucT VII	$C^{68}C^{76}$, $C^{211}C^{214}$, $C^{318}C^{321}$	$C^{68}C^{76}$ [V_s:105;pp:41;pp2:98], $C^{211}C^{214}$ [V_s:100;pp:13;pp2:20], $C^{318}C^{321}$ [V_s:100;pp:31;pp2:70]	$C^{68}C^{76}$ [V_s^*:12;pp:9;pp2:3], $C^{211}C^{214}$ [V_s^*:78;pp:16;pp2:11], $C^{318}C^{321}$ [V_s^*:46;pp:28;pp2:16]
B1,4-GalT	$C^{134}C^{176}$, $C^{247}C^{266}$	$C^{134}C^{176}$ [V_s:100;pp:61;pp2:29], $C^{247}C^{266}$ [V_s:195;pp:88;pp2:177]	$C^{134}C^{176}$ [V_s^*:34;pp:9;pp2:7], $C^{247}C^{266}$ [V_s^*:31;pp:7;pp2:7]
C2GnT-I	$C^{59}C^{413}$, $C^{100}C^{172}$, $C^{151}C^{199}$, $C^{372}C^{381}$	$C^{59}C^{413}$ [V_s:158;pp:237;pp2:61], $C^{151}C^{199}$ [V_s:100;pp:93;pp2:15], $C^{372}C^{381}$ [V_s:100; pp:81;pp2:79]	None
Lysozyme	$C^{24}C^{145}$, $C^{48}C^{133}$	$C^{24}C^{145}$ [V_s:140;pp:65;pp2:88], $C^{48}C^{133}$ [V_s:100;pp:62;pp2:55]	$C^{48}C^{133}$ [V_s^*:135;pp:51;pp2:33]
FT III	$C^{81}C^{338}$, $C^{91}C^{341}$	$C^{81}C^{338}$ [V_s:100;pp:179;pp2:93]	None
Aldolase	None	None	None
Aspa	None	None	None

[a]The scores (V_s) of each disulfide bond and the confidence scores (*pp* and *pp2* values) for the S−S bonds found by the MS-based framework are presented inside brackets.

TABLE 9.7   Sensitivity, Specificity, Accuracy, and Mathew's Correlation Coefficient Values for the Fully Polynomial-Time Method on a Set of Nine Eukaryotic Glycosyltransferases

Protein	Q_c	Q_{nc}	Q_2	c
ST8Sia IV	1.00	1.00	1.00	1.00
β-LG	0.50	1.00	0.95	0.69
FucT VII	1.00	1.00	1.00	1.00
C2GnT-I	0.75	1.00	0.98	0.86
Lysozyme	1.00	1.00	1.00	1.00
B1,4-GalT	1.00	1.00	1.00	1.00
FT III	0.50	1.00	0.94	0.69
Aldolase	X	1.00	1.00	X
Aspa	X	1.00	1.00	X

an overview of results obtained using MS2DB+ on the set of nine eukaryotic glycosyltransferases described earlier. It may be noted that the method failed to identify only three disulfide bonds. Of these cases, one intrabond in the β-LG protein could not be found because of a blind spot caused by the same intrabond, rendering the protein's fragmentation difficult. One cross-linked bond in the FT III protein also could not be identified because this particular connectivity configuration created a large disulfide-bonded structure, which was poorly fragmented by tandem mass spectrometry. One bond in the C2GnT-I protein could not be found, since the precursor ion cannot be formed by chymotryptic digestion, which was the digestion carried for C2GnT-I.

9.5   CONCLUSIONS AND FUTURE DIRECTIONS

This chapter presents a comprehensive introduction to the different algorithmic frameworks available at the state of the art for the determination of disulfide bonds by utilizing data from either protein sequences or tandem mass spectrometry. For the former class of techniques, we identify the different problem formulations, features, and solution frameworks. We also review a number of techniques in the area and show how the aforementioned issues are addressed in them. For MS-based methods, our narrative focuses primarily on two methods that we developed to provide insight into the key challenges and the anatomy of possible solutions and the underlying algorithmic frameworks. The first method is built around the use of hashing functions to efficiently search the space of possible solutions. The second approach presented here uses the framework of approximation algorithms to solve the problem efficiently. Neither of these methods is limited by the disulfide connectivity pattern. Moreover, the fully polynomial time method can also be used to account for the variability of product ion types generated during the fragmentation of precursor ions.

The problem of determining the disulfide connectivity of a molecule continues to be of active interest in structural bioinformatics and structural/functional proteomics, especially with the advent of novel types of mass spectrometric dissociation methods. Since the information available to sequence-based methods and MS-based methods is somewhat different, in some cases one class of methods can determine a specific bond correctly while the other fails to do so. Thus a highly promising, as yet unaddressed challenge lies in the development of methods that can appropriately *fuse* the information from various constituent methods and come up with bond determinations that are more accurate than that possible through the use of any single-constituent method.

ACKNOWLEDGMENTS

This research was supported by funding from NSF Grant IIS-0644418 (CAREER). The authors thank Ten-Yang Yen and Bruce Macher for the data and many discussions.

REFERENCES

1. Angata K, Yen TY, El-Battari A, Macher BA, Fukuda M, Unique disulfide bond structures found in ST8Sia IV polysialyltransferase are required for its activity, *J. Biol. Chem.* **18**:15369–15377 (2001).

2. Ceroni A, Passerini A, Vullo A, Frasconi P, DISULFIND: A disulfide bonding state and cysteine connectivity prediction server, *Nucleic Acids Res.* **34**:177–181 (2006).

3. Chen Y-C, Hwang J-K, Prediction of disulfide connectivity from protein sequences, *Proteins* **61**:507–512 (2005).

4. Chen Y-C, Lin Y-S, Hwang J-K, Prediction of the bonding states of cysteines using the support vector machines based on multiple feature vectors and cysteine state sequences, *Proteins* **55**:1036–1042 (2004).

5. Cormen TH, Leiserson CE, Rivest RL, Stein C, *Introduction to Algorithms*, MIT Press, Cambridge, MA, 2001.

6. Fariselli P, Riccobelli P, Casadio R, Role of evolutionary information in predicting the disulfide-bonding state of cysteine in proteins, *Proteins: Struct., Funct., Genet.* **36**:340–346 (1999).

7. Fariselli P, Casadio R, Prediction of disulfide connectivity in proteins, *Bioinformatics* **17**:957–964 (2001).

8. Ferre F, Clote P, Disulfide connectivity prediction using secondary structure information and diresidue frequencies, *Bioinformatics* **21**:2336–2346 (2005).

9. Ferre F, Clote P, DiANNA: A web server for disulfide connectivity prediction, *Nucleic Acids Res.* **33**:230–232 (2005).

10. Fiser A, Cserzo M, Tudos E, Simon I, Different sequence environments of cysteines and half cystines in proteins: Application to predict disulfide forming residues, *FEBS Lett.* **302**:117–120 (1992).

11. Fiser A, Simon I, Predicting the oxidation state of cysteines by multiple sequence alignment, *Bioinformatics* **16**:251–256 (2000).

12. Forner F, Foster L, Toppo S, Mass spectrometry data analysis in the proteomics era, *Curr. Bioinformatics.* **2**(1):63–93 (2007).

13. Frasconi P, Passerini A, Vullo A, A two-stage SVM architecture for predicting the disulfide bonding state of cysteines, *Proc. IEEE Workshop on Neural Networks for Signal Processing*, 2002, pp. 25–34.

14. Gabow H, *Implementation of Algorithms for Maximum Matching on Nonbipartite Graphs*, PhD thesis, Stanford Univ., 1973

15. Lee T, Singh R, Yen R, Macher B, An algorithmic approach to automated high-throughput identification of disulfide connectivity in proteins using tandem mass spectrometry, *Proc. Computational Systems Bioinformatics Conf.*, 2007, pp. 41–51.

16. Lee T, Singh R, Yen R, Macher B, MS2DB: A mass-based hashing algorithm for the identification of disulfide linkage patterns in protein utilizing mass spectrometric data, *Proc. IEEE Int. Symp. Computer-Based Medical Systems*, 2007, pp. 397–402.

17. Lee TR, Singh R, Yen T-Y, Macher B, MS2DB: An algorithmic approach to determine disulfide linkage patterns in proteins by utilizing tandem mass spectrometric data, *Proc. IEEE Int. Symp. Computer-Based Medical Systems*, 2006, pp. 947–952.

18. Lenffer J, Lai P, El-Mejaber W, Khan AM, Koh JLY, Tan P, Seah S, Brusic V, CysView: Protein classification based on cysteine pairing patterns, *Nucleic Acids Res.* **32**(Suppl 2):W350–W355 (2004).

19. Martelli PL, Fariselli P, Malaguti , Casadio R, Prediction of the disulfide bonding state of cysteines in proteins with hidden neural networks. *Protein Eng.* **15**:951–953 (2002).

20. Mirny LA, Shakhnovich EI, How to derive a protein folding potential? A new approach to an old problem, *J. Mol. Biol.* **264**:1164–1179 (1996).

21. Mucchielli-Giorgi MH, Hazout S, Tuffery P, Predicting the disulfide bonding state of cysteines using protein descriptors, *Proteins* **46**:243–249 (2002).

22. Muskal SM, Holbrook SR, Kim S-H, Prediction of the Disulfide-bonding state of cysteine in proteins, *Protein Eng.* **3**:667–672 (1990).

23. Murad W, Singh R, Yen T-Y, An efficient algorithmic approach for mass spectrometry-based disulfide connectivity determination in proteins using multi-ion analysis, *BMC Bioinformatics* **12**[Suppl. 1 (S12)]: (Feb. 2011).

24. Nesvizhskii A, Vitek O, Aebersold R, Analysis and validation of proteomics data generated by tandem mass spectrometry, *Nat. Methods* **4**(10):787–797 (2007).

25. Sander C, Schneider R, Database of homology-derived protein structures, *Proteins: Struct., Funct., Genet.* **9**:56–68 (1991).

26. Singh R, A review of algorithmic techniques for disulfide-bond determination, *Brief. Funct. Genomics Proteomics* **7**:157–172 (2008).

27. Thomas S, Yen TY, Macher BA, Eukaryotic glycosyltransferases: Cysteines and disulfides, *Glycobiology* **12**:4G–7G (2002).

28. Vitek O, Getting started in computational mass spectrometry-based proteomics, *PLoS Comput Biol*. **5**(5):e1000366 (2009).

29. Vullo A, Frasconi P, Disulfide connectivity prediction using recursive neural networks and evolutionary information, *Bioinformatics* **20**:653–659 (2004).

30. Xu H, Freitas MA, A mass accuracy sensitive probability based scoring algorithm for database searching of tandem mass spectrometry data, *BMC Bionformatics* **8**:133–142 (2007).

31. Xu H, Zhang L, Freitas M, Identification and characterization of disulfide bonds in proteins and peptides from tandem MS data by use of the MassMatrix MS/MS search engine, *J. Proteome Res.* **7**:138–144 (2008).

32. Yen TY, Macher BA, Determination of glycosylation sites and disulfide bond structures using LC/ESI-MS/MS analysis, *Methods Enzymol.* **415**:103–113 (2006).

33. Zhao E, Liu H-L, Tsai C-H, Tsai H-K, Chan C-H, Kao C-Y, Cysteine separation profiles on protein sequences infer disulfide connectivity, *Bioinformatics* **8**:1415–1420 (2005).

CHAPTER 10

PROTEIN CONTACT ORDER PREDICTION: UPDATE

YI SHI, JIANJUN ZHOU, DAVID S. WISHART, and GUOHUI LIN

10.1 INTRODUCTION

Contact order (CO) is the most widely adopted property used to measure the topological complexity of a protein structure. More specifically, contact order quantitatively measures the nonadjacent amino acid proximity within a folded protein. A contact between two distinct amino acid residues in a protein is formed when there is a pair of heavy atoms (C, O, S, or N), one from each residue, whose physical (Euclidean) distance is within a defined threshold [22,36]. The *absolute* contact order (denoted as Abs_CO in this chapter) of a protein is defined as the average number of residues separating the contacts inside the protein (where two sequentially adjacent residues are separated by one residue). The *relative* contact order, or simply the contact order (denoted as CO), is the Abs_CO normalized over the protein length.

Mathematically, given a protein with a primary sequence of length L, we use a_i to denote its ith amino acid residue. For two distinct residues a_i and a_j, if there are two heavy atoms (C, O, S, or N), one from each residue, within 6 Å, then a_i and a_j form a contact. Let L_{ij} denote the number of residues, $|i - j|$, separating this contact. Assuming that there are a total of N contacts in the protein, the Abs_CO of this protein is defined as

$$\text{Abs\_CO} = \frac{1}{N} \sum_{(a_i, a_j)} L_{ij} \qquad (10.1)$$

Algorithmic and Artificial Intelligence Methods for Protein Bioinformatics. First Edition.
Edited by Yi Pan, Jianxin Wang, Min Li.
© 2014 John Wiley & Sons, Inc. Published 2014 by John Wiley & Sons, Inc.

where the summation goes over all contacting residue pairs (a_i, a_j) in the protein [22,36]. The CO is defined as

$$CO = \frac{1}{L} \times Abs\_CO \qquad (10.2)$$

Essentially, Abs_CO measures the average separation between contacting residues in the native state of a protein, while CO is the normalized variant. Abs_CO (CO as well) increases with the proportion of interacting atoms that are far away in the protein sequence.

10.2 CORRELATED PROTEIN PROPERTIES

Since the early 1980s, considerable computational and experimental efforts have been devoted to learning about or predicting how proteins fold. Bulk properties such as protein folding rates [26,32], free energies of folding [43], and hydrogen exchange rates [13] can be measured experimentally to provide insights into protein folding mechanisms. These folding mechanisms are correlated with molecular properties such as secondary structure [23], molecular topology [36], and solvent accessibility [33]. In the past few decades, there were remarkable observations that protein folding rates vary over many orders of magnitude, from microseconds [32] to hours [26]. In combination with theoretical studies, these experimental observations have led to a general agreement that protein folding mechanisms and folding landscapes are determined largely by the topology of the protein native state and are relatively insensitive either to the details of the interatomic interactions [1,7,16,22,36] or to protein length [36].

To quantify the topological complexity and the stability of protein native states, various measurements pertaining to the contacts between amino acid residues in protein 3D structure have been proposed [12,15,20,22,27,29,36–39,48], where the relative contact order CO is the most robust representative. Both positive and negative correlations have been found between CO and several bulk protein properties such as protein folding rate and transition state placements [5,17,18,21,22,31,36].

Using a test dataset containing (only) 12 proteins, Plaxco et al. showed that there is a statistically significant relation between protein folding kinetics and native state topological complexity [36]. As it is proportional to the height of the transition state barrier, the logarithm of the intrinsic refolding rate was found to be well correlated with CO with a coefficient of 0.81 and an associated p value of 0.0001. It was also observed that the correlation coefficient between estimates of folding transition state placement θ_m and CO is 0.68 with an associated p value of 0.01 [36]. Here θ_m is computed from the ratio of the denaturant dependences of the relative free energy of the native folding and folding transition states. It is thought to reflect the fraction of solvent-accessible surface buried in the native state that is also buried in the transition state. Plaxco et al. also found a high correlation coefficient between CO and the helical content of the protein [36]. This observation is not surprising because helices have numerous close contacts characterized by a three-residue periodicity. However, the correlations between helical content or protein folding rate and transition state placement were shown to be much less significant; likewise, relationships between the size or stability of the proteins in the dataset and their refolding kinetics were found to be weak or nonexistent.

Contact order has also been shown to have certain utility in ab initio protein structure prediction [7], in addition to its application in predicting protein folding kinetic properties. Bonneau et al. observed that protein "decoy" (i.e., candidate) structures with higher topological complexity are more likely to be undersampled during the candidate structure generation stage in ab initio structure prediction programs, especially among larger proteins [7]. Such a bias can be alleviated by normalizing the CO distribution of candidate structures, and subsequently better protein structure predictions were generally achieved [7]. CO filtering is now an integral part of the Rosetta protein structure prediction package [10].

10.3 OTHER CONTACT MEASUREMENTS

As shown in early studies, Abs_CO exhibits a weaker correlation with two-state protein folding kinetics than CO does [16,36]. More recently, however, Ivankov et al. showed that Abs_CO is a more appropriate parameter for predicting the folding rate of proteins as it actually spans a wider range of folding state kinetics (i.e., two-state, multistate, and short peptides) [22]. Ivankov et al. summarized CO and protein length (L) into a general parameter called the size-modified contact order (SMCO):

$$SMCO = CO \times L^P \tag{10.3}$$

Apparently, from Eq. (10.3), SMCO reduces to CO when $P = 0$, and reduces to Abs_CO when $P = 1$. It was observed that any $P > 0.7$ results in approximately the same correlation for the totality of proteins and peptides collected [22], with the best correlation achieved at $P \approx 1$, that is, when SMCO $\approx$ Abs_CO. This hints that the more promising applications of CO prediction or calculation lie in the prediction of protein folding rates, folding transition state placements, and other folding properties.

In the literature, there are several other well-studied concepts on residue contacts, such as residuewise contact order (RWCO) [25,28,30,42], effective contact order (ECO) [39], contact number [CN; also known as *residue contact number* or *residue coordination number* (RCN)] [12,15,20,27,29,37,38,48], and Kendall's tau nearest-neighbor topology (K_τ-NN) [39]. These measurements are used largely to characterize the topology or topological complexity of protein native structure, but unlike CO, they are not directly correlated with certain global protein properties such as protein folding rate and folding transition state placements.

The residuewise contact order (RWCO) describes the sequence separations between the residues of interest and its contacting residues in a protein sequence [42]. RWCO provides important information for reconstructing a protein 3D structure from a set of one-dimensional structural properties. RWCO can also assist in protein 3D structure prediction and protein folding rate prediction, as well as providing insights into protein sequence–structure relationships. The *discrete* RWCO value of the ith residue in a length L protein sequence is defined by

$$\mathrm{RWCO}_i = \frac{1}{L} \sum_{j:|j-i|>2}^{L} \sigma(r_{i,j}) \times |j - i|$$

where $\sigma(r_{i,j}) = 1$ if $r_{i,j} < r_d$ and $\sigma(r_{i,j}) = 0$ otherwise. $r_{i,j}$ is the Euclidean distance between the C_β atoms of the ith and the jth residues in the protein sequence. Note that a sequential separation of at least two residues is required. By replacing the step function $\sigma(r_{i,j})$ with a sigmoid function, one obtains the *continuous* RWCO, or simply RWCO [42]. Song et al. developed a (continuous) RWCO prediction method based on PSI-BLAST and support vector regression from protein primary sequences, and achieved a correlation coefficient of 0.60 and a root-mean-square error of 0.82 on a well-curated dataset containing 680 protein sequences [42].

The effective contact order (ECO), as an alternative measurement to contact order, was proposed by Dill and coworkers [11,14] who adjusted the number of residues between a contacts as the number of residues on the shortest path between the two contacting residues. For example, when residues a_i and a_j $(i < j)$ form a contact with $|i - j| = 20$, and in between them residues $a_{i'}$ and $a_{j'}$ $(i < i' < j' < j)$ form an inner contact with $|i' - j'| = 5$, then in ECO L_{ij} is adjusted to be 15 instead of 20, as used in Equation (10.1). The shortest path between residues a_i and a_j in this case is $a_i - a_{i+1} - \cdots - a_{i'} - a_{j'} - a_{j'+1} - \cdots - a_j$. Because of the presence of existing covalent or topological links, ECO operationalizes contacts and scope in terms of shortest pathlengths between residues. ECO is assumed to relate to protein folding rate because it attempts to capture loop size, which is related to the size of the conformational search space necessary to form a conditional contact based on preexisting links.

The contact number (CN) measures how amino acid residues are spatially arranged. It is defined as the number of C_β atoms in other residues and within a sphere centered at the C_β atom of interest [48]. Therefore, CN is a residuewise measure. The same as for RWCO, Yuan et al. defined two kinds of contact number in their study: the *discrete* and the *continuous*. The discrete CN of the ith residue CN_i in a length L protein is defined as

$$\mathrm{CN}_i = \sum_{j:|j-i|>2}^{L} \sigma(r_{i,j})$$

where $\sigma(r_{i,j})$ is the same step function used in the definition of $RWCO_i$, as well as $r_{i,j}$ and the radius r_d. Note again that a sequential separation of at least two residues is required. Also, if one replaces the step function $\sigma(r_{i,j})$ with a sigmoid function, the *continuous* CN of the ith residue is defined. CN can be used to assist in protein fold recognition [24], to describe conserved solvent exposure of similar folds without a common evolutionary origin [19], to determine the energy function allowing molecular dynamics simulations of protein structures [27], and to partly characterize protein 3D structure [48]. Yuan et al. proposed a CN prediction method using PSI-BLAST and support vector regression, and achieved a correlation coefficient of 0.70; furthermore, they showed that if residues are classified as being either "contacted" or "non-contacted" then the correlation coefficient can reach 0.77.

Most recently, Segal et al. proposed a new topological measurement based on a means for operationalizing 3D proximity with respect to the underlying chain [39]. Specifically, the euclidean distances between all pairs of residues are computed and recorded in a distance matrix using their 3D coordinates. Then, for each residue, its Euclidean distances are mapped to a nearest-neighbor ranking. With this ranking, cycle structure can be used to capture topology with respect to the underlying chain. Such a ranking-based approach is insensitive to noise, which is a known concern with regard to structure determination experiments. For each residue a reference ranking is generated to capture the denatured random coil and the Kendall's tau nearest-neighbor (K_τ-NN) approach is used to measure the difference between the ranking of the folded structure's residue and the ranking of the reference residue. To measure the topology of the whole folded structure, Segal et al. took the average over all residues' K_τ-NN values. Compared to CO, the K_τ-NN measurement needs no tuning parameters during the computation; moreover, the chain deformation/structural information between the reference and contacting residues captured by the K_τ-NN measurement is ignored in computing CO. When tested on a set of two-state proteins under standardized conditions, this measurement showed an improved correlation coefficient with folding and unfolding rates. On a selected dataset containing 27 proteins, Segal et al. showed that the correlation coefficient between the folding and the unfolding rates of the proteins and the K_τ-NN values are -0.68 and -0.61, respectively, while the correlation coefficient between the two rates and the CO are only -0.58 and -0.30, respectively.

10.4 CONTACT ORDER CALCULATION

Here and in Sections 10.5 and 10.6, we introduce our work on contact order calculation and prediction. Because of the trivial relationship between Abs_CO and CO, where one can be directly computed from the other, in the sequel, we often refer to Abs_CO and CO interchangeably, unless otherwise explicitly specified.

While a large number of contact order algorithms have been described, the limited accessibility or availability of these algorithms (i.e., lack of downloadable programs or web servers) has prevented their widespread use by protein chemists or structural biologists. To increase the utility and accessibility of contact order calculations for experimentalists, we have developed a web server that both calculates Abs_CO (and CO) from 3D coordinate data and predicts Abs_CO (and CO) from protein sequence data. This public web server (http://www.copredictor.ca) calculates Abs_CO using Equation (10.1), where two distinct residues form a contact if there are two heavy atoms (C, O, S, or N), one from each residue, within 6 Å. It is worth pointing out that in the literature, several different distance thresholds other than 6 Å have been tested with no significant difference found [48]; besides, some constraints on contacting residue sequential separation (such as at least three residues apart from each other) and/or heavy atoms (such as $C\beta$ only) have been suggested [7], but again no essential difference exists as the underlying idea of using CO to quantify the topology of a protein's native state 3D structure remains the same.

The input to our Abs_CO calculator is a three-dimensional structure (uploading either the PDB [6] coordinate file or the PDB ID). The calculator typically returns the Abs_CO value within a few seconds. We note that there is an earlier published CO calculation server [36], and these two calculators returned nearly identical Abs_CO values with a correlation coefficient of 0.999. However, this earlier server failed (tested on May 2, 2007) to recognize 61% of the 933 monomeric PDB files that were successfully processed by our server.

10.5   CONTACT ORDER PREDICTION BY HOMOLOGY

Many protein properties, including tertiary structure, secondary structure, and solvent accessibility, can be predicted via homology [35]. In other words, the properties of a query sequence can be predicted by directly transferring the properties or features of a homologous protein to the query protein. Since CO is a property that is a function of structure, we hypothesized that the calculated CO of known 3D structures could be used to predict the CO of homologous proteins.

This approach has been implemented in our public CO web server http://www.copredictor.ca.

More specifically, the Abs_CO for 16,499 nonredundant proteins obtained from the PDB were calculated. These proteins were selected using the PDB culling/filtering service called PISCES [45]. Structures were initially selected using a 95% identity sequence redundancy cutoff and a requirement for better than 3 Å resolution (for X-ray structures). Structures were further processed by removing disordered structures (i.e., total secondary structure content <10%) as well as all membrane proteins (i.e., membrane β barrel and trans-membrane helix proteins). These 16,499 sequences with their Abs_CO values form the CO database that the server uses for its homology search, via a local copy of BLAST [2].

When the input to our web server is the primary sequence of a query protein, the BLAST search finds a homolog from the web server's CO database of 16,499 sequences. If this homolog is not an exact match to the query sequence but exhibits more than 20% sequence identity (which is computed as the number of identical residues divided by the query sequence length) and the query sequence is ±40% of the length of the homolog, the pre-computed Abs_CO of the homolog is used as the predicted Abs_CO of the query sequence [40].

We performed tests through a *modified* five-fold cross-validation using a random sample of 1,000 sequences on the CO database, using a variety of sequence identity cutoffs and sequence length thresholds to assess their influence on both the accuracy and the coverage (coverage refers to the percentage of query sequences that could be predicted by this homology-based method) [40]. Among other tested settings, the 20% sequence identity cutoff and the 40% length threshold provided the best overall accuracy–coverage tradeoff. Under this specific setting, on average 74.2% (±2.2% standard deviation) of sample sequences found homologs in the CO database. CO prediction by sequence homology turns out to be a surprisingly accurate prediction method, with a correlation coefficient of 0.977 between the 742 pairs of true absolute contact order and predicted absolute contact order values. These Abs_CO predictions are on average 93.4% correct (±0.5% standard deviation) [40].

10.6 CONTACT ORDER PREDICTION FROM SEQUENCE

Obviously not every protein can have its CO calculated from coordinate data or predicted via sequence homology. In the above experiment with 1,000 sequences, 258 of them failed to find a homolog. In order to deal with the situation where no homolog can be found for CO prediction, we have implemented a regression-based prediction method in the `http://www.copredictor.ca` CO web server [40]. As Abs_CO is observed to correlate well with a linear combination of the percentage of residues in α-helices $p(\alpha)$, the percentage of residues in β strands $p(\beta)$ and the protein length L, a linear regression to optimize the correlation between Abs_CO and the protein primary and secondary structures was developed

$$\text{Abs\_CO} = \chi_1 \cdot p(\alpha) + \chi_2 \cdot p(\beta) + \chi_3 \cdot L + c \qquad (10.4)$$

where χ_i, $i = 1, 2, 3$, are the coefficients of the three factors $p(\alpha)$, $p(\beta)$, and L, and c is a constant. During prediction, proteins with unknown three-dimensional structure can have their secondary structures predicted by Proteus [35] (or any other similar programs such as PSIPRED [34]). Proteus is a secondary structure predictor that achieves highly accurate predictions (Q_3 accuracy score of $\geq 81.3\%$) based on VADAR [46] and the PPT-Database [47]. To train the regressor, that is, to determine the values for χ_i, $i = 1, 2, 3$, c, a set of 933 monomeric proteins with an X-ray resolution <1.5 Å were extracted from the PDB [6]. Readers may refer to the study by shi et al. [40] for more detailed statistics on these proteins, such as their SCOP classification [4] and length distribution. Using these 933 high-resolution three-dimensional protein structures through a five-fold cross-validation, the optimal parameters in Equation (10.4) localize at $\chi_1 = -6.8968$, $\chi_2 = 7.6216$, $\chi_3 = 0.0612$, and $c = 8.0397$.

In addition to this three-factor linear CO predictor, denoted as F3-LR, several other linear regressors have also been developed to include more factors that might be strongly correlated to Abs_CO. These factors are the number of β hairpins (two adjacent β-strand segments form a hairpin if they are separated by two to five residues), the number of distant beta strands (two adjacent β-strand segments are considered "distant" if they are separated by at least five residues), the amino acid frequencies, and the hydrophobicity frequencies [40]. Besides linear regression, support vector regression (SVR) [41] and neural network (NN) [3] methods have also been implemented on our web server.

On the training dataset of 933 proteins, the five-fold cross-validation in the study by shi et al. [40] shows that the simplest regression model (F3-LR) actually performed remarkably well, achieving a correlation coefficient of 0.8571. Using more factors was shown to improve the correlation coefficient by a small amount. For instance, using four more factors, the F7-LR model improved the correlation coefficient by 0.0032; and the F27-LR achieved a correlation coefficient of 0.8702.

10.7 THE PUBLIC CONTACT ORDER WEB SERVER

A contact order calculator, the homology-based contact order predictor, and the linear regression–based contact order predictors are implemented as a public web server http://www.copredictor.ca. The input to the server can be either a three-dimensional structure (either the PDB coordinate file or the PDB Id) or the primary sequence of the query protein. When the input is a sequence, our server will first use BLAST to identify a sequence in our CO database that is either identical or the most homologous to the query. There are three possible scenarios: (1) if the input is a 3D structure, or the query sequence matches exactly a known structure in our database of 16,499 proteins, our server will calculate its Abs_CO; (2) if the input is a sequence and the BLAST search finds a homolog that is not an exact match but satisfies certain criteria, the precomputed Abs_CO of the homolog is used as the predicted Abs_CO of the query sequence; (3) if the input is a sequence and has no BLAST match that falls into scenario 2, our server will call Proteus to predict the secondary structure content for the query protein, and then report its Abs_CO predicted by Equation (10.4).

We have used our program to predict the Abs_COs and the derived protein folding rates [22] for all the proteins collected in TrEMBL (http://www.uniprot.org) [44], as of July 21, 2011. The result is available as a downloadable file from the server website.

10.8 CONCLUSIONS

Contact order (CO) is the most widely used approach to quantitatively measure the topological complexity of protein structures. CO can be used to accurately predict protein folding rates and to assist in *de novo* protein structure prediction/generation. However, the utility of the CO method, especially for experimentalists, has been limited by the lack of availability of programs or web servers that either support CO calculation (from coordinate data) or allow CO prediction (from sequence data). For proteins with solved three-dimensional structures, we have developed a public web server (`http://www.copredictor.ca`) that accurately calculates COs, thereby overcoming the limited functionality of an earlier web server. In addition, this server also offers a very effective method for predicting protein contact order from primary sequence data. This latter function is particularly important because of the 3D structure only a tiny fraction of known proteins is known. Many factors, in particular the percentage of residues in alpha helices, the percentage of residues in beta strands, and sequence length, are known to be strongly correlated with the absolute contact order. Tests using a large dataset of high-resolution monomeric proteins showed that our method achieved a correlation coefficient of 0.857–0.870. In addition, we have shown that it is possible to use sequence homology to accurately predict the contact order for proteins for which no 3D structure exists, with a high correlation coefficient of 0.977. This web server has been recognized or used to help in a number of studies in protein folding [8,9,39,49] and to demonstrate the effectiveness of K_τ-NN [39].

REFERENCES

1. Alm E, Baker D, Matching theory and experiment in protein folding, *Curr. Opin. Struct. Biol.* **9**:189–196 (1999).
2. Altschul SF, Gish W, Miller W, Myers EW, Lipman DJ, Basic local alignment search tool, *J. Mol. Biol.* **215**:403–410 (1990).
3. Anderson JA, *An Introduction to Neural Networks*, MIT Press, 1995.
4. Andreeva A, Howorth D, Brenner SE, Hubbard TJP, Chothia C, Murzin AG, SCOP database in 2004: Refinements integrate structure and sequence family data, *Nucleic Acids Res.* **32**:D226–D229 (2004).
5. Baker D, A surprising simplicity to protein folding, *Nature* **405**:39–42 (2000).
6. Berman HM, Westbrook J, Feng Z, Gilliland G, Bhat TN, Weissig H, Shindyalov IN, Bourne PE, The protein data bank, *Nucleic Acids Res.* **28**:235–242 (2000).
7. Bonneau R, Ruczinski I, Tsai J, Baker D, Contact order and ab initio protein structure prediction, *Protein Sci.* **11**:1937–1944 (2002).
8. Campbell K, Kurgan L, Sequence-only based prediction of beta-turn location and type using collocation of amino acid pairs, *Open Bioinformatics J.* **2**:37–49 (2008).

9. Chen K, Stach W, Homaeian L, Kurgan L, iFC2: An integrated web-server for improved prediction of protein structural class, fold type, and secondary structure content, *Amino Acids* **40**:963–973 (2011).

10. Chivian D, Kim DE, Malmstrom L, Schonbrun J, Rohl CA, Baker D, Prediction of CASP6 structures using automated Robetta protocols. (Available at `http://robetta.bakerlab.org/pub/dylan/`).

11. Dill KA, Fiebig KM, Chan HS, Cooperativity in protein-folding kinetics, *Proc. Nat. Acad. Sci. USA* **90**:1942–1946 (1993).

12. Fariselli P, Casadio R, RCNPRED: prediction of the residue co-ordination numbers in proteins, *Bioinformatics* **17**:202–204 (2001).

13. Fezoui Y, Braswell EH, Xian W, Osterhout JJ, Dissection of the de novo designed peptide alpha-t-alpha: Stability and properties of the intact molecule and its constituent helices, *Biochemistry* **38**:2796–2804 (1999).

14. Fiebig KM, Dill KA, Protein core assembly process, *J. Chem. Phys.* **98**:3475–3487 (1993).

15. Flöckner H, Braxenthaler M, Lackner P, Jaritz M, Ortner M, Sippl MJ, Progress in fold recognition, *Proteins* **23**:376–386 (1995).

16. Grantcharova V, Alm EJ, Baker D, Horwich AL, Mechanisms of protein folding, *Curr. Opin. Struct. Biol.* **11**:70–82 (2001).

17. Gromiha MM, Selvaraj S, Comparison between long-range interactions and contact order in determining the folding rate of two-state proteins: Application of long-range order to folding rate prediction, *J. Mol. Biol.* **310**:27–32 (2001).

18. Gromiha MM, Thangakani AM, Selvaraj S, Fold-rate: Prediction of protein folding rates from amino acid sequence, *Nucleic Acids Res.* **34**:W70–W74 (2006).

19. Hamelryck T, An amino acid has two sides: A new 2d measure provides a different view of solvent exposure. *Proteins* **59**:38–48 (2005).

20. Ishida T, Nakamura S, Shimizu K, Potential for assessing quality of protein structure based on contact number prediction, *Proteins* **64**:940–947 (2006).

21. Ivankov DN, Finkelstein AV, Prediction of protein folding rates from the amino acid sequence-predicted secondary structure, *Proc. Nat. Acad. Sci. USA* **101**:8942–8944 (2004).

22. Ivankov DN, Garbuzynskiy SO, Alm E, Plaxco KW, Baker D, Finkelstein AV, Contact order revisited: Influence of protein size on the folding rate, *Protein Sci.* **13**:2057–2062 (2003).

23. Kabsch W, Sander C, Dictionary of protein secondary structure: pattern recognition of hydrogen-bonded and geometrical features, *Biopolymers* **22**:2577–2637 (1983).

24. Karchin R, Cline M, Karplus K, Evaluation of local structure alphabets based on residue burial, *Proteins* **55**:508–518 (2004).

25. Kihara D, On the effect of long range interactions on secondary structure formation in proteins, *Protein Sci.* **14**:1955–1963 (2005).

26. Kim PS, Baldwin RL, Intermediates in the folding reactions of small proteins, *Annu. Rev. Biochem.* **59**:631–660 (1990).

27. Kinjo AR, Horimoto K, Nishikawa K, Predicting absolute contact numbers of native protein structure from amino acid sequence, *Proteins* **58**:158–165 (2005).

28. Kinjo AR, Nishikawa K, Predicting secondary structures, contact numbers, and residue-wise contact orders of native protein structure from amino acid sequence using critical random networks, *Biophysics* **1**:67–74 (2005).

29. Kinjo AR, Nishikawa K, Recoverable one-dimensional encoding of three-dimensional protein structures, *Bioinformatics* **21**:2167–2170 (2005).

30. Kinjo AR, Nishikawa K, CRNPRED: Highly accurate prediction of one-dimensional protein structures by large-scale critical random networks, *BMC Bioinformatics* **7**:401 (2006).

31. Koga N, Takada S, Roles of native topology and chain-length scaling in protein folding: A simulation study with a Go-like model, *J. Mol. Biol.* **313**:171–180 (2001).

32. Kubelka J, Hofrichter J, Eaton WA, The protein folding "speed limit," *Curr. Opin. Struct. Biol.* **14**:76–88 (2002).

33. Lee B, Richards FM, The interpretation of protein structures: Estimation of static accessibility, *J. Mol. Biol.* **55**:379–380 (1971).

34. McGuffin LJ, Bryson K, Jones DT, The PSIPRED protein structure prediction server, *Bioinformatics* **16**:404–405 (2000).

35. Montgomerie S, Sundararaj S, Gallin W, Wishart DS, Improving the accuracy of protein secondary structure prediction using structural alignment, *BMC Bioinformatics* **7**:301 (2006).

36. Plaxco KW, Simons KT, Baker D, Contact order, transition state placement and the refolding rates of single domain proteins, *J. Mol. Biol.* **227**:985–994 (1998). (Available at http://depts.washington.edu/bakerpg/contact_order/).

37. Pollastri G, Baldi P, Fariselli P, Casadio R, Improved prediction of the number of residue contacts in proteins by recurrent neural networks, *Bioinformatics* **17**:S234–S242 (2001).

38. Pollastri G, Baldi P, Fariselli P, Casadio R, Prediction of coordination number and relative solvent accessibility in proteins, *Proteins* **47**:142–153 (2002).

39. Segal MR, A novel topology for representing protein folds, *Protein Sci.* **18**:686–693 (2009).

40. Shi Y, Zhou J, Arndt D, Wishart DS, Lin G, Protein contact order prediction from primary sequences, *BMC Bioinformatics* **9**:255 (2008). (Available at http://www.copredictor.ca/).

41. Smola AJ, Schölkopf B, A tutorial on support vector regression, *Stat. Comput.* **14**:199–222 (2003).

42. Song J, Burrage K, Predicting residue-wise contact orders in proteins by support vector regression, *BMC Bioinformatics* **7**:425 (2006).

43. Tanaka S, Scheraga HA, Model of protein folding: inclusion of short-, medium-, and long-range interactions, *Proc. Nat. Acad. Sci. USA* **72**(10): 3802–3806 (1975).

44. The UniProt Consortium, Ongoing and future developments at the Universal Protein Resource, *Nucleic Acids Res.* **39**:D214–D219 (2011). (Available at http://www.uniprot.org/).

45. Wang G, Dunbrack RL Jr, PISCES: A protein sequence culling server, *Bioinformatics* **19**:1589–1591 (2003).

46. Willard L, Ranjan A, Zhang H, Monzavi H, Boyko RF, Sykes BD, Wishart DS, VADAR: A web server for quantitative evaluation of protein structure quality, *Nucleic Acids Res.* **31**:3316–3319 (2003).

47. Wishart DS, Arndt D, Berjanskii M, Guo AC, Shi Y, Shrivastava S, Zhou J, Zhu Y, Lin G, PPT-DB: The protein property prediction and testing database, *Nucleic Acids Res.* **36**:D222–D229 (2008).

48. Yuan Z, Better prediction of protein contact number using a support vector regression analysis of amino acid sequence, *BMC Bioinformatics* **6**:248 (2005).

49. Zhang H, Zhang T, Chen K, Kedarisetti KD, Mizianty MJ, Bao Q, Stach W, Kurgan L, Critical assessment of high-throughput standalone methods for secondary structure prediction, *Brief. Bioinformatics* **12**:672–688 (2011).

CHAPTER 11

PROGRESS IN PREDICTION OF OXIDATION STATES OF CYSTEINES VIA COMPUTATIONAL APPROACHES

AIGUO DU, HUI LIU, HAI DENG, and YI PAN

11.1 INTRODUCTION

Cysteine is one of the few amino acids that contain sulfur. The free thiol group allows it to bond with another cysteiene residue to form disulfide bond and help maintain the structure of proteins. The thiol group on cysteine residues is nucleophilic and easily oxidized. Because of this reactivity, cysteine residues serve numerous biological functions such as activation of certain biological activities [1], DNA binding [2], and reproductive systems [3] as well as the aging process of proteins [4]. As was shown in Figure 11.1, cysteine residues can be found in two chemical states in proteins: oxidized state and reduced state. The two states are interchangeable when proper conditions are met. When in reduced form, cysteine undergoes chemical reactions such as alkylation [5,6], oxidation [7], or forming complex compounds with metal ions [8]. These chemical reactions play critical biological roles such as activation, deactivation of the active sites of enzymes, and altering the local environment of the proteins. In their oxidized form, two cysteine residues form disulfide bond and enable more complicated protein structures [9,10] and functions [11,12].

The disulfide bond is the covalent bond formed between two cysteine residues on protein chains. The formation of disulfide bonds is a critical step for some of the membrane and secreted proteins in both eukaryotic and prokaryotic cells. Disulfide bonds are considered one of the elements of protein tertiary structure and directly contribute to the stability of the protein [13]. Figure 11.2 illustrates protein in 3D with the disulfide bonds denoted in light green.

Disulfide bonds have been generally classified into three categories: structural disulfide bonds, catalytic disulfide bonds, and allosteric disulfide bonds.

Algorithmic and Artificial Intelligence Methods for Protein Bioinformatics. First Edition.
Edited by Yi Pan, Jianxin Wang, Min Li.
© 2014 John Wiley & Sons, Inc. Published 2014 by John Wiley & Sons, Inc.

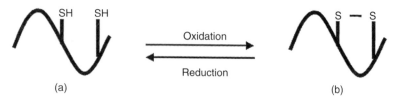

Figure 11.1 Reduced form (a) and oxidized form (b) of cysteine residues (twoStates.png).

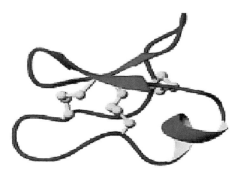

Figure 11.2 Illustration of disulfide bonds (shown in light green) on protein (disulfideBond.png).

An important function of disulfide bonds is that they constrain the distal portions of protein chain and reduces the entropy of the unfolded molecule [14] and hence influence the thermodynamics of protein folding. Disulfide bonds also stabilize the folded state of a protein chain [14]. The stabilization of the protein structure helps in reducing protein damage in the presence of oxidants and proteolytic enzymes. Because of their biological importance, knowing the disulfide connectivity in the protein is essential for studying protein structure. Knowledge of the oxidation states of individual cysteines is the first step toward acquiring knowledge on disulfide bonds connectivity and hence inspired significant interest in developing effective and economical ways of finding the oxidation states of individual cysteines.

The bonding state of cysteines can be obtained both directly via lab methods or indirectly by information derived from sequence information. Experimentally, the determination of bonding states of cysteine and disulfide bonds often involves use of costly biomarker and thiol reagents and techniques such as electrophoresis [15], mass spectroscopy [16], and HPLC [17]. These experimental approaches are normally time-consuming and dependent on expensive equipment. Therefore, many researchers resort to computational approaches. Predicting the oxidation states of cysteines computationally usually involves first extracting commonalities from the available data obtained by observation or statistical analysis, or utilizing artificial intelligence. Then the acquired knowledge is applied to sequences with

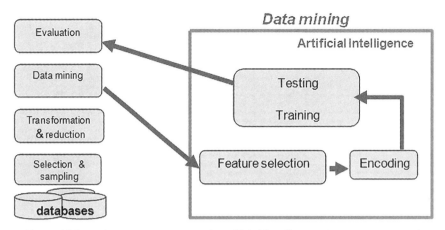

Figure 11.3 Information discovery via artificial intelligence (dataMining.png).

the bonding states unknown. Accuracy as calculation was based on the percentage of correct predictions among all test cases. To date, artificial intelligence achieves the highest accuracy among all computational methods attempted. Figure 11.3 is a flowchart of the prediction process via artificial intelligence. First, known data are extracted from database. Redundancy or over representation of certain protein families were avoided by careful selection and sampling. Then sequence information is transformed and reduced to fit the purpose of the data mining step, where relevant features are encoded and used to train the learning machine. After proper training, the resulted decision rules are used to evaluate to for the test data.

11.2 SURVEY OF PREVIOUS EFFORTS TO PREDICT BONDING STATE OF CYSTEINE RESIDUES ON PROTEIN VIA COMPUTATIONAL APPROACHES

In this chapter we surveyed ∼15 research efforts published since the 1980s in predicting cysteine oxidation states via computational methods, from the initial attempt using neural networks [18] to the present state of the art [19]. Most of these research efforts have reported prediction accuracy, although some of them used datasets that differed from the others. The essential information used for the predictions was first summarized all to determine the factors impacting the problem. In the following paragraphs we discuss prediction efforts in detail.

11.2.1 Major Factors Influencing Prediction of Cysteine Oxidation States

Figure 11.4 shows the information used in cysteine oxidation state prediction. Sequences local to the bonded cysteines provide a local chemical physical

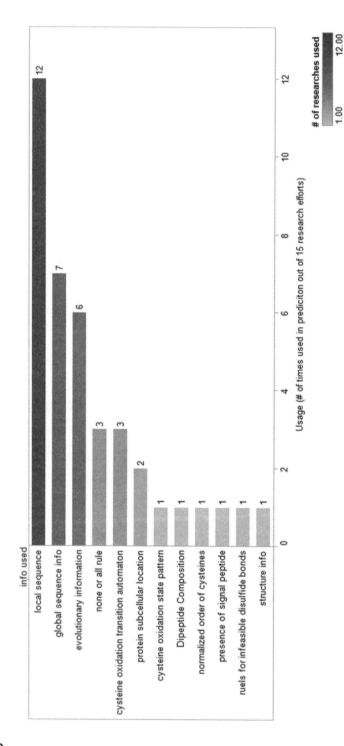

Figure 11.4 Statistics on information used for predicting oxidation states of cysteines (featuresUsedStatistics.png).

environment for the enzyme-mediated process of disulfide bond formation; therefore, it is critical for prediction. Out of the 15 research efforts surveyed, 12 (80%) included local sequence as input to their algorithms. Two of the early research efforts are based exclusively on the local flanking sequence [18,20]. Local sequence information usually consists of amino acid composition, charge, and hydrophobicity of the neighboring amino acids. Except for the flanking amino acids on the protein sequence, spatially neighboring amino acids are also considered as part of the local sequence information in some more recent research efforts [21].

Global sequence information was perceived as a good indicator of the protein type and ranks as the second most popular input feature used in prediction algorithms. Features such as the amino acid composition of the whole chain, chain length, and total number of cysteine on the chain belong to the global sequence information category.

Because of their biological importance, disulfide bonds are considered highly conserved features in proteins. Thus evolution information derived from multiple-sequence alignment is utilized in much of the research on oxidation state prediction. Addition of evolution information has shown improved prediction accuracy by significant percentage [e.g., 22].

Experiments have indicated that subcellular location of proteins is relevant to disulfide bond formation as well as stabilization. For example, disulfide bonds are hardly found in cytoplasm, and for eukaryotes, disulfide bond formation occurs mostly in the lumen of endoplasmic reticulum. By including the subcellular localization information as input, Savojardo et al. improved prediction accuracy was achieved for eukaryotes [19].

Other characteristics have also been explored such as the 'none-or-all rule' derived from direct observations of the test datasets, cysteine oxidation state transition automaton, dipeptide composition calculation, cysteine oxidation state pattern, normalized order of cysteines, the presence of signal peptide, and secondary structure information. Some of these features were used as an additional feature to train the learning machines. Some are used to fine-tune or correct the prediction results, including cysteine oxidation transition automaton [23–25] and the rules for infeasible disulfide bond [25] shown in Figure 11.5. Although not as popularly used as the local and global information and the evolution features mentioned above, each addition of these new features or new rules was reported to contribute to the overall prediction accuracy.

11.2.2 Major Efforts in Prediction of Cysteine Oxidation States

Figure 11.6 summarizes the efforts in predicting cysteine oxidation states. Since the 1980s, various computation techniques have been applied to the oxidation state prediction problem, ranging from single-layer neural networks to multistage support vector machines with increasingly relevant features added to the computation. As a result, prediction accuracy has increased from 71% for relatively

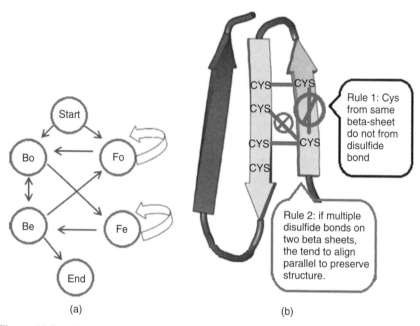

(a)   (b)

Figure 11.5 Fine-tuning steps reported in the literature: (a) *cysteine oxidation transition automaton* to limit the number of oxidized cysteines to even numbers; (b) rules for infeasible bonds (fineTunes.png).

small datasets to 93% for larger and more inclusive datasets. The details of these research are discussed in detail in the following paragraphs.

11.2.2.1 *Predicting Cysteine Bonding State from Local Amino Acid Sequence Only* Muskal et al. [18] trained simple feedforward neural networks with the flanking sequences around cysteine. This is the first effort reported in the literature to tackle the topic. The assumption was that local sequence is the determinant factor for the oxidation states of cysteines. Accuracy of 80% was achieved on 30 randomly selected proteins (15 sequences from sequences surrounding disulfide-bonded cysteines and 15 from non-disulfide-bonded) from a pool of 689. The window size of flanking sequences were also studied, and it was found that with increased window size, accuracy increases, but memorization becomes apparent after window size of 12 (6 before cysteine and 6 after).

Noticing the influence of flanking amino acids, Fiser et al. [20] took a statistical approach and analyzed a larger population of amino acids around cysteine residues (they studied 37,000 flanking residues vs. 9,000 residues studied in a previous effort). For each flanking sequence from −10 to +10 relative to the cysteine residue in consideration, the occurrence of the 20 amino acids were counted, and ratios of appearance as bonded and free cysteines were calculated on the basis of their appearance frequency. Finally, the disulfide forming potential

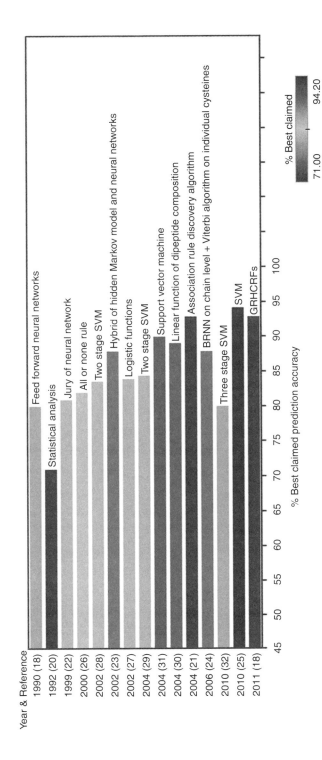

Figure 11.6 Research efforts on prediction of cysteine oxidation states since the 1980s (`methodsSurvey.png`).

for a cysteine containing segment was calculated as the product of the corresponding values of ratio of appearance of all flanking amino acids. The accuracy for prediction is 71% with 1.0 as the threshold of the overall accuracy. This research effort further confirmed that the flanking sequences around bonded and free cysteines differ substantially and are applicable in prediction of bonding state of cysteines.

11.2.2.2 Predicting Cysteine Bonding State from Evolution Information and Local Sequence Information

Fariselli et al. [22] trained a neural network–based predicator to differentiate the bonding states of cysteine in protein chain in terms of both the flanking sequence and the evolution information via multiple-sequence alignment. Eight different encodings were used in this research. With only the local amino acid composition encoded, the prediction accuracy is ~72%. Addition of evolution information such as multiple sequence plus charge, hydrophobicity, conservation weight, and relative entropy gave an improved accuracy of 80.1%. Finally, a jury of neural networks further improved prediction accuracy to 81%.

11.2.2.3 Predicting Cysteine Bonding State by Multiple Sequence Alignment Plus the "All or None" Rule

Fiser et al. [26] examined two datasets (81 protein chains from PDB and 233 protein chains, respectively, both from PDB) and found that only very few (2–4%) of the protein contain cysteines in both bonding states. In the majority of proteins containing cysteine residues, the cysteines are in either all-bonded state or in all-free state. This observation, combined with a conservation score calculated from physicochemical properties of the flanking amino acid, yielded a prediction approach with 82% in prediction accuracy. The dataset used here relatively small (81 protein chains included).

11.2.2.4 Predicting Cysteine Bonding State by Global Sequence Information

Mucchielli-Giorgi et al. [27] used information on either the residues flanking the cysteines or the amino acid content of the whole protein chain to train single logistic function. Two descriptors were used to train the function: (1) the cysteine environment descriptor corresponding to the local flanking sequence and (2) the protein descriptor. The latter was calculated as $P_r = \log \left(f_{l,k}/f_l \right)$, where $f_{l,k}$ is the occurrence frequency of amino acid l in this protein chain and f_l is the total number of occurrences of this amino acid in all protein chains in the DB. The prediction performance rates of the descriptors were compared and the weights associated with the logistic function analyzed. Final results showed that the local sequence environment of the cysteines contains less information than the global amino acid composition of the protein chain. The prediction accuracy in a dataset of 559 protein chains was ~84%.

11.2.2.5 Cysteine Bonding State Prediction via Combined Global and Local Sequence Information

Martelli et al. [23] designed a hybrid system based on the hidden Markov model (HMM) and neural networks (NN).

A standard feedforward neural network was first trained with the local sequence of 27 residue-long input window around the cysteine. Then a Markov model with N states connected by means of transition probabilities is applied. The transition between each possible state is restrained only to those that make sense. (If the chain contains disulfide bonds, then the number of bonded cysteine is bounded to be even. Transitions ending up with odd number of boned cysteines are not possible with the transition chart.) The prediction accuracy was up to 88% with this hybrid system.

11.2.2.6 Cysteine Bonding State Prediction Using a Two-Stage SVM Architecture

Because cysteines and half-cysteines rarely occur simultaneously in the same protein chain, Frasconi et al. [28] designed a system based on SVM architecture with two cascaded classifiers. The first classifier predicts the type of protein (*all*, *none*, or *mix*, indicating all, none, or a mixed number of oxidized cysteines on the protein chain) based on the whole sequence. In this stage the inputs include amino acid composition of the protein chain, the length percentage of the protein chain compared with that of the training set (calculated as length of protein under consideration divided by the average protein length in the training set). Also, a flag is encoded in input features indicating whether the number of cysteine count is odd. According to the output of the first classifier, the second stage classifier further classifies cysteines from those protein chains that were marked as *mix*. The stage 2 classifier uses the multiple-sequence alignment profile of the local input window to predict the bonding states of each individual cysteine on the chain. The prediction accuracy reported was 83.6% for a test set of 716 chains from 2001 PDB database.

11.2.2.7 Cysteine Bonding State Prediction Using a Combination of Kernel Machines

Ceroni et al. [29] extended the two-stage SVM architecture described above with a combination of kernel machines. First, a kernel machine based on the spectrum kernel was adopted and whole-protein sequence characteristics were used as input to this stage. In second stage, evolution information in the form of multiple-sequence alignments around cysteines were used. The accuracy was improved to 84.5% for the same protein dataset described in Section 11.2.2.7.

11.2.2.8 Cysteine Bonding State Prediction Based on Dipeptide Composition

Song et al. [30] implemented a two-class predicator based on dipeptide composition information to improve the bonding state prediction accuracy to 89.1% for 8114 cysteine-containing protein chains selected from PISCES culled PDB. The linear function of the probability of dipeptides P_{ab} (which can be the same or a different amino acid) is used to calculate characteristic index Q_k, specifically, $Q_k = \sum_{ab} V_{ab} P_{ab}^{(k)}$, where V_{ab} is constant for all proteins.

11.2.2.9 Signal Peptide as a Strong Indicator for Cysteine Bonding States in Extracellular Proteins

To gain full understanding of the biological

factors during the process of disulfide bonds formation in cells, Tessier et al. [21] collected sequential and spatial neighborhood information, structural information (such as secondary structure information and the calculated hydrophobic regions on the chain), and evolutionary information as well as other important information about the protein such as the presence of a signal peptide, parity of the cysteines, and the subcellular location of the protein. By applying the associating rule discovery algorithm a priori, it was observed that for extracellular proteins, the presence of a signal peptide is a strong descriptor of the bonding state of cysteines. This rule can be further reinforced when there are an even number of cysteines on the chain. Such an association was only found in extracellular proteins and not valid in membrane proteins and proteins from other compartments.

11.2.2.10 Cysteine Bonding State Prediction Using SVM Based on Local and Global Sequences Combined with Cysteine State Sequence

Chen et al. [31] integrated all the ideas described in earlier research efforts as inputs to a two-stage approach based on SVM. The decision value from the first SVM is normalized by the arctan transfer function before being used to predict the bonding state prediction. The second stage used the branch-and-bound algorithm to optimize the probability of cysteine state sequences (CSSs) while constrain the number of oxidized cysteines to an even number. With the local sequence information and the global amino acid composition alone, with SVM alone, an accuracy of 86% was obtained. Further coupling with the CSS yielded up to 90% in the overall prediction accuracy.

11.2.2.11 Cysteine Bonding State Prediction Using SVM and Bidirectional Recurrent Neural Networks

Ceroni et al. [24] employed SVM binary classifier to predict the overall cysteine bonding states for the whole chain (not on an individual cysteine basis), followed by a refinement step with bidirectional recurrent neural network (BRNN). For each cysteine, the BRNN output was computed using the logistic function. Then the number of the bonded cysteine was enforced to be even using a finite-state automaton. This approach achieved an accuracy of 88%.

11.2.2.12 Cysteine Bonding State Prediction with SVM Based on Protein Types

Lin et al. [25] used a SVM-based two-stage system to bring the prediction accuracy to 94.2%. In the first stage, an iterative protein level "type" (none, mix, or all) classification was performed. Each iteration uses the output probabilities of SVM of the previous iteration as the new feature until the result converges. The second stage is the mix classification using SVM for those chains that were classified as *mix* chain. Inputs to the SVM in this stage include position-specific scoring matrix (PSSM), normalized order of the cysteine in the protein chain, normalized length of protein length. In addition, a procedure called *simple tune* (Fig. 11.5b) is applied on the output from SVM. The *simple tune* step is based on two assumptions: (1) disulfide bonds in one chain do not locate in the same β sheet and (2) in case there are multiple disulfide bonds on two peptide chains of a β sheet, the disulfide bonds that are parallel to each other would be biologically favored so as to preserve the protein structure. The simple tune step consists of four tuning steps: boundary adjustment, oxidized inversion, reduced inversion, and odd–even revision. These fine-tune steps was reported to noticeably improve the prediction accuracy.

11.2.2.13 *Prediction of Cysteine Oxidation States Using Three-Stage SVM* Guang et al. [32] proposed a three-stage SVM to predict the oxidation of cysteines: (1) protein chains are classified into '*none*' or '*have*' categories to indicate whether there are disulfide bonds on the protein chain; (2) the *have* sequences are further classified to *mix* and *all*, indicating whether all cysteines on the chain are in the oxidized form; and (3) cysteiens in the '*mix*' sequences are analyzed with respect to a sliding window centered by cysteine. Features used as input to SVM include amino acid composition, local sequence around cysteines, evolution information, and secondary structure information as well as the existence of signal peptide from protein annotation. Accuracies of 90.05%, 96.36%, and 80% were achieved for the three stages of prediction, respectively.

11.2.2.14 *Cysteine Oxidation State Prediction with Grammatically Restrained Hidden Conditional Random Fields (GRHCRFs) Based on Protein Subcellular Localization and Position-Specific Scoring Matrix (PSSM)* Motivated by the fact that subcellular localization provides a suitable ambient environment for redox reaction of cysteines to occur, Savojardo et al. [19] included predicted protein subcellular localization in addition to other sequence information such as PSSM. It was found that inclusion of protein subcellular localization improves the prediction accuracy by two or three percentage points. The machine learning technique used here is GRHCRFs, which was found to perform better than other machine learning methods [33]. The prediction accuracy reached 93%. At the protein level, the prediction accuracy is reported to be 86%. It's worth noting that the dataset PDBCYS used in this study has excluded the trivial cases and that protein chains containing a single cysteine are not present.

11.3 SUMMARY

Since the 1980s, tremendous progresses have been made in the area of predicting oxidation states of cysteines. From simply utilizing the local sequences and single-layer neural networks to a broad spectrum of protein characteristics combined with multistage machine learning algorithms, researchers have improved the prediction accuracy from 71% for a relatively small dataset containing $\leq 93\%$ accuracy for a larger and more selective dataset excluded proteins with single cysteine (in which case, the oxidation states for those cysteines would have been obvious without performing complicated calculations). Research on the prediction of oxidation states of cysteines is surveyed, and the details of each study are discussed in this chapter. With the rapid advancement in biological research and better understanding of the mechanism of protein oxidative folding [34,35], prediction of oxidation states of cysteines on protein chains is more selective in terms of substrate (eukaryotes vs. prokaryotes or, e.g., whether catalyzed by a certain enzyme family) and focuses more attend on the mechanism of disulfide bond formation. This chapter is intended to serve as a reference source for future developments in the most recent efforts.

REFERENCES

1. Chamberlain LH, Burgoyne RD, Activation of the ATPase activity of heat-shock proteins Hsc70/Hsp70 by cysteine-string protein, *Biochem. J.* **322**(3):853–858 (1997).

2. McBride AA, Klausner RD, Howley PM, Conserved cysteine residue in the DNA-binding domain of the bovine papillomavirus type 1 E2 protein confers redox regulation of the DNA- binding activity in vitro, *Proc. Natl. Aca. Sci*, *USA* **89**(16):7531–7535 (1992).

3. Hatch TP, Allan I, Pearce JH, Structural and polypeptide differences between envelopes of infective and reproductive life cycle forms of Chlamydia spp., *J. Bacteriol.* **157**(1):13–20 (1984).

4. Berlett BS, Stadtman ER, Protein oxidation in aging, disease, and oxidative stress, *J. Biol. Chem.* **272**(33):20313–20316 (1997).

5. Kudo N, Matsumori N, Taoka H, Fujiwara D, Schreiner EP, Wolff B, Yoshida M, Horinouchi S, Leptomycin B inactivates CRM1/exportin 1 by covalent modification at a cysteine residue in the central conserved region, *Proc Natl. Acad. Sci.* **96**(16):9112–9117 (1999).

6. Zhang Z-Y, Dixon JE, Active site labeling of the Yersinia protein tyrosine phosphatase: The determination of the pKa of the active site cysteine and the function of the conserved histidine 402, *Biochemistry* **32**(8):9340–9345 (1993).

7. Arne ES and Holmgren A, Physiological functions of thioredoxin and thioredoxin reductase, *Eur J. Biochem.* **267**(2):6102–6109 (2000).

8. Vallee BL, Auld DS, Zinc coordination, function, and structure of zinc enzymes and other proteins, *Biochemistry* **29**(24):5647–5659 (1990).

9. Lehrer SS, Effects of an interchain disulfide bond on tropomyosin structure: intrinsic fluorescence and circular dichroism studies,. *J Mol. Biol.* **118**(2):209–226 (1978).

10. Wagner DD, Lawrence SO, Ohlsson-Wilhelm BM, Fay PJ, Marder VJ, Topology and order of formation of interchain disulfide bonds in von Willebrand factor, *Blood* **69**(1):27–32 (1987).

11. Reiter Y, Brinkmann U, Webber KO, Jung S-H, Lee B, Pastan I, Engineering interchain disulfide bonds into conserved framework regions of Fv fragments: improved biochemical characteristics of recombinant immunotoxins containing disulfide-stabilized Fv, *Protein Eng.* **7**(5):697–704 (1994).

12. Reiter Y, Brinkmann U, Jung SH, Lee B, Kasprzyk PG, King CR, Pastan I, Improved binding and antitumor activity of a recombinant anti-erbB2 immunotoxin by disulfide stabilization of the Fv fragment, *J. Biol. Chem.* **269**(28):18327–18331 (1994).

13. Horton HR, Moran LA, Ochs RS, Ravn JD, Scrimgeour KG, *Principles of Biochemistry*, 2nd ed., Prentice-Hall, Upper Saddle River, NJ, pp. 102

14. Wedemeyer WJ, Welkler E, Narayan M, et al, Disulfide bonds and protein folding, *Biochemistry* **39**:4207–4216 (2000).

15. Huck CW, Bakry R, Bonn GK, Progress in capillary electrophoresis of biomarkers and metabolites between 2002 and 2005, *Electrophoresis* **27**(1):111–125 (2005).

16. Kim SO, Merchant K, et al, OxyR a molecular code for redox-related signaling, *Cell* **109**(3):383–396 (2002).

17. Toyo'oka T et al, Amino acid composition analysis of minute amounts of cysteinecontaining proteins using 4-(aminosulfonyl)-7-fluoro-2,1,3- benzoxadiazole and 4-fluoro-7-nitro-2,1,3-benzoxadiazole in combination with HPLC, *Biomed Chromatogr.* **1**(1):5–20 (1986).

18. Muskal S, Holbrook S, Kim S, Prediction of the disulfide-bonding state of cysteine in proteins, *Protein Eng.* **3**(8):667–672 (1990).

19. Savojardo C, Fariselli P, Alhamdoosh M, Martelli PL, Pierleoni A, and Casadio R, Improving the prediction of disulfide bonds in eukaryotes with machine learning methods and protein subcellular localization, *Bioinformatics*: **27**(16):2224–2230 (2011).

20. Fiser AM, Cserzo ET, Simon I, Different sequence environments of cysteines and half cystines in proteins, application to predict disulfide forming residues, *FEBS Lett.* **302**:117 (1992).

21. Tessier D, Bardiaux B, Larré C, Popineau Y, Data mining techniques to study the disulfide-bonding state in proteins: signal peptide is a strong descriptor, *Bioinformatics* **20**(16):2509–2512 (2004).

22. Fariselli P, Riccobelli P, Casadio R, Role of evolutionary information in predicting the disulfide-bonding state of cysteine in proteins, *Proteins* **36**:340 (1999).

23. Martelli PL, Fariselli P, Malaguti L, Casadio R, Prediction of the disulfide bonding state of cysteines in proteins at 88% accuracy, *Protein Sci.* **11**:2735–2739 (2002).

24. Ceroni A, Passerini A, Vullo A, Frasconi P, DISULFIND: A disulfide bonding state and cysteine connectivity prediction server, *Nucleic Acids Res.* **34**:W177–W181 (2006).

25. Lin CY, Yang CB, Hor CY, and Huang KS, Disulfide bonding state prediction with SVM based on protein types, *Proc. 5th Int. IEEE Conf., Bio-Inspired Computing: Theories and Applications (BIC-TA)*, Changsha, 2010, pp. 1436–1442.

26. Fiser A, Simon I, Predicting the oxidation state of cysteines by multiple sequence alignment, *Bioinformatics* **16**:251 (2000).

27. Muccielli-Giorgi MH, Hazout S, Tuffery P, Predicting the disulfide bonding state of cysteines using protein descriptors, *Proteins* **46**:243–249 (2002).

28. Frasconi P, Passerini A, Vullo A, A two-stage SVM architecture for predicting the disulfide bonding state of cysteines, *Proc. 12th IEEE Workshop on Neural Networks for Signal Processing*, 2002, pp. 25–34.

29. Ceroni A, Frasconi P, Passerini A, Vullo A, Predicting the disulfide bonding state of cysteines with combinations of kernel machines, *J. VLSI Signal Process.* **35**:287–295 (2003).

30. Song JN, Wang ML, Li WJ, Xu WB, Prediction of the disulfide-bonding state of cysteines in proteins based on dipeptide composition, *Biochem. Biophys. Res. Commun.* **318**:142–147 (2004).

31. Chen YC, Lin YS, Lin CJ, Hwang JK, Prediction of the bonding states of cysteines using the support vector machines based on multiple feature vectors and cysteine state sequences, *Proteins: Struct. Funct. Bioinformatics* **55**(4):1036–1042 (2004).

32. Guang X, Guo Y, Xiao J, Wang X, Sun J, Xiong W, Li M, Predicting the state of cysteines based on sequence information, *J. Theor. Biol.* **267**:312–318 (2010).

33. Savojardo C, Fariselli P, Martelli PL, Shukla P, Casadio R, Prediction of the bonding state of cysteine residues in proteins with machine-learning methods, *Computational Intelligence Methods for Bioinformatics and Biostatistics*, Lecture Notes in Computer Science, **6685**, pp 98–111 (2011).

34. Mamathambika BS, Bardwell JC, Disulfide-linked protein folding pathways, *Annu. Rev. Cell Devel. Biol.* **24**:211–235 (2008).

35. Sevier CS, New insights into oxidative folding, *J. Cell Biol.* **188**:757–758 (2010).

CHAPTER 12

COMPUTATIONAL METHODS IN CRYOELECTRON MICROSCOPY 3D STRUCTURE RECONSTRUCTION

FA ZHANG, XIAOHUA WAN, and ZHIYONG LIU

12.1 INTRODUCTION

Electron cryomicroscopy (cryoEM) is a rapidly emerging tool in structural biology for three-dimensional (3D) structure determination of macromolecular complexes. Single-particle cryoEM allows structural elucidation of macro-molecular assemblies at subnanometer resolution [1,2], and, in some cases, at atomic resolution [3]. Electron cryotomography (ET) allows structural studies of complex speciments at near-molecular resolution as well as visualization of macromolecular complexes in their native cellular context [4]. The integrative combination of these cryoEM modalities with other high-resolution approaches, such as X-ray crystallography or nuclear magnetic resonance (NMR), is expected to provide a comprehensive description of the cellular function in molecular detail [5].

In ET, a series of projection images where structural features from different layers of the 3D structure of the specimen are first superposed along the direction of the electron beam. In general, those images are obtained by tilting the specimen around tilt axes [6]. The 3D structure of the sample can then be derived from those projection images, by means of tomographic reconstruction algorithms [7]. Because of physical limitations of microscopes, the angular tilt range is limited and, as a result, tomographic tilt series have a wedge of missing data corresponding to the uncovered angular range. Moreover, biological material is very sensitive to radiation, so specimens must be imaged at very low electron doses, which makes projection images extremely noisy. In high-resolution structural studies, this poor signal-to-noise ratio (SNR) is in the order of only 0.1 [8].

Algorithmic and Artificial Intelligence Methods for Protein Bioinformatics. First Edition.
Edited by Yi Pan, Jianxin Wang, Min Li.
© 2014 John Wiley & Sons, Inc. Published 2014 by John Wiley & Sons, Inc.

As a consequence, high-resolution electron tomography requires a method of 3D reconstruction from projections able to deal with limited angle conditions and extremely low SNR of the projection images.

In terms of computation, there are several main problems in ET reconstruction: the extremely low SNR of the images, alignment and classification of the images, 3D reconstruction under limited angle conditions, and post-processing and interpretation of the reconstruction results [8]. Also, because of the poor SNR in projection images, the size of tomograms and the number of projection images increase for high-resolution studies, and the computation time for 3D reconstruction also increases, which becomes a bottleneck for routine applicaitons of ET.

Since the demands of huge computational costs and resources derive from the computational complexity of the recontruction algorithms and the large size and number of the projection images involved, this chapter addresses the 3D reconstruction algorithm and its multilevel parallel strategy on GPU platform. We present an adaptive simulatneous algebraic reconstruction technique (ASART) for imcomplete data and noisy conditons. Specifically, we develop three key techniques—*modified multilevel access scheme* (MMAS), *adaptive adjustment of relaxation* (AAR) parameters, and *column sum substitution* (CSS) technique, to improve the reconstruction quality and speed of the reconstruction process. Also, we present a multilevel parallel strategy for iterative reconstruction algorithm in ET on multi-GPUs, and we develop an asynchronous comunication scheme and data structure named blob-ELLR to accelerate reconstruction processing and reduce memory requirements.

The remainder of the chapter is organized as follows Section 12.2 reviews icterative 3D reconstruciton methods for ET. Section 12.3 focuses on the ASART algorithm. Section 12.4 presents a multilevel parallel strategy for iterative reconstruction algorithm. Section 12.5 shows and analyzes the experimental results. Section 12.6 concludes the chapter with a summary.

12.2   ITERATIVE IMAGE RECONSTRUCTION METHODS

In ET, the projection images are acquired from a specimen through so-called single-axis tilt geometry. The specimen is tilted over a range, typically from $-60°$ (or $-70°$) to $+60°$ (or $+70°$) due to physical limitations of microscopes, with small tilt increments ($1°$ or $2°$). An image of the same object area is recorded at each tilt angle, and then the 3D reconstruction of the specimen can be obtained from a set of projection images by reconstruction methods.

Several reconstruciton methods for ET have been proposed. Weighted backprojection (WBP) has been one of the most popular methods in the field of 3D reconstruction of ET, due to its algorithmic simplicity and computational efficiency [9]. The major disadvantage of WBP, however, is that the results may be strongly affected by limited-angle data and noisy conditions [10]. Series expansion methods (i.e., iterative methods) constitute one of the main alternatives to WBP in 3D reconstruction of ET, owing to their good performance in handling incomplete and noisy data. Several traditional iterative methods, such as algebraic reconstruction techniques (ARTs) [11,12], simultaneous iterative reconstruction technique (SIRT) [13], component averaging methods (CAVs) [10], block-iterative CAV (BICAV) [10], and simultaneous algebraic reconstruction technique (SART) [14] have all been utilized to 3D reconstruction of ET. ART enjoys a rapid convergence but exhibits a very noisy salt-and-pepper image characteristic of reconstructed images. SIRT and CAV, on the contrary, produce fairly smooth reconstructed images, but still require a large number of iterations for convergence. SART is characterized by better robustness than ART under noise, and its convergence speed is reported to be faster than that of SIRT and CAV [14].

In this section, we give a brief overview of blob-based iterative reconstruction methods and describe the simultaneous algebraic reconstruction technique (SART).

12.2.1 Blob-Based Iterative Reconstruction Methods

Iterative methods are based on the series expansion approach [15], in which 3D volume f is represented as a linear combination of a limited set of known and fixed basis functions b_j, with appropriate coefficients x_j, that is

$$f(r, \phi_1, \phi_2) \approx \sum_{j=1}^{N} x_j b_j(r, \phi_1, \phi_2) \qquad (12.1)$$

where (r, ϕ_1, ϕ_2) is a spherical coordinate, and N is the total number of the unknown variables x_j. In 3D reconstruction, the basis functions used to represent the object greatly influences the reconstructed results. During the 1990s, spherically symmetric volume elements (called *blobs*) were thoroughly investigated and, as a consequence, the conclusion that blobs yield better reconstructions than the traditional voxels has been drawn in 3D reconstruction [16]. The use of blob basis functions provides iterative methods with better resolution–noise performance than voxel basis functions because of the overlapping nature of their rotational symmetric basis functions. Thus, we consider the blob basis instead of the traditional voxel one. The blob basis discussed in this chapter is constructed using generalized Kaiser–Bessel (KB) window functions

$$b(r) = \begin{cases} \dfrac{(\sqrt{1-(r/a)^2})^m I_m(\alpha\sqrt{1-(r/a)^2})}{I_m(\alpha)}, & 0 \leq r \leq a \\ 0, & \text{otherwise} \end{cases} \qquad (12.2)$$

where $I_m(\cdot)$ denotes the modified Bessel function of the first kind of order m, a is the radius of the blob, and α is a nonnegative real number controlling the shape of the blob. The choice of the parameters m, a, and α will influence the quality of blob-based reconstructions. The basis functions that developed by Matej and

Lewitt are used for the choice of the parameters in our algorithm (i.e., $m = 2$, $a = 2$, $\alpha = 3.6$).

In 3D ET, the model of the image formation process is expressed by the following linear system

$$p_i \approx \sum_{j=1}^{N} w_{ij} x_j, \quad 1 \leq i \leq M \tag{12.3}$$

where p_i denotes the ith measured image of f; $M = BS$ is the dimension of p, where B is the number of projection angles and S the number of projection values per view; and w_{ij} is a weighting factor representing the contribution of the jth basis function to the ith projection. Under such a model, the element w_{ij} can be calculated according to the projected procedure as follows:

$$w_{ij} = 1 - (rf_{ij} - \text{int}(rf_{ij})),$$
$$rf_{ij} = \text{projected}(x_j, \theta_i) \tag{12.4}$$

where rf_{ij} is the projected value of the pixel x_j at an angle θ_i; W is defined as a sparse matrix with M rows and N columns where w_{ij} is the element of W. In general, the storage demand of the weighted matrix W rapidly increases as the size and number of projection images increase. For example, when the size of images is $2k \times 2k$, the storage demand of the matrix approaches 3.5 GB.

Under those assumptions, the image reconstruction problem can be modeled as the inverse problem of estimating the x_j values from the p_i values by solving the system of linear equations given by Equation (12.3). This problem is usually resolved by means of iterative methods.

12.2.2 Simultaneous Algebraic Reconstruction Technique (SART)

The SART algorithm is a basic iterative method designed to solve the linear system in image reconstruction. Typically, the algorithm begins with an arbitrary $X^{(0)}$ and then begins to iterate until convergence [18]. The arbitrary initial value may greatly deviate from the true value. So the number of iterations can be very large. In order to accelerate the process of convergence, SART further adopts a backprojection technique (BPT), a simple WBP without the weighting functions, to estimate the first approximation $X^{(0)}$ [19]. BPT is a simple reconstruction method where the gray level of a pixel can be considered as the weighted average of the projections for all the possible rays passing through the pixel [7,20]. Consequently, the initial solution $X^{(0)}$ is defined by as follows:

$$x_j^{(0)} = \frac{\sum_{i=1}^{M} w_{ij} p_i}{\sum_{i=1}^{M} w_{ij}}, \quad j = 1, 2, \ldots, N \tag{12.5}$$

Then, in an iterative process, SART is described by the following expression

$$x_j^{(k+1)} = x_j^{(k)} + \sum_{s=1}^{S} a_{ij} \left(p_i - \sum_{h=1}^{N} w_{ih} x_h^{(k)} \right)$$

$$a_{ij} = \frac{\lambda w_{ij}}{\sum_{s=1}^{S} w_{ij} \cdot \sum_{h=1}^{N} w_{ih}} \tag{12.6}$$

where k is the number of iterations, a_{ij} is the relaxation parameter, λ is the fixed value (in general, $0 < \lambda < 2$), S is the number of projections per view, and $i = bS + s$ denotes the ith equation of the system; B is the number of all views obtained $b = (k \bmod B)$ is the index of the view, and $x_j^{(k+1)}$ is the next iterative value obtained by updating $x_j^{(k)}$. SART adopts a view-by-view strategy; that is, an approximation is updated simultaneously by all the projections of each view.

As mentioned above, the convergence speed of SART is higher than that of SIRT and CAV; the convergence process of SART is still slow and it is difficult to acquire satisfactory results:

1. SART adopts a sequential accessing scheme (SAS) to update views and thus converges slowly owing to the high correlation between consecutive views [21]. Several methods [e.g., random access scheme (RAS), multilevel access scheme (MAS), weighted distance scheme (WDS)] have been proposed and evaluated to minimize this correlation in the tomography field [21]–[23]. These methods are adopted mostly where projection views are distributed uniformly among $180°$, cannot be directly used in 3D reconstruction of ET.

2. It has been pointed out that careful selections for the relaxation parameters can lead to the better qualities of reconstructions [24,25]. However, SART employs a constant relaxation parameter a_{ij} [since λ is fixed and w_{ij} is invariable during the reconstruction procedure in each iteration, as shown in Eq. (12.6). With the constant relaxation parameter, the pixels with large gray level x_j have the same back-projection of the discrepancies as the pixels with small x_j as seen in Eq. (12.6). So the gray levels of the pixels should be considered for the selection of the relaxation parameters.

3. Computing the column sum for each view is time-consuming and storing it requires massive amount of memory.

12.3 ADAPTIVE SIMULTANEOUS ALGEBRAIC RECONSTRUCTION TECHNIQUE (ASART)

To generate high-quality reconstructions with improved computational speed, we have developed a technique known more popularly by its acronym, ASART. The key techniques developed in ASART include a modified multilevel access scheme (MMAS) to arrange the order of projection data, an adaptive adjustment of relaxation parameters (AAR) to correct the discrepancy between actual and computed projections, and a column sum substitution (CSS) to reduce the memory requirement and computation time.

12.3.1 Modified Multilevel Access Scheme (MMAS)

The SART method adopts SAS to order the views so that there is a high correlation between consecutive views. The convergence can be significantly facilitated if the views are ordered to maximize their orthogonality [21]. Toward this goal, a multilevel access scheme (MAS) is adopted to substantially decrease the correlated error between the consecutive views. A detailed comparison between MAS and SAS shows that MAS yields the most efficient reconstruction [26]. Applications in different situations have shown that MAS can obtain promising results [27,28].

The MAS method is based on the fact that two views of $90°$ apart are minimally correlated, and the third view is set to the angle halving the former two views to minimize the correlation of three views [21]. The MAS ordering applies to any number of views but works best if the number of views is a power of 2. Suppose that the views are indexed as $0, 1, \ldots, B - 1$, where B is the number of views. In MAS, views can be organized in a total of L levels where L is expressed by

$$L = \lceil \log_2 B \rceil \tag{12.7}$$

In level $l = 1$, view 0 $(0°)$ and view $B/2$ $(90°)$ with a maximum orthogonality are accessed first. Then, in level $l = 2$, there are two views: $45°$ and $135°$ (or whose indices are $B/4$ and $3B/4$). Furthermore, in level $l = 3$, the indices of views are respectively $B/8$, $5B/8$, $3B/8$, and $7B/8$. In every level, the views with the odd indices and the following ones with even indices are orthogonal.

As described above, MAS is adapted for the complete projection views distributed uniformly from $0°$ to $180°$. However, the projection views of ET are incomplete and limited in a certain range. We cannot always find two projections whose views are $90°$ apart. If MAS is directly used to arrange the order of the views in ET, some views to which there are no views perpendicular will be left. If these views that remain unprocessed by MAS are then arranged by SAS, there will be a high correlation between the consecutive views. We propose a modified MAS (MMAS) to arrange the order of projections in ASART. Only a series of projections evenly distributed across the whole angle is considered as ET projections. For example, the tilt angle ranges from $-60°$ to $+60°$ with a small tilt increment of $2°$. In MMAS, we adopt the range θ $(\theta = 120°)$ of tilt angles as the selected factor instead of B since the range is $120°$ rather than $180°$. Note that the range for the tilt angles can still vary in different situations. In the first level, we choose view $-60°$ and view $0°$ between whom the angle is the half of the range (but not $90°$). The two views that halve the angles between the first two are in the second level (i.e., view $-30°$ and view $30°$). In such a scheme, views

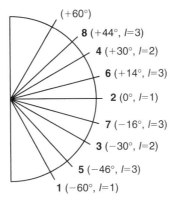

Figure 12.1 The access orders of the first three levels for the example. The left bold numbers on the left denote the index of access, and l denotes the number of the level.

in one level will halve (or almost) the views in all previous levels. Figure 12.1 shows the situation for the example by labeling the order of access in our MMAS scheme on the corresponding view angles. The proposed scheme clearly covers all angular regions evenly over time as shown in Figure 12.1. Table 12.1 summarizes the results of every level for this example. Note that in any level, the computed value of views may not be included in the projected views or may have already been accessed. If so, we search both sides of the computed value until the closest unused value is found and then put it into the sequence. Before the iterative process of ASART is carried out, the order of the overall views is arranged according to MMAS as discussed above.

12.3.2 Adaptive Adjustment of Relaxation Parameters (AARPs)

In SART, the gray level X is corrected by the relaxation parameters a_{ij} and the discrepancies between the actual projections P and the computed projections P'

TABLE 12.1 Access Orders for P Projections Ranging from $-60°$ to $+60°$ ($\theta = 120°$)

$l = 1(\theta/2)$	$-60°, 0°$
$l = 2(\theta/4)$	$-30°, +30°$
$l = 3(\theta/8)$	$-46°, +14°, -16°, +44°$
$l = 4(\theta/16)$	$-54°, +6°, -24°, +36°, -38°, +22°, -8°, +52°$
$l = 5(\theta/32)$	$-58°, +2°, -34°, +26°, -42°, +18°, -12°, +48°, -50°, +10°,$
	$-20°, +40°, -36°, +24°, -4°, +56°$
$l = 6(\theta/64)$	$-56°, +4°, -28°, +32°, -48°, +12°, -18°, +42°, -52°, +8°,$
	$-22°, +38°, -40°, +20°, -6°, +54°, -44°, +16°, -26°, +34°,$
	$-32°, +28°, -10°, +50°, -2°, +58°, +60°$

in each iteration. As shown in Equation (12.6), the relaxation parameters a_{ij} are determined only by the weight w_{ij} and the fixed value λ in the iterative procedure. The convergence process can be faster if the relaxation parameters are adjusted as a function of the number of iterations. The relaxation parameters are determined in such a way that they decrease as the number of iterations increases [19]. In SART, the relaxation parameters are determined only by the weight W while the gray level X is ignored. Thus the pixels with large gray levels will have the same backprojection of the discrepancies as the pixels with small gray levels.

In fact, the pixels with different gray levels make different contributions to the discrepancies. In ASART, a data-driven adjustment of relaxation parameters (AAR) is applied during the reconstruction procedure. In AAR, the relaxation parameters are determined according to the gray levels as well as the weights as shown in the following equation:

$$a_{ij} = \frac{\lambda w_{ij} x_j^{(k)}}{\sum_{s=1}^{S} w_{ij} \cdot \sum_{h=1}^{N} w_{ih} x_h^{(k)}} \tag{12.8}$$

With this approach, the relaxation parameter for each pixel is adjusted according to its gray level obtained in the previous iteration. Note that w_{ij} represents the geometry contribution of the *jth* pixel only to the *ith* ray integral. According to Eq. (12.8), the contribution of the *jth* pixel to the *ith* ray integral includes both the geometry contribution w_{ij} and the contribution of the gray level x_j of the *jth* pixel. This is different from SART, where the gray level x_j of the *jth* pixel is not considered as shown in Equation (12.6).

To illustrate intuitively how the convergence process can be accelerated by AAR, we consider a case with only two variables x_1 and x_2 satisfying the following equations:

$$\begin{cases} x_1 + x_2 = 2.7 \\ x_1 + 2x_2 = 3 \end{cases} \tag{12.9}$$

The computational procedures for locating the solution from an initial guess $(x_1{=}1.5, x_2{=}1.3)$ are displayed in Figure 12.2. The line in red denotes the procedure with the constant relaxation parameter by Eq. (12.6), and the line in blue describes the process with the adaptive relaxation parameter by Eq. (12.8). It is seen that the solution obtained by Eq. (12.8) is closer to the true solution than that obtained by Eq. (12.6) after the same number of iterations.

Note that in fact we don't need to recompute the sum of $w_{ih} x_h$ in Eq. (12.8) since it is equal to p_i, which has been computed in the process of reprojection. Extra computation is needed only for the multiplication of w_{ij} and $x_j^{(k)}$, but it is not time-consuming compared with the total computation.

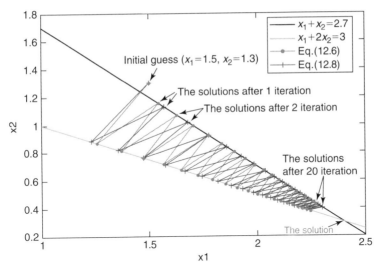

Figure 12.2   Illustration of the computational procedures from an initial guess.

12.3.3   Column Sum Substitution Technique (CSS)

We define c_j as the reciprocal of the sum of the jth column in each view by

$$c_j = \frac{1}{\sum_{s=1}^{S} w_{ij}} \qquad (12.10)$$

Although the column sums remain unchanged in each iteration, large memory space is needed to store each column sum for a SART reconstruction of large images. In fact, it has been proved that c_j has no effect on the final solution to which SART converges [29]. In another iterative method called BICAV (block-iterative component averaging) [10], the relaxation parameters are generated by the following equation

$$a_{ij} = \frac{\lambda w_{ij}}{\sum_{h=1}^{N} s_j^b (w_{ij})^2} \qquad (12.11)$$

where s_h^b denotes the number of times that components x_h of the volume contributes with nonzero value to the equations in the bth block. This is called *oblique projection in BICAV*. SART, on the other hand, is based on orthogonal projections. It has been proved that oblique projections allow iterative methods to have higher convergence speeds, especially during the early stages of iterations [10].

Accordingly, we propose that c_j is replaced by a scalar β denoting the maximum number of the nonzero weight w_{ij} in each view. In this way, the memory requirement and computation time are reduced, and the high qualities of the results are obtained because of this oblique projections. In the blob (if the radius $a=2$), the maximum number of the rays that affect every pixel on its reconstructed gray level in each view is 4. The relaxation parameter a_{ij} with our CSS technique can be expressed by

$$a_{ij} = \frac{\lambda w_{ij} x_j^{(k)}}{4 \sum_{h=1}^{N} w_{ih} x_h^{(k)}} \tag{12.12}$$

This modification can conserve runtime because the algorithm doesn't need to compute each column sum W for each view. The modification can also reduce the memory requirement by using the scalar β instead of the vector c_j, especially when the size of the image is very large.

With the improvements mentioned above, ASART is formulated as follows:

$$\begin{cases} x_j^{(0)} = \dfrac{\sum_{i=1}^{M} w_{ij} p_i}{\sum_{i=1}^{M} w_{ij}}, & j = 1, 2, \dots, N \\[4mm] x_j^{(k+1)} = x_j^{(k)} + \dfrac{\lambda}{4} \sum_{s=1}^{S} \dfrac{w_{ij} x_j^{(k)} (p_i - \sum_{h=1}^{N} w_{ih} x_h^{(k)})}{\sum_{h=1}^{N} w_{ih} x_h^{(k)}} \end{cases} \tag{12.13}$$

12.4 MULTILEVEL PARALLEL STRATEGY FOR ITERATIVE RECONSTRUCTION ALGORITHM

The reconstruction time of blob-based iterative methods is a major challenge in ET because of the large reconstructed data volume. So parallel computing on multiple GPUs is becoming paramount to satisfying the computational requirement. In this section, we present a multilevel parallel strategy for blob-based iterative reconstruction and implement it on the OpenMP-CUDA architecture.

12.4.1 Coarse-Grained Parallel Scheme Using OpenMP

In the first level of the multilevel parallel scheme, a coarse-grained parallelization is straightforward in line with the properties of ET reconstruction. The single-tilt axis geometry allows data decomposition into slabs of slices orthogonal to the tilt axis. For this decomposition, the number of slabs equals the number of GPUs, and each GPU reconstructs its own slab. Consequently, the 3D reconstruction problem can be decomposed into a set of 3D slab reconstruction subproblems. However, the slabs are interdependent because of the overlapping nature of blobs. Therefore, each GPU has to receive a slab that is composed of its corresponding own slices and additional redundant slices reconstructed in neighbor slabs. The number of redundant slices depends on the blob extension. In a slab, its own slices are reconstructed by the corresponding GPU and require information provided by the redundant slices from the neighbor GPUs. During the process of 3DET reconstruction, each GPU has to communicate with other GPUs for the additional redundant slices.

We have implemented the 3DET reconstruction based on the architecture in which a CPU controls several GPUs and the GPUs share the memory. We adopt two GPUs in the different platforms to implement the blob-based reconstruction. Thus the first-level parallel strategy makes use of two GPUs to perform the coarse-grained parallelization of the reconstruction. As shown in Figure 12.3, the 3D volume data are halved into two slabs, and each slab contains its own slices and a redundant slice. According to the shape of the blob adopted (the blob radius is 2 in our experiments), only one redundant slice is included in each slab. Each slab is assigned to and reconstructed on each individual GPU in parallel. A shared-memory parallel programming scheme (OpenMP) is employed to fork two threads to control the separated GPU. Each slab is reconstructed on each individual GPU by each parallel thread. Consequently, the partial results attained by GPUs are combined to complete the final result of the 3D reconstruction. Certainly, the parallel strategy can be applied on GPU clusters. In a GPU cluster, the number of slabs equals the number of GPUs for the decomposition described above.

12.4.2 Fine-Grained Parallel Scheme Using CUDA

In the second level of the multilevel parallel scheme, 3D reconstruction of one slab, as a fine-grained parallelization, is implemented on each GPU using CUDA. In the 3D reconstruction of a slab, the generic iterative process is described as follows:

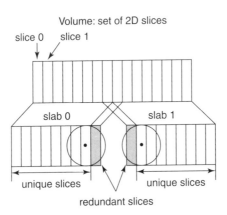

Figure 12.3 Coarse-grained parallel scheme using blob. 3D volume is decomposed into slabs of slices. The number of slabs equals the number of GPUs.

- *Initiation*—compute the wight matrix W and create an initial value for $X^{(0)}$ by BPT.
- *Reprojection*—estimate the computed projection data P' basis of the on the current approximation X.
- *Comparison*—compare and compute the discrepancy ΔP between the real experimental and calculated projections.
- *Backprojection*—backproject the comparison results over the image space and obtain ΔX.
- *Refinement*—update the current approximation X by incorporating the weighted backprojection ΔX.

The interdependence among neighbor slabs implies that, after computation of either the reprojection or backprojection for a given slab, there must be a proper exchange of information between neighboring GPUs.

12.4.3 Asynchronous Communication Scheme

As described above for the multilevel parallel scheme, there must be two communications between neighbor GPUs during one iterative reconstruction process: (1) to exchange the computed projections of the redundant slices after the reprojection process and (2) to exchange the reconstructed pixels of the redundant slices after the backprojection process. CUDA provides a synchronous communication scheme [cudaThreadSynchronize(#)] to accommodate the communication between GPUs. With the synchronous communication scheme, GPUs must sit idle while data are exchanged, which has a negative impact on the performance of the reconstruction in ET.

In the 3DET reconstruction on clusters, the use of blobs as basis functions involves significant additional difficulties in the parallelization and necessitates substantial communications among the processors. In any parallelization project where communication between nodes is involved, latency hiding becomes an issue [30]. An effective strategy stands for overlapping communication and computing so as to keep the processor busy while waiting for the communications to be completed [10]. In this study, a latency hiding strategy has been devised to deal with the communications efficiently. To minimize the idle time on the GPUs, we also present a latency hiding strategy using an asynchronous communication scheme in which different streams are used to perform GPU execution and CPU-GPU memory access asynchronously. The communication scheme splits GPU execution and memory copies into separate streams. Execution in one stream can be performed at the same time as a memory copy from another. In one slab reconstruction, reprojection of the redundant slices, memory copies and backprojection of the redundant slices are performed in one stream. The executions (i.e., reprojection and backprojection) of the slab's own slices are performed in the other stream. This can be extremely useful for reducing the idle time of GPUs.

12.4.4   Blob-ELLR Format with Symmetric Optimization Techniques

In the parallel blob-based iterative reconstruction, another problem is the lack of memory on GPUs for the sparse weighted matrix. Several data structures have been developed to store sparse matrices. Compressed row storage (CRS) and ELLPACK are the most two extended formats to store the sparse matrix on CPUs [31]. ELLPACK-R (ELLR), a variant of the ELLPACK format, has been proved to outperform the most efficient formats for storing the sparse matrix data structure on GPUs. ELLR consists of two arrays, $A[\#]$ and $I[\#]$ of dimension $N \times MaxEntriesbyRows$, and an additional N-dimensional integer array called $rl[\#]$ is included in order to store the actual number of nonzeros in each row [33]. With the size and number of projection images increasing, the memory demand of the sparse weighted matrix rapidly increases. The weighted matrix involved is too large to load into most of GPUs because of the limited available memory, even with the ELLR data structure.

Vazquez et al. proposed a matrix approach and exploited several geometry-related symmetry relationships to reduce the weighted matrix involved in the WBP reconstruction method [32]. In our work, we present a data structure named blob-ELLR and exploit several geometric symmetry relationships to reduce the weighted matrix involved in iterative reconstruction methods. The blob-ELLR data structure decreases the memory requirement and then accelerates the speed of ET reconstruction on GPUs. Compared with the matrix approach [32], our matrix blob-ELLR is adopted to store the weighted matrix W instead of the transpose of the one involved in the original ELLR. As shown in Figure 12.4 (a), the maximum number of rays related to each pixel is four because of the blob radius (viz., $a = 2$). To store the matrix W, the blob-ELLR includes two 2D arrays: one float $A[\#]$ to save the entries, and the other integer $I[\#]$ to save the columns of every entry (see Fig. 12.4b). Both arrays are of dimension $(4B) \times N$, where N is the number of columns of W and $4B$ is the maximum number of nonzeros in the columns (B is the number of the projection angles). Because the percentage of zeros is low in the blob-ELLR, it is not necessary to store

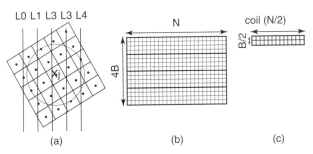

Figure 12.4   Blob-ELLR format with symmetric optimization techniques are exploited to reduce the storage space of A to almost $\frac{1}{16}$th of the original size.

the actual number of nonzeros in each column. Thus the additional integer array $rl[\#]$ is not included in the blob-ELLR.

Although the blob-ELLR without symmetric techniques can reduce the storage of the sparse matrix W, the number of $(4B) \times N$ is rather large, especially when the number of N increases rapidly. The optimization takes advantage of the symmetry relationships as follows:

Symmetry 1. Assume that the jth column elements of the matrix W in each view are $w_{0j}, w_{1j}, w_{2j}, w_{3j}$. The relationship among the adjacent column elements is

$$w_{0j} = 1 + w_{1j}; \quad w_{2j} = 1 - w_{1j}; \quad w_{3j} = 2 - w_{1j} \quad (12.14)$$

So, only w_{1j} need to be stored in the blob-ELLR, whereas the other elements are easily computed from w_{1j}. This scheme can reduce the storage spaces of A and I to 25%.

Symmetry 2. Assume that a point (x, y) of a slice is projected to a point r $[r = \text{project}(x, y, \theta)]$ in the projection image corresponding to the tilt angle θ and project(x, y, θ) is shown as follows:

$$\text{Project}(x, y, \theta) = x \cos \theta + y \sin \theta \quad (12.15)$$

It is easy to see that the point $(-x, -y)$ of a slice is then projected to a point r_1 $(r_1 = -r)$ in the same tilt angle θ. The weighted value of the point $(-x, -y)$ can be computed according to that of the point (x, y). Therefore, it is not necessary to store the weighted value of almost half of the points in the matrix W so that the space requirements for A and I are further reduced by nearly 50%.

Symmetry 3. In general, the tilt angles used in ET are halved by $0°$. Under this condition, a point $(-x, y)$ with a tilt angle $-\theta$ is projected to a point $r2$ $(r2 = -r)$. Therefore, the projection coefficients are shared with the projection of the point (x, y) with the tilt angle θ. This further reduces the storage spaces of A and I by nearly 50% again.

With the three symmetric optimizations mentioned above, the size of the storage for two arrays in the blob-ELLR is almost $(B/2) \times (N/2)$ reducing to nearly $\frac{1}{16}$th of the original size.

12.5   EXPERIMENTAL RESULTS AND DISCUSSION

The objective of this study is to improve the quality and efficiency of 3D ET reconstruction. In this chapter, a reconstruction method ASART and a multilevel parallel strategy are presented. Two experiments have been carried out to evaluate the proposed methods, respectively. To evaluate the performance of ASART, we compare the reconstruction qualities of ASART with those of WBP and SART. To evaluate the performance of the multilevel parallel strategy, two different experimental datasets are reconstructed on Fermi platforms.

12.5.1 Materials and Computing Resources

All the experimental data in our work are the caveolae from the procine aorta endothelial (PAE) cell, collected by FEI Tecnai 20 in China National Key Laboratory of Biomacromolecules [34]. Two different experimental datasetsare used (denoted by small-sized and large-sized) with 112 images of 1024×1024 pixels, and 119 images of 2048×2048 pixels, to reconstruct tomograms of $1024 \times 1024 \times 126$ and $2048 \times 2048 \times 430$, respectively.

The first experiment is carried out on a machine running Ubuntu 9.10 32-bit with an Inter Core 2 Q8200 at 2.33 GHz and 4 GB of DDR2 memory. The second experiment is carried out on Fermi platform. The Fermi platform is composed of the same CPU with GT200, and two NVIDIA Tesla C2050 cards. NVIDIA Tesla C2050 adopts the Fermi architecture and contains 14 SMs of 32 SPs (i.e., 448 SPs) at 1.15 GHz, with 3 GB of memory.

12.5.2 Experimental Results of 3D Data Reconstruction

To evaluate the performance of ASART, we have performed the 3D reconstructions of two datasets of PAE cell using WBP, SART, and ASART, respectively. We use a popular software IMOD [35] to perform the reconstructions of WBP, and adopt the relaxation factor λ with 0.2 and perform the reconstructions with different numbers of iterations.

Montages showing one z section of the volume reconstructed with the large datasets are presented in Figure 12.5. It clear that the quality of the image obtained

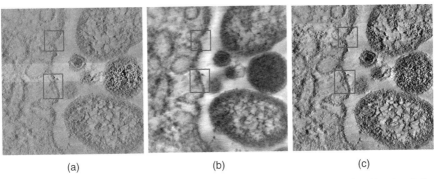

(a)   (b)   (c)

Figure 12.5 In the large dataset (2048×2048), one of slices along the Z axis of the reconstructions of the caveolae by WBP (a), 50 iterations of SART (b), and 50 iterations of ASART (c). Caveolae membrane structures (indicated by the red rectangles) can be clearly observed in the result of ASART (c).

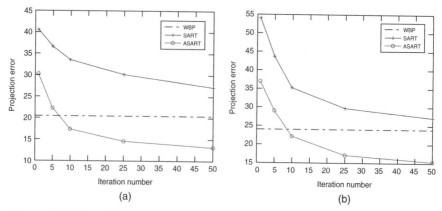

Figure 12.6 Plots of the projection errors ε versus the iteration numbers for the reconstructions of the caveolae using WBP, SART, and ASART at low resolution (a) and high resolution (b).

by ASART is superior to the images obtained by WBP and SART. Since this dataset has a large noise level and no gold markers, the results of WBP and SART are so blurred that we can't catch the legible bilayer outlines of caveolae membrane structure, while the structure–phospholipid bilayer can be clearly observed in the result of ASART, as shown the red rectangles in Figure 12.5.

Also, we adopt a projection error ε criterion for the comparison of WBP, SART, and ASART in a practical situation. ε measures the mean discrepancy between the ray integral p_i and its calculated value p_i', defined as

$$\varepsilon = \left[\frac{1}{M} \sum_{i=1}^{M} \frac{(p_i - p_i')^2}{n_i} \right]^{1/2} \tag{12.16}$$

where $n_i = w_i \times w_i$, and w_i is a J-dimensional vector whose jth component is w_{ij}. In the 3D data reconstruction, the qualities of the reconstructions, with SART and ASART, respectively, have been evaluated using the measure ε. In general, a smaller projection error indicates a better reconstruction. The curves of the measure ε versus the number of iterations are presented in Figure 12.6. As shown in that Figure 12.6, ε of the reconstructions with WBP remain constant, with the value of 20.35 and 23.94 in the small and large datasets, respectively. In the two different experiments, ε of the reconstructions with ASART is smaller than that with SART in the same iterations. For the medium and large datasets, the values of ε become smaller than that of WBP in 10 iterations. Consequently, it is shown that ASART has the advantage in dealing with extremely noisy conditions, and can obtain results better than those with WBP and SART.

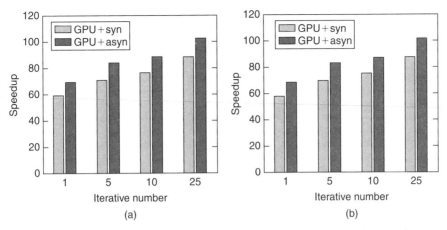

Figure 12.7   Speedup factors of different iterations shown by both implementations on the Tesla C2050 and CPU.

12.5.3   Experimental Results of GPU Platform

To evaluate the multilevel parallel strategy, we have performed two sets of experiments to estimate the performance of an asynchronous communication scheme and the blob-ELLR data structure, respectively.

First, to estimate the performance of the asynchronous communication scheme, we implemented the blob-based iterative reconstruction algorithm (ASART) using the two experimental datasets on the Fermi platform. All the reconstructions adopt two methods separately: multi-GPUs with the synchronous communication scheme (viz., GPU+syn), and multi-GPUs with the asynchronous communication scheme (viz., GPU+asyn). In the experiments, the blob-ELLR developed in our work is used to storage the weighted matrix in the reconstruction. Figure 12.7 shows the speedups of the two communication schemes for different reconstructions iterative numbers (i.e., 1, 5, 10, 25) using the two datasets on the Tesla C2050 versus CPU. As shown in Figure 12.7, the speedups of GPU+asyn are larger than those of GPU+syn for two datasets. The asynchronous communication scheme exhibits excellent acceleration factors, reaching up to $90\times$, $95\times$ and $100\times$ for 25 iterations, on two datasets, respectively. In general, the asynchronous communication scheme provides better performance than the synchronous scheme for the reason of asynchronous overlap of communications and computations.

Further, to evaluate the bolb-ELLR data structure, we implemented and compared the blob-based iterative reconstruction method using standard matrix, ELLR matrix, and blob-ELLR matrix on the Fermi platform, respectively. Figure 12.8 compares the speedups against the method using standard matrix. To ensure a clear and brief description, we show the results of only two datasets for one iteration. Because of the limited memory, the ELLR matrix method for large dataset

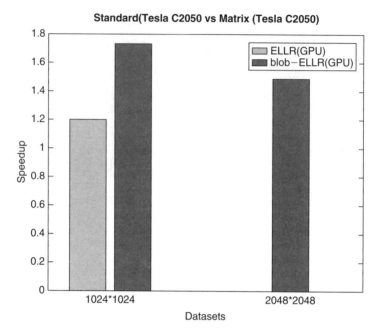

Figure 12.8   Speedup factors of the different matrix methods (ELLR and blob-ELLR) for one iteration over the standard method on the Tesla C2050s.

cannot be implemented on the Tesla C2050s. It is clearly seen that the blob-ELLR matrix method yields better speedups than the ELLR matrix method on the Tesla C2050s. Figure 12.9 compares the speedup factors of different methods on the Tesla C2050s over the standard method on the CPU for one iteration. It is clear that the blob-ELLR matrix method can reduce the memory requirement of the weighted matrix and yield the best performance compared with the ELLR matrix and the standard methods on GPU platforms.

12.6   SUMMARY

In this study, we present an adaptive simulatneous algebraic reconstruction technique, named ASART, to obtain high-quality reconstructions, and developed a multilevel parallel strategy for a blob-based reconstruction algorithm on GPU platform. The contributions of ASART include a scheme MMAS for the organization and sequence of access to projections, a strategy AAR for parameter adjustment to correct the discrepancy between real projections and computed ones in each iteration, and a strategy CSS to process the weights for each view to reduce memory requirement and computation time. Experimental results show than ASART can obtain high-quality 3D reconstruction of ET under the condition of noisy and incomplete data. In the multilevel parallel strategy, the asynchronous

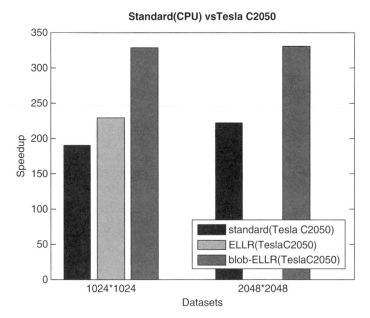

Figure 12.9 Speedup factors of the different matrix methods (standard, ELLR, and blob-ELLR) for one iteration on the Tesla C2050s.

communication scheme is used to minimize the idle GPU time. The blob-ELLR structure only needs nearly $\frac{1}{16}$th of the storage space in comparison with the ELLR storage structure and yields significant acceleration compared to the standard and ELLR matrix methods.

ACKNOWLEDGMENTS

We would like to thank Professor Fei Sun in Institute of Biophysics, Chinese Academy of Sciences for providing the experimental datasets. This work supported by Chinese Academy of Sciences knowledge innovation key project (KGCX1-YW-13), and National Natural Science Foundation of China grant 61232001, 61202210 and 61103139.

REFERENCES

1. Frank J, *Three-Dimensional Electron Microscopy of Macromolecular Assemblies. Visualization of Biological Molecules in Their Native StateNature*, Oxford Univ. Press, New York, 2006.

2. Henderson R, Realising the potential of electron cryomicroscopy, *Q. Rev. Biophys.* **37**:3–13 (2004).

3. Zhou ZH, Towards atomic resolution structural determination by singleparticle cryo-electron microscopy realising the potential of electron cryomicroscopy, *Curr. Opin. Struct. Biol.* **18**:218–228 (2008).

4. Lucic U, Foerster F, Baumeister W, Structural studies by electron tomography: From cells to molecules, *Annu. Rev. Biochem.* **74**:833–865 (2004).

5. Robinson CV, Sali A, Baumeister W, The molecular sociology of the cell, *Nature* **450**:973–982 (2007).

6. Marabini R, Rietzel E, Schroeder E, Herman G, Carazo J, Three-dimensional reconstruction from reduced sets of very noisy images acquired following a single-axis tilt schema: Application of a new three-dimensional reconstruction algorithm and objective comparison with weighted backprojection. The molecular sociology of the cell, *J. Struct. Biol.* **120**:363–371 (1997).

7. Herman GT, *Fundamentals of Computerized Tomography: Image Reconstruction from Projections*, 2nd ed., Springer Press, London, 2009.

8. Fernandez JJ, Sorzano C, Marabini R, Carazo J, Image processing and 3-D reconstruction in electron microscopy, *IEEE Signal Process. Mag.* **23**(3):84–94 (2006).

9. Radermacher M, Weighted back-projection methods, in *Electron Tomography: Methods for Three-Dimensional Visualization of Structures in the Cell*, 2nd ed., Springer, New York, 2006, Chap. 8.

10. Fernandez JJ, Lawrence A, Roca J, Garca J, Ellisman M, Carazo J, High performance electron tomography of complex biological specimens, *J. Struct. Biol.* **138**:6–20 (2002).

11. Marabini R, Herman G, Carazo J, 3D reconstruction in electron microscopy using ART with smooth spherically symmetric volume elements (blobs), *Ultramicroscopy* **72**:53–65 (1998).

12. Bilbao-Castro JR, Marabini R, Sorzano C, Garcia I, Carazo J, Fernandez JJ, Exploiting desktop supercomputing for three-dimensional electron microscopy reconstructions using ART with blobs, *Ultramicroscopy* **165**:19–26 (2009).

13. Sorzano C, Marabini R, Boisset N, Rietzel E, Schroder R, Herman G, Carazo J, The effect of overabundant projection directions on 3D reconstruction algorithms, *J. Struct. Biol.* **133**(2–3):108–118 (2001).

14. Castano-Diez D, Mueller H, Frangakis A, Implementation and performance evaluation of reconstruction algorithms on graphics processors, *J. Struct. Biol.* **157**:288–295 (2007).

15. Censor Y, Finite series-expansion reconstruction methods, *Proc. IEEE* **71**(3):409–419 (1983).

16. Lewitt RM, Alternative to voxels for image representation in iterative reconstruction algorithms, *Phys. Med. Biol.* **37**:705–716 (1992).

17. Matej S, Lewitt RM, Efficient 3D grids for image-reconstruction using spherically-symmetrical volume elements, *IEEE Trans. Nucl. Sci.* **42**:1361–1370 (1995).

18. Andersen AH, Kak AC, Simultaneous algebraic reconstruction technique (SART): A superior implementation of the ART algorithm, *Ultrasonic Imag.* **6**:81–94 (1984).

19. Herman GT, Meyer L, Algebraic reconstruction can be made computationally efficient, *IEEE Trans. Med. Imag.* **12**(3):600–609 (1993).

20. Frank J, *Electron Tomography: Methods for Three-Dimensional Visualization of Structures in the Cell*, 2nd ed., Springer, New York, 2006.

21. Guan H, Gordon R, A projection access order for speedy convergence of ART (algebraic reconstruction technique): A multilevel scheme for computed tomography, *Phy. Med. Biol.* **39**:2005–2022 (1994).

22. Mueller K, Yagel R, Cornhill JF, The weighted-distance scheme: A globally optimizing projection ordering method for ART, *IEEE Trans. Med. Imag.* **16**(2):223–230 (2002).

23. Kazantsev I, Matej S, Lewitt RM, Optimal ordering of projections using permutation matrices and angles between projection subspaces, *Electron. Notes Discrete Math.* **20**:205–216 (2005).

24. Wenkai L, Adaptive algebraic reconstruction technique, *Med. Phys.* **31**:3222–3230 (2004).

25. Wan XH, Zhang F, Liu ZY, Modified simultaneous algebraic reconstruction technique and its parallelization in cryo-electron tomography, *Proc. Int. Conf. Parallel and Distributed Systems* 2009, pp. 384–390.

26. Guan H, Gordon R, Computed tomography using algebraic reconstruction techniques (ARTs) with different projection access schemes: A comparison study under practical situations, *Phys. Med. Biol.* **41**:1727–1743 (1996).

27. Guan H, Gordon R, Zhu Y, Combining various projection access schemes with the algebraic reconstruction technique for low-contrast detection in computed tomography, *Phys. Med. Biol.* **43**:2413–2421 (1998).

28. Guan H, Yin FF, Zhu Y, Kim JH, Adaptive portal CT reconstruction: A simulation study, *Med. Phys.* **27**:2209–2214 (2000).

29. Jiang M, Wang G, Convergence studies on iterative algorithms for image reconstruction, *IEEE Trans. Med. Imag.* **22**:569–575 (2002).

30. Fernandez JJ, Carazo J, Garca I, Three-dimensional reconstruction of cellular structures by electron microscope tomography and parallel computing, *J. Parallel Distrib. Comput.* **64**:285–300 (2004).

31. Bisseling RH, *Parallel Scientific Computation*, Oxford Univ. Press, New York, 2004.

32. Vazquez F, Garzon EM, Fernandez JJ, A new approach for sparse matrix vector product on NVIDIA GPUs, *Concurr. Comput.: Pract. Exper.* **23**:815–826 (2011).

33. Vazquez F, Garzon EM, Fernandez JJ, A matrix approach to tomographic reconstruction and its implementation on GPUs, *J. Struct. Biol.* **170**:146–151 (2010).

34. Sun S, Zhang K, Xu W, Wang G, Chen J, Sun F, 3D structural investigation of caveolae from porcine aorta endothelial cell by electron tomography, *Progress Biochem. Biophys.* **36**(6):729–735 (2009).

35. Kremer JR, Mastronarde DN, McIntosh JR, Computer visualization of three-dimensional image data using IMOD, *J. Struct. Biol.* **116**:71–76 (1996).

PART III

PROTEIN STRUCTURE ALIGNMENT AND ASSESSMENT

CHAPTER 13

FUNDAMENTALS OF PROTEIN STRUCTURE ALIGNMENT

MARK BRANDT, ALLEN HOLDER, and YOSI SHIBBERU

13.1 INTRODUCTION

The central dogma of molecular biology asserts a one-way transfer of information from a cell's genetic code to the expression of proteins. Proteins are the functional workhorses of a cell, and studying these molecules is at the foundation of much of computational biology. Our goal here is to present a succinct introduction to the biological, mathematical, and computational aspects of making pairwise comparisons between protein structures. The presentation is intended to be useful for those who are entering this research area. The chapter begins with a brief introduction to the biology of protein comparison, which is followed by a brief taxonomy of the different mathematical frameworks for protein structure alignment. We conclude with a couple of more recent pairwise comparison techniques that are at the forefront of efficiency and accuracy. Such methods are becoming important as structural databases grow.

13.2 BIOLOGICAL MOTIVATION OF PROTEIN STRUCTURE ALIGNMENT

Proteins are crucially important molecules that are responsible for a large variety of biological functions required for life to exist. The DNA sequence of the genome provides a one-dimensional descriptive code; proteins are self-organizing systems that allow expansion of this one-dimensional code into complex three-dimensional structures possessing a great diversity of functions. Understanding the types of protein structures that are possible is an important part of understanding the existing biological systems, of understanding the

Algorithmic and Artificial Intelligence Methods for Protein Bioinformatics. First Edition.
Edited by Yi Pan, Jianxin Wang, Min Li.
© 2014 John Wiley & Sons, Inc. Published 2014 by John Wiley & Sons, Inc.

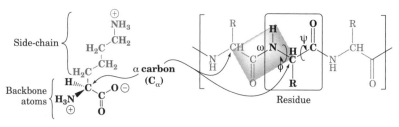

Figure 13.1 The structure of one type of amino acid (lysine) is shown on the left, with the sidechain and backbone atoms indicated. Proteins consist of amino acid residues, where the backbone atoms are linked together to form the chain, and the sidechains determine the folded structure and much of the function of the protein. In the partial protein shown on the right, the sidechains are denoted as R, and the three types of dihedral angles (the specific angle formed by the atoms bonded at each position along the backbone) are shown. The ϕ and ψ angles may vary, within geometric limits imposed by the surrounding atoms; the ω angle is fixed, with the six atoms forming the planar structure shown.

aberrant processes that result in genetic disorders, and in the engineering of proteins with novel functions.

Proteins are synthesized as linear polymers of amino acids (Fig. 13.1); the vast majority of proteins consist of a set of 20 different types of amino acids, in defined sequences that, depending on the protein, vary from about 50 to more than 28,000 amino acid residues. Although there are exceptions, in general, the specific sequence of amino acids is specified by the genome; this linear sequence determines the 3D structure of the protein.

The 3D structure of a protein is an emergent property of the linear sequence. Predicting the 3D structure entirely on the basis of the linear sequence has proved to be challenging because the defined structure exhibited by most proteins is a consequence of a large number of relatively weak interactions. The existence of a defined structure is possible because of geometric constraints imposed by the backbone atoms, and because of geometry-dependent hydrogen bonding, electrostatic, and nonpolar interactions between the atoms of the backbone and sidechains.

Prior to the experimental determination of the first protein structures, Linus Pauling predicted the formation of regular repeating structures (especially α helices and β sheets), based on a theoretical understanding of the geometric constraints inherent in the backbone structure. The increasing number of experimentally determined protein structures has confirmed that most proteins consist of arrangements of α helices and β sheets, along with regions of less well-defined structural elements. Because proteins are such large molecules, and because the secondary structural elements are important parts of the overall structure, most proteins are represented in ways that emphasize the arrangement of secondary structural elements (see Fig. 13.2).

Analysis of protein structures has revealed that many proteins consist of one or more separate domains, which are regions within the protein that fold

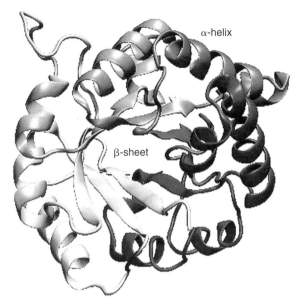

Figure 13.2   An α-carbon trace emphasizing the secondary structure of one monomer of the enzyme triose phosphate isomerase (from PDB ID 2YPI). This protein folds into an α/β barrel structure, with a multistrand β sheet (the thick arrows near the center of the structure) surrounded by α-helical elements. A number of other proteins exhibit this α/β barrel structure, despite considerable difference in both their sequence and function.

independently of the remainder of the protein. Protein domains are currently considered to be units of evolution; one major constraint on tolerated mutations is the result of the requirement to maintain the folded structure of the domain.

Comparison of different proteins is crucial to an understanding of the relationships between protein amino acid sequences, protein structure, and protein function. Protein sequence information can be obtained from the genome sequencing projects, and protein sequences can be readily compared. However, many proteins are known to have limited sequence similarity and yet have structures that appear visually similar. This raises the question of how to compare complex 3D structures both quantitatively and in ways that will allow a better understanding of the relationships between their structure and function.

Many proteins exhibit generally similar structures and similar functions. For example, a considerable number of serine protease enzymes have been discovered from species as widely divergent as mammals and bacteria. Although the two proteins shown in Figure 13.3 have very different amino acid sequences, portions of the structure match rather closely. However, in analyzing the structures, it is less clear how important the structural differences are in the subtle differences in function between these proteins. In addition, it is less clear how to best represent the structural differences in a manner that is both consistent and informative.

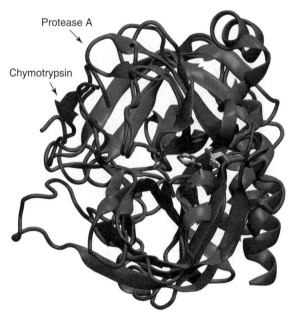

Figure 13.3   An overlay of two proteins with similar function: protease A from the bacterium *Streptomyces griseus* (PDB ID 3SGA) and *Bos taurus* chymotrypsin (PDB ID 1YPH). The two proteins share limited sequence identity (~20%), but similar catalytic mechanisms, and considerable structural similarity, especially in the core of the protein. In contrast, another protein, subtilisin from *Bacillus amyloliquefaciens*, also exhibits a similar catalytic mechanism but has a very different structure.

Another example of the importance of structure is provided by the prion proteins (see Fig. 13.4). Prions are monomeric proteins normally found on the surface of a variety of cells; however, these proteins are capable of undergoing an incompletely understood conformational change that results in oligomerization, with lethal effects to the affected individual. The spongiform encephalopathy diseases are one of a significant number of diseases caused by protein misfolding. An improved understanding of protein structure and protein folding processes might allow intervention in disease processes that are currently untreatable. In addition, many genetic disorders result from altered protein structure and function. While it is apparent that the changes in one of a small number of residues within a large protein cause disease, only a better understanding of the elaboration of sequence information into an overall structure will allow insight into possible approaches for treatment.

A final purpose of studying protein structure is to allow the design of novel proteins. Enzymes are phenomenal catalysts, which generally exhibit both high reaction rates and high levels of specificity. While biological enzymes catalyze a large range of reactions, no enzymes exist to catalyze many industrially useful reactions. The ability to design new enzyme mechanisms is extremely attractive

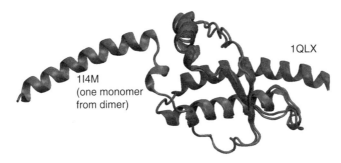

Figure 13.4 The same protein in two different conformations: a fragment from the human prion protein. The 1I4M structure is part of a dimer, which may represent a stage in the structural transformation from the largely helical protein shown here to the toxic β-sheet conformation thought to cause the lethal spongiform encephalopathy diseases such as Creutzfeldt–Jakob disease and kuru.

as a method for carrying out reactions at higher rates, with less expense from heating costs and waste product formation. Current methods for protein design are inefficient and essentially entirely empirical and are largely limited to minor alterations to existing proteins.

We have an increasing database of protein structures; however, we still lack a full understanding of how protein sequence, structure, and function are related. Comparing the structures of existing proteins of different sequences provides important data that will likely lead to an improved understanding of the mechanisms by which existing protein sequences give rise to their corresponding functional protein structures.

13.3 MATHEMATICAL FRAMEWORKS

The two main mathematical frameworks studied in the protein alignment literature are the contact map overlap (CMO) problem and the largest common point set (LCP) problem under bottleneck distance constraint [17]. Figure 13.5 illustrates a 2D version of each framework.

Let $A = \{a_1, a_2, \ldots, a_m\}$ and $B = \{b_1, b_2, \ldots, b_n\}$ be the sets of C_α atom coordinates of two proteins, proteins A and B, that we wish to align. (These are the carbon atoms in Fig. 13.1 that bind to the sidechains.) For a given distance cutoff value $\kappa > 0$, define $E_A = \{(a_i, a_j) : \|a_i - a_j\| \leq \kappa \text{ for } i < j\}$ and $E_B = \{(b_i, b_j) : \|b_i - b_j\| \leq \kappa \text{ for } i < j\}$ to be the sets of edges in the contact graphs of proteins A and B, respectively. (Edges are represented by arcs in Fig. 13.5.) Define $\Pi : A' \to B'$ to be a bijection (one-to-one, onto map) from a subset $A' \subset A$ to a subset $B' \subset B$. Define $T : B \to B'$ to be a rigid-body transformation of the fold of protein B. (In Figure 13.5, T is simply a translation of fold B onto fold A.) Then solve the two problems as follows:

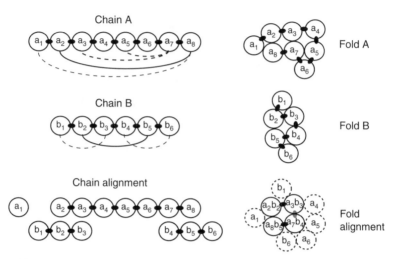

Figure 13.5   A 2D depiction of protein alignment. Chain A collapses into fold A, creating long-range contact depicted by arcs on chain A. Likewise, chain B collapses into fold B. Then a rigid-body transformation, in this case a vertical translation, superimposes folds A and B to create a fold alignment. In the CMO problem, the arcs on chains A and B are aligned directly (solid arcs) without reference to the superimposed folds. (The consecutive chain contacts are not considered.) In the LCP problem, the superimposed folds determine the chain alignment.

CMO Problem. Determine the bijection $\Pi : A' \rightarrow B'$ that maximizes the size of the matched subsets of edges $E'_A \subset E_A$ and $E'_B \subset E_B$, where an edge $(a_i, a_j) \in E_A$ is considered a match if $(\Pi(a_i), \Pi(a_j))$ is an edge in E_B.

LCP Problem. For all rigid-body transformations $T : B \rightarrow B'$, determine the largest subset $A^* \subset A$ for which there exists a bijection $\Pi : A^* \rightarrow B$ such that $\|a_i - T(\Pi(a_i))\| \leq \kappa$ for all $a_i \in A^*$.

Goldman et al. [9] proved that the CMO problem is NP-hard. Caprara et al. [6] apply linear integer programming methods to obtain exact solutions to the CMO problem for proteins that are similar to one another. Their methods have been improved significantly by Andonov et al. [1] (see Section 13.4). By imposing a proximity requirement for aligned residues and employing packing constraints satisfied by actual protein folds, Xu et al. [25] and Li and Ng [17] have developed polynomial time approximation schemes for the CMO problem. The CMO problem is discussed further in Section 13.4.

The LCP problem appears to be easier to solve than the CMO problem. The LCP problem is more geometric in character, whereas the CMO problem is graph-theoretic in nature. A possible disadvantage of the LCP problem, however, is that it treats proteins as rigid objects. In reality proteins are quite flexible. Hasegawa and Holm [10] claim that alignment methods that allow for flexibility give the most biologically meaningful results.

The main ideas used to develop a polynomial time algorithm for the LCP problem are due to Kolodny and Linial [13] and Poleksic [19,20]. We describe next a polynomial time algorithm for solving the LCP problem. The basic ideas were developed by Kolodny and Linial [13] and extended by Poleksic [20]. Although their analyses [13,20] pertain to the 3D alignment problem, here, for simplicity of exposition, we describe the algorithm for the 2D alignment problem.

In two dimensions, we can parametrize rigid-body transformations by $r = (\theta, x, y)$ as

$$T_r(b_i) = \begin{pmatrix} \cos\theta & -\sin\theta \\ \sin\theta & \cos\theta \end{pmatrix} b_i + \begin{pmatrix} x \\ y \end{pmatrix}$$

where b_i is the coordinates of a Cα atom in protein fold B. For a prescribed distance cutoff value, $\kappa > 0$, and for a given rigid-body transformation $T_r(b)$, define A_r to be the largest subset of A for which there exists a bijection $\Pi_r : A_r \to B$ such that

$$\|a_i - T_r(\Pi(a_i))\| \leq \kappa \text{ for all } a_i \in A_r.$$

The set A_r and the bijection Π_r can easily be computed in $O(m\,n)$ time by applying dynamic programming, see Section 13.4 for the score matrix $[C]_{ij}$, where

$$C_{ij} = \begin{cases} 1, & \text{if } \|a_i - T_r(b_j)\| \leq \kappa \\ 0, & \text{otherwise} \end{cases}$$

The solution to the LCP problem is then given by $A_r^* = \max_r \{A_r\}$.

A key observation by Kolodny and Linial [13] is that only a finite set of rigid-body transformations needs to be considered in order to optimize commonly used alignment scoring functions. To demonstrate this, first observe that only the compact subset, $R = \{r : |\theta| \leq \pi, |x| \leq \gamma, |y| \leq \gamma\}$ of rigid-body transformations needs to be considered because if protein B is translated by $|x| > \gamma$ or $|y| > \gamma$, where γ is sufficiently large, A_r will be the empty set since proteins A and B will have no points in common. Since $T_r(b)$ is continuous and R is compact, $T_r(b)$ is uniformly continuous on R. Uniform continuity implies that there exists a $\delta_\varepsilon > 0$ such that for any $r_1 \in R$ and $r_2 \in R$ satisfying $\|r_1 - r_2\| < \delta_\varepsilon$ we have that $\|T_{r_1}(b_i) - T_{r_2}(b_i)\| < \varepsilon$ for all $b_i \in B$. Now, consider the open balls $B(r_0, \delta_\varepsilon) = \{r : \|r - r_0\| < \delta_\varepsilon\}$ where $r_0 \in R$. The open balls $B(r_0, \delta_\varepsilon)$ cover R, that is, $R \subset \cup_{r_0 \in R} B(r_0, \delta_\varepsilon)$. Since R is compact, a finite subset of these open balls also covers R; that is, there exist $r_i \in R$ for $i = 1, 2, \ldots, N$ such that $R \subset \cup_{i=1}^N B(r_i, \delta_\varepsilon)$. Thus, all the rigid-body transformations in the compact set R can be approximated to within a distance of ε by the finite set of rigid-body transformations $\{r_1, r_2, \ldots, r_N\}$.

The alignment scoring functions considered by Kolodny and Linial [13] must satisfy a Lipschitz condition. Their algorithm only computes an ε approximation of the optimal solution. Poleksic [20] extended Kolodny and Linial's approach to the LCP problem. Moreover, Poleksic's extension computes the exact solution to the LCP problem in expected polynomial time $O(n^{11})$ for globular proteins of size n [19,20]. We describe Poleksic's algorithm next.

Let $r_* \in \arg \max_{r \in R}\{A_r\}$. Also, for $\kappa > 0$, define the function $S_r(\kappa) = |A_r|$, where $|A_r|$ is the number of elements in A_r. Since $r_* \in R \subset \cup_{i=1}^{N} B(r_i, \delta_\varepsilon)$, there exists an i_* such that $r_* \in B(r_{i_*}, \delta_\varepsilon)$, which implies

$$\|T_{r_*}(b_j) - T_{r_{i_*}}(b_j)\| < \varepsilon \text{ for all } b_j \in B$$

From this inequality, we can conclude that

$$S_{r_*}(\kappa) \leq S_{r_{i_*}}(\kappa + \varepsilon)$$

because if a_i and $T_{r_*}(b_j)$ are in contact for cutoff κ, then a_i and $T_{r_{i_*}}(b_j)$ remain in contact for cutoff $\kappa + \varepsilon$. We also have that

$$S_{r_{i_*}}(\kappa - \varepsilon) \leq S_{r_{i_*}}(\kappa) \leq S_{r_*}(\kappa)$$

Combining these inequalities, we have

$$S_{r_{i_*}}(\kappa - \varepsilon) \leq S_{r_*}(\kappa) \leq S_{r_{i_*}}(\kappa + \varepsilon).$$

The LCP problem can be solved exactly in a finite number of steps if we can determine an $\varepsilon > 0$ for which

$$S_{r_{i_*}}(\kappa - \varepsilon) = S_{r_{i_*}}(\kappa + \varepsilon)$$

since this would imply that $S_{r_*}(\kappa) = S_{r_{i_*}}(\kappa - \varepsilon) = S_{r_{i_*}}(\kappa + \varepsilon)$. Poleksic [20] showed that such an ε exists for all except a finite set of cutoff values $\kappa_1, \kappa_2, \ldots, \kappa_{|A|}$ as follows. The function $S_r(\kappa) = |A_r|$ is a nondecreasing function of κ having integer values in the range from 0 to $|A|$. The function $S_r(\kappa)$ is therefore piecewise constant except for possible jump discontinuities at cutoff values $\kappa_1, \kappa_2, \ldots, \kappa_{|A|}$. If we avoid this finite set of cutoff values, then we can choose an $\varepsilon > 0$ such that $S_{r_{i_*}}(\kappa - \varepsilon) = S_{r_{i_*}}(\kappa + \varepsilon)$. The size of the finite set of rigid-body transformations $T_{r_i}(b)$ that we need to search to determine i_* is determined by how small ε is. The size of ε is determined by how close κ is to one of the jump discontinuity points κ_i, $i = 1, 2, \ldots, |A|$. These jump discontinuity points are not known in advance. However, Poleksic [20] provides a proof that the overall expected complexity of the algorithm is polynomial in time.

13.3.1 Spectral Methods

Spectral methods have emerged as a new mathematical framework for the protein structure alignment problem. An advantage of spectral methods over CMO methods pointed out by Bhattacharya et al. [4] is that comparisons with spectral methods are based on two residues (one from each protein) rather than the four residues (two from each protein to define an edge) required by CMO methods. Another advantage over CMO pointed out by Lena et al. [15] is that unlike CMO, spectral methods scale well with the size of the distance cutoff parameter κ.

In 1988, Umeyama [23] published a spectral, polynomial-time algorithm for computing a bijection between two weighted graphs that are isomorphic. The adjacency matrix of each graph is assume to have distinct eigenvalues. Umeyama's algorithm also works well if the graphs are nearly isomorphic. We describe the details of Umeyama's algorithm next.

Let C_A and C_B be the adjacency matrices of two undirected, weighted graphs with the same number of nodes and distinct eigenvalues. The goal is to determine a permutation matrix Ω that minimizes $\|\Omega C_A \Omega^\top - C_B\|$. Let $C_A = U_A D_A U_A^\top$ and $C_B = U_B D_B U_B^\top$ be the eigensystem decomposition of C_A and C_B. It is possible to prove that

$$\|C_A - C_B\|^2 \geq \sum_{i=1}^{n} (\lambda_i^A - \lambda_i^B)$$

where λ_i^A and λ_i^B, $i = 1, 2, \ldots, n$, are the ordered eigenvalues of C_A and C_B. Umeyama showed that there exists an orthogonal matrix $U^* = U_B D U_A^\top$ for some diagonal matrix D, where D has diagonal elements -1 or 1, for which

$$\|U^* C_A (U^*)^\top - C_B\| = \min_U \|U C_A U^\top - C_B\| = \sum_{i=1}^{n} (\lambda_i^A - \lambda_i^B)$$

For isomorphic graphs, Umeyama proved that U^* is a permutation matrix Ω^*. Moreover, Ω^* can be computed in polynomial time by solving the assignment problem

$$\Omega^* = \operatorname*{argmax}_{\Omega} \operatorname{trace}(\Omega |U_A| |U_B^\top|)$$

using the Hungarian algorithm. (The entries of the matrices $|U_A|$ and $|U_B|$ are the absolute values of the entries in U_A and U_B.) Umeyama also observed that the optimal solution can often be obtained for nonisomorphic graphs by using the solution to the assignment problem above as an initial guess and then applying a local optimization algorithm.

Umeyama's algorithm for the graph isomorphism problem does not apply directly to the protein structure alignment problem, which is a subgraph isomorphism problem. In other words, Umeyama's algorithm cannot handle insertions and deletions. In addition, the weighted graphs of protein structures may not be similar to one another, a requirement for Umeyama's algorithm to work reliably.

Bhattacharya et al. [4] attempt to overcome the limitations of Umeyama's algorithm by considering local alignments to identify similar neighborhoods of the same size and then piecing these neighborhoods together. Rather than apply Umeyama's algorithm directly, Bhattacharya et al. normalize each eigenvector by the size of the protein and then compare the eigenvectors without taking absolute values. (Like Umeyama, they do not use the eigenvalues in their algorithm.) A complication arising in the approach used by Bhattacharya et al. is the fact that the eigenvector decomposition of an adjacency matrix does not specify an orientation of the eigenvectors. In other words, if v_i is an eigenvector, so is $-v_i$. This requires 2^k eigenvector orientations to be checked, where k equals the number of eigenvectors compared. The time complexity of the resulting algorithm, called Matchprot, is $O(2^k \max \{m^3, n^3\})$. Bhattacharya et al. point out that empirical observations suggest that $k = 3$ eigenvectors is sufficient for good results. However, Matchprot has difficulty with alignments involving large insertions and deletions.

Lena et al. [15] introduced a spectral algorithm called Al-Eigen. Unlike Matchprot, Al-Eigen uses a global alignment. Al-Eigen scales eigenvectors by the square root of the corresponding eigenvalues. Like Matchprot, Al-Eigen searches through the 2^k orientations of the k eigenvectors it compares, starting with comparing just one eigenvector from each protein, up to t eigenvectors. The complexity of Al-Eigen is $O(2^{t+1} m \, n)$.

In this section we have tersely reviewed the primary mathematical models associated with optimally aligning protein structures. The intent of the CMO, the LCP, and the spectral frameworks is to discern biologically relevant alignments between two proteins. Each paradigm has advantages and disadvantages, and continued research is important. The algorithmic complexity and resulting solution times were substantial enough that, until quite recently, undertaking the task of completing numerous pairwise comparisons was a weighty computational burden. However, a host of modern algorithms is emerging that hasten the comparison procedure. These are discussed in the next section.

13.4   MORE RECENT ADVANCES WITH DATABASE QUERIES

Protein databases contain tens of thousands of structures and continue to grow. One of the research fronts in computational biology is the design of algorithms that can efficiently search and organize these databases. For example, a researcher may want to find those proteins whose structure is similar to one under investigation, or may want to navigate a database by functionally similar proteins. Such queries require comparisons against an entire database. As protein databases grow, undertaking these numerous comparisons requires efficient and accurate comparison algorithms.

We review three methods that are designed for making efficient structural comparisons: (1) a geometric approach that encodes each residue with angle and distance information called globa structure superposition of proteins (GOSSIP) [12] (2) a spectral approach called EIGAS that assigns each residue an eigenvalue associated with a high-dimensional feature [22], and (3) a solution procedure to the CMO problem called A_purva [1]. While these methods represent protein chains differently, they share the common algorithmic solution procedure of dynamic programming (DP). The emerging literature on protein structure alignment points to the important role that DP is fulfilling as an efficient algorithmic framework. Our specific goal here is to highlight this observation and develop the use of DP in each of these alignment procedures.

Dynamic programming was invented by Bellman in the 1940s [3], and its use in biological applications began in 1970 [18]. The discrete version we consider calculates an optimal match between two sequences, say, $r_1, r_2, \ldots, r_n$ and $r'_1, r'_2, \ldots, r'_m$. The algorithm requires that each possible match be scored, and we let $S_{ij} = S(r_i, r'_j)$ be the score associated with matching element i of the first sequence with element j of the second. Dynamic programming follows a recursion to calculate an optimal match between the two sequences

$$
V(i,j) = \text{opt} \begin{cases} V(i-1,k) + \rho \\ V(i,j-1) + \rho \\ V(i-1,j-1) + S(r_i, r'_j) \end{cases} \tag{13.1}
$$

where ρ is a gap penalty. The gap penalty can depend on whether a gap is being initiated or continued; in the former the penalty is called a *gap opening penalty* and in the latter, a *gap extension penalty*. Completing this recursion over i and j calculates the optimal value of the matching, and backtracing the optimal iterations lists the optimal matching. The optimal match depends not only on the scoring matrix S but also on the penalties to open and continue a gap, and hence, the use of DP to optimally align sequences requires parameter tuning. The computational complexity of calculating an optimal matching is $O(mn)$, showing that DP is an efficient polynomial algorithm.

The coordinates of the $C\alpha$ atoms of each residue are used to describe the protein in each of the techniques presented below. Because of the lack of an absolute coordinate system, a protein is commonly abstracted into pairwise comparisons between $C\alpha$ atoms, which provides a coordinate and rotation free description of the protein. Each of A_purva, GOSSIP, and EIGAS assigns different information to each $C\alpha$ atom, and hence, each imposes a different pairwise relationship between residues. In what follows, we briefly describe each technique so as to highlight the similarities and dissimilarities between the algorithms. In particular, we show how to construct the scoring matrices used for DP so that each method is seen as an application of DP applied to sequence similarity.

13.4.1 GOSSIP

The GOSSIP algorithm uses DP with a scoring matrix created by local 3D geometry. A residue is encoded with eight characteristics that depend on a parameter q that defines the local geometry. The characteristics for residue r_i depend on the polygon created by residues r_i, r_{i+2}, r_{q-2}, and r_q. Five of the characteristics are distances, and we use $d(r_i, r_j)$ to denote the Euclidean distance between the $C\alpha$ atoms of residues i and j. The characteristics are

Characteristic	1	2	3	4
	$d(r_i, r_{i+2})$	$d(r_{i+2}, d_{i+q-2})$	$d(r_{i+q-2}, r_{i+q})$	$d(r_{i+q}, r_i)$
Characteristic	5	6	7	8
	$d(r_i, r_{i+q-2})$	θ_i	i	$n-i+1$

The angle θ_i is created by the line segments (r_i, r_{i+q}) and (r_i, C), where C is the centroid of the protein structure and n is the number of residues in the protein chain. See Figure 13.6 for an example. All but the last $n-q$ residues are encoded.

The score assigned to matching residue i of the first protein to residue j of the second is

$$S_{ij} = 3 - 2|d(r_i, r_{i+q}) - d(r_j, r_{i+q})| - 0.1|\theta_i - \theta_j|$$

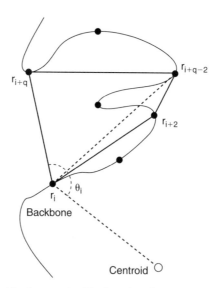

Figure 13.6 Residue i is characterized by lengths of a polygon, the length of a diagonal, the angle θ_i, and two indices.

where the coefficients 2 and 0.1 are experimentally decided. DP is applied to the scoring matrix $[S]_{ij}$, but with a few adaptations. First, an indicator function $\delta(i,j)$ is used to decide if the characteristics of residues i and j are similar enough to consider a match. Each characteristic is compared, and agreement is decided based on a threshold value that is characteristic dependent. If enough characteristics agree, then $\delta(i,j) = 1$, but if not $\delta(i,j) = 0$. This adaptation alters the recursion in 13.1 to

$$
V(i,j) = \max \begin{cases} V(i-1,k) + \rho \\ V(i,j-1) + \rho \\ \delta(i,j)(V(i-1,j-1) + S(r_i, r'_j)) \end{cases}
$$

A second adaptation is that $V(i,j)$ is not calculated if the difference between i and j exceeds a threshold indicating the maximum number of gaps allowed in a match. GOSSIP further limits the number of the protein chains that are compared by associating with each chain a collection of chains of similar lengths.

Numerical work for GOSSIP is promising. Two datasets described by Kifer et al. [12] were used for testing, one containing 2,930 protein structures from CATH and one containing 3,613 structures from Astral. An all-against-all comparison requires 4,290,985 alignments in the CATH dataset and 6,525,078 comparisons in the Astral dataset. To gauge the effectiveness of GOSSIP, 267 proteins from the CATH dataset and 348 from the Astral dataset were selected, and all-against-all comparisons were made on these smaller datasets. Runtimes were then scaled to the larger datasets. The GOSSIP adaptations to DP were estimated to complete all pairwise comparisons in the large datasets in the range from 9 (17.3) h to 5.1 (9.1) min on CATH (Astral), depending on how similar the lengths of the protein chains needed to be to consider an alignment. The longest runtimes were for comparisons in which the chain lengths need to be within only 60% of each other, and the shortest times required the chain lengths to be within 95% of each other. The accuracy of the method lies between the results of MultiProt [21] and YAKUSA [7], and while MultiProt better identifies structural similarity, it requires several hundred hours of computational time. GOSSIP bests YAKUSA's results while comparing reasonably with regard to run time.

13.4.2   Eigensystem Alignment with a Spectrum

As with the other methods described in this section, the central theme of aligning protein chains by *EIG*ensystem *A*lignment with the *S*pectrum (EIGAS) is to align the residues so that the matching is as similar as possible with regard to a measure of intra-similarity between the residues of the individual proteins. EIGAS uses a scaled version of the Euclidean distance between the Cα atoms of any two residues, a measure called smooth contact. A smooth-contact matrix C has as its

ijth element the smooth contact between residues i and j,

$$[C]_{ij} = \begin{cases} 1 - d(r_i, r_j)/\kappa, & d(r_i, r_j) \leq \kappa \\ 0, & \text{otherwise} \end{cases}$$

where $d(r_i, r_j)$ is the Euclidean distance between the Cα atoms of residues i and j. Euclidean distances less than the cutoff parameter κ are scaled linearly between the maximum smooth-contact value of 1, which occurs if $i = j$, and the minimum value of 0, which occurs if the distance between the residues exceeds κ. The smooth-contact measure is an assessment of the proximity of the residues. So the smooth contact between a residue and itself is 1. If κ is small, then the smooth contact between most residues is zero, but if κ is large, then more values are nonzero.

Smooth-contact matrices have the favorable mathematical property that they are positive definite, that is, that all eigenvalues are positive, for suitably small κ values. This follows from the fact that the diagonal elements are independent of the value of κ since a C_α atom is always in contact with itself, whereas the off-diagonal elements can be made arbitrarily small as κ decreases. Hence the sum of the off-diagonal elements of any row is guaranteed to be less than the diagonal element itself for sufficiently small κ, a property called *diagonal dominance*. A well-known result in linear algebra is that a diagonally dominant matrix is positive definite. The positive definite property guarantees that a smooth-contact matrix can be factored as

$$C = UDU^T = (U\sqrt{D})(U\sqrt{D})^T = R^T R \qquad (13.2)$$

where the columns of U form an orthonormal set of eigenvectors of C and D is a diagonal matrix of the positive eigenvalues. Moreover, a smooth-contact matrix imposes an inner product, and subsequently a norm and a metric, on $\mathbb{R}^n$, where n is the number of residues in the protein chain. So, each protein chain coincides with a geometric rendering of $\mathbb{R}^n$.

To illustrate the mathematical and geometric properties induced by a smooth-contact matrix, we consider a three-residue protein chain whose smooth-contact matrix is located in Figure 13.7. The inner product of the vectors v and w induced by the smooth-contact matrix is $<v, w>_C = v^T C w$, which has the following properties:

- $\sqrt{v^T C v} = \|v\|_C$ is the norm of v relative to C.
- $v^T C w / \|v\|_C \|w\|_C$ is the cosine of the angle between v and w.
- $\sqrt{(v-w)^T C (v-w)} = \|v - w\|_C$ is the distance between v and w relative to C.

The inner product supports an embedding of the residues in an n-dimensional space so that the smooth contact between any two residues is the result of an inner

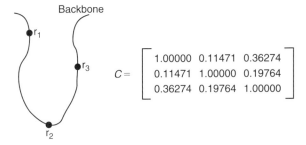

Figure 13.7   The path of the backbone indicates that the Euclidean distances between residues 1 and 3 and between 2 and 3 are shorter than the distance between residues 1 and 2. This is seen in the smooth-contact matrix since both $C_{13} = 0.36274$ and $C_{23} = 0.19764$, both of which are greater than $C_{12} = 0.11471$.

product calculation. Let the first residue be associated with $e_1 = (1, 0, 0, \ldots, 0)^T$, the second with $e_2 = (0, 1, 0, \ldots, 0)^T$, and so on. Then $e_i^T C e_j = C_{ij}$, which is the smooth contact between residues i and j, for example, $e_1^T C e_3 = C_{13} = 0.36274$ for the smooth-contact matrix in Figure 13.7.

The vector space $\mathbb{R}^n$ with the inner product $< v, w >_C$ is called a *contact space*, and the geometry induced by C is, in some sense, a "skewed" Euclidean geometry. As an illustration we note that a sphere is the collection of unit length vectors, which in contact space means that v is on the sphere only if $\|v\|_C = 1$. Such a collection is an ellipsoid because the metric is scaled by C. The unit ellipsoid with respect to the contact matrix in Figure 13.7 is depicted in Figure 13.8. The residues are represented by the thick dark vectors e_1, e_2, and e_3, which lie along the standard axes. The angle between e_i and e_j is not as it appears in the figure. For example, in Euclidean geometry the angle between e_1 and e_3 is $90°$, but in contact space the angle is $\cos^{-1}(0.36274) = 68.731°$. Also, in Euclidean geometry the distance between between e_1 and e_3 is $\sqrt{2} \approx 1.4142$, but in contact space the distance is $\sqrt{(e_1 - e_3)^T C (e_1 - e_3)} = 1.1289$.

The motivation behind EIGAS is that each protein is associated with an n-dimensional geometry, and this perspective allows the problem of aligning protein structures to be restated as a question of optimally aligning the geometries of contact spaces. However, contact spaces vary in dimension just as protein chains vary in length, and the algorithmic design question is to create a method of matching the residues so that the lower-dimensional geometries of the two contact spaces are as similar as possible.

Contact geometries are defined by the eigenvectors and eigenvalues, which give the direction and length of the unit ellipsoid's principal axes. Moreover, the eigenvectors are linear combinations of the e_i vectors. So, in terms of the protein, each eigenvector represents a weighted sum of the residues in contact space. In some research communities these weighted sums would be called "features" of the protein. Each residue is associated with its nearest eigenvector and is assigned

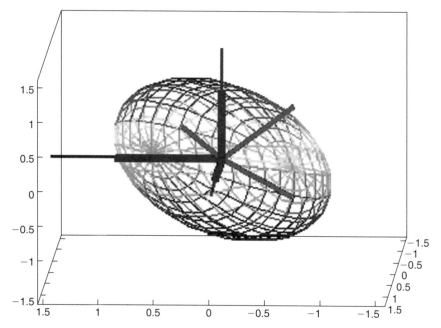

Figure 13.8   The ellipsoid is the collection of all unit length vectors with respect to the contact matrix in Figure 13.7. The thick dark vectors represent the residues and are e_1 (pointing to the left), e_2 (pointing out from the page), and e_3 (pointing upward). The thin vectors are the orthonormal eigenvectors that form the columns of U in Equation (13.2). The eigenvectors lie along the principal axes of the ellipsoid, and the length of each axis is $2/\sqrt{\lambda}$.

its corresponding eigenvalue. Formally, residue r_i is assigned the eigenvalue λ_k, where the associated eigenvector u_k of the smooth-contact matrix solves

$$\max_t \left| \frac{u_t^T C e_i}{\|u_t\|_C \|e_i\|_C} \right| = \max_t |R_{ti}|$$

where u_t denotes the eigenvectors that comprise the columns of U and $R = \sqrt{D}U^T$ from Equation (13.2). This eigenvalue assignment associates each residue with one of the principal axes of the ellipsoid defined by the smooth-contact map. A matching of the residues between the protein chains is scored by comparing the eigenvalues associated with the corresponding principal axes.

Consider the problem of matching the protein chain in Figure 13.7 with the chain in Figure 13.9. The middle three residues of the chain in Figure 13.9 are in the same configuration as the residues in Figure 13.7, and one would expect an alignment technique to match r_1 with r_2', r_2 with r_3', and r_3 with r_4'. The eigenvalues of the smooth-contact matrix in Figure 13.7 are 1.47, 0.91, and 0.63, and the eigenvalues of the smooth-contact matrix in Figure 13.9 are 1.62, 1.05,

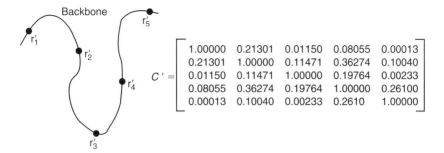

Figure 13.9 Residues r_2', r_3', and r_4' are in the same geometric configuration with r_1, r_2, and r_3, respectively, in Figure 13.7

0.99, 0.76, and 0.57. Assigning the residues the eigenvalues of their nearest eigenspaces leads to the matching problem depicted below:

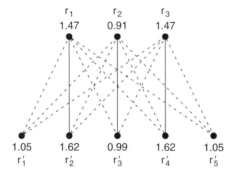

The optimal three-residue matching is shown by the solid edges. The optimal value is the combined eigenvalue difference, $|1.47 - 1.62| + |0.91 - 0.99| + |1.47 - 1.62| = 0.38$, which is the lowest possible among all matchings of three residues. Note that this is the anticipated alignment.

The value of matching residue i with residue j is estimated by $S_{ij} = |\lambda_i - \lambda_j|$. If the eigenvalues are similar, then the principal axes of the unit ellipsoids associated with the residues are of approximately the same length. Hence the contact geometries are similar along these particular axes. EIGAS uses the scoring matrix $[S]_{ij}$ and DP to find an optimal matching between the residues. EIGAS was reported [22] to correctly identify the SCOP classification of the Skolnick40 dataset by completing all 780 comparisons in about ~58 s. On Proteus300 EIGAS completed all 44,850 comparisons in about ~1.2 h. The best results in terms of quality were achieved with $\kappa = 14$ Å and a gap penalty of 1. More recent results [11] show that EIGAS can complete all 44,850 comparisons in 137 seconds if the DP is coded in C++ and the computational effort is distributed over eight cores. This more recent numerical work shows that if $\kappa = 17$ Å, the

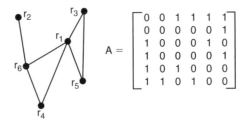

Figure 13.10 A graphical representation of a protein chain of six residues along with its adjacency matrix.

gap opening penalty is 0.9, and the gap extension penalty is 0.4, then EIGAS correctly identifies the SCOP classifications of Proteus300 (perfect classifications were reported for many parameter combinations).

13.4.3 A_purva

As is often the case in applied mathematics, the concept of structure can be represented in terms of graph theory, and this is the manner in which contact map overlap (CMO) is derived. The backbone of each protein chain is represented as a graph, say, (V, E). The vertices in V represent the Cα atoms, and two Cα atoms are adjacent, meaning that they form an edge in E, if the distance between them satisfies a contact criteria. For example, if $0 < d(r_i, r_j) < \kappa$, then residues i and j are in contact and (r_i, r_j) induces an edge in E. We let V be the index set $\{1, 2, \ldots, |V|\}$ and E be the collection of edges (i, j) such that $d(r_i, r_j)$ satisfies the contact criteria. A_purva [1] uses an upper bound of $\kappa = 7.5$ Å, and edges for consecutive residues along the protein backbone are not permitted. If we let A_{ij} form a binary matrix with a value of 1 if residues i and j satisfy the contact criteria, then we have represented the protein chain as a graph associated with this adjacency matrix (see Fig. 13.10).

The goal of CMO is to optimize a pairing between the graphical representations of the two proteins, meaning that we want to pair residues so that their contact structures match as well as possible. This question is similar to the classic NP-hard problem of finding a maximum induced subgraph, which is to find the largest possible subgraph of one graph that is a subgraph of the other. However, CMO adds the constraint that the sequential ordering of the nodes must be preserved in the vertex matching. For example, if r_1 of the first protein is matched with r_3' of the second, then r_2 of the first protein cannot be matched to r_2' of the second since this would violate the linear ordering inherited from a protein's backbone. Residue r_2 could be matched to any r_k' of the second protein as long as $k > 3$.

To accomplish the residue matching, the graphs of two proteins are joined to create a bipartite graph. Let (V^1, E^1) and (V^2, E^2) be the graphs of two proteins and A and A' be their respective adjacency matrices. Form the complete bipartite graph between the two vertex sets, meaning that every possible edge between V^1

and V^2 is included. The edge sets E^1 and E^2 are used to weight every possible pair of matches, indexed by (i,j,k,l) to indicate that r_i of the first protein is matched with r'_k of the second and that r_j of the first is matched with r'_l of the second. Each (i,j,k,l) is assigned the product of the corresponding elements of the adjacency matrices:

$$A_{ij}A'_{kl} = \begin{cases} 1, & (i,j) \in E^1 \text{ and } (k,l) \in E^2 \\ 0, & \text{otherwise} \end{cases}$$

We say that the paired residue matches (r_i, r'_k) and (r_j, r'_l) share a common contact provided that $A_{ij}A'_{kl}$ is 1. As an example, if we are trying to align the protein depicted in Figure 13.10 with a four-residue protein in which the only contacts are between r'_1 and r'_3 and between r'_2 and r'_4, then $A_{13}A'_{13} = 1$ but $A_{26}A'_{12} = 0$. A schematic is depicted in Figure 13.11.

The bipartite weights are used to score matchings between the residue sets by adding all possible weights in the matching. If r_i is matched with r'_i, for $i = 1, 2, 3, 4$, in the example above, then this matching has a contact score of

$$A_{12}A'_{12} + A_{13}A'_{13} + A_{14}A'_{14} + A_{23}A'_{23} + A_{24}A'_{24} + A_{34}A'_{34}$$
$$= 0 + 1 + 0 + 0 + 0 + 0 = 1$$

This value indicates that the only overlap of this residue matching is due to the fact that matching r_1 to r'_1 and r_3 to r'_3 yields a common contact. In matrix terms, the score is half of $\|(A_{I,R} \circ A'_{I,R})\|_1$, where I denotes the residues from the first protein; R, the residues from the second protein; the set subscripts, the submatrices whose rows and columns are listed in the sets; and $\circ$, the Hadamard (elementwise) product. The 1-norm is the elementwise norm and not the operator

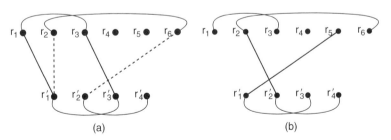

(a)   (b)

Figure 13.11   Diagram (a) depicts two possible pairs of matchings between two proteins. The pair depicted with solid lines is weighted with a one since r_1 is in contact with r_3 and r'_1 is in contact with r'_3. The pair depicted by dashed lines is weighted with a zero since r'_1 is not in contact with r'_2. Note that not all edges from Figure 13.10 are shown for the top protein. Diagram (b) shows a pairing that would not be allowed since it violates the residue ordering imposed by the proteins' backbones.

norm. To see the preceding calculation in this matrix form, let $I = R = \{1, 2, 3, 4\}$, which gives

$$A_{I,R} \circ A'_{I,R} = A_{I,R} \circ A'$$

$$= \begin{bmatrix} 0 & 0 & 1 & 1 \\ 0 & 0 & 0 & 0 \\ 1 & 0 & 0 & 0 \\ 1 & 0 & 0 & 0 \end{bmatrix} \circ \begin{bmatrix} 0 & 0 & 1 & 0 \\ 0 & 0 & 0 & 1 \\ 1 & 0 & 0 & 0 \\ 0 & 1 & 0 & 0 \end{bmatrix} = \begin{bmatrix} 0 & 0 & 1 & 0 \\ 0 & 0 & 0 & 0 \\ 1 & 0 & 0 & 0 \\ 0 & 0 & 0 & 0 \end{bmatrix}$$

As above, the only nonzero elements result from residues r_1 and r_3 being in contact in the first protein and residues r'_1 and r'_3 being in contact in the second. The symmetry of the adjacency matrices doubles the score. The matrix description shows that we are looking for ordered index sets of the residues from both proteins so that the elementwise product of the resulting adjacency submatrices has as many ones as possible.

The combinatorial problem of maximizing the contact overlap can be stated as a binary optimization problem. For the ith residue in V^m, with m indicating either the first or second protein, let $\delta_m^+(i) = \{j : j > i, (i,j) \in E^m\}$ and $\delta_m^-(i) = \{j : j < i, (i,j) \in E^m\}$. We let y_{ijkl} be a binary variable indicating that if we match r_i of the first protein with r'_k of the second and r_j of the first with r'_l of the second. We also let x_{ik} be a binary variable indicating if r_i of the first protein is matched with r'_k of the second. With this notation, the standard formulation of the CMO problem is

$$\max \sum_{\substack{(i,j) \in E^1 \\ (k,l) \in E^2}} y_{ijkl} \qquad = \max \sum_{(ijkl)} A_{ij} A'_{kl} y_{ijkl}$$

subject to

$$\sum_{j \in \delta_1^+(i)} y_{ijkl} \leq x_{ik}, \qquad \forall\, i \in V^1,\, (k,l) \in E^2$$

$$\sum_{i \in \delta_1^-(j)} y_{ijkl} \leq x_{jl}, \qquad \forall\, j \in V^1,\, (k,l) \in E^2$$

$$\sum_{l \in \delta_2^+(k)} y_{ijkl} \leq x_{ik}, \qquad \forall\, k \in V^2,\, (i,j) \in E^1 \tag{13.3}$$

$$\sum_{k \in \delta_2^-(l)} y_{ijkl} \leq x_{jl}, \qquad \forall\, l \in V^2,\, (i,j) \in E^1$$

$$x_{ik} + x_{jl} \leq 1, \qquad \begin{aligned} &\forall\, 1 \leq i \leq j \leq |V^1|,\, i \neq j \\ &\forall\, 1 \leq k \leq l \leq |V^2|,\, k \neq l \end{aligned}$$

$$x_{ik} \in \{0,1\}, \qquad \forall\, i \in V^1,\, k \in V^2$$

$$y_{ijkl} \in \{0,1\}, \qquad \forall\, (i,j) \in E^1,\, (k,l) \in E^2$$

Solving the CMO problem has drawn much attention, and many have argued favorably for this alignment method. However, the combinatorial complexity of

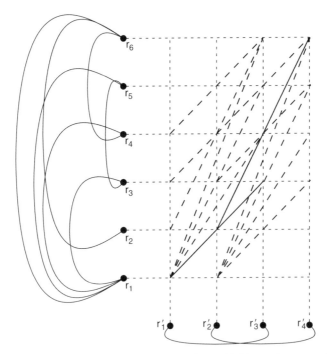

Figure 13.12   The contacts of the protein from Figure 13.11 are shown on the left, and the contacts for the second protein are shown at the bottom. The new graph links pairs of residue matches if they share a contact. All edges of the new graph are shown as either dashed or solid lines, with the solid lines indicating an optimal solution of (r_1, r'_1), (r_2, r'_2), (r_3, r'_3), and (r_6, r'_4). The optimal value of the CMO problem is 2 because this is the maximum number of noncrossing edges.

the problem has challenged it with becoming an efficient model for working with entire databases. More recent work [11] shows otherwise. The insight is to reformulate the problem so that the new formulation lends itself to DP.

The reformulation is interpreted on a new graph $(V^1 \times V^2, \mathcal{E})$, where $\mathcal{E} = \{(i, k, j, l) : A_{ij} A'_{kl} = 1\}$. In this new graph each vertex is an ordered pair of vertices, and each edge corresponds to a matched pair of residues that share a contact. In terms of the protein chains, each vertex of this graph is a possible match between the residues of the different proteins, and an edge exists between a pair of possible residue matches only if they share a common contact. A depiction of this graph is found in Figure 13.12.

The reformulation hints at how DP can be used to solve the CMO problem. The central concept is to move from the lower left corner toward the upper right corner in an optimal fashion. Unlike the other alignment algorithms discussed in this section, which require a single application of DP, the method of A_purva requires a coupling of two DP algorithms. The two decisions are (1) where to link any possible match, called the *local problem*; and (2) how to construct on optimal sequence from the local decisions, called the *global problem*. The example in Figure 13.12 illustrates the decisions. From the match (r_1, r_1') we could have selected any of (r_3, r_3'), (r_4, r_3'), (r_5, r_3') or (r_6, r_3'). In all but (r_6, r_3') we could have found a second nonintersecting edge that would have given a CMO score of 2. For example, if we had instead used the edge from (r_1, r_1') to (r_5, r_3'), then we could have added the edge from (r_4, r_2') to (r_6, r_4'). The local decision has to assess which edges should be considered. Once we know the optimal local solutions for each (r_i, r_k'), we use this information to select the global collection of edges so as to maximize the number of edges while maintaining that edges don't cross.

The forward-looking perspective means that we are always making decisions for indices in δ_m^+, and hence we need to account for the constraints whose summands are over δ_m^-. Andonov et al. [1] use a classic Lagrangian relaxation that moves these constraints to the objective and penalizes them with multipliers. The relaxed problem maximizes

$$\sum_{\substack{(i,j)\in E^1 \\ (k,l)\in E^2}} y_{ijkl}$$

$$+ \sum_{\substack{j\in V^1 \\ (k,l)\in E^2}} \lambda_{jkl} \left(x_{jl} - \sum_{i\in\delta_1^-(j)} y_{ijkl} - \sum_{\substack{s=k+1\ldots l-1 \\ t=1 \\ (t,s)\in E^1}} y_{tskl} - \sum_{\substack{s=1\ldots k-1 \\ t=j-1 \\ (t,s)\in E^1}} y_{tskl} \right)$$

$$+ \sum_{\substack{l\in V^2 \\ (i,j)\in E^1}} \sigma_{ijl} \left(x_{jl} - \sum_{k\in\delta_2^-(l)} y_{ijkl} - \sum_{\substack{s=k+1\ldots j-1 \\ t=1 \\ (s,t)\in E^2}} y_{stkl} - \sum_{\substack{s=1\ldots k-1 \\ t=l-1 \\ (s,t)\in E^2}} y_{stkl} \right)$$

subject to

$$\sum_{j\in\delta_1^+(i)} y_{ijkl} \le x_{ik}, \qquad \forall\, i \in V^1,\ (k,l) \in E^2$$

$$\sum_{l\in\delta_2^+(k)} y_{ijkl} \le x_{ik}, \qquad \forall\, k \in V^2,\ (i,j) \in E^1$$

$$x_{ik} + x_{jl} \le 1, \qquad \forall\, 1 \le i \le j \le |V^1|,\ i \ne j$$

$$\qquad\qquad\qquad\qquad \forall\, 1 \le k \le l \le |V^2|,\ k \ne l$$

$$x_{ik} \in \{0, 1\}, \qquad \forall\, i \in V^1,\ k \in V^2$$

$$y_{ijkl} \in \{0, 1\}, \qquad \forall\, (i,j) \in E^1,\ (k,l) \in E^2$$

We note that this is not directly a Lagrangian relaxation of (13.3) because of a tighter description of the feasible region. Specifically, the authors make the following replacements in (13.3):

$$\sum_{i \in \delta_1^-(j)} y_{ijkl} \le x_{jl} \Rightarrow \sum_{i \in \delta_1^-(j)} y_{ijkl} + \sum_{\substack{s=k+1 \dots l-1 \\ t=1 \\ (t,s) \in E^1}} y_{tskl} + \sum_{\substack{s=1 \dots k-1 \\ t=j-1 \\ (t,s) \in E^1}} y_{tskl} \le x_{jl}$$

$$\sum_{k \in \delta_2^-(l)} y_{ijkl} \le x_{jl} \Rightarrow \sum_{k \in \delta_2^-(l)} y_{ijkl} + \sum_{\substack{s=k+1 \dots j-1 \\ t=1 \\ (s,t) \in E^2}} y_{stkl} + \sum_{\substack{s=1 \dots k-1 \\ t=l-1 \\ (s,t) \in E^2}} y_{stkl} \le x_{jl}$$

The additional terms continue to satisfy the noncrossing property, but they give a more accurate description of the search space.

The Lagrange multipliers λ_{jkl} and σ_{ijl} are restricted to be nonnegative, and through the application of DP, the relaxed problem can be solved in polynomial time for any collection of Lagrange multipliers, as the complexity is no worse than $O(|V^1||V^2| + |\mathcal{E}|)$. The local use of DP creates a scoring matrix for each (i,k) in $V^1 \times V^2$. Specifically, let S_{ik}^L be the matrix whose rows are indexed by $\delta_1^+(i)$ and whose columns are indexed by $\delta_2^+(k)$. The score at each position is $[S_{ik}^L]_{jl} = 1 - \lambda_{jkl} - \sigma_{ijl}$, which corresponds to the coefficient of the y_{ijkl} variable in the objective. Let c_{ik}^* be the optimal value of applying DP to S_{ik}^L.

The global problem uses the local scores to create an optimal solution to the relaxed problem. Specifically, let S^G be the scoring matrix whose components for each $i \in V^1$ and $k \in V^2$ are

$$[S^G]_{ik} = c_{ik}^* + \sum_{j \in \delta_1^-(i)} \lambda_{jkl} + \sum_{k \in \delta_2^-(l)} \sigma_{ijl}$$

Note that the last two summations are the coefficients for the x_{jl} variables, and that the remaining portion of the objective collapses into c_{ik}^*. Hence, an optimal solution to the Lagrangian relaxation for any nonnegative collections of λ_{jkl} and σ_{ijl} can be calculated with a double application of DP.

While the relaxation can be solved efficiently, the relaxed solution is not a solution to the original CMO problem unless the Lagrange multipliers satisfy an optimality condition of their own. The optimization problem that defines a collection of multipliers for which the relaxed problem actually solves the CMO problem is called the *dual-optimization problem*, which is a minimization problem over the Lagrange multipliers for a fixed collection of x and y variables. A discussion of this topic is outside the scope of this chapter, but interested readers can find descriptions in most nonlinear programming texts [2]. The Lagrangian process is iterative in that starting with initial Lagrange multipliers, the relaxation is solved with DP, and then the Lagrange multipliers are updated by (nearly) solving the dual problem. The process repeats and is stopped once the value of the CMO problem is sufficiently close to the optimal value of the dual problem or due to a time limitation. For details about how A_purva updates the Lagrange multipliers, see the paper by Andonov et al. [1].

Iterative Lagrangian algorithms are a mainstay in the nonlinear programming community, and a common sentiment among experts in optimization is that problems either do or do not lend themselves to this tactic. The numerical tests for A_purva show that the relaxation of CMO lends itself nicely to this solution procedure. A_purva was tested as a database comparison algorithm on both Skolnick40 [6] and Proteus300 [1]. Reported solution times were 357 s for all 780 pairwise comparisons for Skolnick40 (approximately 0.46 s per comparison) and 13 h and 38 min for all 44,850 comparisons for Proteus300 (approximately 1.09 s per comparison). The comparisons were perfect in their agreement with the SCOP classification via clustering with Chavl [16]. Although not as fast as either of the other techniques discussed in this section, the results are significant advances for CMO, which before A_purva would have been impractical for a dataset like Proteus300.

13.4.4 Comments on Dynamic Programming and Future Research Directions

The application of DP to align protein structures is not restricted to the more recent literature on database applications, and in particular, DP was one of the early solution methods for the CMO problem, [6,14]. However, the more recent literature indicates that DP is becoming a central algorithmic method to efficiently align protein structures well enough for classification across a sizable database. Other research groups are arriving at the same conclusion about DP [24]. Indeed, as the authors were preparing this document they found additional examples in the more recent literature [5].

With the emerging success that DP is having, we feel compelled to note a few of its limitations. First, DP is a sequential decision process that is optimal only under the Markov property, that is, that the current decision does not depend on past decisions. All the applications of DP discussed here use the natural sequence of the backbone to order the decisions process, but using DP in this fashion does not allow for the possibility of nonsequential alignments. The ability to identify nonsequential alignments is argued by some as a crucial element to identifying protein families [8]. Adapting the DP framework to consider nonsequential alignments is a promising and important avenue for future research.

One of the concerns about three-dimensional alignment methods is that they don't easily adapt to a protein's natural flexibility. Many proteins have several confirmations, and an alignment method that can correctly classify the different confirmations would be beneficial. Moreover, the crystallography and NMR experiments from which we gain three-dimensional coordinates are not without error, and the alignment methods should be robust enough to correctly classify proteins under coordinate perturbations. Whether methods based on DP provide the robustness to handle a protein's flexibility and experimental error is not yet well established. Hasegawa and Holm [10] suggest that more attention should be focused on the robustness of the optimization procedures used to align protein structures.

Finally, DP requires tuning that is experimental in nature. The gap opening and gap extension penalties need to be experimentally set to achieve agreement with biological classifications. Parameter tuning has not been shown to be database-independent, and without such experimental validation, we lack the confidence that DP-based methods can be used to organize a database without an a priori biological classification, which somewhat defeats the purpose of automating database classification.

REFERENCES

1. Andonov R, Malod-Dognin N, Yanev N, Maximum contact map overlap revisited, *J. Comput. Biol.* **18**(1):27–41 (Jan. 2011).

2. Bazaraa M, Sherali H, Shetty C, *Nonlinear Programming: Theory and Algorithms*, 3rd ed., Wiley-Interscience, 2006.

3. Bellman R, *Dynamic Programming*, Princeton Univ. Press, Princeton, NJ, 1957.

4. Bhattacharya S, Bhattacharyya C, Chandra N, Projections for fast protein structure retrieval, *BMC Bioinformatics* **7**(Suppl. 5):S5 (2006).

5. Bonnel N, Marteau P, *LNA: Fast Protein Classification Using a Laplacian Characterization of Tertiary Structure*, Technical Report, Univ. Bretagne Sud, France, 2011.

6. Caprara A, Carr R, Istrail S, Lancia G, Walenz B, 1001 optimal pdb structure alignments: Integer programming methods for finding the maximum contact map overlap, *J. Comput. Biol.* **11**(1):27–52 (2004).

7. Carpentier M, Brouillet S, Pothier J, Yakusa: A fast structural database scanning method, *Proteins* **61**(1):137–151 (Oct. 2005).

8. Chen L, Wu L, Wang Y, Zhang S, Zhang X, Revealing divergent evolution, identifying circular permutations and detecting active-sites by protein structure comparison, *BMC Struct Biol.* **6**:18 (2006).

9. Goldman D, Istrail S, Papadimitriou C, Algorithmic aspects of protein structure similarity. *Proc. 40th Annual Symp. Foundations of Computer Science*, 1999, pp. 512–521.

10. Hasegawa H, Holm L, Advances and pitfalls of protein structural alignment, *Curr. Opin. Struct. Biol.* **19**(3):341–348 (June 2009).

11. Holder A, Simon J, Strauser J, Shibberu Y, *An Investigation into the Robustness of Algorithms Designed for Efficient Protein Structure Alignment across Databases*, Technical Report, Rose-Hulman Inst. Technology, 2012.

12. Kifer I, Nussinov R, Wolfson H, Gossip: A method for fast and accurate global alignment of protein structures, *Bioinformatics* **27**(7):925–932 (2011).

13. Kolodny R, Linial N, Approximate protein structural alignment in polynomial time, *Proc Natl Acad Sci USA* **101**(33):12201–12206 (Aug. 2004).

14. Lancia G, Carr R, Walenz B, Istrail S, 101 optimal pdb structure alignments: A branch-and-cut algorithm for the maximum contact map overlap problem, *Proc. 5th Annual Int. Conf. Computational Biology*, ACM Press, New York, 2001, pp. 143–202.

15. Di Lena P, Fariselli P, Margara L, Vassura M, Casadio R, Fast overlapping of protein contact maps by alignment of eigenvectors, *Bioinformatics* **26**(18):2250–2258 (Sept. 2010).

16. Lerman I, Likelihood linkage analysis (lla) classification method, *Biochimie* **75**:379–397 (1993).

17. Cheng Li S, Kaow Ng Y, On protein structure alignment under distance constraint, *Theor. Comput. Sci.* **412**(32):4187–4199 (2011) (algorithms and computation).

18. Needleman S, Wunsch C, A general method applicable to the search for similarities in the amino acid sequence of two proteins, *J. Mol. Biol.* **48**(3):443–453 (March 1970).

19. Poleksic A, Algorithms for optimal protein structure alignment, *Bioinformatics*, **25**(21):2751–2756 (Nov. 2009).

20. Poleksic A, Optimizing a widely used protein structure alignment measure in expected polynomial time, *IEEE/ACM Trans. Comput. Biol. Bioinform.* **8**(6):1716–1720 (2011).

21. Shatsky M, Nussinov R, Wolfson H, A method for simultaneous alignment of multiple protein structures, *Proteins* **56**(1):143–156 (July 2004).

22. Shibberu Y, Holder A, A spectral approach to protein structure alignment, *IEEE/ACM Trans. Comput. Biol. Bioinform.* **8**:867–875 (Feb. 2011).

23. Umeyama S, An eigendecomposition approach to weighted graph matching problems, *IEEE Trans. Pattern Anal. Machine Intell.* **10**(5):695–703 (1988).

24. Wohlers I, Andonov R, Klau G, *Algorithm Engineering for Optimal Alignment of Protein Structure Distance Matrices*, Technical Report, CWI, Life Sciences Group, Netherlands, 2011.

25. Xu J, Jiao F, Berger B, A parameterized algorithm for protein structure alignment, *J. Comput. Biol.* **14**(5):564–577 (June 2007).

CHAPTER 14

DISCOVERING 3D PROTEIN STRUCTURES FOR OPTIMAL STRUCTURE ALIGNMENT

TOMÁŠ NOVOSÁD, VÁCLAV SNÁŠEL, AJITH ABRAHAM, and
JACK Y. YANG

14.1 INTRODUCTION

Analyzing three-dimensional protein structures is a very important task in molecular biology. Nowadays, the solution for protein structures often stems from the use of the state-of-the-art technologies such as nuclear magnetic resonance (NMR) spectroscopy techniques or X-ray crystallography as seen in the increasing number of PDB [34] entries. The Protein Data Bank (PDB) is a database of 3D structural data of large biological molecules, such as proteins and nucleic acids. It was proved that structurally similar proteins tend to have similar functions even if their amino acid sequences are not similar to one another. Thus, it is very important to find proteins with similar structures (even in part) from the growing database to analyze protein functions. Yang et al. [47] exploited machine learning techniques, including variants of self-organizing global ranking, a decision tree, and support vector machine (SVM) algorithms to predict the tertiary structure of transmembrane proteins. Hecker et al. [14] developed a state-of-the-art protein disorder predictor and tested it on a large protein disorder dataset created from the PDB. The relationship between of sensitivity and specificity is also evaluated. Habib et al. [11] presented a new SVM-based approach to predict the subcellular locations based on amino acid and amino acid pair composition. More protein features can be factored in to improve the accuracy significantly. Wang et al. [45] discussed an empirical approach to specify the localization of protein binding regions utilizing information including the distribution pattern of the detected RNA fragments and the sequence specificity of RNase digestion.

Algorithmic and Artificial Intelligence Methods for Protein Bioinformatics. First Edition.
Edited by Yi Pan, Jianxin Wang, Min Li.
© 2014 John Wiley & Sons, Inc. Published 2014 by John Wiley & Sons, Inc.

Another important aproach of protein structural similarity is based on database indexing methods. Gao and Zaki [9] proposed a method for indexing protein tertiary structure by extracting a protein local feature vectors and suffix trees. Shibuya [43] developed a structure called *geometric suffix tree*, which indexes protein 3D structures based on their Cα atoms' 3D coordinates.

These studies are often targeted mainly at some kind of selection of the PDB database. In our past work [28,29] we focused on the task of computing all-to-all protein similarities, which appear in the current PDB database, based on their 3D structural features. The structural similarity defined between any two proteins in PDB can be calculated using information retrieval methods and schemes and suffix trees. These methods were previously widely studied and are commonly used these days [5,13,21,23,49]. To be able to evaluate the precision of the methods used to determine the protein structural similarity, it is important to compare the results toward the existing state-of-the-art techniques or databases. The existing state-of-the-art databases of protein structural similarities include DALI [15], SCOP [42], and CATH [3].

14.2   PROTEIN STRUCTURE

Proteins are large molecules that provide structure and control reactions in all cells. In many cases only a small part of the structure—*an active site*—is directly functional, and the remainder exists only to create and fix the spatial relationship among the active site residues [19]. Chemically, protein molecules are long polymers typically containing several thousand atoms, composed of a uniform repetitive backbone (or mainchain) with a particular sidechain attached to each residue. The amino acid sequence of a protein records the succession of sidechains. There are 20 different amino acids that make up essentially all protein molecules on Earth. Every amino acid has its own original design composed of a central carbon (also called the *alpha carbon*, Cα), which is bonded to hydrogen, carboxylic acid group, amino group and unique sidechain or R group (e.g., see Fig. 14.1). The chemical properties of the R group are what give an amino acid its character.

The Danish protein chemist K. U. Linderstrøm-Lang described the protein structure in three different levels: primary structure, secondary structure, and tertiary structure. For proteins composed of more than one subunit, J. D. Bernall called the assembly of the monomers the *quaternary structure*.

14.2.1   Primary Structure

The unique sequence of amino acids in a protein is termed the *primary structure*. When amino acids form a protein chain, a unique bond, termed the *peptide bond*, exists between two amino acids. The sequence of a protein begins with the amino of the first amino acid and continues to the carboxyl end of the last amino acid. Each amino acid has its own unique one-letter abbreviation (e.g., alanine—A,

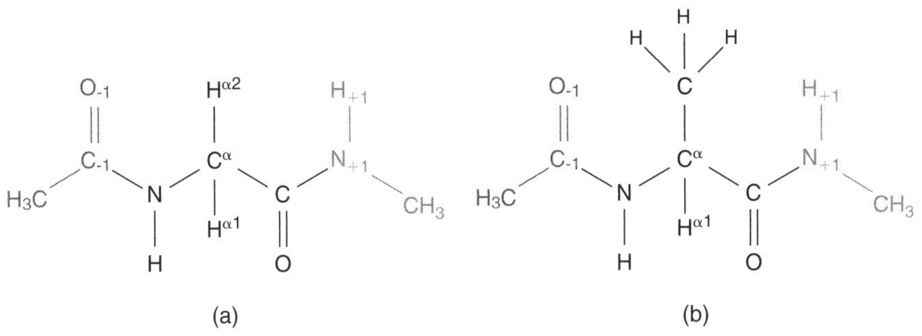

Figure 14.1 Chemical structure of two amino acids: (a) glycine; (b) alanine.

methionine—M, arginine—R). Thus the primary structure of the protein can be expressed as a string of these letters. Examples of protein primary structure encoding are as follows:

```
MVLSEGEWQLVLHVWAKVEADVAGHGQDILIRLFKSHPETLEKFDRVKHL...
MNIFEMLRIDEGLRLKIYKDTEGYYTIGIGHLLTKSPSLNAAKSELDKAI...
AYIAKQRQISFVKSHFSRQLEERLGLIEVQAPILSRVGDGTQDNLSGAEK...
```

14.2.2 Secondary Structure

The second level in the hierarchy of protein structure consists of the various spatial arrangements resulting from the folding of localized parts of a polypeptide chain; these arrangements are referred to as *secondary structures* [20]. These foldings are either in a helical shape, called the *alpha helix* (α helix) (which was first proposed by Linus Pauling et. al in 1951 [32]), or a *beta-pleated sheet* (β sheet) shaped similar to the zigzag foldings of an accordion. The turns of the α helix are stabilized by hydrogen bonding between every fourth amino acid in the chain. The β-pleated sheet is formed by folding successive planes [35]. Each plane is five to eight amino acids long. Both α helices and β sheets are linked by less structured loop regions to form domains (Fig. 14.2). The domains can potentionaly form fully functional proteins.

14.2.3 Tertiary Structure

The term *tertiary structure* (Fig. 14.3) refers to the overall conformation of a polypeptide chain, that is, the 3D arrangement of all its amino acid residues. Each atom of amino acid residue has its own 3D x, y, z coordinates. In contrast with secondary structures, which are stabilized by hydrogen bonds, tertiary structure is stabilized primarily by hydrophobic interactions between the nonpolar sidechains, hydrogen bonds between polar sidechains, and peptide bonds. These stabilizing forces hold elements of secondary structure α helices, β strands, turns,

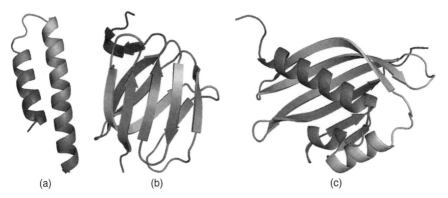

Figure 14.2   Secondary structure elements and domain example: (a) α helix; (b) β sheet; (c) domain.

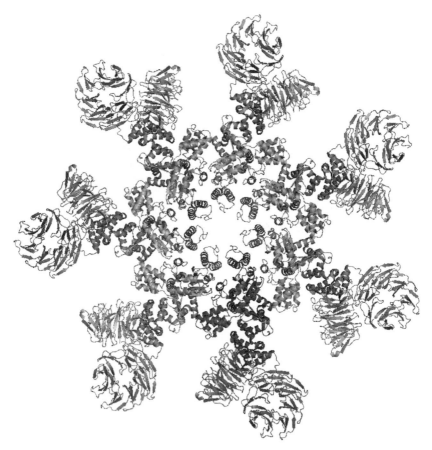

Figure 14.3   Tertiary structure of an apoptosome–procaspase 9 CARD complex.

and random coils compactly together. The most the protein structures ($\sim$90%) available in the Protein Data Bank have been resolved by X-ray crystallography. This method allows one to measure the 3D density distribution of electrons in the protein (in the crystallized state) and thereby infer the 3D coordinates of all the atoms to be determined to a certain resolution. Only $\sim$9% of the known protein structures have been obtained by nuclear magnetic resonance techniques (NMR spectroscopy) [2].

14.2.4 Quaternary Structure

Some proteins need to functionally associate with others as subunits in a multimeric structure. This is called the *quaternary structure* of the protein. This can also be stabilized by disulfide bonds and by noncovalent interactions with reacting substrates or cofactors. An excellent example of quaternary structure is hemoglobin. Adult hemoglobin consists of two alpha (α) subunits and two beta (β) subunits, held together by noncovalent interactions [35].

14.3 PROTEIN DATABASES

Currently there exist several protein databases publicly available online. These databases assembles various data about proteins, protein structures, protein functions, protein relationships, and other information. Probably the main and most valuable database is the PDB, which consists of protein 3D structures resolved by state-of-the-art techniques such as X-ray crystallography or NMR spectroscopy. Other online databases are generated by automated computer methods or by biologists themselves.

14.3.1 Protein Data Bank (PDB)

The PDB was established in 1971 at Brookhaven National Laboratory and originally contained seven structures. Nowadays the PDB archive contains almost 80,000 resolved structures and is still growing practically every day. The PDB archive is the single worldwide repository that contains information about experimentally determined structures of proteins, nucleic acids, and complex assemblies. The structures in the archive range from tiny proteins and bits of DNA to complex molecular machines like the ribosome. The structures in this archive is resolved by the state-of-the-art methods X-ray crystallography and NMR spectroscopy. As a member of the wwwPDB, the RCSB PDB curates and annotates PDB data according to established standards [34]. The PDB archive freely available to everyone and is updated each week at target time of Wednesday 00:00 UTC (Coordinated Universal Time). This database can be accessed online at http://www.pdb.org. The structures can also be downloaded from their FTP service at ftp://ftp.wwpdb.org/pub/pdb/.

14.3.2 Structural Classification of Proteins (SCOP)

This database provides a detailed and comprehensive description of the structural and evolutionary relationships of proteins whose 3D structures have been determined by X-ray crystallography or NMR spectroscopy (PDB entries). The most recent version 1.75 (June 2009) of this database includes 38,221 PDB entries. Classification of protein structures in the database is based on evolutionary relationships and on the principles that govern their 3D structure. The method used to construct the protein classification in SCOP is essentially the visual inspection and comparison of structures, although various automatic tools are used to make the task manageable and help provide generality [24–27,42]. Each protein entry in the SCOP database (each chain of protein, respectively) is classified into the class, folding pattern, superfamily, family, domain, and species categories. These categories are hierarchically arranged from class to species. The SCOP database is accessible at no cost for the user at `http://scop.mrc-lmb.cam.ac.uk/scop/`.

14.3.3 CATH Protein Structure Classification

The CATH is a database constructed using a semiautomatic method for hierarchical classification of protein domains [31]. The CATH stands for *c*lass, *a*rchitecture, *t*opology and *h*omologous superfamily. CATH shares many broad features with its main rival, SCOP; however there are also many areas in which the detailed classification differs greatly. CATH defines four classes: mostly α, mostly β, α and β and a few secondary structures. Much of the work in the CATH database is done by automatic methods toward the SCOP, although there are important manual tasks in the classification. The most important step in CATH classification is to separate the proteins into domains. The domains are next automatically sorted into classes and clustered on the basis of sequence similarities. These clusters (groups) form the *H levels* of the classification (homologous superfamily groups). The topology level is formed by structural comparisons of the homologous groups. Finally, the architecture level is assigned manually [31]. For more detailed descriptions of the CATH database building process and comparison with SCOP and other databases, please see References 6 and 12. The CATH database can be accessed and searched at `http://www.cathdb.info/`.

14.3.4 Distance Matrix Alignment (DALI)

The DALI database is based on exhaustive all-against-all 3D structure comparison of protein structures currently in the PDB. The structural neighborhoods and alignments are automatically maintained and regularly updated using the DALI search engine. The DALI algorithm works with 3D coordinates of each protein that are used to calculate residue-to-residue ($C\alpha$—$C\alpha$) distance matrices. The distance matrices are first decomposed into elementary contact patterns, such as hexapeptide–hexapeptide submatrices. Then, similar contact patterns in the two matrices are paired and combined into larger consistent sets of pairs. This method is fully automatic and identifies structural resemblances and common structural cores accurately and sensitively, even in the presence of geometric distortions [15,16]. The DALI database can be accessed from the DALI server at `http://ekhidna.biocenter.helsinki.fi/dali`.

14.4 VECTOR SPACE MODEL

The vector model [1] of documents was established in the 1970s [37,38]. A document in the vector model is represented as a vector. Each dimension (element) of this vector corresponds to a separate term appearing in document collection. If a term occurs in the document, its value in the vector is nonzero. The vector model is a widely used information retrieval scheme for measuring similarity between documents or between user query and documents in the collection [7,17,18,23,28,29,39,41].

In the vector model there are m different terms $t_1, \ldots, t_m$ for indexing N documents. Then each document d_i is represented by a vector

$$d_i = (w_{i1}, w_{i2}, \ldots, w_{im})$$

where w_{ij} is the weight of the term t_j in the document d_i. These term *weights* is ultimately used to compute the degree of similarity between all documents stored in the system and the user query. The weight of the term in the document vector can be determined in many ways. A common approach uses the so-called (term frequency × inverse document frequency (TF × IDF)) method [40], in which the weight of the term is determined by the frequency with which the term t_j occurs in the document d_i (the term frequency TF_{ij}) and how often it occurs in the whole document collection (the document frequency DF_j). Precisely, the weight of the term t_j in the document d_i is [8]

$$w_{ij} = TF_{ij} \times IDF_j = TF_{ij} \times \log \frac{n}{DF_j} \qquad (14.1)$$

where IDF stands for the inverse document frequency. This method assigns high weights to terms that appear frequently in a small number of documents in the document set.

An index file of the vector model is represented by the matrix

$$D = \begin{pmatrix} w_{11} & w_{12} & \cdots & w_{1m} \\ w_{21} & w_{22} & \cdots & w_{2m} \\ \vdots & \vdots & \ddots & \vdots \\ w_{n1} & w_{n2} & \cdots & w_{Nm} \end{pmatrix}$$

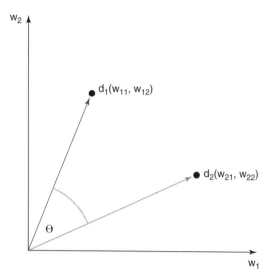

Figure 14.4   Geometric representation of cosine similarity.

where the ith row matches the ith document and the jth column matches the jth term.

The similarity between two documents in the vector model is usually expressed by the following formula (termed the *cosine similarity measure*):

$$sim(d_i, d_j) = \cos \theta = \frac{\sum_{k=1}^{m} (w_{ik} w_{jk})}{\sqrt{\sum_{k=1}^{m} (w_{ik})^2 \sum_{k=1}^{m} (w_{jk})^2}} \qquad (14.2)$$

Suppose that we have two documents $d_1 = (w_{11}, w_{12})$ and $d_2 = (w_{21}, w_{22})$, where w_{11}, w_{12} represent the weights of terms $t_1; t_2$, in document d_1; and w_{21}, w_{22}, the weights of terms t_1, t_2 in document d_2. Then the geometric representation of cosine similarity is as shown in Figure 14.4.

For more information about the vector space model, please consult the literature [1,22,33,37–39].

14.5   SUFFIX TREES

A *suffix tree* is a data structure that allows efficient string matching and querying. Suffix trees have been studied and used extensively, and have been applied to fundamental string problems such as finding the longest repeated substring [46], string comparisons [8], and text compression [36]. Following this, we describe the suffix tree data structure—its definition, construction algorithms, and main characteristics.

14.5.1 Definitions

The following description of the suffix tree was taken from Gusfield's book *Algorithms on Strings, Trees and Sequences* [10]. Suffix trees commonly deal with strings as a sequence of characters. One major difference is that we treat documents as sequences of words, not characters. A suffix tree of a string is simply a compact trie (a *trie* is also termed a *digital tree* or a *prefix tree*) of all the suffixes of that string. Zamir [48] provides the following definition.

Definition 14.1 A suffix tree T for an m-word string S is a rooted directed tree with exactly m leaves numbered from 1 to m. Each internal node, other than the root, has at least two children, and each edge is labeled with a nonempty substring of words of S. No two edges out of a node can have edge labels beginning with the same word. The key feature of the suffix tree is that for any leaf i, the concatenation of the edge labels on the path from the root to leaf i exactly spells out the suffix of S that starts at position i; that is, it spells out $S[i \cdots m]$.

In cases where one suffix of S matches a prefix of another suffix of S, then no suffix tree obeying Definition 14.1 is possible since the path for the first suffix would not end at a leaf. To avoid this, we assume that last word of S does not appear anywhere else in the string. This prevents any suffix from being a prefix to another suffix. To achieve this, we can add a terminating character, which is not in the language that S is taken from, to the end of S.

Suppose that we have a short protein sequence MALAGA that is a combination of four amino acids: methionine, alanine, leucine and glycine. An example of a suffix trie of the string MALAGA# is shown in Figure 14.5a. A corresponding suffix tree of the string MALAGA# is presented in Figure 14.5b. There are six leaves in this example, marked as rectangles and numbered from 1 to 6. The terminating characters are also shown in this figure.

In a similar manner, a suffix tree of a set of strings, called a *generalized suffix tree* [10], is a compact trie of all the suffixes of all the strings in the set [48], defined as follows.

Definition 14.2 A generalized suffix tree T for a set S of n strings S_n, each of length m_n, is a rooted directed tree with exactly $\sum m_n$ leaves marked by a two-number tuple (k, l), where k ranges from 1 to n and l ranges from 1 to m_k. Each internal node, other than the root, has at least two children, and each edge is labeled with a nonempty substring of words of a string in S. No two edges out of a node can have edge labels beginning with the same word. For any leaf (i, j), the concatenation of the edge labels on the path from the root to leaf (i, j) exactly spells out the suffix of S_i that starts at position j; that is, it spells out $S_i[j \ldots m_i]$.

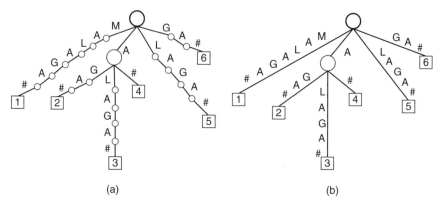

(a)   (b)

Figure 14.5   Simple example of suffix trie and suffix tree of string MALAGA#: (a) suffix trie; (b) suffix tree.

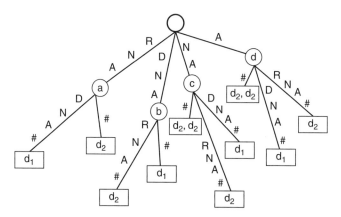

Figure 14.6   Example of the generalized suffix tree.

Figure 14.6 is an example of a generalized suffix tree of the set of two strings: RNADNA# and DNARNA#. The internal nodes of the suffix tree are drawn as circles, and are labeled from a to d. Leaves are drawn as rectangles, and numbers $d_i = (d_1, \ldots, d_n)$ in each rectangle indicate the string from which that suffix originates—a unique number that identifies the string. Each string is considered to have a unique terminating symbol.

14.5.2 Suffix Tree Construction Algorithms

The naive, straightforward method for building a suffix tree for a string S of length L takes $O(L^2)$ time. The naive method first enters a single edge for the suffix $S[1 \cdots L]$ into the tree. Then it successively enters the suffix $S[i \cdots L]$ into the growing tree for i increasing from 2 to L. The details of this construction method are beyond the scope of this chapter. Various suffix tree construction algorithms can be found in Gusfield's text [10] (a good source on suffix tree construction algorithms in general).

Several linear time algorithms for constructing suffix trees exist [30,44,46]. To be precise, these algorithms also exhibit a time dependence on the size of the vocabulary (or the alphabet when dealing with character-based trees); they actually have a time bound of $O(L \times \min(\log |V|, \log L))$, where L is the length of the string and $|V|$ is the size of the language. These methods are more difficult to implement than the naive method, which is sufficiently suitable for our purpose.

Some implementation improvements of the naive method can also be made to improve the $O(L^2)$ worst-case time bound. With these improvements, it can achieve constant access time for finding an appropriate child of the root (this is important because the root node has the same *count* or number of child nodes as the number of letters in the alphabet—count of terms in document collection) and logarithmic time needed to find an existing child or to insert a new child node in any other internal nodes of the tree [10,23].

14.6 INDEXING 3D PROTEIN STRUCTURES

As was mentioned above, the data for protein 3D structures indexing are retrieved from PDB database, which consists of proteins, nucleic acids, and complex assemblies. Before indexing protein structures, we consider only complete protein structures. We filter out all nucleic acids and complex assemblies from the entire PDB database. Next we filter out proteins, which have incomplete N—Cα—C—O backbones (e.g., some of the files have C atoms in the protein backbone missing). After this cleaning step, we have a collection of files containing a description of a specific protein and its 3D structure and containing only amino acid residues with complete a N—Cα—C—O atom sequence. Each retrieved file has at least one mainchain (some proteins have more than one mainchain) of at least one model (some PDB files contained more models of 3D protein structure). In cases when the PDB file contained multiple chains or models, we took into account all of those (all mainchains of all models).

To be able to measure 3D protein structure similarity using suffix trees and the vector space model, we need to encode protein 3D structure into a vector representation. This can be achieved in various ways [4,9,16,28,50].

14.6.1 Torsion Angles

Any plane can be defined by two noncollinear vectors lying in that plane; taking their crossproduct and normalizing yields the normal unit vector to the plane. Thus, a torsion angle can be defined by four pairwise noncollinear vectors.

The backbone torsion angles of proteins are called ϕ (phi, involving the backbone atoms C—N—Cα—C), ψ (psi, involving the backbone atoms N—Cα—C—N) and ω (omega, involving the backbone atoms Cα—C—N—Cα). Thus, ϕ controls the C—C distance, ψ controls the N—N distance and ω controls the Cα—Cα distance.

The planarity of the peptide bond usually restricts ω to be $180°$ (the typical trans case) or $0°$ (the rare cis case). The ϕ and ψ torsion angles tend to range from $-180°$ to $180°$.

14.6.2 Encoding the 3D Protein Mainchain Structure for Indexing

To be able to index proteins by information retrieval (IR) techniques, we need to encode the 3D structure of the protein backbone into some sequence of characters, words, or integers (as in our case). The area of protein 3D structure encoding has been widely studied [e.g., [4,9,50]. Since the protein backbone is the sequence of the amino acid residues (in 3D space), we are able to encode this backbone into the sequence of integers in the following manner.

For example, let us say that the protein backbone consists of six amino acid residues RNADNA (abbreviations for arginine, asparagine, alanine, and aspartic acid). The relationship between the two following residues can be described by their torsion angles ϕ, ψ, and ω. Since ϕ and ψ take values from the interval $-180°, 180°$, this must be done with some normalization. From this interval we can obtain discrete values by dividing the interval into equal-sized subintervals (e.g., into 36 subintervals; e.g., $-180°$, $-170°$, $\ldots$, $0°$, $10°$, $\ldots$, $180°$). Each of these values was labeled with nonnegative integers as follows: 00, 01, $\ldots$, 36 where 00 stands for $-180°$. Now, let's say that ϕ is $-21°$; the closest discrete value is $-20°$, which has the label 16, so we have encoded this torsion with the string 16. The same holds true for ψ. Torsion angle ω was encoded as either of the two characters A or B since the ω tends to be almost in every case $0°$ or $180°$. After concatenation of these three parts we obtain a string that looks something like A0102, which means that $\omega \approx 180°$, $\phi \approx -170°$, $\psi \approx -160°$. Concatenation was done in the following manner: $\omega\phi\psi$.

The suffix tree can index sequences of characters, numbers, words, and so on. To conserve computer memory space, it is better to represent the sequence of words with a sequence of nonnegative integers. For example, let's say that we have a protein with a backbone consisting of six residues, such as RNADNA with its 3D properties. The resulting encoded sequence can be, for example; {A3202, A2401, A2603, A2401, A2422, A2422, A2220}.

After obtaining this six-word sequence, we create a dictionary of these words (each unique word receives its own unique nonnegative integer identifier). The translated sequence appears as {0, 1, 2, 1, 3, 3, 4}.

In this way, we can encode each mainchain of each model contained into one PDB file. This task is done for every protein included in our filtered PDB collection. Now we are ready to index proteins using suffix trees.

14.7 PROTEIN SIMILARITY ALGORITHM

We describe the algorithm for measuring protein similarity on the basis of their tertiary structure [28,29]. A brief description of the algorithm follows:

1. Encode 3D protein structure into the vectors presented in Section 14.6.
2. Insert all encoded mainchains of all proteins in the collection into the generalized suffix tree data structure.
3. Find all maximal substructure clusters in the suffix tree.
4. Construct a vector model of all proteins in our collection.
5. Build proteins similarity matrix.
6. For each protein find the top N similar proteins.

14.7.1 Inserting All Mainchains into the Suffix Tree

At this stage of the algorithm, we construct a generalized suffix tree of all encoded mainchains. As mentioned in Section 14.6, we obtain the encoded forms of 3D protein mainchains—sequences of positive numbers. All of these sequences are inserted into the generalized suffix tree data structure (Section 14.5).

14.7.2 Finding All Maximal Substructure Clusters

To build a vector model of proteins, we have to find all maximal phrase clusters. Recall the example given in Section 14.6, namely, that the phrases can be RNADNA#, RNA#, DNA#, and so on (just imagine that phrase RNA# is equal to A3202 A2401 A2603 #). The *phrase* in the present context is an encoded protein mainchain or any of its parts. The document in our context can be seen as a set of encoded mainchains of the protein. Now we can define a maximal phrase cluster (the longest common substructure; see Fig. 14.7) [49].

Definition 14.3 A phrase cluster is a phrase that is shared by at least two documents, and the group of documents that contain the phrase. A maximal phrase cluster is a phrase cluster whose phrase cannot be extended by any word in the language without changing (reducing) the group of documents that contain it. Maximal phrase clusters are those that we are interested in.

Now we simply traverse the generalized suffix tree and identify all maximal phrase clusters (i.e., all of the longest common substructures). *A maximal phrase cluster can be seen as a kind of 3D structural alignment—common parts of 3D protein structure shared between two or more proteins.* Figure 14.7 displays the example of maximal phrase cluster.

14.7.3 Building a 3D Protein Structure Vector Model

We describe the procedure for building the matrix representing the vector model index file (Section 14.4). In a classical vector space model, the document is represented by the terms (which are words), respectively, and by the weights of the terms. *In our model the document is represented not by the terms but by the*

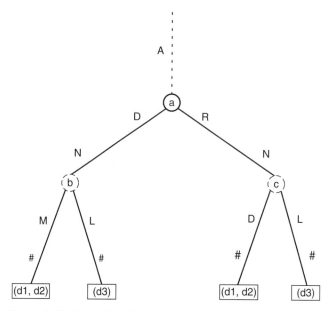

Figure 14.7   Example of maximal phrase cluster: nodes *b* and *c*.

common phrases (maximal phrase clusters)! The term in our context is a common phrase, that is, a maximal phrase cluster.

In the previous stage of the algorithm, we identified all maximal phrase clusters—all the longest common substructures. From the definition of the phrase cluster, we know that the phrase cluster is the group of documents sharing the same phrase (group of proteins sharing the same substructure). Now we can obtain the matrix representing the vector model index file directly from the generalized suffix tree. Each document (protein) is represented by the maximal phrase clusters in which it is contained. For computing the weights of the phrase clusters, we are using a TF × IDF weighting schema as given by Equation (14.1).

Let us say consider a simple example that we have a phrase cluster containing documents d_i. These documents share the same phrase t_j. We compute w_{ij} values for all documents appearing in a phrase cluster sharing the phrase t_j. This task is done for all phrase clusters identified by the previous stage of the algorithm.

Now we have a complete matrix representing the index file in a vector space model (see Section 14.4).

14.7.4   Building a Similarity Matrix

In the previous stage of the algorithm, we constructed a vector model index file. To build a protein similarity matrix, we use standard information retrieval techniques for measuring the similarity in a vector space model. As mentioned in Section 14.4, we have used cosine similarity, which appears to be quite suitable for our purpose. The similarity matrix is given by the following documents (proteins) similarity matrix:

$$S = \begin{pmatrix} 1 & sim(d_1, d_2) & \cdots & sim(d_1, d_n) \\ sim(d_2, d_1) & 1 & \cdots & sim(d_2, d_n) \\ \vdots & \vdots & \ddots & \vdots \\ sim(d_n, d_1) & sim(d_n, d_2) & \cdots & 1 \end{pmatrix},$$

Here, the ith row matches the ith document (protein, respectively), and the jth column matches the jth document (protein). The similarity matrix is diagonally symmetric.

14.7.5 Finding Similar Proteins

This step is quite simple. When we have computed the similarity matrix S, we simply sort the documents (proteins) on each row according to their similarity scores. The higher the score, the more similar the two proteins are. We do this for each protein in our protein collection. The results of the algorithm can be found in [28].

14.8 SUMMARY

Analysis of 3D protein structures is an important part of current bioinformatics. It is a key part of discovering protein–protein interactions, necessitating efficient algorithms. Since the current protein databank (PDB) is growing almost every week and new structures have been discovered by NMR or X-ray crystallography very successfully, algorithms that can process large amounts of data are essential. Protein indexing algorithms can very efficiently discover the protein interactions on the basis of their tertiary structures and can be useful for building protein interactions networks, prediction of protein functions, fold recognition, homology detection, alignment of 3D protein structures, drug discovery, and other purposes.

REFERENCES

1. Baeza-Yates R, Ribeiro-Neto B, *Modern Information Retrieval*, Adison-Wesley, 1999.
2. Bünger AT, *X-PLOR, Version 3.1. A System for X-ray Crystallography and NMR*, Yale Univ. Press, New Haven, CT, 1992.
3. *CATH: Protein Structure Classification* http://www.cathdb.info/; last accessed 7/10/09.
4. Chew LP, Huttenlocher D, Kedem K, Kleinberg J, Fast detection of common geometric substructure in proteins, *J. Comput. Biol.* **6**(3/4):313–326 (1999).

5. Chim H, Deng X, A new suffix tree similarity measure for document clustering, *Proc. 16th Int. Conf. World Wide Web* (WWW 2007), ACM, New York, 2007, pp. 121–130.

6. Day R, Beck DA, Armen RS, Daggett V, A consensus view of fold space: Combining SCOP, CATH, and the Dali Domain Dictionary, *Sci.* **12**(10):2150–2160 (2003).

7. Dráždilová P, Dvorský J, Martinovič J, Snášel V, Search in documents based on topical development, in AWIC 2009, Amazon.ca, 2009.

8. Ehrenfeucht A, Haussler D, A new distance metric on strings computable in linear time, *Appl. Math.* **20**(3):191–203 (1988).

9. Gao F, Zaki MJ, PSIST: Indexing protein structures using suffix trees, *Proc. IEEE Computational Systems Bioinformatics Conference (CSB)*, 2005, pp. 212–222.

10. Gusfield D, *Algorithms on Strings, Trees and Sequences: Computer Science and Computational Biology*, Cambridge Univ. Press, 1997.

11. Habib T, Zhang C, Yang JY, Yang MQ, Deng Y, Supervised learning method for the prediction of subcellular localization of proteins using amino acid and amino acid pair composition, *BMC Genomics* **9**(Suppl. 1):S16 (2008).

12. Hadley C, Jones DT, A systematic comparison of protein structure classifications: SCOP, CATH and FSSP, *Structure* **7**(9):1099–1112 (1999).

13. Hammouda KM, Kamel MS, Efficient phrase-based document indexing for web document clustering, *IEEE Trans. Knowl. Data Eng.* **16**(10):1279–1296 (2004).

14. Hecker J, Yang JY, Cheng J, Protein disorder prediction at multiple levels of sensitivity and specificity, *BMC Genomics* **9**(Suppl. 1):S9 (2008).

15. Holm L, Sander C, Dali: A network tool for protein structure comparison, *Trends Biochem. Sci.* **20**(11):478–480 (1995).

16. Holm L, Sander C, Protein structure comparison by alignment of distance matrices, *J. Mol. Biol.* **233**:123–138 (1993).

17. Hruška P, Martinovič J, Dvorský J, Snášel V, *XML Compression Improvements Based on the Clustering of Elements*, CISIM, Poland, 2010.

18. Lee DL, Chuang H, Seamons KE, Document ranking and the vector-space model, *IEEE Software*, 1997, pp. 67–75.

19. Lesk AM, *Introduction to Bioinformatics*, Oxford Univ. Press, 2008.

20. Lodish H, Berk A, Matsudaira P, Kaiser AC, Krieger M, Scott PM, Zipursky L, Darnell J, *Molecular Cell Biology*, 6th ed. Freeman WH, 2007.

21. Lexa M, Snášel V, Zelinka I, Data-mining protein structure by clustering, segmentation and evolutionary algorithms, in *Data Mining: Theoretical Foundations and Applications*, Springer-Verlag, Studies in Computational Intelligence Series, vol. 204, 2009, pp. 221–248.

22. Manning CD, Raghavan P, Schütze H, *Introduction to Information Retrieval*, Cambridge Univ. Press, 2008.

23. Martinovič J, Novosád T, Snášel V, *Vector Model Improvement Using Suffix Trees*, IEEE, ICDIM, 2007, pp. 180–187.

24. Murzin AG, Brenner SE, Hubbard T, Chothia C, SCOP: A structural classification of proteins database for the investigation of sequences and structures, *J. Mol. Biol.* **247**:536–540 (1995).

25. Lo Conte L, Brenner SE, Hubbard TJP, Chothia C, Murzin A, SCOP database in 2002: Refinements accommodate structural genomics, *Nucleic Acids Res.* **30**(1):264–267 (2002).

26. Andreeva A, Howorth D, Brenner SE, Hubbard TJP, Chothia C, Murzin AG, SCOP database in 2004: Refinements integrate structure and sequence family data, *Nucleic Acids Res.* **32**:D226–D229 (2004).

27. Andreeva A, Howorth D, Chandonia J-M, Brenner SE, Hubbard TJP, Chothia C, Murzin AG, Data growth and its impact on the SCOP database: New developments. *Nucleic Acids Res.* **36**:D419–D425 (2008).

28. Novosád T, Snášel V, Abraham A, Yang JY, Prosima—protein similarity algorithm, *Proc. World Congress on Nature and Biologically Inspired Computing*, 2009, pp. 84–91.

29. Novosád T, Snášel V, Abraham A, Yang JY, Searching protein 3-D structures for optimal structure alignment using intelligent algorithms and data structures, *IEEE Trans. Inform. Technol. Biomed.* **14**(6):1378–1386 (2010).

30. McCreight E, A space-economical suffix tree construction algorithm, *J. ACM* **23**:262–272 (1976).

31. Orengo CA, Michie AD, Jones S, Jones DT, Swindells MB, Thornton JM, CATH—a hierarchic classification of protein domain structures, *Structure* **5**(8):1093–1108 (1997).

32. Pauling L, Corey RB, Branson HR, The structure of proteins; two hydrogen-bonded helical configurations of the polypeptide chain, *Proc. Natl. Acad. Sci. USA* **4**:205–211 (1951).

33. van Rijsbergen CJ, *Information Retrieval*, 2nd ed., Butterworths, London, 1979.

34. RCSB Protein Databank—PDB (http://www.pdb.org)

35. Robinson R, *Genetics*, Macmillan Reference USA (2002).

36. Rodeh M, Pratt VR, Even S, Linear algorithm for data compression via string matching, *J. ACM* **28**(1):16–24 (1981).

37. Salton G, *The SMART Retrieval System—Experiments in Automatic Document Processing*, Prentice-Hall, Englewood Cliffs, NJ, 1971.

38. Salton G, Lesk ME, Computer evaluation of indexing and text processing, *J. ACM* **15**(1):8–36 (1968).

39. Salton G, Wong A, Yang CS, A vector space model for automatic indexing, *Commun. ACM* **18**(11): (1975).

40. Salton G, Buckley C, Term-weighting approaches in automatic text retrieval, *Inform. Process. Manage.* **24**(5):513–523 (1988).

41. Sarkar IN, A vector space model approach to identify genetically related diseases, *J. Am. Med. Inform. Assoc.* **19**(2):249–254 (2012).

42. *SCOP: A Structural Classification of Proteins Database for the Investigation of Sequences and Structure* http://scop.mrc-lmb.cam.ac.uk/scop/; last accessed 7/10/09.

43. Shibuya T, Geometric suffix tree: A new index structure for protein 3D structures, in *Combinatorial Pattern Matching*, LNCS series, vol. 4009, 2006, pp. 84–93.

44. Ukkonen E, On-line construction of suffix trees, *Algorithmica* **14**:249–260 (1995).

45. Wang Xin, Wang G, Shen C, Li L, Wang Xinguo, Mooney SD, Edenberg HJ, Sanford JR, Liu Y, Using RNase sequence specificity to refine the identification of RNA-protein binding regions, *BMC Genomics* **9**(Suppl. 1):S17 (2008).

46. Weiner P, Linear pattern matching algorithms, *Proc. 14th Annual Sympo. Foundations of Computer Science*, 1973, pp. 1–11.

47. Yang JY, Yang MQ, Dunker AK, Deng Y, Huang X, Investigation of transmembrane proteins using a computational approach, *BMC Genomics* **9**(Suppl. 1):S7 (2008).

48. Zamir O, *Clustering Web Documents: A Phrase-Based Method for Grouping Search Engine Results*, doctoral dissertation, Univ. Washington, 1999.

49. Zamir O, Etzioni O, Web document clustering: A feasibility demonstration, *Proc. Special Interest Group on Information Retrieval Conf.*, (SIGIR'98), 1998, pp. 46–54.

50. Ye J, Janardan R, Liu S, Pairwise protein structure alignment based on an orientation-independent backbone representation, *J. Bioinformatics Comput. Biol.* **2**:699–718 (2004).

CHAPTER 15

ALGORITHMIC METHODOLOGIES FOR DISCOVERY OF NONSEQUENTIAL PROTEIN STRUCTURE SIMILARITIES

BHASKAR DASGUPTA, JOSEPH DUNDAS, and JIE LIANG

15.1 INTRODUCTION

An increasing number of protein structures are becoming available that either have no known function or whose functional mechanism is unknown or incomplete. Using experimental methods alone to explore these proteins in order to determine their functional mechanism is unfeasible. For this reason, much research has been put into computational methods for predicting the function of proteins [5,14,31,34,44,53]. One such computational method is functional inference by homology, where annotations from a protein with known function are transferred onto another protein on the basis of sequence or structural similarities.

Protein sequence comparisons have been used as a straightforward method for functional inheritance. If two proteins have a high level of sequence identity, frequently the two proteins have the same or related biological functions. This observation has been used as a basis for transferring annotations from a protein that is well characterized to a protein with unknown function when the two proteins have high sequence similarity [3,4,45]. Frequently, only the protein residues that are near the functional region of the protein are under evolutionary pressure for conservation. Therefore, the global sequence similarity may be relatively low while local regions within the two sequences maintain a higher level of sequence similarity. In this case, probabilistic models such as profiles have been constructed using only the local regions of high sequence similarity [3,32,28].

Algorithmic and Artificial Intelligence Methods for Protein Bioinformatics. First Edition.
Edited by Yi Pan, Jianxin Wang, Min Li.
© 2014 John Wiley & Sons, Inc. Published 2014 by John Wiley & Sons, Inc.

Sequence comparison methods have the advantage that large numbers of sequences are deposited into sequence databases such as Swiss-Prot [11], which provides adequate information for constructing probabilistic models. However, a relatively high level of sequence similarity is needed in order to accurately transfer protein function. In fact, problems begin to arise when the sequence identity between a pair of proteins is < 60% [57].

Because proteins often maintain structural similarities even when sequence identity falls as low as 30% [6], making protein structure more strongly correlated with protein function than protein sequence [24], many researchers have begun to compare the three-dimensional structure of proteins in an attempt to uncover more distant evolutionary relationships among proteins. The SCOP [40] and CATH [43] databases have organized protein structures hierarchically into different classes and folds on the basis of their overall similarity in topology and fold. Classification of protein structures relies heavily on the reliable protein structure comparison methods. Common structural comparison methods include DALI (see Section 14.3.4) [27] and CE [47]. However, structural alignment methods cannot guarantee optimal results and do not have an interpretability comparable to sequence alignment methods.

Several challenges arise when trying to compare protein structures:

1. When searching for global structural similarity, similar to sequence alignment methods, one can search for global similarity or similarity within local surface regions of interest. Unlike sequence alignment scoring methods, which are heavily based on models of protein evolution [13,25], scoring systems for structural alignment must account for both the 3D positional deviations between the aligned residues or atoms, and other biologically important shared characteristics. Defining a robust quantitative measure of similarity is challenging. This difficulty is illustrated by the variety of structural alignment scoring methods that have been proposed [23].

2. Many alignment methods assume that the ordering of the residues follows that of the primary sequence [47,51]. This sequence order dependence can lead to problems when comparing local surface regions that often contain residues and atoms from different locations on primary sequence fold together to form functional regions in 3D space. On the global backbone level, the existence of permuted proteins, such as the circular permutation [17,37] also poses significant problems for sequence order–dependent alignment methods.

3. Proteins may undergo small sidechain structural fluctuations or larger backbone fluctuations *in vivo* that are not represented in a single static snapshot of a crystallized structure in the Protein Data Bank (PDB) [9]. Many structural alignment methods assume rigid bodies and cannot factor in structural changes.

In this chapter, we will discuss several issues of structural alignment and then discuss methods that we have implemented for sequence order–independent structural alignment at the global and local surface levels. We illustrate the utility of our methods by showing how our sequence order–independent global structural alignment method detects circular permuted proteins. We then show how our local surface sequence order–independent structural alignment method can be used to construct a basis set of signature pockets of binding surfaces for a specific biological function. The signature pocket represents structurally conserved surface regions. A set of signature pockets can then be used to represent a functional family of proteins for protein function prediction.

15.2   STRUCTURAL ALIGNMENT

Comparing the structure of two proteins is an important problem [23] that may detect evolutionary relationships between proteins even when sequence identity between two proteins is relatively low. A widely used method for measuring structural similarity is the root-mean-squared distance (RMSD) between the equivalent atoms or residues of two proteins. If the equivalence relationship is known, a rotation matrix R and a translation vector T that when applied to one of the protein structures will minimize the RMSD can be found by solving the minimization problem

$$min \sum_{i=1}^{N_B} \sum_{j=1}^{N_A} |T + RB_i - A_j|^2, \tag{15.1}$$

where N_A is the number of points in structure A and N_B is the number of points in structure B. If $N_A = N_B$, then the least-squares estimation of the parameters R and T in this equation can be found using singular value decomposition.

The equivalence relationship is rarely known a priori when aligning to protein structures. In this case, the structural alignment method consists in minimizing RMSD while maximizing the number of aligned points. Heuristics must be used to solve this multiobjective optimization problem.

A number of heuristic methods have been developed [1,22,48,49,52,56,59] that can be divided into two main categories. *Global* methods are used to detect similarities between the overall fold of two proteins, and *local* alignment methods are used to detect similarities within local regions of interest within the two proteins. Most current methods are restricted to finding structural similarities only where the order of the structural elements within the alignment follows the order of the elements within the primary sequence. Sequence order–independent methods ignore the sequential ordering of the atoms or residues in primary sequence. These methods are better suited for finding more complex global similarities and can also be employed for finding all atoms local comparisons. We have implemented both sequence order–independent methods for both global and local structural alignments.

15.3   GLOBAL SEQUENCE ORDER–INDEPENDENT STRUCTURAL ALIGNMENT

Looking for similarities between the overall fold can elucidate evolutionary or functional relationships between two proteins. However, most of the current methods for structural comparison are sequence order–dependent and are restricted to comparison of similar topologies between the two backbones. It has been discovered that throughout evolution, a genetic event can rearrange the topology of the backbone. One such example is regarded circular permutation. Conceptually, a circular permutation can be as a ligation of the N and C termini of a protein and cleavage somewhere else on the protein backbone. It has been observed that circular permutations often maintain a similar 3D spatial arrangement of secondary structures. In addition to circular permutations, research has shown that more complex topological rearrangements are possible [37]. Detection of these permuted proteins will be valuable for studies in homology modeling, protein folding, and protein design.

15.3.1   Sequence Order–Independent Global Structural Alignment

We have developed a sequence order–independent structural alignment algorithm for detecting structural similarities between two proteins that have undergone topological rearrangement of their backbone structures [17]. Our method is based on fragment assembly where the two proteins to be aligned are first exhaustively fragmented. Each fragment $\lambda_{i,k}^{A}$ from protein structure S_A is pairwise superimposed onto each fragment $\lambda_{j,k}^{B}$ from protein structure S_B. The result is a set of fragment pairs $\chi_{i,j,k}$, where $i \in S_A$ and $j \in S_B$ are the indices in the primary sequence of the first residue of the two fragments. The variable $k \in \{5, 6, 7\}$ is the length of the fragment. Each fragment pair is assigned a similarity score

$$\sigma(\chi_{i,j,k}) = \alpha \left[C - s(\chi_{i,j,k}) \cdot \frac{\text{cRMSD}}{k^2} \right] + \text{SCS} \qquad (15.2)$$

where cRMSD is the measured RMSD value after optimal superposition, α and C are two constants, $s(\chi_{i,j,k})$ is a scaling factor to the measured RMSD values that depends on the secondary structure of the fragments, and SCS is a BLOSUM (*blocks substitution matrix*)-like measure of similarity in sequence of the matched fragments [25]. Details of the scoring method can be found in an earlier study [17].

The goal of the structural alignment is to find a consistent set of fragment pairs $\Delta = \{\chi_{i_1,j_1,k_1}, \chi_{i_2,j_2,k_2}, \ldots, \chi_{i_t,j_t,k_t}\}$ that minimizes the overall RMSD. Finding the optimal combination of fragment pairs is a special case of the well-known maximum-weight-independent set problem in graph theory. This problem is MAX-SNP-hard. We employ an approximation algorithm that was originally described for the scheduling of split-interval graphs [8] and is itself based on a fractional version of the local ratio approach.

To begin, a conflict graph $G = (V, E)$ is created, where a vertex is defined for each aligned fragment pair. Two vertices are connected by an edge if any of the fragments $(\lambda_{i,k}^A, \lambda_{i',k'}^B)$ or $(\lambda_{j,k}^B, \lambda_{j',k'}^B)$ from the fragment pair is not disjoint, that is, if both fragments from the same protein share one or more residues. For each vertex representing aligned fragment pairs, we assign three indicator variables $x_\chi, y_{\chi\lambda_A}$, and $x_\chi, y_{\chi\lambda_B} \in \{0, 1\}$, and a closed neighborhood $Nbr[\chi].x_\chi$ indicates whether the fragment pair should be used ($x_\chi = 1$) or not ($x_\chi = 0$) in the final alignment. $x_\chi, y_{\chi\lambda_A}$ and $x_\chi, y_{\chi\lambda_B}$ are artificial indicator values for λ_A and λ_B, which allow us to encode consistency in the selected fragments. The closed neighborhood of a vertex χ of G is $\{\chi' | \chi, \chi' \in E\} \cup \{\chi\}$, which is simply χ and all vertices that are connected to χ by an edge.

The sequence order–independent structural alignment algorithm can be described as follows. To begin, initialize the structural alignment Δ equal to the entire set of aligned fragment pairs. We then

1. Solve a linear programming (LP) formulation of the problem:

Maximize
$$\sum_{\chi \in \Delta} \sigma(\chi) \cdot x_\chi \tag{15.3}$$

subject to
$$\sum_{a_t \in \lambda^A} y_{\chi\lambda_A} \le 1 \qquad \forall a_t \in S_A \tag{15.4}$$

$$\sum_{b_t \in \lambda^B} y_{\chi\lambda_B} \le 1 \qquad \forall b_t \in S_B \tag{15.5}$$

$$y_{\chi\lambda_A} - x_\chi \le 1 \qquad \forall \chi \in \Delta \tag{15.6}$$

$$y_{\chi\lambda_B} - x_\chi \le 1 \qquad \forall \chi \in \Delta \tag{15.7}$$

$$x_\chi, y_{\chi\lambda_A}, y_{\chi\lambda_B} \le 1 \qquad \forall \chi \in \Delta \tag{15.8}$$

2. For every vertex $\chi \in V_\Delta$ of G_Δ, compute its *local conflict number* $\alpha_\chi = \sum_{\chi' \in Nbr_\Delta[\chi]} x_{\chi'}$. Let $\chi_{\min}$ be the vertex with the *minimum* local conflict number. Define a new similarity function σ_{new} from σ as follows:

$$\sigma_{\text{new}}(\chi) = \begin{cases} \sigma(\chi), & \text{if } \chi \notin Nbr_\Delta[\chi_{\min}] \\ \sigma(\chi) - \sigma(\chi_{\min}), & \text{otherwise} \end{cases}$$

3. Create $\Delta_{\text{new}} \subseteq \Delta$ by removing from Δ every substructure pair χ such that $\sigma_{\text{new}} \le 0$. Push each removed substructure on to a stack in arbitrary order.

4. If $\Delta_{\text{new}} \ne 0$ then repeat from step 1, setting $\Delta = \Delta_{\text{new}}$ and $\sigma = \sigma_{\text{new}}$. Otherwise, continue to step 5.

5. Repeatedly pop the stack, adding the substructure pair to the alignment as long as the following conditions are met:

   a. The substructure pair is consistent with all other substructure pairs that already exist in the selection.

   b. The cRMSD of the alignment does not change beyond a threshold. This condition bridges the gap between optimizing a local similarity between substructures and optimizing the tertiary similarity of the alignment. It guarantees that each substructure from a substructure pair is in the same spatial arrangement in the global alignment.

15.3.2 Detecting Permuted Proteins

This algorithm was implemented in a large-scale study to search for permuted proteins in the Protein Data Bank (PDB) [9]. A subset of 3336 protein structures taken from the PDBSELECT90 dataset [26] are structurally aligned in a pairwise fashion. From the subset of 3336 proteins, we aligned two proteins if they met the following conditions (see Ref. 17 for details):

1. The difference in their lengths was no more than 75 residues.
2. The two proteins shared approximately the same secondary structure content.

Within the approximately 200,000 structural alignments performed, we found many known circular permutations and three novel circular permutations, as well as a more complex pair of noncyclic permuted proteins. Here we describe the details of the circular permutation that we found between a neucleoplasmin core and an auxin binding protein, as well as details of the more complex noncyclic permutation.

15.3.2.1 Nucleoplasmin Core and Auxin Binding Protein   We found a novel circular permutation between the nucleoplasmin core protein in *Xenopu laevis* (PDB ID 1k5j, chain E) [19] and the auxin binding protein in maize (PDB ID 11rh, chain A, residues 37–127) [58]. The structural alignment between 1k5jE (Fig. 15.1, top) and 11rhA (Fig. 15.1, bottom) consisted of 68 equivalent residues superimposed with a RMSD of 1.36 Å. This alignment is statistically significant with a p value of 2.7×10^{-5} after Bonferroni correction. Details of the p value calculation can be found in our earlier study [17]. The short loop connecting two antiparallel strans in nucleoplasmin core protein (in circle, top of Fig. 15.1b) becomes disconnected in auxin binding protein 1 (in circle, bottom of Fig. 15.1b), and the N and C termini of the nucleoplasmin core protein (in square, top of Fig. 15.1b) are connected in auxin binding protein 1 (square, bottom of Fig. 15.1b). For details of other circular permutations we found, including permutations between microphage migration inhibition factor and the C-terminal domain of arginine repressor, please see our earlier study [17].

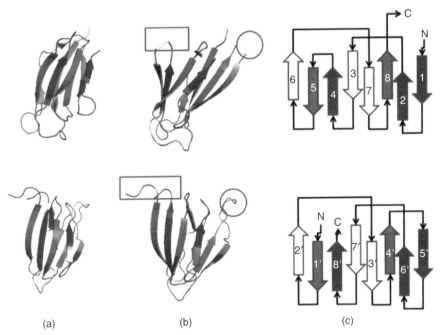

(a)   (b)   (c)

Figure 15.1 A newly discovered circular permutation between nucleoplasmin core [1k5j, chain E, *top panel*), and a fragment of auxin binding protein 1 (residues 37–127) (11rh, chain A, *bottom panel*). (a) These two proteins align well with a RMSD value of 1.36 Å over 68 residues, with a significant p value of 2.7×10^{-5} after Bonferroni correction. (b) The loop connecting strands 4 and 5 of nucleoplasmin core (in *rectangle*, top) becomes disconnected in auxin binding protein 1. The N and C termini of nucleoplasmin core (in *rectangle*, top) become connected in auxin binding protein 1 (in *rectangle*, bottom). To facilitate visualization of the circular permutation, residues in the N-to-C direction before the cut in the nucleoplasmin core protein are colored by the lighter shade, and residues after the cut are colored by the darker shade. (c) The topology diagram of these two proteins. In the original structure of nucleoplasmin core, the electron density of the loop connecting strands 4 and 5 is missing in the PDB structure file. (This figure is modified from Hruška et al. [17].)

15.3.2.2 Complex Protein Permutations

Because of their relevance in understanding the functional and folding mechanism of proteins, circular permutations have received much attention [37,55]. However, the possibility of more complex backbone rearrangements were experimentally verified by artificially rearranging the topology of the ARC repressor and were found to be thermodynamically stable [50]. Very little is known about this class of permuted proteins, and the detection of noncyclic permutations is a challenging task [2,15,29,46].

Our database search uncovered a naturally occurring noncyclic permutation between chain F of AML1/core binding factor (AML1/CBF, PDB ID 1e50, Fig. 15.2a, *top*) and chain A of riboflavin synthase (PDB ID 1pkv, Fig. 15.2a, *bottom*).

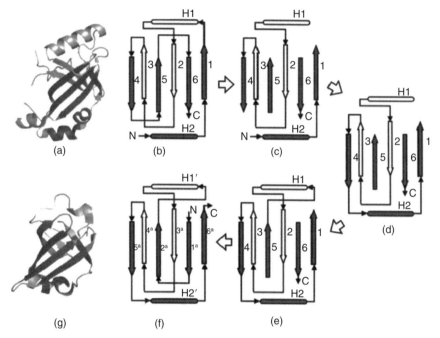

Figure 15.2 A noncyclic permutation discovered between AML1/core binding factor (AML1/CBF PDB ID 1e50, chain F, *top*) and riboflavin synthase (PDB ID 1pkv, chain A, *bottom*). (a) These two proteins structurally align with an RMSD of 1.23 Å over 42 residues and have a significant *p*value of 2.8×10^{-4} after Bonferroni correction. The residues that were assigned equivalences from the structural alignment are colored by the darker shade. (b) These proteins are structurally related by a complex permutation. The steps to transform the topology of AML1/CBF (*top*) to riboflavin (*bottom*) are as follows: (c) Remove the loops connecting strand 1 to helix 2, strand 4 to strand 5, and strand 5 to helix 6; (d) Connect the *C*-terminal end of strand 4 to the original *N* termini; (e) connect the *C*-terminal end of strand 5 to the *N*-terminal end of helix 2; (f) connect the original *C*-termini to the *N*-terminal end of strand 5. The *N*-terminal end of strand 6 becomes the new *N* termini, and the *C*-terminal end of strand 1 becomes the new *C* termini. We now have the topology diagram of riboflavin synthase. (This figure is modified from Hruska et al. [17]).

The two structures align well with an RMSD of 1.23 Å at an alignment length of 42 residues, with a significant *p* value of 2.8×10^{-4} after Bonferroni correction.

The topology diagram of AML1/CBF (Fig. 15.2b) can be transformed into that of riboflavin synthase (Fig. 15.2f) by the following steps. Remove the loops connecting strand 1 to helix 2, strand 4 to strand 5, and strand 5 to strand 6 (Fig. 15.2c). Connect the *C*-terminal end of strand 4 to the original *N* terminal (Fig. 15.2d). Connect the *C*-terminal end of strand 5 to the *N*-terminal end of helix 2 (Fig. 15.2e). Connect the original *C* termini to the *N*-terminal end of strand 5. The *N*-terminal end of strand 6 becomes the new *N* termini, and the *C*-terminal end of strand 1 becomes the new *C* termini (Fig. 15.2f).

15.4 LOCAL SEQUENCE ORDER–INDEPENDENT STRUCTURAL ALIGNMENT

Comparison of the global backbone can lead to discovery of distant evolutionary relationships between proteins. However, when attempting to detect similar functions or functional mechanisms between two proteins, global backbone similarity is not a robust indicator [20,36,41]. It can be assumed that the physicochemical properties of the local region where function takes place (i.e., substrate binding) is under more evolutionary pressure to be conserved. This assumption has been backed up by several studies [21,30,38,42,53,54].

A typical protein contains many concave surface regions, commonly referred to as *surface pockets*. However, only a few of the surface pockets supply a unique physiochemical environment that is conducive to the protein carrying out its function. The protein must maintain this surface pocket throughout evolution in order to conserve its biological function. For this reason, shared structural similarities between *functional surfaces* among proteins may be a strong indicator of shared biological function. This has led to a number of promising studies, in which protein functions can be inferred by similarity comparison of local binding surfaces [7,10,21,35,39]

The inherent flexibility of the protein structure makes the problem of structural comparison of protein surface pockets challenging. A protein is not a static structure as represented by a PDB [9] entry. The whole protein as well as the local functional surface may undergo various degrees of structural fluctuations. The use of a single surface pocket structure as a representative template for a specific protein function can lead to many false negatives. This is due to the inability of a single representative to capture the full functional characteristics across all conformations of a protein.

We have addressed this problem by developing an algorithm that can identify the atoms of a surface pocket that are structurally preserved across a family of protein structures that have similar functions. Using a sequence order–independent local surface alignment method to pairwise-align the functional pockets across a family of protein structure, we automatically find the structurally conserved atoms and measure their fluctuations. We call these structurally conserved atoms the *signature pocket*. More than one signature pocket may result for a single functional class. In this case, our method can automatically create a *basis set* of signature pockets for that functional family. We can then use these signature pockets as representatives for scanning a structure database for functional inference by structural similarity.

15.4.1 Bipartite Graph Matching Algorithm for Local Surface Comparison

We have modified and implemented a sequence order–independent local structural alignment algorithm based on the maximum-weight bipartite graph matching formulation developed by Chen et al. [12].

As mentioned earlier, the structural alignment problem boils down to a problem of finding an equivalence relation between residues of a reference protein S_R and a query protein S_Q that when applied will optimize the superposition of the two structures. The formulation here does this in an iterative two-step process: (1) an optimal set of equivalent atoms are determined under the current superposition using a bipartite graph representation and (2) the new equivalence relation is used to determine a new optimal superposition. The two steps are then repeated until a stopping condition is met.

The equivalence relationship is found between the two atoms of the functional pocket surfaces by representing the atoms the atoms of S_R and S_Q as nodes in a graph. This graph is *bipartite*, meaning that edges exist only between atoms of S_R and atoms of S_Q. A directed edge is drawn between two nodes if a similarity threshold is met. In our implementation, the measure of similarity takes into account both spatial distances and the chemical property similarities between the two corresponding atoms.

Each edge $e_{i,j}$ connecting nodes i and j is assigned a weight $w(i,j)$ equal to the similarity score between the two corresponding atoms (see [12] for details). The optimal equivalence relationship given the current superposition is a subset of the edges within this bipartite graph that have maximum combined weight, where at most one edge can be selected per atom, making this a maximum-weight bipartite graph matching problem. The solution to this problem can be found using the Hungarian algorithm [33].

The Hungarian method is as follows. Initially, an overall score $F_{all} = 0$ is set. Additionally, an artificial source node s and an artificial destination node d are added to the bipartite graph. A directed edge es,i with zero weight is added for each of the atom nodes i from S_R and similarly, directed edges ej,d with zero weight are drawn from each of the atoms nodes of S_Q. The algorithm then proceeds as follows:

1. Find the shortest distance $F(i)$ from the source node s to every other node i using the Bellman–Ford algorithm.
2. Assign a new weight $w'(i,j)$ to each edge that does not originate from the source node s as follows:

$$w'(i,j) = w(i,j) + [F(i) - F(j)] \qquad (15.9)$$

3. Update F_{all} as $F_{all}' = F_{all} - F_d$.
4. Reverse the direction of the edges along the shortest path from s to d.
5. If $F_{all} > F_d$ and a path exists between s and d, then repeat step 1.

The iterative process of the Hungarian algorithm stops when either there is no path from s to d or the shortest distance from the source node to the destination node $F(d)$ is greater than the current overall score F_{all}. At the end of the process, the graph will consist of a set of directed edges that have been reversed (they now point from nodes of S_Q to nodes from S_R. These reversed edges represent the new equivalence relationships between the atoms of S_Q and the atoms of S_R.

The equivalence relationship found by the bipartite matching algorithm can now be used to superimpose the two proteins using the singular value decomposition. After superpositioning the new equivalent atoms, a new bipartite graph is created and the process is iterated until the change in RMSD on superposition falls below a threshold.

15.4.2 A Basis Set of Binding Surface Signature Pockets

The ability to compare structural similarities between to protein surface regions can provide insight into shared biological functions. As mentioned earlier, when dealing with local surface regions, one has to be careful when choosing a functional representative pocket because of the inherent flexibility of the binding surfaces. We have developed a method that automatically generates a set of functional pocket templates, called *signature pockets* of local surface regions that can be used as a representative a functional surface for structural comparison. These signature pockets contain broad structural information and have discriminating ability.

A signature pocket is derived from sequence order–independent structural alignments of precomputed surface pockets. Our signature pocket method does not require the atoms of the signature pocket to be present in all member structures. Instead, signature pockets can be created at varying degrees of partial structural similarity and can be hierarchically organized according to their structural similarity.

The input of our signature pocket algorithm is a set of functional pockets from the CASTp database [18]. All versus all pairwise sequence order–independent local surface alignment is performed on the input functional surface pockets. A distance is calculated on the basis of the RMSD and the chemistry of the paired atoms of the structural alignment [16]. The resulting distance matrix is used by an agglomerative clustering method. The signature of the functional pocket is then derived using a recursive process following the hierarchical tree.

The recursive process begins by finding the two closest siblings (pockets S_A and S_B), and combining them into a single structure S_{AB}. During the recursive process, S_A or S_B may themselves already be a combination of several structures. When combining two structures, we follow these criteria:

1. If two atoms were considered equivalent in a structural alignment, a single coordinate is created in the new structure to represent both atoms. The new coordinate is calculated as the average of the two underlying atom coordinates.

2. If no equivalence was found for an atom during the structural alignment, the coordinates of that atom are transferred directly into the new pocket structure.

A count of the number of times that an atom at the position i was present in the underlying set of pockets (N) is recorded during each step in the recursive process. A *preservation ratio* $\rho(i)$ is calculated for each atom of the signature pocket by dividing N by the total number of constituent pockets. In addition, the mean distance of the coordinates of the aligned atoms to their geometric center is recorded as the *location variation* v. At the end of each step, the new structure S_{AB} replaces the two structures S_A and S_B in the hierarchical tree and the process is repeated on the updated hierarchical tree.

The recursive process can be stopped at any point during its traversal of the hierarchical tree by selecting a ρ threshold. Depending on the choice of the ρ threshold, a single or multiple signature pockets can be created. Figure 15.3a shows a low ρ threshold that results in a set of three signature pockets. As the threshold is raised, fewer signature pockets are created (Fig. 15.3b). A single signature pocket representing all surface pockets in the dataset can be generated by raising the threshold even further (Fig. 15.3). The set of signature pockets from different clusters in the hierarchical tree form a *basis set* that represents an ensemble of differently sampled conformations of the surface pockets in the PDB. The basis set of signature pockets can be used to accurately classify and predict enzymatic function.

15.4.2.1 Signature Pockets of NAD Binding Proteins

To illustrate how signature pockets and the basis set help identify structural elements that are important for binding and to show their accuracy in functional inference, we discuss a study performed on the nicotinamide adenine dinucleotide (NAD) binding proteins. NAD plays essential roles in metabolisms where it acts as a coenzyme in redox reactions, including glycolysis and the citric acid cycle.

We obtained a set of 457 NAD binding proteins of diverse fold and diverse evolutionary origin. We extracted the NAD binding surfaces from the CASTp database of protein pockets [18]. We obtained the hierarchical tree using the

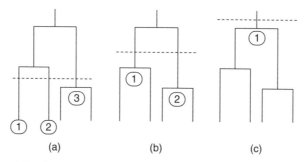

(a)	(b)	(c)

Figure 15.3 Different basis sets of signature pockets can be produced at different levels of structural similarity by raising or lowering the similarity threshold (*vertical dashed line*): (a) a low threshold will produce more signature pockets; (b) as the threshold is raised, fewer signature pockets will be created; (c) a single signature pocket can, in principle, be created to represent the full surface pocket dataset by raising the threshold.

results of our sequence order–independent surface alignments. The resulting nine signature pockets of the NAD binding pocket form a basis set, shown in Figure 15.4.

The signature pockets of NAD contain biological information. The signature pocket show in Figure 15.4j is based on a cluster of NAD binding proteins that act on the aldehyde group of donors, the signature pockets in (Fig. 15.4f,g) are for oxioreductases that act on the CH–CH group of donors, and the signature pockets of Figure 15.4e, h, and i are for clusters of alcohol oxioreductases that act on the CH–OH group of donors. The NAD–binding lyase family is represented in two signature pockets. The first represents lyases that cleave both C–O and P–O (Fig. 15.4d) and the second, containing lyases that cleave both C–O and CC bonds (Fig. 15.4b). These two signature pockets from two clusters of lyase conformations have a different class of conformations of the bound NAD cofactor (extended and compact).

In addition to the structural fold, the signature pockets are also determined by the conformation of the bound NAD cofactor (Fig. 15.4a). It can be seen in Fig. 15.4b–j that there are two general conformations of the NAD coenzyme. The coenzymes labeled C (Fig. 15.4b,c,f,g,h,j) have a closed conformation, while the conenzymes labeled X (Fig. 15.4d,e,i) have an extended conformation. This indicates that the binding pocket may take multiple conformations yet bind the same substrate in the same general structure. For example, the two structurally distinct signature pockets shown in Fig. 15.4f,g are derived from proteins that have the same biological function and SCOP fold. All of these proteins bind to the same NAD conformation.

We further evaluated the effectiveness of the NAD basis set by determining its accuracy at correctly classifying enzymes as either NAD binding or non-NAD-binding. We constructed a testing dataset of 576 surface pockets from the CASTp database [18]. This dataset is independent of the 457 NAD binding proteins that we used to create the signature pockets. We collected the 576 surface pockets by selecting the top three largest pockets by volume from 142 randomly chosen proteins and 50 proteins that have NAD bound in the PDB structure. We then structurally aligned each signature pocket against each of the 576 testing pockets. The testing pocket was assigned to be an NAD binding pocket if it structurally aligned to one of the nine NAD signature pockets with a distance under a pre-defined threshold. Otherwise it was classified as non-NAD-binding. The results show that the basis set of nine signature pockets can classify the correct NAD binding pocket with sensitivity and specificity of 0.91 and 0.89, respectively. We performed further testing to determine whether a single representative NAD bind-ing pocket, as opposed to a basis set, is sufficient for identifying NAD binding enzymes. We chose a single pocket representative from one of the nine clusters at random and attempted to classify our testing dataset by structural alignment. We used the same predefined threshold used in the basis set study. This was repeated 9 times using a representative from each of the nine clusters. We found that the results deteriorated significantly with an average sensitivity and speci-ficity of 0.36 and 0.23, respectively. This strongly indicates that the construction

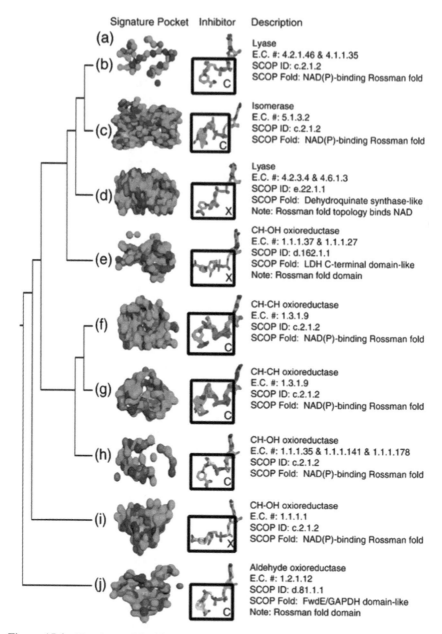

Figure 15.4   Topology of the hierarchical tree and signature pockets of the NAD binding pockets: (a) the resulting hierarchical tree topology; (b–j) the resulting signature pockets of the NAD binding proteins, along with the superimposed NAD molecules that were bound in the pockets of the member proteins of the respective clusters. The NAD coenzymes have two distinct conformations. Those in an extended conformation are marked with an X, and those in a compact conformation are marked with a C.

of a basis set of signature pockets to be used as a structural template provides significant improvement for functional inference of a set of evolutionarily diverse proteins.

15.5 CONCLUSION

We have discussed methods that provide solutions to the problems that arise during functional inference by structural similarity at both the global and at local surface levels. Both of our methods disregard the ordering of residues in the protein's primary sequence, making them sequence order–independent. The global method can be used to address the challenging problem of detecting structural similarities even after topological rearrangements of the proteins backbone. The fragment assembly approach based on the formulation of a relaxed integer programming problem and an algorithm based on scheduling split-interval graphs is guaranteed by an approximation ratio. We showed that this method is capable of discovering circularly permuted proteins and other more complex topological rearrangements.

We also described a method for sequence order–independent alignment of local surfaces on proteins. This method is based on a bipartite graph matching problem. We further show that the surface alignments can be used to automatically construct a basis set of signature pockets representing structurally preserved atoms across a family of proteins with similar biological functions.

ACKNOWLEDGMENTS

DasGupta and Liang was partially supported by NSF grant DBI-1062328.

REFERENCES

1. Aghili AS, Agrawal D, El Abbadi A, PADS: Protein structure alignment using directional shape signatures, *Proc. Database Systems for Advanced Applications (DASFAA) Conf.*, 2004.

2. Alexandrov NN, Fischer D, Analysis of topological and nontopological structural similarities in the PDB: New examples from old structures, *Proteins* **25**:354–365 (1996).

3. Altschul SF, Madden TL, Schaffer AA, Zhang J, Zhang Z, Miller W, Lipman DJ, Gapped BLAST and PSI-BLAST: A new generation of protein database search programs, *Nucleic Acids Res.* **25**:3389–3402 (1997).

4. Altschul SF, Warren G, Miller W, Myers EW, Lipman DJ, Basic local alignment search tool, *J. Mol. Biolo.*, **215**:403–410 (1990).

5. Andrade MA, Brown NP, Leroy C, Hoersch S, de Daruvar A, Reich C, Franchini J, Tamames A, Valencia A, Ouzounis C, Sander C, Automated genome sequence analysis and annotation, *Bioinformatics*, **15**:391–412 (1999).

6. Rost B, Twilight zone of protein sequence alignments, *Protein Eng.* **12**:85–94 (1999).

7. Bandyopadhyay D, Huan J, Liu J, Prins J, Snoeyink J, Wang W, Tropsha A, Functional neighbors: Inferring relationships between nonhomologous protein families using family-specific packing motifs, *IEEE Trans. Inf. Technol. Biomed.* **14**(5):1137–1143 (2010).

8. Bar-Yehuda R, Halldorsson MM, Naor J, Shacknai H, Shapira I, Scheduling split intervals, *Proc. 14th ACM-SIAM Symp. Discrete Algorithms*, 2002, pp. 732–741.

9. Berman HM, Westbrook J, Feng Z, Gilliland G, Bhat TN, Weissig H, Shindyalov IN, Bourne PE, The protein data bank, *Nucleic Acids Res.* **28**:235–242 (2000).

10. Binkowski TA, Joachimiak A, Protein functional surfaces: Global shape matching and local spatial alignments of ligand binding sites, *BMC Struct. Biol.* **8**:45 (2008).

11. Boeckmann B, Bairoch A, Apweiler R, Blatter MC, Estreicher A, Gasteiger E, Martin MJ, Michoud K, O'Donovan C, Phan I, Pilbout S, Schneider M, The SWISS-PROT protein knowledgebase and its supplement TrEMBL in 2003, *Nucleic Acids Res.* **31**:365–370 (2003).

12. Chen L, Wu LY, Wang R, Wang Y, Zhang S, Zhang XS, Comparison of protein structures by multi-objective optimization, *Genome Inform.* **16**(2):114–124 (2005).

13. Dayhoff MO, Schwartz RM, Orcutt BC, A model of evolutionary change in proteins, *Atlas Protein Seq. Struct.* **5**(3):345–352 (1978).

14. Deng M, Zhang K, Mehta S, Chen T, Sun F, Prediction of protein function using protein-protein interaction data, *J. Comput. Biol.* **10**(6):947–960 (2009).

15. Dror O, Benyamini H, Nussinov R, Wolfson HJ, MASS: Multiple structural alignment by secondary structures, *Bioinformatics* **19**:i95–i104 (2003).

16. Dundas J, Adamian L, Liang J, Structural Signatures of Enzyme Binding Pockets from Order-Independent Surface Alignment: A Study of Metalloendopeptidase and NAD Binding Proteins, *J. Mol. Biol.* **406**(5):713–729 (2011).

17. Dundas J, Binkowski TA, DasGupta B, Liang J, Topology independent protein structural alignment, *BMC Bioinformatics* **8**:388 (2008).

18. Dundas J, Ouyang Z, Tseng J, Binkowski TA, Turpaz Y, Liang J, CASTp: Computed atlas of surface topography of proteins with structural and topographical mapping of functionally annotated residues, *Nucleic Acids Res.*, **34**:W116–W118 (2006).

19. Dutta S, Akey IV, Dingwall C, Hartman KL, Laue T, Nolte RT, Head JF, Akey CW, The crystal structure of nucleoplasmin-core implications for histone binding and neucleosome assembly, *Mol. Cell* **8**:841–853 (2001).

20. Fischer D, Norel R, Wolfson H, Nussinov R, Surface motifs by a computer vision technique: Searches, detection, and implications for protein-ligand recognition, *Proteins* **16**:278–292 (1993).

21. Binkowski TA, Adamian L, Liang J, Inferring functional relationship of proteins from local sequence and spatial surface patterns, *J. Mol. Biol.* **332**:505–526 (2003).

22. Gold ND, Jackson RM, Fold independent structural comparisons of protein-ligand binding sites for exploring functional relationships, *J. Mol. Biol.* **355**:1112–1124 (2006).

23. Hasegawa H, Holm L, Advances and pitfalls of protein structural alignment, *Curr. Opin. Struct. Biol.* **19**:341–348 (2009).

24. Hegyi H, Gerstein M, The relationship between protein structure and function: A comprehensive survey with application to the yeast genome, *J. Mol. Biol.*, **288**:147–164 (1999).

25. Henikoff S, Henikoff JG, Amino acid substitution matrices from protein blocks, *Proc. Natl. Acad. Sci. USA* **89**(22):10915–10919 (1992).

26. Hobohm U, Sander C, Enlarged representative set of protein structures, *Protein Sci.* **3**:522 (1994).

27. Holm L, Sander C, Protein structure comparison by alignment of distance matrices, *J. Mol. Biol.* **233**:123–138 (1993).

28. Hulo N, Sigrist CJA, Le Saux V, Recent improvements to the PROSITE database, *Nucleic Acids Res.* **32**:D134–D137 (2004).

29. Ilyin VA, Abyzov A, Leslin CM, Structural alignment of proteins by a novel TOPOFIT method, as a superimposition of common volumes at a topomax point, *Protein Sci.* **13**:1865–1874 (2004).

30. Jeffery C, Molecular mechanisms for multi-tasking; recent crystal structures of moonlighting proteins, *Curr. Opin. Struct. Biol.* **14**:663–668 (2004).

31. Jensen LJ, Gupta R, Blom N, Devos D, Tamames J, Kesmir C, Nielsen H, Staerfeldt HH, Rapacki K, Workman C, Andersen CAF, Knudsen S, Krogh A, Valencia A, Brunak S, Prediction of human protein function from post-translational modifications and localization features, *J. Mol. Biol.* **319**:1257–1265 (2002).

32. Karplus K, Barret C, Hughey R, Hidden Markov models for detecting remote protein homologues, *Bioinformatics* **14**:846–856 (1998).

33. Kuh HW, The Hungarian method for the assignment problem, *Nav. Res. Logist. Q.* **2**:83–97 (1995).

34. Laskowski RA, Watson JD, Thornton JM, ProFunc: A server for predicting protein function from 3D structure, *Nucleic Acids Res.* **33**:W89–W93 (2005).

35. Lee S, Li B, La D, Fang Y, Ramani K, Rustamov R, Kihara D, Fast protein tertiary structure retrieval based on global surface shape similarity, *Proteins* **72**:1259–1273 (2008).

36. Lichtarge O, Bourne HR, Cohen FE, An evolutionary trace method defines binding surfaces common to protein families, *J. Mol. Biol.* **7**:39–46 (1994).

37. Lindqvist Y, Schneider G, Circular permutations of natural protein sequences: Structural evidence, *Curr. Opin. Struct. Biol.* **7**:422–477 (1997).

38. Meng E, Polacco B, Babbitt P, Superfamily active site templates, *Proteins*, **55**:962–967 (2004).

39. Moll M, Kavraki L, LabelHash, *A Flexible and Extensible Method for Matching Structural Motifs*, available from Nature Precedings (`http://dx.doi.org/10.1038/npre.2008.2199.1`) (2008).

40. Murzin AG, Brenner SE, Hubbard T, Chothia C, SCOP: A structural classification of proteins database for the investigation of sequences and structures, *J. Mol. Biol.* **247**:536–540 (1995).

41. Norel R, Fischer H, Wolfson H, Nussinov R, Molecular surface recognition by computer vision-based technique, *Protein Eng.* **7**(1):39–46 (1994).

42. Orengo C, Todd A, Thornton J, From protein structure to function, *Curr. Opin. Struct. Biol.* **9**:374–382 (1999).

43. Orengo CA, Michie AD, Jones DT, Swindells MB, Thornton JM, CATH: A hierarchical classification of protein domains structures, *Structure* **5**:1093–1108 (1997).

44. Pal D, Eisenberg D, Inference of protein function from protein structure, *Structure* **13**:121–130 (2005).

45. Shah I, Hunterm L, Predicting enzyme function from sequence: A systematic appraisal, *Intell. Syst. Mol. Biol.* **5**:276–283 (1997).

46. Shih ES, Hwang MJ, Alternative alignments from comparison of protein structures, *Proteins* **56**:519–527 (2004).

47. Shindyalov IN, Bourne PE, Protein structure alignment by incremental combinatorial extension (CE) of the optimal path, *Protein Eng.* **11**(9):739–747 (1998).

48. Standley DM, Toh H, Nakamura H, Detecting local structural similarity in proteins by maximizing the number of equivalent residues, *Proteins: Struct., Funct., Genet.* **57**:381–391 (2004).

49. Szustakowski JD, Weng Z, Protein structure alignment using a genetic algorithm, *Proteins: Struct., Func., Genet.* **38**:428–440 (2000).

50. Tabtiang RK, Cezairliyan BO, Grant RA, Chochrane JC, Sauer RT, Consolidating critical binding determinants by noncyclic rearrangement of protein secondary structure, *Proc. Natl. Acad. Sci. USA* **7**:2305–2309 (2004).

51. Teichert F, Bastolla U, Porto M, SABERTOOTH: Protein structure comparison based-on vectorial structure representation, *BMC Bioinformatics* **8**:425 (2007).

52. Teyra J, Paszkowski-Rogacz M, Anders G, Pisabarro MT, SCOWLP classification: structural comparison and analysis of protein bindign regions, *BMC Bioinformatics* **9**:9 (2008).

53. Tseng YY, Dundas J, Liang J, Predicting protein function and binding profile via matching of local evolutionary and geometric surface patterns, *J. Mol. Biol.* **387**(2):451–464 (2009).

54. Tseng YY, Liang J, Estimation of amino acid residue substitution rates at local spatial regions and application in protein function inference: A Bayesian Monte Carlo approach, *Mol. Biol. Evol.* **23**:421–436 (2006).

55. Uliel S, Fliess A, Amir A, Unger R, A simple algorithm for detecting circular permutations in proteins, *Bioinformatics* **15**(11):930–936 (1999).

56. Veeramalai M, Gilbert D, A novel method for comparing topological models of protein structures enhanced with ligand information, *Bioinformatics* **24**(23):2698–2705 (2008).

57. Weidong T, Skolnick J, How well is enzyme function conserved as a function of pairwise sequence identity, *J. Mol. Biol.* **333**:863–882 (2003).

58. Woo EJ, Marshall J, Bauly J, Chen JG, Venis M, Napier RM, Pickersgill RW, Crystal structure of the auxin-binding protein 1 in complex with auxin, *EMBO J.* **21**:2877–2885 (2001).

59. Zhu J, Weng Z, A novel protein structure alignment algorithm, *Proteins: Struct., Funct., Bioinform.* **58**:618–627 (2005).

CHAPTER 16

FRACTAL RELATED METHODS FOR PREDICTING PROTEIN STRUCTURE CLASSES AND FUNCTIONS

ZU-GUO YU, VO ANH, JIAN-YI YANG, and SHAO-MING ZHU

16.1 INTRODUCTION

The molecular function of a protein can be inferred from the protein's structure information [1]. It is well known that an amino acid sequence partially determines the eventual three-dimensional structure of a protein, and the similarity at the protein sequence level implies similarity of function [2,3]. The prediction of protein structure and function from amino acid sequences is one of the most important and challenge problems in molecular biology.

Protein secondary structure, which is a summary of the general conformation and hydrogen bonding pattern of the amino acid backbone [4,5], provides some knowledge to further simplify the complicated 3D structure prediction problem. Hence an intermediate but useful step is to predict the protein secondary structure. Since the 1970s, many methods have been developed for predicting protein secondary structure (see the more recent references cited in Ref. [6]).

Four main classes of protein structures, based on the types and arrangement of their secondary structural elements, were recognized [7]: (1) the α helices, (2) the β strands, and (3) those with a mixture of α and β shapes denoted as $\alpha + \beta$ and α/β. This structural classification has been accepted and widely used in protein structure and function prediction. As a consequence, it has become an important problem and can help build protein database and predict protein function. In fact, Hou et al. [1] (see also a short report published in *Science* [8]) constructed a map of the protein structure space using the pairwise structural similarity of 1898 protein chains. They found that the space has a defining feature showing these four classes clustered together as four elongated arms emerging

Algorithmic and Artificial Intelligence Methods for Protein Bioinformatics. First Edition.
Edited by Yi Pan, Jianxin Wang, Min Li.
© 2014 John Wiley & Sons, Inc. Published 2014 by John Wiley & Sons, Inc.

from a common center. A review by Chou [9] described the development of some existing methods for prediction of protein structural classes. Proteins in the same family usually have similar functions. Therefore family identification is an important problem in the study of proteins.

Because similarity in the protein sequence normally implies similarity of function and structure, the similarities of protein sequences can therefore be used to detect the biological function and interaction of proteins [10]. It is necessary to enrich the concept and context of similarity, because some proteins with low sequence identity may have similar tertiary structure and function [11].

Fractal geometry provides a mathematical formalism for describing complex spatial and dynamical structures [12,13]. Fractal methods are known to be useful for detection of similarity. Traditional multifractal analysis is a useful way to characterize the spatial heterogeneity of both theoretical and experimental fractal patterns [14]. More recently it has been applied successfully in many different fields, including time series analysis and financial modeling [15]. Some applications of fractal methods to DNA sequences are provided in References [16–18] and references cited therein.

Wavelet analysis, recurrence quantification analysis (RQA), and empirical mode decomposition (EMD) are related to fractal methods in nonlinear sciences. Wavelet analysis is a useful tool in many applications such as noise reduction, image processing, information compression, synthesis of signals, and the study of biological data. Wavelets are mathematical functions that decompose data into different frequency components and then describe each component with a resolution matched to its scale [19,20]. The recurrence plot (RP) is a purely graphical tool originally proposed by Eckmann et al. [21] to detect patterns of recurrence in the data. RQA is a relatively new nonlinear technique introduced by Zbilut and Webber [22,23] that can quantify the information supplied by RP. The traditional EMD for data, which is a highly adaptive scheme serving as a complement to Fourier and wavelet transforms, was originally proposed by Huang et al. [24]. In EMD, a complicated dataset is decomposed into a finite, often small, number of components called *intrinsic mode functions* (IMFs). Lin et al. [25] presented a new approach to EMD. This method has been used successfully in many applications in analyzing a diverse range of datasets in biological and medical sciences, geophysics, astronomy, engineering, and other fields [26,27].

Fractal methods have been used to study proteins. Their applications include fractal analysis of the proton exchange kinetics [28], chaos game representation of protein structures [29], sequences based on the detailed HP model [30,31], fractal dimension of protein mass [32], fractal properties of protein chains [33], fractal dimensions of protein secondary structures [34], multifractal analysis of the solvent accessibility of proteins [35], and the measure representation of protein sequences [36]. The wavelet approach has been used for prediction of secondary structures of proteins [37–45]. Chen et al. [41] predicted the secondary structure of a protein by the continuous wavelet transform (CWT) and Chou–Fasman method. Marsolo et al. [42] combined the pairwise distance with wavelet decomposition to generate a set of coefficients and capture some features of proteins.

Qiu et al. [43] used the continuous wavelet transform to extract the position of the α helices and short peptides with special scales. Rezaei et al. [44] applied wavelet analysis to membrane proteins. Pando et al. [45] used the discrete wavelet transform to detect protein secondary structures. Webber et al. [46] defined two independent variables to elucidate protein secondary structures based on the RQA of coordinates of α-carbon atoms. The variables can describe the percentage of α carbons that are composed of an α helix and a β sheet, respectively. The ability of RQA to deal with protein sequences was reviewed by Giuliani et al. [47]. The IMFs obtained by the EMD method were used to discover similarities of protein sequences, and the results showed that IMFs may reflect the functional identities of proteins [48,49].

More recently, the authors used the fractal methods and related wavelet analysis, RQA and EMD methods to study the prediction of protein structure classes and functions [50–54]. In this chapter, we review the methods and results in these studies.

16.2 METHODS

16.2.1 Measure Representation Based on the Detailed HP Model and Six-Letter Model

The detailed HP model was proposed by Yu et al. [30]. In this model, 20 different kinds of amino acids are divided into four classes: nonpolar, negative polar, uncharged polar, and positive polar. The nonpolar class consists of the eight residues ALA, ILE, LEU, MET, PHE, PRO, TRP, and VAL; the negative polar class consists of the two residues ASP and GLU; the uncharged polar class is made up of the seven residues ASN, CYS, GLN, GLY, SER, THR, and TYR; and the remaining three residues ARG, HIS, and LYS designate the positive polar class.

For a given protein sequence $s = s_1 \cdots s_L$ with length L, where s_i is one of the 20 kinds of amino acids for $i = 1, \cdots, L$, we define

$$
a_i = \begin{cases}
0, & \text{if } s_i \text{ is nonpolar} \\
1, & \text{if } s_i \text{ is negative polar} \\
2, & \text{if } s_i \text{ is uncharged polar} \\
3, & \text{if } s_i \text{ is positive polar}
\end{cases}
\tag{16.1}
$$

This results in a sequence $X(s) = a_1 \cdots a_L$, where a_i is a letter of the alphabet $\{0, 1, 2, 3\}$. The mapping (16.1) is called the detailed HP model [30].

According to Chou and Fasman [55], the 20 different kinds of amino acids are divided into six classes: strong β, former (H_β); β former (h_β); weak β, former (I_β); β indifferent (i_β); β breaker (b_β); and strong β breaker (B_β). The H_β class consists of the three residues Met, Val, and IIE; the h_β class consists of the seven residues Cys, Tyr, Phe, Gln, Leu, Thr, and Trp; the I_β class consists of the residue

Ala; the i_β class consists of the three residues Arg, Gly, and Asp; the b_β class is made up of the five residues Lys, Ser, His, Asn, and Pro; and the remaining residue Glu constitutes the B_β class.

For a given protein sequence $s = s_1 \cdots s_L$ with length L, where s_i is one of the 20 kinds of amino acids for $i = 1 \cdots L$, we define

$$
a_i = \begin{cases}
0, & \text{if } s_i \text{ is in the } B_\beta \text{ class} \\
1, & \text{if } s_i \text{ is in the } b_\beta \text{ class} \\
2, & \text{if } s_i \text{ is in the } i_\beta \text{ class} \\
3, & \text{if } s_i \text{ is in the } I_\beta \text{ class} \\
4, & \text{if } s_i \text{ is in the } h_\beta \text{ class} \\
5, & \text{if } s_i \text{ is in the } H_\beta \text{ class}
\end{cases}
\tag{16.2}
$$

This results in a sequence $X(s) = a_1 \cdots a_L$, where a_i is a letter of the alphabet $\{0, 1, 2, 3, 4, 5\}$. The mapping (16.2) is called the *six-letter model* [51].

Here we call any string made up of K letters from the set $\{0, 1, 2, 3\}$ (for the detailed HP model) or $\{0, 1, 2, 3, 4, 5\}$ (for the six-letter model) a K-string. For a given K, there are in total 4^K or 6^K different K strings. In order to count the number of K strings in a sequence $X(s)$ from a protein sequence s, we need 4^K or 6^K counters. We divide the interval $[0, 1]$ into 4^K or 6^K disjoint subintervals, and use each subinterval to represent a counter. For $r = r_1 \cdots r_K, r_i \in \{0, 1, 2, 3\}, i = 1, \cdots, K$, which is a substring with length K, we define

$$
x_{\text{left}}(r) = \sum_{i=1}^{K} \frac{r_i}{4^i}, \qquad x_{\text{right}}(r) = \frac{1}{4^K} + \sum_{i=1}^{K} \frac{r_i}{4^i}
\tag{16.3}
$$

For $r = r_1 \cdots r_K$, $r_i \in \{0, 1, 2, 3, 4, 5\}$, $i = 1, \cdots, K$, which is a substring with length K, we define

$$
x_{\text{left}}(r) = \sum_{i=1}^{K} \frac{r_i}{6^i}, \qquad x_{\text{right}}(r) = \frac{1}{6^K} + \sum_{i=1}^{K} \frac{r_i}{6^i}.
\tag{16.4}
$$

We then use the subinterval $[x_{\text{left}}(r), x_{\text{right}}(r))$ to represent substring r. Let $N_K(r)$ be the number of times that a substring r with length K appears in the sequence $X(s)$ (when we count these numbers, we open a reading frame with width K and slide the frame one amino acid each time). We define

$$
F_K(r) = \frac{N_K(r)}{L - K + 1}
\tag{16.5}
$$

to be the frequency of substring r. It follows that $\sum_{\{r\}} F_K(r) = 1$. We can now define a measure μ_K on $[0, 1)$ by $d\mu_K(x) = Y(x)dx$, where

$$
Y_K(x) = 4^K F_K(r),
\tag{16.6}
$$

when $x \in [x_{\text{left}}(r), x_{\text{right}}(r))$ defined by (16.3). We define a measure ν_K on $[0, 1)$ by $d\nu_K(x) = Y_K'(x)dx$, where

$$Y_K'(x) = 6^K F_K(r), \tag{16.7}$$

when $x \in [x_{\text{left}}(r), x_{\text{right}}(r))$ defined by (16.4). We see that $\int_0^1 d\mu_K(x) = 1$ and $\int_0^1 d\nu_K(x) = 1$. We call μ_K and ν_K the *measure representation* of the protein sequence corresponding to the given K based on the detailed HP model and the six-letter model, respectively.

16.2.2 Measures and Time Series Based on the Physicochemical Features of Amino Acids

Measured in kcal/mol, the *hydrophobic free energies* of the 20 amino acids are $A = 0.87$, $R = 0.85$, $N = 0.09$, $D = 0.66$, $C = 1.52$, $Q = 0.0$, $E = 0.67$, $G = 0.0$, $H = 0.87$, $I = 3.15$, $L = 2.17$, $K = 1.65$, $M = 1.67$, $F = 2.87$, $P = 2.77$, $S = 0.07$, $T = 0.07$, $W = 3.77$, $Y = 2.76$, and $V = 1.87$ [39].

The *solvent accessibility* (SA) values for solvent exposed area > 30 Å are $S = 0.70$, $T = 0.71$, $A = 0.48$, $G = 0.51$, $P = 0.78$, $C = 0.32$, $D = 0.81$, $E = 0.93$, $Q = 0.81$, $N = 0.82$, $L = 0.41$, $I = 0.39$, $V = 0.40$, $M = 0.44$, $F = 0.42$, $Y = 0.67$, $W = 0.49$, $K = 0.93$, $R = 0.84$, and $H = 0.66$ [56].

The *Schneider–Wrede scale* (SWH) values of the 20 kinds of amino acids are $A = 1.6$, $R = -12.3$, $N = -4.8$, $D = -9.2$, $C = 2$, $Q = -1.1$, $E = -8.2$, $G = 1$, $H = -3$, $I = 3.1$, $L = 2.8$, $K = -8.8$, $M = 2.4$, $F = 3.7$, $P = -0.2$, $S = 0.6$, $T = 1.2$, $W = 1.9$, $Y = -0.7$, and $V = 2.6$ [47]. Yang et al. [51] added a constant 12.30 to these values to make all the 20 values nonnegative, yielding the *revised Schneider–Wrede scale hydrophobicity* (RSWH).

Rose et al. [57] proposed different measures of hydrophobicity of proteins. They gave four kinds of values for surface area and hydrophobicity of each amino acid. We use A^0, the stochastic standard state accessibility, that is, the *solvent accessible surface area* (SASA) of a residue in standard state. The SASA of the 20 kinds of amino acids are $A = 118.1$, $R = 256.0$, $N = 165.5$, $D = 158.7$, $C = 146.1$, $Q = 193.2$, $E = 186.2$, $G = 88.1$, $H = 202.5$, $I = 181.0$, $L = 193.1$, $K = 225.8$, $M = 203.4$, $F = 222.8$, $P = 146.8$, $S = 129.8$, $T = 152.5$, $W = 266.3$, $Y = 236.8$, and $V = 164.5$.

Each amino acid can also be represented by the value of the *volume of sidechains* of amino acids [58]. These values are $A = 27.5$, $C = 44.6$, $D = 40$, $E = 62$, $F = 115.5$, $G = 0$, $H = 79$, $I = 93.5$, $K = 100$, $L = 93.5$, $M = 94.1$, $N = 58.7$, $P = 41.9$, $Q = 80.7$, $R = 105$, $S = 29.3$, $T = 51.3$, $V = 71.5$, $W = 145.5$, and $Y = 117.3$.

We convert each amino acid according to hydrophobic free energy, SA, RSWH, SASA, and volume of sidechains along the protein sequence to calculate five different numerical sequences, and view them as time series.

Let T_t, $t = 1, 2, \ldots, N$, be the time series with length N. First, we define $F_t = T_t / (\sum_{j=1}^{N} T_j)$, $(t = 1, 2, \ldots, N)$ as the frequency of T_t. It follows that

$\sum_{t=1}^{N} F_t = 1$. Now we can define a measure ν_t on the interval $[0, 1)$ by $d\nu_t(dx) = Y_1(x)dx$, where

$$Y_1(x) = N \times F_t = \frac{T_t}{\frac{1}{N} \sum_{j=1}^{N} T_j}, \quad x \in \left[\frac{t-1}{N}, \frac{t}{N} \right) \tag{16.8}$$

We denote the interval $[(t-1)/N, t/N)$ by I_t. It is seen that $\nu_t([0, 1)) = 1$ and $\nu_t(I_t) = F_t$. We call $\nu_t(x)$ the *measure* for the time series.

16.2.3   Z-Curve Representation of Proteins

The concept of Z-curve representation of a DNA sequence was first proposed by Zhang and Zhang [59]. We propose a similar concept for proteins [50]. Once we get the sequence $X(s) = a_1 \cdots a_L$ for a protein, where a_i is a letter of the alphabet $\{0, 1, 2, 3\}$ as in Section 16.2.1, we can define the *Z-curve representation* of this protein as follows. This Z curve consists of a series of nodes Q_i, $i = 0, 1, \ldots, L$, whose coordinates are denoted by x_i, y_i and z_i. These coordinates are defined as

$$\begin{cases} x_i = 2(\text{num}_i^0 + \text{num}_i^2) - i \\ y_i = 2(\text{num}_i^0 + \text{num}_i^1) - i, \quad i = 0, 1, 2, \ldots, L \\ z_i = 2(\text{num}_i^0 + \text{num}_i^3) - i \end{cases} \tag{16.9}$$

where $\text{num}_i^0, \text{num}_i^1, \text{num}_i^2, \text{num}_i^3$ denote the number of occurrences of the symbols 0,1,2,3 in the prefix $a_1 a_2 \cdots a_i$, respectively, and $\text{num}_0^0 = \text{num}_0^1 = \text{num}_0^2 = \text{num}_0^3 = 0$. The connection of nodes $Q_0, Q_1, \ldots, Q_L$ to one another by straight lines is defined as the *Z-curve representation* of this protein. We then define

$$\begin{cases} \Delta x_i = x_i - x_{i-1} \\ \Delta y_i = y_i - y_{i-1}, \quad i = 1, 2, \ldots, L \\ \Delta z_i = z_i - z_{i-1} \end{cases} \tag{16.10}$$

where Δx_i, Δy_i, and Δz_i can only have values 1 and -1.

16.2.4   Chaos Game Representation of Proteins and Related Time Series

Chaos game representation (CGR) of protein structures was first proposed by Fiser et al. [29]. We denote this CGR by 20-CGR as 20 kinds of letters are used to represent protein sequences. Later Basu et al. [60] and Yu et al. [31] proposed other kinds of CGRs for proteins, in which 12 and 4 kinds of letters were used for protein sequences, respectively. We denote them by 12-CGR and 4-CGR.

16.2.4.1 Reverse Encoding for Amino Acids It is known that there are several kinds of coded methods for some amino acids. As a result, there should be many possible nucleotide sequences for one given protein sequence. We have used [52], the encoding method proposed by Deschavanne and Tufféry [61], which is listed in Table 1 of our study [52]. Deschavanne and Tufféry [61] explained that the rationale for the choice of this fixed code is to keep a balance in base composition so as to maximize the difference between the amino acid codes.

After one protein sequence is transformed into nucleotide sequences, we can use the CGR of nucleotide sequences [62] to analyze it; the CGR obtained is abbreviated AAD-CGR (amino acids to DNA CGR). The CGR for a nucleotide sequence is defined on the square $[0, 1] \times [0, 1]$, where the four vertices correspond to the four letters A, C, G, and T: the first point of the plot is placed half way between the center of the square and the vertex corresponding to the first letter of the nucleotide sequence; the ith point of the plot is then placed half way between the $(i - 1)$th point and the vertex corresponding to the ith letter. The plot is then called the CGR of the nucleotide sequence, or the AAD-CGR of the protein sequence.

We can decompose the AAD-CGR plot into two time series [52]. Any point in the AAD-CGR plot is determined by two coordinates: x and y coordinates. Because the AAD-CGR plot can be uniquely reconstructed from these two time series, all the information stored in the AAD-CGR plot is contained in the time series, and the information in the AAD-CGR plot comes from the primary sequence of proteins. Therefore, any analysis of the two time series is equivalent to an indirect analysis of the protein primary sequence. It is possible that such analysis provides better results than direct analysis of the protein primary sequences.

16.2.5 Time Series Based on 6-Letter Model, 12-Letter Model, and 20-Letter Model

According to the 6-letter model, the protein sequence can be represented by a numerical sequence $\{a_i\}_{i=1}^{L}$; here $a_i \in \{0, 1, 2, 3, 4, 5\}$ for each $i = 1, 2, \ldots, L$.

We now analogously define a 12-letter model and a 20-letter model. With the idea of chaos game representation based on a 12-sided regular polygon [60], we define the 12-letter model as $A = 0$, $G = 0$, $P = 1$, $S = 2$, $T = 2$, $H = 3$, $Q = 4$, $N = 5$, $D = 6$, $E = 6$, $R = 7$, $K = 7$, $I = 8$, $L = 8$, $V = 8$, $M = 8$, $W = 9$, $F = 10$, $Y = 10$, and $C = 11$ according to the order of vertices on the 12-sided regular polygon to represent these amino acids.

The 20-letter model can be similarly defined as $A = 0$, $R = 1$, $N = 2$, $D = 3$, $C = 4$, $Q = 5$, $E = 6$, $G = 7$, $H = 8$, $I = 9$, $L = 10$, $K = 11$, $M = 12$, $F = 13$, $P = 14$, $S = 15$, $T = 16$, $W = 17$, $Y = 18$, and $V = 19$ according to the dictionary order of the 3-letter representation of each amino acid listed in Brown's treatise [63].

These three models can be used to convert a protein sequence into three different numerical sequences (and also can be viewed as time series).

16.2.6 Iterated Function Systems Model

In order to simulate the measure representation of a protein sequence, we proposed use of the *iterated function systems* (IFS) model [30]. IFS is the acronym assigned by Barnsley and Demko [64] originally to a system of contractive maps $w = \{w_1, w_2, \ldots, w_N\}$. Let E_0 be a compact set in a compact metric space, $E_{\sigma_1 \sigma_2 \cdots \sigma_n} = w_{\sigma_1} \circ w_{\sigma_2} \circ \cdots \circ w_{\sigma_n}(E_0)$ and

$$E_n = \bigcup_{\sigma_1, \ldots, \sigma_n \in \{1, 2, \ldots, N\}} E_{\sigma_1 \sigma_2 \cdots \sigma_n}$$

Then $E = \bigcap_{n=1}^{\infty} E_n$ is called the *attractor* of the IFS. The attractor is usually a fractal set and the IFS is a relatively general model to generate many well-known fractal sets such as the Cantor set and the Koch curve. Given a set of probabilities $P_i > 0$, $\sum_{i=1}^{N} P_i = 1$, we pick an $x_0 \in E$ and define the iteration sequence

$$x_{n+1} = w_{\sigma_n}(x_n), \qquad n = 0, 1, 2, 3, \ldots$$

where the indices σ_n are chosen randomly and independently from the set $\{1, 2, \ldots, N\}$ with probabilities $P(\sigma_n = i) = P_i$. Then every orbit $\{x_n\}$ is dense in the attractor E [64]. For n sufficiently large, we can view the orbit $\{x_0, x_1, \ldots, x_n\}$ as an approximation of E. This process is called *chaos game*.

Let χ_B the characteristic function for the Borel subset $B \subset E$, then, from the ergodic theorem for IFS [64], the limit

$$\mu(B) = \lim_{n \to \infty} \left[\frac{1}{n+1} \sum_{k=0}^{n} \chi_B(x_k) \right]$$

exists. The measure μ is the invariant measure of the attractor of the IFS. In other words, $\mu(B)$ is the relative visitation frequency of B during the chaos game. A histogram approximation of the invariant measure may then be obtained by counting the number of visits made to each pixel.

The coefficients in the contractive maps and the probabilities in the IFS model are the parameters to be estimated for a real measure that we want to simulate. A moment method [30,65] can be used to perform this task.

From the measure representation of a protein sequence based on the detailed HP model, it is logical to choose $N = 4$ and

$$w_1(x) = \frac{x}{4}, \qquad w_2(x) = \frac{x}{4} + \frac{1}{4},$$

$$w_3(x) = \frac{x}{4} + \frac{1}{2}, \qquad w_4(x) = \frac{x}{4} + \frac{3}{4}$$

in the IFS model. For a given measure representation of a protein sequence based on the detailed HP model, we obtain the estimated values of the probabilities P_1, P_2, P_3, P_4 by solving an optimization problem [65]. Using the estimated values of the probabilities, we can use the chaos game to generate a histogram approximation of the invariant measure of the IFS that can be compared with the real measure representation of the protein sequence.

16.2.7 Detrended Fluctuation Analysis

The exponent in a detrended fluctuation analysis can be used to characterize the correlation of a time series [17,18]. We view Δx_i, Δy_i, and Δz_i, $i = 1, 2, \ldots, L$, in the Z-curve representation of proteins as time series. We denote this time series by $F(t), t = 1, \ldots, L$. First, the time series is integrated as $T(k) = \sum_{t=1}^{k}[F(t) - F_{av}]$, where F_{av} is the average over the whole time period. Next, the integrated time series is divided into boxes of equal length n. In each box of length n, a linear regression is fitted to the data by least squares, representing the trend in that box. We denote the T coordinate of the straight-line segments by $T_n(k)$. We then detrend the integrated time series $T(k)$ by subtracting the local trend $T_n(k)$ in each box. The root-mean-square fluctuation of this integrated and detrended time series is computed as

$$\mathcal{F}(n) = \sqrt{\frac{1}{N} \sum_{k=1}^{N} [T(k) - T_n(k)]^2} \tag{16.11}$$

Typically, $\mathcal{F}(n)$ increases with box size n. A linear relationship on a log–log plot indicates the presence of scaling $\mathcal{F}(n) \propto n^\lambda$. Under such conditions, the fluctuations can be characterized by the scaling exponent λ, the slope of the line in the regression $\ln \mathcal{F}(n)$ against $\ln n$. For uncorrelated data, the integrated time series $T(k)$ corresponds to a random walk, and therefore, $\lambda = 0.5$. A value of $0.5 < \lambda < 1.0$ indicates the presence of long memory so that, for example, a large value is likely to be followed by large values. In contrast, the range $0 < \lambda < 0.5$ indicates a different type of power-law correlation such that positive and negative values of the time series are more likely to alternate. We consider the exponents λ for the Δx_i, Δy_i, and Δz_i, $i = 1, 2, \ldots, L$, of the Z-curve representation of protein sequences as candidates constructing parameter spaces for proteins in this chapter. These exponents are denoted by λ_x, λ_y, and λ_z respectively.

16.2.8 Ordinary Multifractal Analysis

The most common algorithms of multifractal analysis are the so-called *fixed-size box counting algorithms* [16]. In the one-dimensional case, for a given measure μ with support $E \subset \mathbb{R}$, we consider the *partition sum*

$$Z_\epsilon(q) = \sum_{\mu(B) \neq 0} [\mu(B)]^q \tag{16.12}$$

with $q \in \mathbb{R}$, where the sum runs over all different nonempty boxes B of a given side ϵ in a grid covering of the support E, that is, $B = [k\epsilon, (k+1)\epsilon)$. The exponent $\tau(q)$ is defined by

$$\tau(q) = \lim_{\epsilon \to 0} \frac{\ln Z_\epsilon(q)}{\ln \epsilon} \tag{16.13}$$

and the generalized fractal dimensions of the measure are defined as

$$D_q = \frac{\tau(q)}{q-1} \qquad \text{for } q \neq 1 \tag{16.14}$$

$$D_q = \lim_{\epsilon \to 0} \frac{Z_{1,\epsilon}}{\ln \epsilon} \qquad \text{for } q = 1 \tag{16.15}$$

where $Z_{1,\epsilon} = \sum_{\mu(B) \neq 0} \mu(B) \ln \mu(B)$. The generalized fractal dimensions are numerically estimated through a linear regression of $(\ln Z_\epsilon(q))/(q-1)$ against $\ln \epsilon$ for $q \neq 1$, and similarly through a linear regression of $Z_{1,\epsilon}$ against $\ln \epsilon$ for $q = 1$. The value D_1 is called the *information dimension* and D_2, the *correlation dimension*.

The concept of phase transition in multifractal spectra was introduced in studies of logistic maps, Julia sets, and other simple systems. By following the thermodynamic formulation of multifractal measures, Canessa [66] derived an expression for the analogous specific heat as

$$C_q \equiv -\frac{\partial^2 \tau(q)}{\partial q^2} \approx 2\tau(q) - \tau(q+1) - \tau(q-1) \tag{16.16}$$

He showed that the form of C_q resembles a classical phase transition at a critical point for financial time series.

The singularities of a measure are characterized by the Lipschitz–Hölder exponent α, which is related to $\tau(q)$ by

$$\alpha(q) = \frac{d}{dq}\tau(q) \tag{16.17}$$

Substitution of Equation (16.13) into Equation (16.17) yields

$$\alpha(q) = \lim_{\epsilon \to 0} \frac{\sum_{\mu(B) \neq 0} [\mu(B)]^q \ln \mu(B)}{Z_\epsilon(q) \ln \epsilon}. \tag{16.18}$$

Again the exponent $\alpha(q)$ can be estimated through a linear regression of

$$\sum_{\mu(B) \neq 0} \frac{[\mu(B)]^q \ln \mu(B)}{Z_\epsilon(q)}$$

against $\ln \epsilon$ [35]. The multifractal spectrum $f(\alpha)$ versus α can be calculated according to the relationship $f(\alpha) = q\alpha(q) - \tau(q)$.

16.2.9 Analogous Multifractal Analysis

The analogous multifractal analysis (AMFA) is similar to multiaffinity analysis, and can be briefly sketched as follows [51]. We denote a time series as $X(t)$, $t = 1, 2, \ldots, N$. First, the time series is integrated as

$$y'_q(k) = \sum_{t=1}^{k} (X(t) - X_{av}), \quad (q > 0) \tag{16.19}$$

$$y_q(k) = \sum_{t=1}^{k} |X(t) - X_{av}|, \quad (q \neq 0) \tag{16.20}$$

where X_{av} is the average over the whole time period. Then two quantities $M_q(L)$ and $M'_q(L)$ are defined as

$$M'_q(L) = [\langle |y'(j) - y'(j+L)|^q \rangle_j]^{1/q}, \quad (q > 0) \tag{16.21}$$

$$M_q(L) = [\langle |y(j) - y(j+L)|^q \rangle_j]^{1/q}, \quad (q \neq 0) \tag{16.22}$$

where $\langle \rangle_j$ denotes the average over j, $j = 1, 2, \ldots, N - L$; L typically varies from 1 to N_1 for which the linear fit is good. From the $\ln L$–$\ln M_q(L)$ and $\ln L$–$\ln M'_q(L)$ planes, one can find the following relations:

$$M'_q(L) \propto L^{h'(q)} \quad \text{for} \quad q > 0 \tag{16.23}$$

$$M_q(L) \propto L^{h(q)} \quad \text{for} \quad q \neq 0 \tag{16.24}$$

Linear regressions of $\ln M_q(L)$ and $\ln M'_q(L)$ against $\ln L$ will result in the exponents $h(q)$ and $h'(q)$, respectively.

16.2.10 Wavelet Spectrum

As the wavelet transform of a function can be considered as an approximation of the function, wavelet algorithms process data at different scales or components. At each scale, many coefficients can be obtained and the wavelet spectrum is calculated on the basis of these coefficients. Hence the wavelet spectrum provides useful information for analyzing data. Given a function $f(t)$, one defines its wavelet transform as [19]

$$W_f(a, b) = |a|^{-(1/2)} \int_{-\infty}^{\infty} f(t) \psi\left(\frac{t - b}{a}\right) dt \tag{16.25}$$

where b is the position and a is the scale. The scale a in wavelet transform means the ath resolution of the data. Taking $a = j, j = 2^0, 2^1, 2^2, \ldots$, and $b = k, k \in \mathbb{R}$, we get the wavelet spectrum as

$$\text{Spectrum } [j] = \sum_k C_{j,k}^2, \qquad k = 2^0, 2^1, 2^2, \ldots$$

where $C_{j,k} = W_f(j, k)$.

For simplicity, the scale j can be selected as $j = 1, \frac{3}{2}, 2, \ldots, 20$, which are more adjacent and can be used to capture more details of the data. The wavelet spectrum is calculated by summing the squares of the coefficients in each scale j. The local wavelet spectrum is defined through the modulus maxima of the coefficients [67] as $local \; spectrum \; [j] = \sum_k \tilde{C}_{j,k}^2$, where

$$\tilde{C}_{j,k} = \begin{cases} |C_{j,k}|, & \text{if } |C_{j,k}| > |C_{j,k-1}| \text{ and } |C_{j,k}| > |C_{j,k+1}| \\ 0, & \text{otherwise.} \end{cases}$$

The maximum of the wavelet spectrum and the maximum of the local wavelet spectrum were applied in the prediction of structural classes and families of proteins [53].

In our work, we chose the Daubechies wavelet, which is commonly used as a signal processing tool. These wavelet functions are compactly supported wavelets with extremal phase and highest number of vanishing moments for a given support width. They are orthogonal and biorthogonal functions. The Daubechies wavelets can improve the frequency domain characteristics of other wavelets [19].

16.2.11 Recurrence Quantification Analysis

The *recurrence plot* (RP) is a purely graphical tool originally proposed by Eckmann et al. [21] to detect patterns of recurrence in the data. For a time series $\{x_1, x_2, \ldots, x_N\}$ with length N, we can embed it into the space $\mathbb{R}^m$ with embedding dimension m and a time delay τ. We write $\vec{y}_i = (x_i, x_{i+\tau}, x_{i+2\tau}, \ldots, x_{i+(m-1)\tau}), i = 1, 2, \ldots, N_m$, where $N_m = N - (m-1)\tau$. In this way we obtain N_m vectors (points) in the embedding space $\mathbb{R}^m$. We gave some numerical explanations for the selection of m and τ in our earlier paper [52].

From the N_m points, we can calculate the *distance matrix* (DM), which is a square $N_m \times N_m$ matrix. The elements of DM are the distances between all possible combinations of i points and j points. They are computed according to the norming function selected. Generally, the Euclidean norm is used [47]. DM can be rescaled by dividing each element in the DM by a certain value as this allows systems operating on different scales to be statistically compared. For such a value, the maximum distance of the entire matrix DM is the most commonly used (and recommended) rescaling option, which redefines the DM over the unit interval (0.0–100.0%).

Once the rescaled $DM = (D_{i,j})_{N_m \times N_m}$ is calculated, it can be transformed into a *recurrence matrix* (RM) of distance elements within a *threshold* ε (namely, radius). $RM = (R_{i,j}(\varepsilon))_{N_m \times N_m}$ and $R_{i,j}(\varepsilon) = H(\varepsilon - D_{i,j}), i, j = 1, 2, \dots, N_m$ where H is the Heaviside function

$$
H(x) = \begin{cases} 0, & \text{if } x < 0 \\ 1, & \text{if } x \geq 0 \end{cases} \tag{16.26}
$$

RP is simply a visualization of RM by plotting the points on the ij plane for those elements in RM with values equal to 1. If $R_{i,j}(\varepsilon) = 1$, we say that j points recur with reference to i points. For any ε, since $R_{i,i}(\varepsilon) \equiv 1, (i = 1, 2, \dots, N_m)$, the RP has always a black main diagonal line. Furthermore, the RP is symmetric with respect to the main diagonal as $R_{i,j}(\varepsilon) = R_{j,i}(\varepsilon), (i, j = 1, 2, \dots, N_m)$. ε is a crucial parameter of RP. If ε is chosen too small, there may be almost no recurrence points and we will not be able to learn about the recurrence structure of the underlying system. On the other hand, if ε is chosen too large, almost every point is a neighbor of every other point, which leads to a large number of artifacts [68]. Selection of ε was discussed numerically in [52].

Recurrence quantification analysis (RQA) is a relatively new nonlinear technique proposed by Zbilut and Webber [22,23] that can quantify the information supplied by RP. Eight recurrence variables are usually used to quantify RP [68]. It should be pointed out that the recurrence points in the following definitions consist only of those in the upper triangle in RP (excluding the main diagonal line). The first recurrence variable is *%recurrence* (%REC). %REC is a measure of the density of recurrence points in the RP. This variable can range from 0% (no recurrent points) to 100% (all points are recurrent). The second recurrence variable is *%determinism* (%DET). %DET measures the proportion of recurrent points forming diagonal line structures. For this variable, we have to first decide at least how many adjacent recurrent points are needed to define a diagonal line segment. Obviously, the minimum number required (and commonly used) is 2. The third recurrence variable is *linemax* (L_{max}), which is simply the length of the longest diagonal line segment in RP. This is a very important recurrence variable because it inversely scales with the largest positive Lyapunov exponent. The fourth recurrence variable is *entropy* (ENT), which is the Shannon information entropy of the distribution probability of the length of the diagonal lines. The fifth recurrence variable is *trend* (TND), which quantifies the degree of system stationarity. It is calculated as the slope of the least squares regression of %local recurrence as a function of the displacement from the main diagonal. It should be made clear that the so called %local recurrence is in fact the proportion of recurrent points on certain line parallel to the main diagonal over the length of this line. %recurrence is calculated on the whole upper triangle in RP while %local recurrence is computed on only certain lines in RP, so it is termed as *local*. Multiplying by 1000 increases the gain of the TND variable. The remaining three variables are defined on the basis of the vertical line structure. The sixth recurrence variable is %*laminarity* (%LAM). %LAM is analogous to %DET but is calculated with recurrent points constituting vertical line structures. Similarly, we also select 2 as the minimum number of adjacent recurrent points to form a vertical line segment. The seventh variable, *trapping time* (TT), is the average length of vertical line structures. The eighth recurrence variable is *maximal length of the vertical lines* in RP (V_{max}), which is similar to L_{max}.

16.2.12 Empirical Mode Decomposition and Similarity of Proteins

Empirical mode decomposition (EMD) was originally designed for non-linear and nonstationary data analysis by Huang et al. [24]. The traditional EMD decomposes a time series into components called *intrinsic mode functions* (IMFs) to define meaningful frequencies of a signal.

Lin et al. [25] proposed a new algorithm for EMD. Instead of using the envelopes generated by spline, a lowpass filter is used to generate a moving average to replace the mean of the envelopes. The essence of the shifting algorithm remains. Let $\mathcal{L}$ be a lowpass filter operator, for which $\mathcal{L}(X)(t)$ represents a moving average of X. We now define $\mathcal{T}(X) = X - \mathcal{L}(X)$. In this approach, the lowpass filter $\mathcal{L}$ is dependent on the data X. For a given $X(t)$, we choose a lowpass filter $\mathcal{L}_1$ accordingly and set $\mathcal{T}_1 = I - \mathcal{L}_1$, where I is the identity operator. The first IMF in the new EMD is given by $\lim_{n \to \infty} \mathcal{T}_1^n(X)$, and subsequently the kth IMF I_k is obtained first by selecting a lowpass filter $\mathcal{L}_k$ according to the data $X - I_1 - \cdots - I_{k-1}$ and iterations $I_k = \lim_{n \to \infty} \mathcal{T}_k^n(X - I_1 - \cdots - I_{k-1})$, where $\mathcal{T}_k = I - \mathcal{L}_k$. The process stops when $Y = X - I_1 - \cdots - I_K$ has at most one local maximum or local minimum. Lin et al. [25] suggested using the filter $Y = \mathcal{L}(X)$ given by $Y(n) = \sum_{j=-m}^{m} a_j X(n+j)$. We selected the mask

$$a_j = \frac{m - |j| + 1}{m + 1}, j = -m, \ldots, m$$

in our work [53].

Let $r(t) = X(t) - I_1(t) - \cdots - I_{K_1}(t)$. The original signal can be expressed as $X(t) = \sum_{i=1}^{K_1} I_i(t) + r(t)$, where the number K_1 can be chosen according to a standard deviation. In our work, the number of components in IMFs was set as 4 due to the short length of some amino acid sequences [53].

The similarity value of two proteins at each component (IMF) is obtained as the maximum absolute value of the correlation coefficient. In our work [53], a new cross-correlation coefficient $C^{12}(j)$ is defined by

$$C^{12}(j) = \frac{\sum_{n=0}^{N-1} S_1(n) S_2(n-j)}{\left[\sum_{n=0}^{N_1-1} S_1^2(n) \sum_{n=0}^{N_2-1} S_2^2(n) \right]^{1/2}}, \quad j = 0, \pm 1, \pm 2, \ldots \quad (16.27)$$

where N is the length of the intersection of two signals with lag j, N_1 is the length of signal S_1, and N_2 is the length of signal S_2. *The maximum absolute value C of all the correlation coefficients of the components is considered as the similarity value for two proteins.*

16.3 RESULTS AND CONCLUSIONS

In our earlier paper [50], we selected the amino acid sequences of 43 large proteins from the RCSB Protein Data Bank (`http://www.rcsb.org/pdb/index.html`). These 43 proteins belong to four structural classes according to their secondary structures:

1. We converted the amino acid sequences of these proteins into their measure representations based on the detailed HP model with $K = 5$. We found that the IFS model corresponding to $K = 5$ is a good model for simulating the measure representation of protein sequences, and the estimated value of the probability P_1 from the IFS model contains information useful for the secondary structural classification of proteins [30]. We performed an IFS simulation for the proteins selected and adopted the estimated parameter P_1 as one parameter to construct the parameter space for proteins.

2. We converted the amino acid sequences of these proteins to their Z curve representations and performed their detrended fluctuation analysis. The exponents $\lambda_x, \lambda_y, \lambda_z$ were estimated and used as candidate parameters to construct the parameter space.

3. We computed the generalized fractal dimensions D_q and the related spectra C_q, multifractal spectra $f(\alpha)$ of hydrophobic free energy sequences and solvent accessibility sequences of all 43 proteins.

4. For a structural classification of proteins, we considered the following parameters: P_1 from the IFS estimations of the measure representations; the exponents $\lambda_x, \lambda_y, \lambda_z$ from the detrended fluctuation analysis of the Z curve representations; the range of D_q (i.e. the value $D_{-15}-D_{15}$ in our frame); the maximum value of C_q (denoted $\text{Max}C_q$); the value q_0 of q that corresponds to the maximum value of C_q; the maximum value of α (denoted $\alpha_{\max}$), the minimum value of α (denoted $\alpha_{\min}$) and $\Delta\alpha$ (defined by $\alpha_{\max} - \alpha_{\min}$) from the multifracal analysis of the hydrophobic free-energy sequences and solvent accessibility sequences of proteins as candidates for constructing parameter spaces.

In a parameter space, one point represents a protein. We wanted to determine whether the proteins can be separated from four structural classifications in these parameter spaces. We found that we can propose a method which consists of three components to cluster proteins [50]. We used Fisher's linear discriminant algorithm to give a quantitative assessment of our clustering on the selected proteins. The discriminant accuracies are satisfactory. In particular, they reach 94.12% and 88.89% in separating β proteins from $\{\alpha, \alpha + \beta, \alpha/\beta\}$ proteins in a 3D space.

We [51], considered a set of 49 large proteins that included the 43 proteins studied earlier [50]. Given an amino acid sequence of one protein, we first converted it into its measure representation μ_K based on the six-letter model with length $K = 5$. Then we calculated $D_q, \tau(q), C_q, \alpha$, and $f(\alpha)$ for the measures μ_K of the 49 selected proteins. We then converted the amino acid sequences of proteins into their RSWH sequences according to the revised Schneider–Wrede hydrophobicity scale. We used such sequences to construct the measures ν. The ordinary multifractal analysis was then performed on these measures. The AMFA was also performed on the RSWH sequences. Then nine parameters from these analyses were selected as candidates for constructing parameter spaces. We proposed another three steps to cluster protein structures [51]. Fisher's linear discriminant algorithm was used to assess our clustering accuracy on the 49 selected large proteins. The discriminant accuracies are satisfactory. In particular, they reach 100.00% and 84.21% in separating the α proteins from the $\{\beta, \alpha + \beta, \alpha/\beta\}$ proteins in a parameter space; 92.86% and 86.96%, in separating the β proteins from the $\{\alpha + \beta, \alpha/\beta\}$ proteins in another parameter space; and 91.67% and 83.33%, in separating the α/β proteins from the $\alpha + \beta$ proteins in the last parameter space.

We [52], intended to predict protein structural classes (α, β, $\alpha + \beta$, or α/β) for low-similarity datasets. Two datasets were used widely: *1189* (containing 1092 proteins) and *25PDB* (containing 1673 proteins) with sequence similarity values of 40% and 25%, respectively. We proposed decomposing the chaos game representation of proteins into two kinds of time series. Then we applied recurrence quantification analysis to analyze these time series. For a given protein sequence, a total of 16 characteristic parameters can be calculated with RQA, which are treated as feature representations of the protein. On the basis of such feature representation, the structural class for each protein was predicted with Fisher's linear discriminant algorithm. The overall accuracies with *step-by-step* procedure are 65.8% and 64.2% for *1189* and *25PDB* datasets, respectively. With *one-against-others* procedure used widely, we compared our method with five other existing methods. In particular, the overall accuracies of our method are 6.3% and 4.1% higher for the two datasets, respectively. Furthermore, only 16 parameters were used in our method, which is less than that used by other methods.

Family identification is helpful in predicting protein functions. Since most protein sequences are relatively short, we first randomly linked the protein sequences from the same family or superfamily together to form 120 longer protein sequences [53], and each structural class contains 30 linked protein sequences. Then we used, the 6-letter model, 12-letter model, 20-letter model, the revised Schneider–Wrede scale hydrophobicity, solvent accessibility, and stochastic standard state accessibility values to convert linked protein sequences to numerical sequences. Then we calculated the generalized fractal dimensions D_q, the related spectra C_q, the multifractal spectra $f(\alpha)$, and the $h(q)$ curves of the six kinds of numerical sequences of all 120 linked proteins. The curves of $D_q, C_q, f(\alpha), h(q)$ showed that the numerical sequences from linked proteins are multifractal-like and sufficiently smooth. The C_q curves resemble the phase transition at a certain point, while the $f(\alpha)$ and $h(q)$ curves indicate the multifractal scaling features of proteins. In wavelet analysis, the choice of a wavelet function should be carefully considered. Different wavelet functions represent a given function with different approximation components. We [53], chose the commonly used Daubechies wavelet db2 and computed the maximum of the wavelet spectrum and the maximum of the local wavelet spectrum for the six kinds of numerical sequences of all 120 linked proteins. The parameters from the multifractal and wavelet analyses were used to construct parameter spaces where each linked protein is represented by a point. The four classes of proteins were then distinguished in these parameter spaces. The discriminant accuracies obtained through Fisher's linear discriminant algorithm are satisfactory in separating these classes. We found that the linked proteins from the same family or superfamily tend to group together and can be separated from other linked proteins. The methods are also helpful to identify the family of an unknown protein.

Zhu et al. [54] applied component similarity analysis based on EMD and the new cross-correlation coefficient formula (16.27) to protein pairs. They then considered maximum absolute value C of all the correlation coefficients of the components as the similarity value for two proteins. They also created the threshold of correlation [54]. Two signals are considered strongly correlated if the correlation coefficient exceeds ± 0.7 and weakly correlated if the coefficient is between ± 0.6 and ± 0.7. The results showed that the functional relationships of some proteins may be revealed by component analysis of their IMFs. Compared with those traditional alignment methods, component analysis can be evaluated and described easily. It illustrates that EMD and component analysis can complement traditional sequence similarity approaches that focus on the alignment of amino acids.

From our analyses, we found that the measure representation based on the detailed HP model and six-letter model, time series representation based on physicochemical features of amino acids, Z-curve representation, the chaos game representation of proteins can provide much information for predicting structure classes and functions of proteins. Fractal methods are useful to analyze protein sequences. Our methods may play a complementary role in the existing methods.

ACKNOWLEDGMENT

This work was supported by the Natural Science Foundation of China (Grant 11071282); the Chinese Program for Changjiang Scholars and Innovative Research Team in University (PCSIRT) (Grant No. IRT1179); the Research Foundation of Education Commission of Hunan Province, China (Grant 11A122); the Lotus Scholars Program of Hunan Province of China; the Aid program for Science and Technology Innovative Research Team in Higher Educational Institutions of Hunan Province of China; and the Australian Research Council (Grant DP0559807).

REFERENCES

1. Hou J, Jun S-R, Zhang C, Kim S-H, Global mapping of the protein structure space and application in structure-based inference of protein function, *Natl. Acad. Sci. USA* **102**:3651–3656 (2005).

2. Anfinsen C, Principles that govern the folding of protein chains, *Science* **181**:223–230 (1973).

3. Chothia C, One thousand families for the molecular biologists, *Nature (Lond.)* **357**:543–544 (1992).

4. Frishman D, Argos P, Knowledge-based protein secondary structure assignment, *Proteins* **23**:566–579 (1995).

5. Crooks GE, Brenner SE, Protein secondary structure: Entropy, correlation and prediction, *Bioinformatics* **20**:1603–1611 (2004).

6. Adamczak R, Porollo A, Meller J, Combining prediction of secondary structure and solvent accessibility in proteins, *Proteins* **59**:467–475 (2005).

7. Levitt M, Chothia C, Structural patterns in globular proteins, *Nature* **261**:552–558 (1976).

8. Service., A dearth of new folds, *Science* **307**:1555–1555 (2005).

9. Chou KC, Progress in protein structural class prediction and its impact to bioinformatics and proteomics, *Curr. Protein Peptide Sci.* **6**(5):423–436 (2005).

10. Trad CH, Fang Q, Cosic I, Protein sequence comparison based on the wavelet transform approach, *Protein Eng.* **15**(3):193–203 (2002).

11. Lesk AM, *Computational Molecular Biology: Sources and Methods for Sequence Analysis*, Oxford Univ. Press, 1988.

12. Mandelbrot BB, *The Fractal Geometry of Nature*, Academic Press, New York, 1983.

13. Feder J, *Fractals*, Plenum Press, New York, 1988.

14. Grassberger P, Procaccia I, Characterization of strange attractors, *Rev. Lett.* **50**:346–349 (1983).

15. Yu ZG, Anh V, Eastes R, Multifractal analysis of geomagnetic storm and solar flare indices and their class dependence, *J. Geophys. Res.* **114**:A05214 (2009).

16. Yu ZG, Anh VV, Lau KS, Measure representation and multifractal analysis of complete genome, *Phys. Rev. E* **64**:031903 (2001).

17. Yu ZG, Anh VV, Wang B, Correlation property of length sequences based on global structure of complete genome, *Phys. Rev. E* **63**:011903 (2001).

18. Peng CK, Buldyrev S, Goldberg AL, Havlin S, Sciortino F, Simons M, Stanley HE, Long-range correlations in nucleotide sequences, *Nature* **356**:168–170 (1992).

19. Chui CK, *An Introduction to Wavelets*, Academic Press Professional, San Diego, 1992.

20. Daubechies I, *Ten Lectures on Wavelets*, SIAM, Philadelphia, 1992.

21. Eckmann JP, Kamphorst SO, Ruelle D, Recurrence plots of dynamical systems, *Europhys. Lett.* **4**:973–977 (1987).

22. Zbilut JP, Webber CL Jr, Embeddings and delays as derived from quantification of recurrence plots, *Phys. Lett. A* **171**:199–203 (1992).

23. Webber CL Jr, Zbilut JP, Dynamical assessment of physiological systems and states using recurrence plot strategies, *J. Appl. Physiol.* **76**:965–973 (1994).

24. Huang N, Shen Z, Long SR, Wu ML, Shih HH, Zheng Q, Yen NC, Tung CC, Liu HH, The empirical mode decomposition and Hilbert spectrum for nonlinear and nonstationary time series analysis, *Proc. Roy. Soc. Lond. A* **454**:903–995 (1998).

25. Lin L, Wang Y, Zhou H, Iterative filtering as an alternative for empirical mode decomposition, *Adv. Adapt. Data Anal.* **1**(4):543–560 (2009).

26. Janosi IM, Muller R, Empirical mode decomposition and correlation properties of long daily ozone records, *Phys. Rev. E* **71**:056126 (2005).

27. ZG Yu, Anh V, Wang Y, Mao D, Wanliss J, Modeling and simulation of the horizontal component of the geomagnetic field by fractional stochastic differential equations in conjunction with empirical mode decomposition, *J. Geophys. Res.* **115**:A10219 (2010).

28. Dewey TG, Fractal analysis of proton-exchange kinetics in lysozyme, *Proc. Natl. Acad. Sci. USA* **91**:12101–12104 (1994).

29. Fiser A, Tusnady GE, Simon I, Chaos game representation of protein structure, *J. Mol. Graphies* **12**:302–304 (1994).

30. Yu ZG, Anh VV, Lau KS, Fractal analysis of large proteins based on the detailed HP model, *Physica A* **337**:171–184 (2004).

31. Yu ZG, Anh VV, Lau KS, Chaos game representation, and multifractal and correlation analysis of protein sequences from complete genome based on detailed HP model, *J. Theor. Biol.* **226**:341–348 (2004).

32. Enright MB, Leitner DM, Mass fractal dimension and the compactness of proteins, *Phys. Rev. E* **71**:011912 (2005).

33. Moret MA, Miranda JGV, Nogueira E, et al, Self-similarity and protein chains, *Phys. Rev. E* **71**:012901 (2005).

34. Pavan YS, Mitra CK, Fractal studies on the protein secondary structure elements, *Indian J. Biochem. Biophys.* **42**:141–144 (2005).

35. Balafas JS, Dewey TG, Multifractal analysis of solvent accessibilities in proteins, *Phys. Rev. E* **52**:880–887 (1995).

36. Yu ZG, Anh VV, Lau KS, Multifractal and correlation analysis of protein sequences from complete genome, *Phys. Rev. E* **68**:021913 (2003).

37. Mandell AJ, Selz KA, Shlesinger MF, Mode maches and their locations in the hydrophobic free energy sequences of peptide ligands and their receptor eigenfunctions, *Proc. Natl. Acad. Sci. USA* **94**:13576–13581 (1997).

38. Mandell AJ, Selz KA, Shlesinger MF, Wavelet transformation of protein hydrophobicity sequences suggests their memberships in structural families, *Physica A* **244**:254–262 (1997).

39. Selz KA, Mandell AJ, Shlesinger MF, Hydrophobic free energy eigenfunctions of pore, channel, and transporter proteins contain β-burst patterns, *Biophys. J.* **75**:2332–2342 (1998).

40. Hirakawa H, Muta S, Kuhara S, The hydrophobic cores of proteins predicted by wavelet analysis, *Bioinformatics* **15**:141–148 (1999).

41. Chen H, Gu F, Liu F, Predicting protein secondary structure using continuous wavelet transform and Chou–Fasman method, *Proc. 27th Annual IEEE, Engineering in Medicine and Biology Conf.* 2005.

42. Marsolo K, Ramamohanarao K, Structure-based on querying of proteins using wavelets, *Proc.15th Int. ACM Conf. Information and Knowledge Management*, 2006, pp. 24–33.

43. Qiu JD, Liang RP, Zou XY, Mo JY, Prediction of protein secondary structure based on continuous wavelet transform, *Talanta* **61**(3):285–293 (2003).

44. Rezaei M, Abdolmaleki P, Jahandideh S, Karami Z, Asadabadi EB, Sherafat MA, Abrishami-Moghaddam H, Fadaie M, Foroozan M, Prediction of membrane protein types by means of wavelet analysis and cascaded neural networks, *J. Theor. Biol.* **254**(4):817–820 (2008).

45. Pando J, Sands L, Shaheen SE, Detection of protein secondary structures via the discrete wavelet transform, *Phys. Rev. E* **80**:051909 (2009).

46. Webber CL Jr, Giuliani A, Zbilut JP, Colosimo A, Elucidating protein secondary structures using alpha-carbon recurrence quantifications, *Proteins: Struct., Funct., Genet.* **44**:292–303 (2001).

47. Giuliani A, Benigni R, Zbilut JP, Webber CL Jr., Sirabella P, Colosimo A, Signal analysis methods in elucidation of protein sequence-structure relationships, *Chem. Rev.* **102**:1471–1491 (2002).

48. Shi F, Chen Q, Niu X, Functional similarity analyzing of protein sequences with empirical mode decomposition, *Proc. 4th Int. Conf. Fuzzy Systems and Knowledge Discovery*, 2007.

49. Shi F, Chen QJ, Li NN, Hilbert Huang transform for predicting proteins subcellular location, *J. Biomed. Sci. Eng.* **1**:59–63 (2008).

50. Yu ZG, Anh VV, Lau KS, Zhou LQ, Fractal and multifractal analysis of hydrophobic free energies and solvent accessibilities in proteins, *Phys. Rev. E.* **73**:031920 (2006).

51. Yang JY, Yu ZG, Anh V, Clustering structure of large proteins using multifractal analyses based on 6-letters model and hydrophobicity scale of amino acids, *Chaos, Solitons, Fractals* **40**:607–620 (2009).

52. Yang JY, Peng ZL, Yu ZG, Zhang RJ, Anh V, Wang D, Prediction of protein structural classes by recurrence quantification analysis based on chaos game representation, *J. Theor. Biol.* **257**:618–626 (2009).

53. Zhu SM, Yu ZG, Anh V, Protein structural classification and family identification by multifractal analysis and wavelet spectrum, *Chin. Phys. B* **20**:010505 (2011).

54. Zhu SM, Yu ZG, Anh V, Yang SY, Analysing the similarity of proteins based on a new approach to empirical mode decomposition, *Proc. 4th Int. Conf. Bioinformatics and Biomedical Engineering* (ICBBE2010), vol. 1, (2010).

55. Chou PY, Fasman GD, Prediction of protein conformation, *Biochemistry* **13**:222–245 (1974).

56. Bordo D, Argos P, Suggestions for safe residue substitutions in site-directed mutagenesis, *J. Mol. Biol.* **217**:721–729 (1991).

57. Rose GD, Geselowitz AR, Lesser GJ, Lee RH, Zehfus MH, Hydrophobicity of amino acid residues in globular proteins, *Science* **229**:834–838 (1985).

58. Krigbaum WR, Komoriya A, Local interactions as a structure determinant for protein molecules: II, *Biochim. Biophys. Acta* **576**:204–228 (1979).

59. Zhang R, Zhang CT, Z curves, an intuitive tool for visualizing and analyzing the DNA sequences, *J. Biomol. Struct. Dyn.* **11**:767–782 (1994).

60. Basu S, Pan A, Dutta C, Das J, Chaos game representation of proteins, *J. Mol. Graphics* **15**:279–289 (1997).

61. Deschavanne P, Tufféry P, Exploring an alignment free approach for protein classification and structural class prediction, *Biochimie* **90**:615–625 (2008).

62. Jeffrey HJ, Chaos game representation of gene structure, *Nucleic Acids Res*, **18**:2163–2170 (1990).

63. Brown TA, *Genetics*, 3rd ed., Chapman & Hall, London, 1998.

64. Barnsley MF, Demko S, Iterated function systems and the global construction of fractals, *Proc. Roy. Soc. (Lond.)* **399**:243–275 (1985).

65. Vrscay ER, Iterated function systems: Theory, applications and the inverse problem, in Belair J, Dubuc S. (eds.), *Fractal Geometry and Analysis*, NATO ASI series, Kluwer, 1991.

66. Canessa E, Multifractality in time series, *J. Phys. A: Math. Genet.* **33**:3637–3651 (2000).

67. Arneodo A, Bacry E, Muzy JF, The thermodynamics of fractals revisited with wavelets, *Physica A* **213**:232–275 (1995).

68. Marwan N, Romano MC, Thiel M, Kurths J, Recurrence plots for the analysis of complex systems, *Phys. Reports* **438**:237–329 (2007).

CHAPTER 17

PROTEIN TERTIARY MODEL ASSESSMENT

ANJUM CHIDA, ROBERT W. HARRISON, and YAN-QING ZHANG

17.1 INTRODUCTION

Protein structure prediction has been an important conundrum in the field of bioinformatics and theoretical chemistry because of its importance in medicine, drug design, biotechnology, and other areas. In structure biology, protein structures are often determined by techniques such as X-ray crystallography, NMR spectroscopy, and electron microscopy. A repository of these experimentally determined structures is organized as a centralized, proprietary databank called the Protein Data Bank (PDB). This databank is freely accessible on the Internet [1]. The generation of a protein sequence is much easier than the determination of protein structure. The structure of the protein gives much more insight about its function than its sequence. Therefore computational methods for the prediction of protein structure from its sequence have been developed. Ab initio prediction methods employ only the sequence of the protein based on the physical principles governing any molecular structure. Threading and homology modeling methods can build a 3D model for a protein of unknown structure from experimental structures of evolutionary related proteins. As long as a detailed physicochemical description of protein folding principles does not exist, structure prediction is the only method available to researchers to view the structure of some proteins. Experts agree that it is possible to construct high-quality full-length models for almost all single-domain proteins by using best possible template structure in PDB and state-of-the-art modeling algorithm [1–3]. This suggests that the current PDB structure universe may be approaching completion. So it all comes down to selecting that model in a pool of models.

We aim to obtain a learning algorithm that studies known structures from PDB and when given a protein model predicts whether it belongs to the same class

Algorithmic and Artificial Intelligence Methods for Protein Bioinformatics. First Edition.
Edited by Yi Pan, Jianxin Wang, Min Li.
© 2014 John Wiley & Sons, Inc. Published 2014 by John Wiley & Sons, Inc.

as PBD structures. Since using a whole primary protein sequence to determine a 3D protein structure is very difficult, it is necessary to design new intelligent algorithms to find key features from a large pool of relevant features in biology and geometry to effectively evaluate 3D protein models. The central focus of this study is to develop and implement new granular decision machines to find biologically meaningful features for assessing 3D protein structures accurately and efficiently. This effort will lead to a better understanding of internal mechanism governing 3D protein structures such as how and why the key biological features and geometric features can dominate a 3D protein structure, and identify these critical sequence features and geometric features.

Solving this problem will help us study problems from different domains that have the same intensity of information. There are many complex and important application problems with huge geometric factors. A short list of common problems where geometry is a critical factor would include social and computer network structure, traffic analysis, and computer vision. Biomedical examples include 3D structural features of a protein that are directly related to basic functionality and are crucial for drug design.

17.2 OVERVIEW OF PROTEIN MODEL ASSESSMENT

Protein structure prediction methods are generally classified into three categories according to the necessity of a template structure used as a scaffold of a model of a target sequence: (1) homology modeling, (2) threading or fold recognition, and (3) ab initio methods. Method 1 is based on the observation that proteins with homologous sequence fold to almost identical structure. Therefore, when a highly homologous template structure for a target sequence is available in the PDB, the method can produce an accurate model with a root-mean-squared distance (RMSD) of 1–2 Å to its native structure. Conversely, the range of applications of homology modeling is relatively narrow because a template structure is necessary for calculation. Method 2 seeks a well-fitting known structure for a given target sequence, sometimes from a range of beyond-detectable sequence similarity.

An important task in both structure prediction and application is to evaluate the quality of a structure model. Half a century has passed since it was shown that an amino acid sequence of a protein determines its shape, but a method for reliable translation into the 3D structure still remains to be developed. So it is important to develop methods that determine the quality of a model. Since the early 1990s, a number of approaches have been developed to analyze correctness of protein structures and models. Traditional model evaluation methods use stereochemistry checks, molecular mechanical energy-based functions, and statistical potentials to tackle the problem. More recently, machine learning methods using algorithms such as neural networks (NNs) and support vector machines (SVMs) that are trained on structure models to predict model quality have been introduced [4]. There are various techniques available for determining the quality of a predicted model, either by comparing it with the native structure or with no knowledge of known structure. In the following paragraphs, the most familiar assessment techniques are categorized and the importance of each category is discussed.

These techniques can be divided into three basic categories according to their scoring strategy: local versus global, absolute versus relative, or single versus multiple (consensus or ranking methods). Some methods predict the quality of local regions such as distance between the position of a residue in a protein model and its native structure as supposedly predicting an overall score of a model. Some methods predict both local and global quality, such as Pcons [5]. Wallner and Elofsson's [6] Pcons is a consensus-based method capable of a quite reliable ranking of model sets for both easy and difficult targets. Pcons uses a metaserver approach (i.e., it combines results from several available well-established quality assessment methods) to calculate a quality score reflecting the average similarity of a model to the model ensemble, under the assumption that recurring structural patterns are more likely to be correct than those observed only rarely. It should be underscored that, while the consensus-based methods are useful in model ranking, they can be biased by the composition of the set and, in principle, are incapable of assessing the quality of a single model. This brings us to another category based on scoring: absolute score versus relative score. Relative scoring methods discriminate near-native structure from decoys; these methods are different from methods that produce absolute score. A relative score can only select or rank models but does not indicate the quality of a model, which is critical for using the model. The techniques could also be grouped according to the information needed for quality assessment. In prominent assessment approaches, 3D co-ordinates, sequence information, sequence alignment, alignment information, template, secondary structure information, and other features are generally used to judge quality. Model evaluation methods can be classified into single-model approach such as ProQ, Proq-LG, ProQ-MX, and MODCHECK and multimodel approaches such as clustering methods whose output depends on the number of input models. We can also group these techniques according to prediction accuracy, machine learning tools such as NNS and SVM, clustering, and consensus approaches. Some of these methods are used in critical assessment of structure prediction (CASP), as one of many analyses involved in assessment phase [7–9]. There are many methods that aim at finding the model quality, but very few come up with an absolute score using a single model and information from only its primary sequence and 3D coordinates [6,7,10,11].

In the 2 years following CASP7, a considerable increase in method development in the area of model quality assessment can be observed. More than a dozen papers have been published on the subject, and 45 quality assessment methods, almost double the CASP7 number, have been submitted for evaluation to CASP8 [4,9]. CASP evaluation is based on comparison of each model with the corresponding experimental structure. A GDT_TS score [12] is used in several CASP competitions, which is defined as average coverage of the target sequence of the substructure with four different distance thresholds. Other similar techniques obtain an absolute scoring by comparing the model to its experimental structure. A strikingly different domain involves assessment of the models with no known structure. Several methods have been proposed to solve this problem. Single-model approaches, including ProQ [5], ProQ-LG, ProQ-MX [10], and MODCHECK [13] assign a score to a single model, whereas multimodel approaches, such as clustering and consensus methods, require a large pool of models as inputs. These methods cannot be used to assess the quality of a single model. They may not reliably evaluate the quality of a small number of input models [4]. Machine learning methods such as neural networks and SVM that are trained on structure models predict model quality [11,14,15] differ by including the consensus-based features (i.e., incorporating in the analysis information from multiple models on the same target).

MODCHECK [13] places emphasis on benchmarking individual methods and also offers NN-based metatechniques that combine them. ModFOLD merges four orginal approaches in a program. Some of the more recent methods that make use of single-model, 3D coordinate information, and primary sequence to evaluate an absolute score for model quality assessment are ModelEvaluator [11] and Undertaker [16]. In ModelEvaluator [11] they use a normalized GDT_TS score with SVM regression to train SVM to learn a function that accurately maps input features. For a general overview of available techniques, please refer Table 17.1 [3,5,11–13,16–19].

Since models are not experimental structures determined with known accuracy but provide only predictions, it is vital to present the user with the corresponding estimates of model quality. Much is being done in this area, but further development of tools for reliable assessment of model quality is needed. Our approach is quite different from any recent study; we aim to classify the models into two classes: proteins and nonproteins. With thousands of protein structures available in the Protein Data Bank, it is possible to train a machine learning algorithm to study protein structure and predict whether a given model closely resembles these structures. From initial results we can say with some assurance that it is possible to achieve such a learning curve.

TABLE 17.1 Overview of Current Model Assessment Methods

Method	Year	Scoring	Remark	Reference
GDT_TS	1999	Single score	Compares to native structure	12
ProQ	2003	Single score	Uses neural networks	5
3D-Jury	2003	Ranking	Consensus method	17
SPICKER	2004	Ranking	By clustering	3
MODCHECK	2005	Single score	Classical threading potentials	13
Undertaker	2005	Single score	Uses full 3D information	16
ModFOLD	2008	Single score	TM score is used	18
ModelEvaluators	2008	Single score	Support Vector Regression using GDT_TS	11
TASSER	2008	Ranking	Structure feature and statistical potential	19

The amount and nature of information given to the machine learning system will have an impact on the final output regarding the quality measure of given 3D structure. There are various ways of representing a protein 3D structure, including a backbone sketch of the protein, the entire distance matrix of α-carbon atoms, a fractal dimension of the structure, and 3D information with its sequence data. These methods of representing protein structure are used mostly in comparison and classification problems and are widely studied and researched fields [20].

17.3 DESIGN AND METHOD

In order to classify whether a 3D object is a protein structure, the structure should be represented in machine-understandable format. In this methodology we represent each protein as one data vector. Each data vector should contain both structural and sequence information on that protein structure. For training and testing cycles using the machine learning algorithm, both positive and negative data vectors are needed. Positive vectors can be structures from the PDB database, as these structures are experimentally determined ones. Negative vectors are generated by misaligning the sequence and structure information, so that we have the wrong structure for a particular sequence. Different kernel methods and encoding schemes are used to observe their effectiveness in classifying proteins as either correct or incorrect. The goal here is to encode protein information in numerical form understandable by machine learning technique. The encoding is performed in the following order:

Sequence information + structure information

In the following two paragraphs, different methods for representing sequence and structure information are discussed. These are not the only methods for encoding protein information, but they are commonly used in other research domains, such as structure alignment, protein function classification, and protein secondary structure classification [21].

Protein sequence is a one-dimensional string of 20 different amino acids. To represent each amino acid, we can use one of the two very popular matrices. BLOSUM [blocks of (aminoacid) substitution matrix] is a substitution matrix. The scores measure the logarithm for the ratio of the likelihood of two amino acids appearing with a biological sense and the likelihood of the same amino acids appearing by chance. A positive score is given to the more likely substitutions; a negative score, to the less likely substitutions. The elements in this matrix are used as features for data vectors. For each amino acid there are 20 features to consider. Profile or position specific scoring matrix (PSSM) is a table that lists the frequencies of each amino acid in each position of protein sequence. Highly conserved positions receive high scores, and weakly conserved positions receive scores near zero. Profile, similar to the BLOSUM matrix, provides 20 features per amino acid. In preliminary studies both methods were used to encode sequence

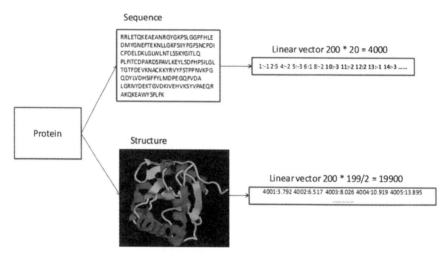

Figure 17.1   Features of vector formation.

information. For IFID3 only BLOSUM matrix is used. This method is further illustrated in Figure 17.1.

The distance matrix containing all pairwise distances between Cα atoms is one commonly used rotationally and translationally invariant representation of protein structure. This technique is used in DALI [20] for protein structure comparison by detecting spatial similarities. The major difficulty with distance matrices is that they cannot distinguish between right-handed and left-handed structures. Another evident problem with this method is computability, as there are too many parameters or attributes to optimize in the case of feature selection or optimization, which are important steps in the machine learning process. Two different simulations are performed for implementation of the design. The first simulation is the direct implementation of a larger dataset performed using support vectors technique. Because of some shortcomings in computational domain and poor prediction accuracy, the second simulation is considered. The second simulation uses a fuzzy decision tree to obtain better prediction accuracy.

The *single positive vector* is a single protein with its sequence information followed by its own structure information. The *single negative vector* has one protein's sequence information followed by another protein's structure information. For initial implementation we have considered two kernels: linear and Gaussian. Sequence information is represented using both BLOSUM and Profile to observe their individual performance. In case of structural information, only the distance matrix is considered to represent protein 3D structure. For example, to encode protein chain 1M56D of sequence length 51 using the Profile + distance matrix encoding scheme, its complete sequence and structure information has to be included. For every amino acid in the sequence we need to input 20 features corresponding to its position-specific score (PSSM or Profile), so the example protein will have 1020 (51*20) features to represent its sequence. For structure information we have to consider the (upper or lower) half of distance matrix, this will result in 1275 (51*50/2) features to represent its structure. In total, 2295 features are used to represent the protein chain. (*Note:* The entire sequence and structure details are considered; thus, for a protein of length 200 we will have 4000 features for sequence information and 19,900 for structure.) This will be a positive vector as it is from the PDB database. Negative vectors are generated by choosing sequence and structure information of two random proteins in a similar manner. For the BLOSUM matrix + distance matrix encoding scheme, the BLOSUM matrix is used instead of Profile.

The PDB entries are culled on the basis of their sequence length and relative homology using the PISCES server [22]. The culled list has $\leq 25\%$ homology among different protein sequences. This will ensure that negative vectors are not false negative with highest probability.

17.4   IMPLEMENTATION USING SVM

Support vector machines (SVMs) are learning systems that use a hypothesis space of linear function in a high-dimensional feature space, trained with a learning algorithm from optimization theory that implements a learning bias derived from statistical learning theory. In supervised learning the learning machine is given a training set of examples (or inputs) with associated labels (or output values). Once the attributes vectors are available, a number of sets of hypotheses can be chosen for the problem. Among these, linear functions are best understood and simplest to apply. The development of learning algorithm became an important subfield of artificial intelligence, eventually forming the separate subject area of machine learning [21,24,23].

In this section, we discuss implementation of the proposed method using support vector machines. Different simulations are done to study the effectiveness of the selected machine learning technique in this data scenario. A specific set of PDB entries are culled according to their sequence length (200) and homology. Positive and negative data are obtained from the same set as discussed in the previous section.

17.4.1   Simulation 1

For this simulation, approximately 2000 PDB entries are culled from the entire PDB databank. These entries form the positive vectors for the learning system. The same number of negative vectors is generated by randomly selecting two PDB entries, one for sequence and other for structure information. The total number of training vectors hence obtained is 4670, and the number of testing vectors is 780. Results after the implementation are shown in Table 17.2.

TABLE 17.2 Encoding Scheme

Linear Kernel		RBF Kernel	
Test Case	Accuracy (%)	Test Case	Accuracy (%)
a. Profile–Distance Matrix			
1	70.52	1	50.58
2	64.74	2	50.43
3	63.29	3	50.58
4	64.45	4	50.00
5	66.18	5	50.72
6	65.32	6	50.87
7	71.82	7	50.29
Average	66.62	Average	50.50
b. BLOSUM Matrix–Distance Matrix			
1	71.11	1	53.08
2	63.59	2	52.95
3	70.77	3	53.95
4	72.31	4	52.18
5	73.21	5	52.44
6	71.41	6	52.82
7	75.51	7	53.08
Average	71.13	Average	52.93

These results show sevenfold testing. From the tables we note that the BLOSUM matrix has better accuracy than does Profile. However, with the BLOSUM matrix for encoding, we note that Gaussian kernels are unable to give results comparable to those of the linear kernel. This might be due to incorrect optimization parameters. These results are not sufficient to warrant recommendation of any one encoding scheme or kernel; more simulations are required. Simulation 2 is performed to determine the effect of using all features as opposed to some randomly selected ones.

17.4.2 Simulation 2

From the simulation 1 results we note that the machine learning algorithm suffers from poor dimensionality, which affects computational efficiency and final accuracy. This could be due to the huge number of features considered in representing protein 3D structure. Feature reduction and selection techniques such as redesigning the feature, selecting an appropriate subset of features, or combining features could be considered to solve this problem. The training and testing datasets are constructed similarly to simulation 1.

To obtain this we will adopt a static scheduling algorithm that will schedule each training vector in a different processor. This scheduling will continue until the desired accuracy (equal to or greater than linear kernel accuracy with all features) or maximum number of tries is attained.

TABLE 17.3   Accuracy Before and After Feature Selection

Test Case	BLOSUM Matrix Encoding (%)	Profile Encoding (%)
a. Before Feature Selection		
1	58.24	59.72
2	65.29	66.67
3	59.41	63.89
4	60.59	63.19
5	60.00	52.78
6	62.94	66.67
7	64.12	58.33
Average	61.51	61.60
b. After Feature Selection		
1	60.50	64.58
2	66.47	68.75
3	62.55	66.67
4	65.29	65.28
5	63.53	58.33
6	65.29	69.44
7	67.06	63.89
Average	64.37	64.69

For effective analysis of the feature selection procedure, a different dataset was culled similar to one shown in previous section but with only 600 PDB entries. The number of training vectors thus obtained is 1030, and the number of testing vectors is 170. The results show the effectiveness of feature selection. The accuracies have also increased after feature selection.

Since the dataset considered here is different from that of simulation 1, we have calculated the sevenfold accuracy for this dataset. These results are shown in Table 17.3a. There is a drop in average percentage accuracies; this might be due to a lower number of training vectors.

17.4.3   Feature Selection Algorithm

A simple algorithm is devised for purposes of feature selection. For a number of features to be selected, several percentages were tested to compare their performance with vectors that have all the features. After several trails 2% proved to be sufficient to obtain the same accuracy. To improve the speed of the algorithm, we used multiple processors. Each processor was scheduled to perform first the feature selection, followed by SVM training and then SVM testing. Once completed, the processor repeated the same task until the desired accuracy was obtained, or for a maximum number of attempts. The algorithm that we used consists in the following steps:

TABLE 17.4 Comparison of Accuracies Before and After Feature Selection

Encoding Scheme	Before Feature Selection (%)	After Feature Selection (%)
BLOSUM matrix	61.51	64.37
Profile	61.60	64.69

1. Select 2% of features from the training set.
2. Schedule a processor to train this training set using SVM light software.
3. Repeat steps 1 and 2 to generate 10 such training sets.
4. Schedule the processors that have completed the training with testing.
5. Check testing accuracy of each set with the testing accuracy of the set with 100% features (previous result from Table 17.3a).
   a. If the testing accuracy is better than previous results, then record the feature numbers used and quit (terminate the procedure)
   b. Otherwise, repeat steps 1–5 until the desired results are obtained or a maximum number of attempts is reached.

Table 17.3b lists the results obtained by using this above algorithm. The average has improved in both encoding schemes. Table 17.4 clearly shows the average accuracies of both encoding schemes before and after feature selection. This emphasizes the fact that all that features are not needed to make the binary decision. This leads us to consider other encoding schemes and representations of protein sequence and structure information. Other kernels should also be considered, as only the linear kernel has shown any real prediction ability [25].

17.5 IMPLEMENTATION USING IFID3

Decision trees are one of the most popular machine learning techniques. They are known for their ability to represent the decision support information in a human-comprehensible form; however, they are recognized as a highly unstable classifier with respect to small changes in training data [26,27]. One of the most popular algorithms for building decision trees is the Interactive Dichotomizer3 (ID3) algorithm proposed by Quinian in 1979 [26]. Generally, trees produced by ID3 (known as "crisp" decision trees) are sensitive to small changes in feature values and cannot handle data uncertainties caused by noise and/or measurement errors [27].

Nael Abu-halaweh and coworkers proposed an improved FID3 algorithm (IFID3) [28], the IFID3 integrates classification ambiguity and fuzzy information gain to select the branching attribute. The IFID3 algorithm outperformed the existing FID3 algorithm on a wide range of datasets. They also introduced an extended version of the IFID3 algorithm (EIFD3). EIFID3 extends IFID3 by introducing a new threshold on the membership value of a data instance to propagate down the decision tree from a parent node to any of its children nodes during the tree construction phase. Using the new threshold, a significant reduction in the number of rules produced, an improved accuracy, and a huge reduction in execution time are achieved. They automate the generation of the membership functions by two simple approaches. In the first approach the ranges of all numerical features in a dataset are divided evenly into an equal number of fuzzy sets. In the second approach, the dataset is clustered and the resulting cluster centers are used to generate fuzzy membership functions. These fuzzy decision trees were applied to the micro-RNA prediction problem; their results showed that fuzzy decision trees achieved a better accuracy than other machine learning approaches such as support vector machines (SVMs) and random forest (RF) [27].

With experimental results, they [27,28] showed that the modified version of IFID3 produces better accuracy and achieves significant reduction in the number of resulting fuzzy rules. Overall, with their new fuzzy decision tree, they have improved the accuracy and execution time of induction algorithms by integrating fuzzy information gain and classification ambiguity to select the branching feature. By introducing a new threshold on the membership value of a data object to propagate down the decision tree from parent node to any of its child nodes, they have significantly reduced the number of fuzzy rules generated [28].

Both these features appeal to our dataset and objective of assessing models. The main reason for using this machine learning technique is the rule set that it generates. The rules will help in understanding the concepts and rules governing protein structure formation. Using these rules, we should be able to map out the path for correct protein structure models.

Three different datasets are considered. Each is a subset of the same dataset with a different number of proteins. Proteins from PDB are culled as discussed in Section 17.3. The proteins within a specific length range (150–200) are considered. Since there is a length variation among different proteins, for smaller proteins, a questionmark (?) is listed as an attribute value for positions where there is no amino acid. This kind of attribute definition is acceptable with IFID3 algorithms. This representation simply means that the attribute has no value or no meaning in the case considered here.

As mentioned earlier, IFID3 uses attribute classification ambiguity to select the branching attribute at the root node, and fuzzy information gain elsewhere. Given a dataset D with attributes $A_1, A_2, \ldots, A_n$, based on the given parameter values, different fuzzy sets are formed for each attribute. The fuzzy ID3 algorithm requires the given dataset to be in a fuzzy form. In the present case, the dataset is not in fuzzy form but in continuous numerical form, so it needs to be fuzzified first. To obtain the optimal number of fuzzy sets, the number of fuzzy sets can be given as a parameter that needs to be tuned. The tree is built according to the given conditional parameters, and each node becomes a leaf node if the number of the dataset is less than a given threshold, if proportion of any class in the

TABLE 17.5 Sevenfold Results Using IFID3

Test Case	100 Proteins (%)	200 Proteins (%)	700 Proteins (%)
1	82.14	87.72	80.50
2	78.57	78.95	82.50
3	85.71	80.70	77.50
4	75.43	78.95	81.50
5	82.14	85.96	85.00
6	78.57	85.96	80.50
7	78.12	84.48	79.50
Average	80.10	83.25	81.00

node is greater than the given fuzziness condition threshold, or if no additional attributes are available for classification [27,28].

For our dataset we considered 10 fuzzy sets and triangular membership function for each attribute. The performance ratings of the tests are shown in Table 17.5. About 20 rules are generated for these datasets. There are three datasets, each with a different number of proteins. The first one has 100 proteins and hence 100 positive vectors and 100 negative vectors. Similarly, dataset 200 and 700 proteins have 200 positive vectors and 700 negative vectors, respectively. For sequence information, only BLOSUM matrix encoding is used. Table 17.7 shows sevenfold test results and their averages [29].

The prediction accuracy of IFID3 is much better when compared to SVM results. More simulations can be done with an increased number of proteins to check whether there is any improvement in prediction results.

17.6 CONCLUSION

Most aspects of experimental protein structure predictions process are difficult, time-consuming, expensive, labor-intensive, and problematic. Scientists have agreed that it is an impossible task to determine a complete set of all protein structures found in nature, since the number of proteins is much larger than the number of genes in an organism. On the other hand, scientists also believe that there are only a limited number of single-domain topologies, such that at some point the library of solved protein structure in PDB would be sufficiently complete and that the likelihood of finding a new fold is minimal. Earlier, although there were several thousand structures in PDB, most of these structures were not unique but rather were multiple variants of identical structure and sequence. So these models did not significantly expand our knowledge of protein structure space. Now experts believe that we have sufficient knowledge of protein structure space. This information is critical because it suggests that PDB structures provide a set from which other proteins can be modeled using computational techniques. These facts lead to the important task of estimating correctness of the prediction techniques and quality of protein models

Evaluating the accuracy of predicted models is critical for assessing structure prediction methods. This problem is not trivial; a large number of assessment measures have been proposed by various groups and have already become an active subfield of research. Most of these methods are normalized scoring functions that compare the given model to experimental structure. In this research we aim to obtain a binary classifier that studies structures from the PDB and classifies models as good or bad. The sheer volume of known structures available makes it possible to develop a machine learning system that studies protein structures and eventually predicts the quality of any new structure model. The most important task in this approach is represent to the protein 3D structure in the best possible manner and use an appropriate machine learning algorithm to obtain good assessment accuracy. The machine learning techniques considered in this chapter are support vector machines and fuzzy decision trees. To solve the protein model assessment problem, we employed attributes from the protein's sequence and structure.

To reduce the computational complexity of the program, we employed feature selection and parallel processing. We have implemented kernels to understand a complex 3D object and to determine whether the object represents a protein structure. By using an improved model of the fuzzy decision tree (IFID3), we could obtain prediction accuracy of >80%. The results look promising, but improvements in dataset a parameters could further improve the accuracy of prediction. Improvements such as making use of graph kernels, string kernels, kernel fusion methods, and decision fusion methods could further enhance the learning system. Also, these machines could be used to predict the results of previous CASP targets to test their accuracy in predicted models.

REFERENCES

1. Berman HM, Westbrook J, Feng Z, Gilliland G, Bhat TN, Weissig H, Shindyalov IN, Bourne PE, The Protein Data Bank, *Nucleic Acids Res.* **28**:235–242 (2000).

2. Berman HM, The Protein Data Bank: A historical perspective, *Acta Crystallogr. A* **64**:88–95 (2008).

3. Zhang Y, Skolnick J, The protein structure prediction problem could be solved using current PDB library, *Proc. Natl. Acad. Sci. USA* **102**:1029–1034 (2005).

4. Cozzetto D, Kryshtafovych A, Ceriani M, Tramontano A, Assessment of predictions in the model quality assessment category, *Proteins* **69**(S8):175–183 (2007).

5. Wallner B, Fang H, Elofsson A, Automatic consensus-based fold recognition using pcons, proq, and pmodeller, *Proteins* **53**:534–541 (2003).

6. Wallner B, Elofsson A, Can correct protein models be identified? *Protein Sci.* **12**:1073–1086 (2003).

7. Moult J, A decade of CASP: Progress, bottlenecks and prognosis in protein structure prediction, *Sci. Direct* **15**:285–289 (2005).

8. Siew N, Elofsson A, Rychlewski L, Fisher D, MaxSUb: An automated measure for the assessment of protein structure prediction quality, *Bioinformatics* **16**(9):776–785 (2000).

9. Kihara D, Chen H, Yang YD, Quality assessment of protein structure models, *Curr. Protein Peptide Sci.* **10**:216–228 (2009).

10. Wallner B, Elofsson A, Can correct regions in protein models be identified? *Protein Sci.* **15**:900–913 (2006).

11. Wang Z, Tegge AN, Cheng J, Evaluating the absolute quality of a single protein model using structural features and support vector machines, *Proteins: Struct., Funct., Bioinformatics* **75**(3):638–647 (2008).

12. Zemla A, Venclovas C, Moult J, Fidelis K, Processing and analysis of CASP3 protein structure prediction, *Proteins* (Suppl. 3):22–29 (1999).

13. Pettitt CS, Improving sequence-based fold recognition by using 3D model quality assessment, *Bioinformatics* **21**(17):3509–3515 (2005).

14. Zhou H, Skolnick J, Protein model quality assessment prediction by combining fragment comparison and a consensus ca contact potential, *Proteins* **71**:1211–1218 (2007).

15. Zhang Y, Skolnick J, SPICKER: A clustering approach to identify near-native protein folds, *J. Comput. Chem.* **25**:865–871 (2004).

16. Karplus K, Katzman S, Shackleford G, Koeva M, Draper J, Barnes B, Soriano M, Hughey R, SAM-T04: What is new in protein structure prediction for CASP6, *Proteins*; **61**:135–142 (2005).

17. Kajan L, Rychlewski L, Evaluation of 3D-jury on casp7 models, *BMC Bioinformatics* **8**:304 (2007).

18. McGuffin LJ, The ModFOLD server for the quality assessment of protein structural models, *Bioinformatics* **24**:586–587 (2008).

19. Zhou H, Skolnick J, Ab initio protein structure prediction using chunk—TASSER, *Biophys. J.* **93**(5):1510–1518 (2007).

20. Holm L, Sander C, Protein structure comparison by alignment of distance matrices, *J. Mol. Biol.* **233**:123–138 (1993).

21. Reyaz-Ahmed (Chida) A, Zhang YQ, Harrison R, Evolutionary neural SVM and complete SVM decision tree for protein secondary structure prediction, *Int. J. Comput. Intell. Syst.* **2**(2):343–352 (2009).

22. Wang G, Dunbrack RL Jr, PISCES: A protein sequence culling server, *Bioinformatics* **19**:1589–1591 (2003).

23. Vapnik V, Corter C, Support vector networks, *Machine Learn.* **20**:273–293 (1995).

24. Shawe-Taylor J, Cristianini N, *Kernel Method for Pattern Analysis*, Cambridge Univ. Press, (2004).

25. Joachims T, Making large-Scale SVM learning practical, in Schölkopf B, Burges C, Smola A, eds., *Advances in Kernel Methods—Support Vector Learning*, MIT Press, Cambridge, MA, 1999.

26. Reyaz-Ahmed (Chida) A, Harrison R, Zhang Y-Q, 3D protein model assessment using geometric and biological features, *Proceedings of SEDM*, Chengdu, 2010, June 23–25.

27. Quinian JR, Discovering rules by induction from large collection of examples, in Michi D, ed.: *Expert Systems in Micro Electronics Age*, Edinburgh Univ. Press, 1979.

28. Abu-Halaweh N, Harrison RW, Prediction and classifiction of real and pseudo microRNA precursors via data fuzzification and fuzzy decision tree. *Proc. Int.*

Symp. Bioinformatics Research on Applications (*ISBRA*), Ft. Lauderdale 2009, pp. 323–334.

29. Abu-Halaweh N, Harrison RW, Rule set reduction in fuzzy decision trees, *Proc. North American Fuzzy Information Processing Society Conf.* (*NAFIPS*), Cincinnati 2009, pp. 1–4.

30. Reyaz-Ahmed (Chida) A, Abu-halaweh N, Harrison R, Zhang YQ, Protein model assessment via improved fuzzy decision tree, *Proc. Int. Conf. Bioinformatics* (*BIOCOMP*), Las Vegas, July 2010, pp. 12–15.

BIBLIOGRAPHY

1. Abu-halaweh N, Harrison RW, Practical fuzzy decision trees, *Proc. IEEE Symp. Computational Intelligence and Data Mining* (*ICTAI*), Nashville 2000, pp. 203–206.

2. Chen XJ, Harrison R, Zhang Y-Q, Genetic fuzzy classification fusion of multiple SVMs for biomedical data, *J. Intell. Fuzzy Syst.* (special issue on evolutionary computing in bioinformatics) **18**(6):527–541 (2007).

3. Fischer D, 3D-SHOTGUN: A novel, cooperative, fold-recognition meta-predictor, *Proteins* **51**:434–441 (2003).

4. Lee K, Lee K, Lee J, Lee-Kwang H, A fuzzy decision tree induction method for fuzzy data, *Proc. IEEE Conf. Fuzzy Systems* (*FUZZ-IEEE 99*), Seoul, 1999, vol. **1**, pp. 16–25.

5. McGuffin L, Bryson K, Jones D, What are the baselines for protein fold recognition? *Bioinformatics* **17**:63–72 (2001).

6. Qiu J, Sheffler W, Baker D, Noble WS, Ranking predicted protein structures with support vector regression, *Proteins* **71**:1175–1182 (2008).

7. Quinlan JR, Introduction of decision trees, *Machine Learn.* **1**:81–106 (1986).

8. Tang YC, Zhang Y-Q, Huang Z, Development of two-stage SVM-RFE gene selection strategy for microarray expression data analysis, *IEEE/ACM Trans. Comput. Biol. Bioinformatics* **4**(3):365–381 (July–Sept. 2007).

9. Zhang Y, Progress and challenges in protein structure prediction, *Curr. Opin. Struct. Biol.* **18**(3):342–348 (June 2008).

PART IV

PROTEIN–PROTEIN ANALYSIS
OF BIOLOGICAL NETWORKS

CHAPTER 18

NETWORK ALGORITHMS FOR PROTEIN INTERACTIONS

SUELY OLIVEIRA

18.1 INTRODUCTION

Graphs or networks are a fundamental way of representing connections between objects or concepts. Connections between proteins can identify functional groups of proteins, and how various proteins work together. Studies of the function of proteins are fundamental in current biological research [40]. We have been able to sequence entire genomes and can identify large numbers of individual genes. However, while the *syntax* of the genes is rapidly becoming clearer, the *semantics* or meaning of those genes is still mostly shrouded in mystery. This mystery has deepened in recent years as it has become apparent hat there is no one-to-one connection between genes and the proteins that actually perform functions in organisms.

In order to unlock the information about how proteins carry out their function, we first need to understand which proteins work together. High-throughput experiments have been able to create interaction networks for large numbers of proteins. One particular method is tandem affinity purification (TAP), which was developed in the late 1990s [31], and has been used to obtain large-scale interaction networks. For example, a large-scale protein–protein interaction (PPI) network was constructed for baker's yeast (*Saccharomyces cerevisiae*) [21] using TAP combined with mass spectrometry to identify the proteins in the complexes. The study [21] identified 7123 interactions among a set of 2708 proteins. Note that this makes the network of interaction quite sparse: only 7123 interactions are identified out of a maximum of $2708 \times (2708 - 1)/2 \approx 3.6 \times 10^6$ possible interactions.

The task that is considered in this chapter is to cluster the set of proteins into natural groups that operate together. These groups should be functional groups

Algorithmic and Artificial Intelligence Methods for Protein Bioinformatics. First Edition.
Edited by Yi Pan, Jianxin Wang, Min Li.
© 2014 John Wiley & Sons, Inc. Published 2014 by John Wiley & Sons, Inc.

and can often be identified as serving a particular purpose in the life of a cell [37].

From the data mining perspective, numerous issues arise in dealing with these PPI networks. Many datasets have numeric values for a number of attributes of each data item (such as the well-known "iris" dataset of Fisher) from which measures *similarity* or *nearness* are computed. In PPI networks, on the other hand, the data are given directly in the form of a network. A second issue is that with biological systems and large-scale experiments, a relatively high error rate is expected. Since the PPI network is fairly sparse, even if the error rate is kept reasonably low, the number of false positives is likely to be at least a significant percentage of the identified interactions. Oliveira and Seok [24,27,28] have addressed these issues.

In this chapter we look at algorithms for clustering that use optimization methods, often combined with hierarchical methods, as exemplified by the author's work [24,27–29] and the work of others, [e.g., 40].

18.2   OPTIMIZATION APPROACHES TO CLUSTERING

Anyone can cluster a dataset. Simply split the items wherever you please, and you have a cluster. The problem is that the clusters so created are unlikely to have any significant coherence. What we really need are high-quality clusters. If we can define the quality of a cluster, then the problem of clustering becomes an optimization problem.

18.2.1   Similarities and Distances

The basic data needed for a clustering then are a measure of the similarity between two data items. Since data items themselves may be given as vectors of numbers or as a collection of attributes, the usual first step is to define the *similarity* between two data items by a function of the entries or attributes of the data items. If the data items are given as vectors of numbers where the ith entry is the strength of a certain attribute, then we can represent the similarity in terms of the distance between the two vectors in a certain norm; for data items k and ℓ represented by vectors $\mathbf{v}_k$ and $\mathbf{v}_\ell \in \mathbb{R}^m$, we take the distance between them to be $\|\mathbf{v}_k - \mathbf{v}_\ell\|$, where $\|\mathbf{z}\|$ is a measure of the size of $\mathbf{z}$. The most common norm is the Euclidean norm, which is given by $\|\mathbf{z}\|_2 = \sqrt{\mathbf{z}^T \mathbf{z}} = [\sum_{i=1}^m z_i^2]^{1/2}$. Other norms include the Manhattan matrix or 1-norm: $\|\mathbf{z}\|_1 = \sum_{i=1}^m |z_i|$, and the max-norm or ∞-norm: $\|\mathbf{z}\|_\infty = \max_i |z_i|$. Norms have a number of basic properties:

- $\|\mathbf{z}\| \geq 0$, and if $\|\mathbf{z}\| = 0$ is possible only if $\mathbf{z} = 0$.
- $\|\alpha \mathbf{z}\| = |\alpha| \, \|\mathbf{z}\|$ for any scale factor α.
- $\|\mathbf{y} + \mathbf{z}\| \leq \|\mathbf{y}\| + \|\mathbf{z}\|$ for any $\mathbf{y}$ and $\mathbf{z}$; this is called the *triangle inequality*.

For clustering applications it is important that the different components of the data vectors $\mathbf{v}_k$ be scaled similarly. If, for example, the ith component of the $\mathbf{v}_k$ vectors is scaled to be much larger than the other components of $\mathbf{v}_k$, then the distance measurement will mainly reflect differences in that component.

Often it is better to think of *weights* or *dissimilarities* instead of distances. For example, we could take $w_{k\ell} = \|\mathbf{v}_k - \mathbf{v}_\ell\|^2$, which may be more appropriate; doubling the distance quadruples the weight in this example. This might be appropriate where outliers should be removed from clusters, but not appropriate where a chain of connections might connect apparently distant data items.

The values $w_{k\ell}$ represent dissimilatiries, and the greater the dissimilarity, the less similar the data items are. If we need to obtain similarities, we will treat then as functions of the distances: $s_{k\ell} = \phi(w_{k\ell})$ is the similarity between data item k and data item ℓ. The function ϕ should be a *decreasing* function of the distance; after all, the greater the distance, the less similar. We will assume that similarity, like distance, must be a nonnegative quantity.

A desirable property of the collection of weights $w_{k\ell}$ or similarities $s_{k\ell}$ is that the array of these values $[w_{k\ell}]_{k,\ell=1}^N$ or $[s_{k\ell}]_{k,\ell=1}^N$ should be *data-sparse*; that is, the arrays should be representable in some way by many fewer than the N^2 entries that appear in the arrays. This is perhaps easier to do with the matrix of similarities if we set $s_{k\ell} = \max(0, w_{\max} - w_{k\ell})$ so that $w_{k\ell} \geq w_{\max}$ results in zero similarity. This can result in a *sparse matrix* (one in which all but a small fraction of the N^2 entries are zero) if $w_{\max}$ is suitably chosen. This can be a reasonable approach, as the degree of similarity between data items is usually important only if the data items are close. Sparse matrices can be stored and used for computation in a memory-efficient way by storing only the nonzero entries along with some additional data structures to navigate the sparsity structure [38]. If the matrix of distances is needed, then the values $w_{k\ell} = \min(w_{\max}, |\mathbf{v}_k - \mathbf{v}_\ell|)$ can also be stored in a data-sparse manner, perhaps by storing $[w_{\max} - w_{k\ell}]_{k,\ell=1}^N$ as a sparse matrix.

18.2.2 Objective Functions

However, to measure the similarities or dissimilarities between data items, we need a way of measuring the quality of the clustering. We will focus on just a few objective functions; there is considerable variation in the objective functions that can be used for this task. In general, there are two objective functions:

1. We want high similarity (or *coherence*) within each cluster.
2. We want strong dissimilarity or distance between different clusters.

Phrased in this way, the problem is a multiobjective optimization problem [7]. As with most multiobjective optimization problems, there is strong tension between the two objectives; the clustering that has the highest coherence within clusters is the clustering in which each data item forms its own cluster, and maximizing distance between different clusters tends to result in few clusters, or perhaps just one. The theory of multiobjective optimization has a conceptual remedy to this tension between objectives, which is the concept of *Pareto optima*; a Pareto optima is a solution where an improvement in one objective can only be made by worsening another objective. There is typically a large set of Pareto optima. The user or application decides how the tradeoff between the objectives should be carried out.

In practice, a multiobjective problem is replaced by a single-objective function that in some way captures the competing objectives. The tradeoff is built into this objective. Often we can incorporate weights or other parameters that allow us to modify the tradeoff between the objectives.

The first objective function that we will consider is a well-known objective for graph bisection: splitting a graph $G = (V, E)$ with weighted edges into two disjoint sets of vertices V_1 and V_2 where $V = V_1 \cup V_2$. The objective to be minimized is the sum of weights of edges connecting V_1 and V_2:

$$f(V_1, V_2) = \sum_{e=\{k,\ell\}\in E,\ k\in V_1,\ \ell\in V_2} w_{k\ell} \tag{18.1}$$

Minimizing this objective without any further constraints leads to either $V_1 = \emptyset$ and $V_2 = V$, or $V_2 = V$ and $V_2 = \emptyset$, both with $f(V_1, V_2) = 0$. Clearly this is not a very useful result. However, if we add the constraint that the number of vertices in V_1 and in V_2 are at least similar in magnitude, the problem becomes much more interesting. For applications in parallel computing, if V_1 and V_2 represent the tasks to be completed and the edge weights represent the communication needed between the associated tasks, then $f(V_1, V_2)$ represents the communication needed between a pair of processors with tasks in V_1 executed on processor 1, and V_2 the tasks executed on processor 2. Minimizing $f(V_1, V_2)$ corresponds to minimizing interprocessor communication. However, in the parallel computing application, it is also important to *balance* the load between the processors. The standard balance condition is that the number of vertices in V_1 (denoted $|V_1|$) differs from the number of vertices in V_2 ($|V_2|$) by no more than one:

$$-1 \le |V_1| - |V_2| \le +1 \tag{18.2}$$

This optimization problem can be put into matrix–vector form by creating a *decision variable* or vector $\mathbf{z}$ with $|V|$ components where $z_k = +1$ if $k \in V_1$ and $z_k = -1$ if $k \in V_2$. Then the objective and constraints can be represented by the following integer optimization (or *integer programming*) problem:

$$\min \sum_{k,\ell \in V} w_{k\ell} \tfrac{1}{4}(z_k - z_\ell)^2 \quad \text{subject to} \tag{18.3}$$

$$-1 \le \sum_{k \in V} z_k \le +1 \tag{18.4}$$

$$z_k \in \{-1, +1\} \quad \text{for all } k \tag{18.5}$$

For clustering, it is not essential that $|V_1| \approx |V_2|$. However, we can impose a condition such as $\max(|V_1|/|V_2|, |V_2|/|V_1|) \le \alpha$ instead of the balance condition [Eq. (18.2)] to prevent clusters from becoming excessively small. In the next section, we will see how we can obtain approximate solutions of these problems with reasonable computational effort.

Splitting a graph into two clusters can be the start of a general clustering algorithm; split a graph into two parts. For each part, if the coherence of the individual part is higher than some threshold, then split the part again. Repeating recursively is a way obtain a clustering of a dataset with any number of clusters. This is a divisive algorithm for creating clusters.

But a dataset might not naturally split into pairs of clusters. Perhaps there are three natural clusters. Then splitting the graph into two parts would hopefully result in two clusters in one part, and the third cluster in the other. A further splitting of the larger part should reveal the natural clustering. But it is difficult to guarantee that the initial splitting would respect the natural clusters. So it is important to have algorithms and objective functions for splitting into more than two parts.

Most multisplitting algorithms assume that we have a fixed number of clusters K to find. One objective function is due to Rao [33] from the 1960s; the cost to be minimized is the sum of the weights of the edges between different clusters, and each data item is assigned to one of K clusters. The decision variables are $z_{jr} = 1$ if data item j is in cluster r, and $z_{jr} = 0$ otherwise. Then z_{jr} form a matrix $Z = [z_{jr}]$ with N rows (for the data items) and K columns (for the clusters). Rao's formulation is then

$$\min_{Z} \sum_{i,j=1}^{N} w_{ij} \sum_{r=1}^{K} z_{ir} z_{jr} \qquad \text{subject to} \qquad (18.6)$$

$$\sum_{r=1}^{K} z_{ir} = 1 \qquad \text{for all } i \qquad (18.7)$$

$$\sum_{i=1}^{N} z_{ir} \ge 1 \qquad \text{for all } r \qquad (18.8)$$

$$z_{ir} \in \{0, 1\} \qquad \text{for all } i, r \qquad (18.9)$$

Constraint (18.7) implies that each data item i belongs to exactly one cluster; constraint (18.8) implies that each cluster r contains at least one data item; constraint (18.9) ensures that each decision variable can be only zero or one. This can be represented in matrix terms. Let $\mathbf{e} = [1, 1, \ldots, 1]^T$ be the column vector of ones of the appropriate size for the context in which it appears. Then constraints (18.6)–(18.9) are equivalent to the following matrix problem:

$$\min_{Z} \operatorname{trace}(WZZ^T) \qquad \text{subject to} \qquad (18.10)$$

$$Z\mathbf{e} = \mathbf{e}, \qquad (18.11)$$

$$Z^T\mathbf{e} \geq \mathbf{e}, \qquad (18.12)$$

$$z_{ir} \in \{0, 1\} \qquad \text{for all } i, r \qquad (18.13)$$

The trace of a matrix X is the sum of its diagonal entries: $\operatorname{trace}(X) = \sum_i x_{ii}$. A basic property of the trace of a matrix is that for any matrices A and B, $\operatorname{trace}(AB) = \operatorname{trace}(BA)$. From this, it can be shown that if X is a symmetric matrix ($X^T = X$), the trace of X is the sum of its eigenvalues. Note that constraint (18.8) and its matrix equivalent [Eq. (18.12)] are very nearly redundant as they only prevents clusters with exactly zero data items. Removing these constraints does not greatly change the optimization problem and its solution.

18.2.3 Spectral Bisection

It has been shown that graph bisection as given by Equations (18.1) and (18.2) is a computationally intractable problem [6,14]; that is, there is no polynomial time algorithm that can solve these equations, nor is there ever likely to be such an algorithm. More precisely, if there ever were a polynomial time algorithm for Equations (18.1) and (18.2); then there would be polynomial time algorithms for a very large collection of problems known as NP. The set of problems for which there are polynomial time algorithms is known as P. The question "Is $P = NP$?" is perhaps the biggest unsolved question in computer science.

Research has then focused on algorithms that give a good but not optimal solution to the problem. Spectral algorithms are based on eigenvalues of matrices, and so spectral bisection is based on a matrix–vector representation of Equations (18.1) and (18.2):

$$\min_{\mathbf{z}} \tfrac{1}{4} \mathbf{z}^T L \mathbf{z} \qquad \text{subject to}$$

$$-1 \leq \mathbf{e}^T \mathbf{z} \leq +1$$

$$z_i \in \{-1, +1\} \qquad \text{for all } i$$

The matrix L is given by

$$L_{ij} = \begin{cases} \sum_{\ell} w_{i\ell}, & \text{if } i = j \\ -w_{ij}, & \text{otherwise} \end{cases} \qquad (18.14)$$

and is called the *graph Laplacian* matrix. Note that $w_{i\ell} = 0$ if vertices i and ℓ are not connected in the graph.

Note that the fact that $z_i^2 = 1$ for all i implies that $\sum_{i=1}^N z_i^2 = \mathbf{z}^T \mathbf{z} = N$. The constraint $\mathbf{z}^T \mathbf{z} = N$ can be added to the problem without changing it. If we now *relax* the problem by removing the restriction that $z_i = \pm 1$ for all i, we obtain the continuous optimization problem

$$\min_{\mathbf{z}} \mathbf{z}^T L \mathbf{z} \quad \text{subject to}$$

$$-1 \le \mathbf{e}^T \mathbf{z} \le +1$$

$$\mathbf{z}^T \mathbf{z} = N$$

If we consider N to be large, then the constraint $-1 \le \mathbf{e}^T \mathbf{z} \le +1$ can reasonably be approximated by the constraint $\mathbf{e}^T \mathbf{z} = 0$. This leads to the following problem:

$$\min_{\mathbf{z}} \mathbf{z}^T L \mathbf{z} \quad \text{subject to}$$

$$\mathbf{e}^T \mathbf{z} = 0$$

$$\mathbf{z}^T \mathbf{z} = N$$

The solution to this problem is given directly in terms of eigenvalues and eigenvectors of L; the minimum value is $N \lambda_2(L)$ and $\mathbf{z}$ is an eigenvector of the eigenvalue $\lambda_2(L)$, where $\lambda_2(L)$ is the second smallest eigenvalue of L. The smallest eigenvalue of L is zero for any graph or weights. The eigenvalue $\lambda_2(L)$ is known as the *Fiedler value* and the corresponding eigenvector, the *Fiedler vector* for the graph in recognition of the the fundamental work of Miroslav Fiedler [12]. The spectral bisection is determined by taking the median value of the components of the Fiedler vector $\mathbf{v}$; if v_{med} is the median value of the components of $\mathbf{v}$, then we assign vertex i to V_1 if $v_i > v_{\text{med}}$ and to V_2 if $v_i \le v_{\text{med}}$. If there is more flexibility in the sizes of V_1 and V_2, we can take a *cut value* v_{cut}, and assign vertex i to V_1 if $v_i > v_{\text{cut}}$ and to V_2 if $v_i \le v_{\text{cut}}$.

Variants of the spectral bisection method for clustering have been developed by a number of authors [9,16,36], but based on similarities s_{ij}, rather than weights or dissimilarities. Two-way spectral clustering algorithms start by constructing optimization problems. These three problems are described as follows.

- *MinMaxCut:* Minimize

$$J_{\text{MMC}}(A, B) = \frac{s(A,B)}{s(A,A)} + \frac{s(A,B)}{s(B,B)} = \frac{s(A,\overline{A})}{s(A,A)} + \frac{s(B,\overline{B})}{s(B,B)} \quad (18.15)$$

- *RatioCut:* Minimize

$$J_{\text{R}}(A, B) = \frac{s(A,B)}{|A|} + \frac{s(A,B)}{|B|} = \frac{s(A,\overline{A})}{|A|} + \frac{s(B,\overline{B})}{|B|} \quad (18.16)$$

- *NormalizedCut:* Minimize

$$J_N(A,B) = \frac{s(A,B)}{s(A,A) + s(A,B)} + \frac{s(A,B)}{s(B,B) + s(A,B)} \tag{18.17}$$

$$= \frac{s(A,\overline{A})}{s(A,A) + s(A,\overline{A})} + \frac{s(B,\overline{B})}{s(B,B) + s(B,\overline{B})} \tag{18.18}$$

where $s(A,B) = \sum_{i \in A, j \in B} s_{ij}$ and $\overline{A} = \{ i = 1, 2, \ldots, n | i \notin A \}$.

In a continuous approximation to this problem [19], the solution is the eigenvector q_2 associated with the second smallest eigenvalue of the system $(D - S)q = \lambda Dq$, where $D = \text{diag}(d_1, d_2, \ldots, d_n)$ and $d_i = \sum_j s_{ij}$. The partition (A, B) is calculated by finding index i^* such that the corresponding objective function gets optimum value with the partition, $A = \{i | q_2(i) < q_2(i^*)\}$ and $B = \{i | q_2(i) \geq q_2(i^*)\}$.

Objective functions for two-way partitioning optimization formulations can be easily generalized for K-way partitioning such as

$$J_{\text{MMC}}(A_1, \ldots, A_k) = \sum_{i=1}^{k} \frac{s(A_i, \overline{A_i})}{s(A_i, A_i)} \tag{18.19}$$

Direct partitioning algorithms compute $k - 1$ eigenvectors, $q_2, \ldots, q_k$ of the same generalized eigenvalue system for two-way formulations and then use (18.19) to create k clusters instead of (18.15) to create two clusters. This objective function (18.19) is also used for recursive bipartitioning during the refinement phase.

The optimum value of two-way MinMaxCut is called the *cohesion* of the cluster and can be an indicator to show how closely vertices of the current cluster are related [9]. This value can be used for the cluster selection algorithm. The cluster that has the least cohesion is chosen for partitioning. Another selection criterion considered in this research is the average similarity, $\overline{s}_i := s(A_i, A_i)/|A_i|^2$. Both algorithms were reported earlier to work very well [9].

18.2.4 Matrix Optimization Methods

There has been a great deal of work on applying matrix optimization methods to combinatorial optimization problems [10,15]. These problems involve matrices as the decision variables in an essential way. The reason for this is that linear constraints on the matrix variables plus certain matrix constraints can represent very good approximations to some hard combinatorial optimization problems while requiring only a modest computational effort to solve. One such approach is *semidefinite programming* (SDP). This is a generalization of linear programming where the variable is a symmetric matrix, and must be semidefinite. To be precise, an SDP has the form

$$\min_{X} C \bullet X := \sum_{i,j} c_{ij} x_{ij} \qquad \text{subject to} \qquad (18.20)$$

$$A_{\ell} \bullet X = b_{\ell}, \qquad \ell = 1, 2, \ldots, m, \qquad (18.21)$$

$$X^T = X \qquad (18.22)$$

$$\text{and } X \text{ is positive semidefinite.} \qquad (18.23)$$

The condition "X is positive semidefinite" (18.23) means that "$\mathbf{z}^T X \mathbf{z} \geq 0$ for all $\mathbf{z}$." This is a convex optimization problem in X; the objective is linear, and all constraints except (18.23) are linear. The set of positive semidefinite matrices is a convex set, as can be readily verified. Thus the problem (18.20)–(18.23) is a convex optimization problem.

The approximation of hard combinatorial optimization problems using SDPs has been done for some important classes of problems [e.g., 34]. SDP algorithms have been developed for various clustering problems as well [e.g., 8].

An alternative approach [29] is described below, which is closely related to the SDP approach. In this approach the final problem was not an SDP, and was not even a convex optimization problem. The starting point for this approximation is Rao's formulation of the general clustering problem [Eqs. (18.6)–(18.9)]. This is a combinatorial problem because of the *zero–one* constraint that each variable $z_{k\ell}$ be zero or one [Eq. (18.9)]. The objective function [Eq. (18.6)], trace$(WZZ^T) =$ trace$(Z^T WZ)$, is not a convex function because W is not a positive semidefinite matrix. This is easily seen because the diagonal entries of W are all zero, and W has nonzero off-diagonal entries. Nevertheless, it is possible to obtain a method that performs reasonably well at clustering by relaxing the zero–one constraint; instead, we require that $z_{k\ell} \geq 0$ for all k, ℓ and $\sum_{\ell} z_{k\ell} = 1$ for all k [Eq. (18.7)]. This gives a problem where we try to minimize a nonconvex function over a convex set. Simple gradient-type methods give effective algorithms, even for large problems [29]. There are a substantial number of local minima, but the algorithms given do not appear to get stuck in irrelevant local minima.

18.3   HIERARCHICAL ALGORITHMS

There are many algorithms for the clustering of networks, especially if the edges have weights denoting the strength of the connection. Practically all of these suffer from a steep increase in computational cost for modest increases in the size of the network under consideration. This is natural, especially when it is realized that certain simplified problems of this type are NP-hard, such as splitting a network into two halves with nearly equal numbers of nodes in each half while minimizing the total number of edges between the two halves [17–19,30,41]. The computational cost of computing a clustering can therefore be reduced by decreasing the size of the network to which it is applied. Combining nodes of a graph into *supernodes* of a quotient graph gives a way of reducing the size of a graph. A clustering algorithm can then be applied to the quotient graph, and after the quotient graph is clustered, the supernodes of each group in the cluster can be expanded in terms of nodes in the original graph, giving a clustering of the original graph.

More formally, the process can be described as follows. Let $G = (V, E)$ be the original graph with V the set of vertices, and E the set of edges of G. We assume that G is an undirected graph, so that each edge $e \in E$ is actually a set of two vertices $e = \{x, y\} \subset V$. Often we assign a weight to each edge e; w_e is a nonnegative real number for each edge e. To create the supernodes for the quotient graph, we need a partitioning P of V. This partition P is a collection of sets $P = \{S_1, S_2, \ldots, S_M\}$, where each S_k is a set of nodes $S_k \subset V$. The collection P of sets must have the following properties:

1. The union of sets in P must be the set of all vertices: $V = \cup_{k=1}^{M} S_k$.
2. The sets in P must be disjoint: $k \neq \ell$ implies $S_k \cap S_\ell = \emptyset$.

Each set S_k becomes a vertex of the quotient graph $\hat{G} = (\hat{V}, \hat{E})$, and there is an edge $\hat{e} \in \hat{E}$ between S_k and S_ℓ if and only if there is an edge $e = \{x, y\} \in E$ in G with $x \in S_k$ and $y \in S_\ell$. We can assign weights to the edges $\hat{e} = \{S_k, S_\ell\}$ of $\hat{E}$ by adding the weights of all edges in G connecting S_k and S_ℓ:

$$\hat{w}_{\hat{e}} = \sum_{x \sim y:\ x \in S_k,\ y \in S_\ell} w_{\{x, y\}}$$

Even if the original graph is *unweighted* (which is equivalent to $w_e = 1$ whenever $e \in E$), the quotient graph has weights that should not be disregarded.

However, the quality of the clustering of the original graph is highly dependent on the way the supernodes were created in the first place. Creating the supernodes is also a kind of clustering, but we do not wish to use complex or expensive algorithms for this part of the process. Simple heuristics such as *heavy edge matching* [25,26] or even just *random edge matching* might be used. But using crude methods for creating the supernodes will result in poor clusterings for the original graph, even if the clustering for the quotient graph is optimal.

The process of coarsening a graph is analogous to some of the operations of multigrid methods for solving discrete approximations to partial differential equations [5,22]. Multigrid methods do not use a single step to go from a fine approximation to a coarse approximation. Rather, there is a sequence of coarsenings where the ratio of the number of coarse variables to the number of fine variables at each stage is not allowed to become too small. More formally, a sequence of graphs $G^{(0)}, G^{(1)}, \ldots, G^{(p)}$ is generated starting with the original graph $G = G^{(0)}$. Each graph $G^{(k+1)}$ is a quotient graph of $G^{(k)}$. The final graph $G^{(p)}$ is the coarsest, and might contain only a handful of vertices.

As noted above, the construction of the nodes of $G^{(k+1)}$ from $G^{(k)}$ by simple heuristics might result in a poor clustering for G even if the clustering of $G^{(p)}$ is optimal. To prevent this deterioration of clustering quality as we move from $G^{(p)}$ to $G = G^{(0)}$, at each stage we use a local search method to improve the quality of the clustering. Suppose that we have a clustering $C^{(k+1)} = \{C_1^{(k+1)}, C_2^{(k+1)}, \ldots, C_r^{(k+1)}\}$ of $G^{(k+1)}$. Note that $C^{(k+1)}$ is a partition of the vertices $V^{(k+1)}$ of $G^{(k+1)}$. Also note that each vertex of $G^{(k+1)}$ is actually a set of vertices of $G^{(k)}$. From $C^{(k+1)}$ we create an initial clustering $C_0^{(k)} := \{C_{0,1}^{(k)}, C_{0,2}^{(k)}, \ldots, C_{0,r}^{(k)}\}$ of $G^{(k)}$ by setting $C_{0,i}^{(k)}$ to be the union of all the supernodes $x \in C_i^{(k+1)}$. We can then use a local method such as the Kenighan–Lin algorithm [20] or the Fiduccia–Mattheyses algorithm [11] to $C_0^{(k)}$ to obtain a locally improved clustering $C^{(k)}$. These local improvements can overcome imperfections in the initial creation of the supernodes of $G^{(k+1)}$.

The details of these algorithms and how they are performed are given in following sections.

18.4 FEATURES OF PPI NETWORKS

Graph theory is commonly used as a method for analyzing PPIs in computational biology. Each vertex represents a protein, and edges correspond to experimentally identified PPIs. Proteomic networks have two important features [4]. One is that the degree distribution function $P(k)$ (the number of nodes with degree k) follows a power law $P(k) \approx$ constant $k^{-\alpha}$ (and so is considered a scale-free network). This means that most vertices have low degrees, called *low-shell proteins*, and a few are highly connected, called *hub proteins*. Figure 18.1 shows the degree distributions of seven organisms in the DIP database [1]. The other feature is the *small-world* property, which is also known as *6 degrees of separation*. This means that the diameter of the graph is small compared with the number of nodes.

The standard tools to understand these networks are the clustering coefficient (Cc), the average pathlength, and the diameter of the network. The clustering coefficient (Cc_i) is defined in terms of $E(G(v_i))$, the set of edges in the neighborhood of v_i. The clustering coefficient is the probability that a pair of randomly chosen neighbors of v_i are connected; that is

$$\text{Cc}_i = \frac{2}{\deg(v_i)[\deg(v_i) - 1]} \cdot |E(G(v_i))| \tag{18.24}$$

where $G(v_i)$ is the neighborhood of v_i and $E(G(v_i))$ are the edges in $G(v_i)$.

Since the denominator is the maximum possible number of edges between vertices connected to v_i, $0 \le \text{Cc}_i \le 1$. The global clustering coefficient can be simply the average of all individual clustering coefficients (Cc_i) like

$$\overline{\text{Cc}} = \sum_{i=1}^{n} \frac{\text{Cc}_i}{n} \tag{18.25}$$

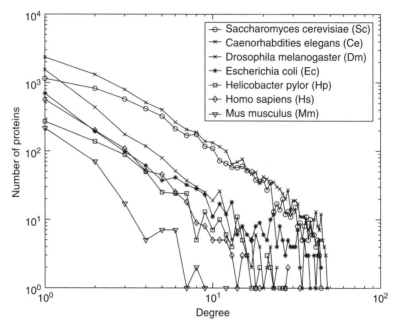

Figure 18.1 The degree distribution of 7 organisms in DIP database.

But this "average of an average" is not very informative [4]; one alternative is to weight each local clustering coefficient

$$Cc = \sum_{i=1}^{n} \frac{\deg(v_i)}{\text{MaxDeg}} \frac{Cc_i}{n} \qquad (18.26)$$

where MaxDeg is the maximum degree in the network. We use the latter Cc as our clustering coefficient for the rest of the chapter.

The pathlength of two nodes v_i and v_j is the smallest sum of edge weights of paths connecting v_i and v_j. For an unweighted network, it is the smallest number of edges to go through. The average pathlength is the average of pathlengths of all pairs (v_i, v_j). The diameter of the network is the maximum pathlength.

Because of the particular characteristics of PPI networks, a two-level approach has been proposed [32]. The main idea is derived from the k-core concept introduced by Batagelj and Zaversnik [3]. If we repeatedly remove vertices of degree less than k from a graph until there are no longer any such vertices, the result is the k-core of the original graph. The vertices removed are called the *low-shell vertices*. Then we remove the hub vertices; we choose a threshold m, and remove all vertices with degree $\geq m$. Pothen et al. [32] used $m = 15$. The two-level approach factors in three assumptions in protein–protein interaction networks:

- The hub proteins interact with many other proteins, so it is difficult to limit them to only one cluster, and the computational complexity increases when they are included.
- There are many low-shell proteins, which increases the size of network. These nodes are easy to cluster when the nodes they are connected to are clustered first.
- Proteomic networks consist mostly of one large component and several small components.

Disregarding hub proteins and low-shell proteins, and limiting attention to the biggest component of proteomic networks leaves us to focus on the nodes that are most meaningful to cluster. Another advantage of this approach is that this architecture favors the size of the residual network, which requires less computational time.

18.5 IMPLEMENTATION OF HIERARCHICAL METHODS

The hierarchical methods discussed here have three main phases:

1. An *aggregation phase*, where we create a hierarchy of quotient graphs
2. A clustering phase where a suitable clustering algorithm (such as spectral clustering) is applied to the coarsest graph
3. A disaggregation phase where the clustering is successively transfered down the hierarchy of graphs, and optionally, a local method is used to improve the clustering at each level before futher disaggregation

The aggregation phase has traditionally been carried out using matching algorithms. This was the case with the early work of Oliveira and Seok on document clustering [26,35]. Rather than use the more expensive maximal or maximum matching algorithms, cheaper greedy or random matching algorithms were used. Because of the high false positive rates in many PPI datasets, matchings can generate lower-quality coarsenings, which can yield lower-quality sets of clusters.

For PPI networks, because of their density and the lack of significant weighting, clique-based aggregation methods were developed. Cliques are sets of vertices in a graph where each pair of vertices in the set is connected by an edge of the graph. Cliques involve larger collections of edges, and so are less affected by high false positive rates. Below we describe some methods based on the use of triangular cliques, and also maximal cliques. As we look for larger cliques for performing the aggregation, both the complexity and the quality of the clusterings increases. How to balance the tradeoff between these aspects is a matter for future research.

After the clustering has been carried out for the coarsest graph in the hierarchy, the clusters must be disaggregated, possibly followed by application of a local method to refine the clustering. The use of a local method typically does not produce many changes, as they cannot "see" the effects of more radical changes to the clustering. However, local methods applied to quotient graphs can be much more effective: moving a vertex from one cluster to another in a quotient graph may represent the transfer of many nodes in the original graph between clusters. Applying refinement at each level of a hierarchy has the effect of "polishing" the cluster at all levels of coarsness. This can overcome problems of low quality in computationally cheap aggregation methods used to generate the hierarchy of graphs.

18.5.1 Matching-Based Methods

A matching in a graph is a set of edges of which no two are incident to the same node. Matchings provide a way of aggregating vertices into supernodes.

A matching is maximal when any edge in the graph that is not in the matching has at least one of its endpoints matched. Some algorithms aim to match as many nodes as possible, and some aim to maximize the sum of all edge weights [13,39]; this is often referred to as *maximum matching*. These algorithms are too time-intensive and are designed for weighted graphs [23]. Instead, the algorithms below try to find a compromise between speed and quality.

The simplest matching for unweighted graphs is random matching. One node is randomly visited, and one of unmatched node is randomly chosen to be merged with the node [random vertex random merge (RVRM)]. A drawback is that the low-degree nodes have a higher chance of remaining unmatched than do high-degree nodes. In order to avoid this problem we can pick the lowest degree node among unmerged nodes and choose one of the unmerged nodes randomly to merge [lowest-degree vertex random merge (LVRM)]. Thus this algorithm tends to merge more nodes than RVRM.

We define the weights of edges as follows. The edge weights are initially all 1s to start but become the sum of the number of edges combined after one matching step. A node weight is defined as the total number of nodes merged into it.

When we have different edge weights we can apply the sorted matching (SM) concept for coarsening in subsequent levels. SM has been used for weighted graphs and merged nodes in order of decreasing edge weight [26]. In the PPI network, at first we have equal edge weights. We perform the first level of coarsening by combining nodes with each other, as long as they are not matched. The results are similar for any order that we select for this step. After this matching we will have groups of edges that share the same weight (the maximum resulting edge weight will be 4 for a clique with four nodes/vertices). We consider these groups in order of decreasing edge weight. Within each group we give higher priority to the edge with lower combined node weights; we take the edge with maximum $1/w(n_i) + 1/w(n_j)$ as a tiebreak specifically, rule, where $w(n_i)$ and $w(n_j)$ are the node weights, that is, the number of nodes of supernodes n_i and n_j. We call this matching scheme *heavy edge small node* (HESN).

Karypis et al. also present heuristic matching-based algorithms for unweighted networks [2]. Their heuristic algorithms were tested for power-law networks. Various algorithms are presented and experimentally compared. They reported that fewer within cluster edges are expected to be deleted when vertices are visited randomly, and one of the unmerged nodes is chosen in a greedy strategy. We include one of their coarsening algorithms in this research and compare it with ours. This *random visit and merge greedy* (RVMG) algorithm visits nodes randomly and a local greedy strategy is applied. In their greedy strategy, vertices that have connected edges with bigger edge weights are considered first. Smaller node weights are used to break ties for the same edge weights.

18.5.2   Clique-Based Methods

Triangular clique (TC)-based algorithms have been developed that merge highly connected triples of nodes [28]. A *clique* is a set of nodes in a graph where each node in the clique is connected to every other node in the clique by an edge of the graph. A *triangular clique* (TC) is a clique of three nodes (i.e., three nodes whose edges form a triangle). Our TC-based multilevel algorithm was inspired by Spirin and Mirny's use of cliques to identify highly connected clusters [37]. Our TC-based algorithm showed more proteins correctly merged into supernodes than any other matching based algorithm. This is because all three vertices in a TC have a very high chance of being part of the same functional module. A weakness of the TC-based algorithms is that there are many TCs in even a moderately sized clique. For example, there are 560 TCs in a clique of 16 nodes. Since we do not have efficient "matching" algorithms for TCs that avoid overlap, there are several choices as to how an algorithm treats a pair of TCs (see Ref. [25] and Fig. 18.2).

The various choices range from never combining connected TCs to form a single supernode (TC_ONLY) to always combining TCs that are connected (TC_ALL). In general, the more conservative approach (TC_ONLY and TC_ONE) gives more accurate clusters, but takes more time, than the more aggressive approaches (TC_TWO and TC_ALL).

Another more recent approach for identifying protein complexes used maximal cliques to create subgraphs with high densities [42]. Cliques are called *maximal* when they are not completely contained in another. In general, enumerating all maximal cliques takes much more time than finding all TCs. Fortunately, PPI networks are quite sparse, so all maximal cliques are enumerated quickly.

Our experimental results show that the quality of maximal cliques for finding protein complexes is very high. The bigger the maximal clique, the higher the quality of the results. This strongly motivates the use of maximal cliques in conjunction with multilevel algorithms. We can generalize TC-based multilevel algorithms to include maximal cliques. Note that the maximal cliques themselves do not identify clusters completely because cliques may have overlaps. Instead, they are used to quickly identify highly connected disjoint subgraphs. We call these approaches *structure-based multilevel algorithms*.

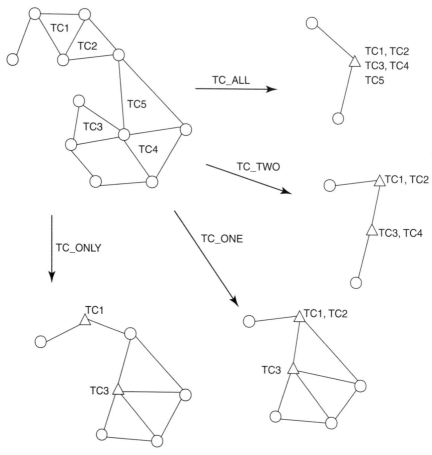

Figure 18.2 Four different TC-based coarsening algorithms. Each circle represents a node, and a triangle represents a supernode after coarsening.

18.5.3 Refinement and Disaggregation

A traditional Kernighan–Lin (KL)-type refinement algorithm can be applied to improve the quality at each level [20], which has $O(N^2)$ complexity. KL starts with an initial partition; it iteratively searches for nodes from each cluster of the graph if moving that node to one of the other clusters leads to a better partition. For each node, there may be more than one cluster giving a smaller objective function value than the current cut. So the node moves to the cluster that gives the biggest improvement. The iteration terminates when it does not find any node to improve the partition. However, this scheme has many redundant computations. For a given node u, all clusters are considered as possible candidates to which the node u moves. Moving an edge to a cluster to which it is not already connected will always increase the number of edges between clusters. So we calculate the improvements for only those clusters that have edges with node u. This modified scheme works much faster than traditional KL, especially for the sparse networks with large numbers of clusters. It should be mentioned that there are possibilities of certain objective functions that may improve when a node u moves to a cluster that does have any edge with u. Note that it would be a good idea to find a faster refinement algorithm for multiway clustering such as the Fiduccia–Mattheyses linear time heuristic, which was used for bipartitioning problems [11].

The choice of the objective function may become important, as the structure of the objective function may make it possible to easily identify optimal vertices to swap, while other objective functions may make this task much harder. For example, if the objective function (to minimize) is the number of edges crossing between clusters, then the test for moving a vertex from cluster 1 to cluster 2 depends on whether the vertex has more edges to cluster 1 or to cluster 2. Efficient data structures can be created to track these numbers efficiently as the clusters are changed. However, if the objective function is more complex, such as J_{MMC} from Equation (18.19), then determining suitable changes to the clustering may require substantially more computational effort.

18.6   CONCLUSION

Clustering problems, like other combinatorial optimization problems, are best tackled using a combination of discrete and continuous tools. Discrete methods (e.g., Kernighan–Lin methods and matching algorithms) are good for working with the local structure of a graph, while continuous methods (spectral clustering and SDP-based methods) are better at seeing the overall or global structure of the graph. The way to obtain optimal performance is likely to be combining them carefully to retain their strengths rather than their weaknesses. Continuous methods (such as spectral clustering) tend to be expensive on large graphs, while discrete methods (such as Kernighan–Lin) tend to be relatively cheap. Hierarchical methods where a graph is coarsened to create a sequence of quotient graphs, and where the coarsest of these is clustered using a continuous method, appear to offer the best compromise between computational cost and quality. Refinement of the clustering during the decoarsening phase of these algorithms seems to be especially useful in obtaining high-quality clusterings in reasonably computation time, even for very large graphs. Note that refinement should be guided by an objective function that is chosen to represent the task at hand, and not because it is convenient.

While there are different coarsening, decoarsening, and clustering algorithms, this framework of optimization-directed hierarchical methods has found success. Graphs with different structure may require different algorithms, but these algorithms have the potential to solve problems far beyond the ones for which they have already been used.

REFERENCES

1. Database of Interacting Proteins (DIP) (available at `http://dip.doe-mbi.ucla.edu/`).

2. Abou-Rjeili A, Karypis G, Multilevel algorithms for partitioning power-law graphs, *Proc. IEEE Int. Parallel & Distributed Processing Symp. (IPDPS)*, 2006.

3. Batagelj V, Zaversnik M, Generalized cores, in *Computing Research Repository (CoRR)*, cs.DS/0202039, Feb. 2002 (available at `http://arxiv.org/abs/cs.DS/0202039`).

4. Bornholdt S, Schuster HG, eds., *Handbook of Graphs and Networks*, Wiley VCH, 2003.

5. Briggs WL, *A Multigrid Tutorial*. SIAM, Philadelphia, 1987.

6. Nguyen Bui TN, Jones C, Finding good approximate vertex and edge partitions is NP-hard, *Inform. Process. Lett.* **42**(3):153–159 (1992).

7. Collette Y, Siarry P, Multiobjective optimization, in *Decision Engineering*, Springer-Verlag, Berlin, 2003 (principles and case studies).

8. De Bie T, Cristianini N, Fast SDP relaxations of graph cut clustering, transduction, and other combinatorial problems, *J. Mach. Learn. Res.* **7**:1409–1436 (2006).

9. Ding C, He X, Zha H, Gu M, Simon H, *A MinMaxCut Spectral Method for Data Clustering and Graph Partitioning*, Technical Report 54111, Lawrence Berkeley National Laboratory (LBNL), Dec. 2003.

10. Dukanovic I, Rendl F, Semidefinite programming relaxations for graph coloring and maximal clique problems, *Math. Program. B* **109**(2–3):S345–365 (2007).

11. Fiduccia CM, Mattheyses RM, A linear time heuristic for improving network partitions, *Proc. 19th IEEE Design Automation Conf.*, Miami Beach, FL, pp. 175–181.

12. Fiedler M, Algebraic connectivity of graphs, *Czech. Math. J.* **23**(98):298–305 (1973).

13. Gabow HN, Data structures for weighted matching and nearest common ancestors with linking, *Proc. ACM-SIAM Symposium on Discrete Algorithms*, 1990, pp. 434–443.

14. Garey MR, Johnson DS, Stockmeyer L, Some simplified NP-complete graph problems, *Theor. Comput. Sci.* **1**:237–267 (1976).

15. Goemans MX, Semidefinite programming in combinatorial optimization, *Math. Program.* **B79**(1–3):143–161 (1997) [lectures on mathematical programming (ismp97) (Lausanne, 1997)].

16. Hagen L, Kahng A, Fast spectral methods for ratio cut partitioning and clustering, *Proc. IEEE Int. Conf. Computer Aided Design*, IEEE, 1991, pp. 10–13.

17. Jerrum M, Sorkin GB, Simulated annealing for graph bisection, *Proc. 34th Annual Symp. Foundations of Computer Science*, IEEE Comput. Soc. Press, Los Alamitos, CA, 1993, pp. 94–103.

18. Jerrum M, Sorkin GB, The Metropolis algorithm for graph bisection, *Discrete Appl. Math.* **82**(1–3):155–175 (1998).

19. Karisch SE, Rendl F, Clausen J, Solving graph bisection problems with semidefinite programming, *INFORMS J. Comput.* **12**(3):177–191 (2000).

20. Kernighan BW, Lin S, An efficient heuristic procedure for partitioning graphs, *Bell Syst. Tech. J.* **49**(1):291–307 (1970).

21. Krogan N, et al, Global landscape of protein complexes in the yeast saccharomyces cerevisiae, *Nature* **440**(7084):637–643 (2006).

22. McCormick SF, ed., *Multigrid Methods*, SIAM Frontiers in Applied Mathematics, Philadelphia, 1987.

23. Monien B, Preis R, Diekmann R, Quality matching and local improvement for multilevel graph-partitioning, *Parallel Comput.* **26**(12):1609–1634 (2000).

24. Oliveira S, Seok SC, A matrix-based multilevel approach to identify functional protein models, *Int. J. Bioinformatics Res. Appl.* (in press).

25. Oliveira S, Seok SC, Multilevel approaches for large-scale proteomic networks, *Int. J. Comput. Math.* **84**(5):683–695 (2007).

26. Oliveira S, Seok SC, A multi-level approach for document clustering, *Lect. Notes Comput. Sci.* **3514**:204–211 (Jan. 2005).

27. Oliveira S, Seok SC, A multilevel approach for identifying functional modules in protein-protein interaction networks, *Proc. 2nd Int. Workshop on Bioinformatics Research and Applications* (*IWBRA*), Atlanta, GA, LNCS Series, Vol. 3992, 2006, pp. 726–773.

28. Oliveira S, Seok SC, Triangular clique based multilevel approaches to identify functional modules, *Proc. 7th Int. Meeting on High Performance Computing for Computational Science* (VECPAR), 2006.

29. Oliveira S, Stewart DE, Clustering for bioinformatics via matrix optimization, *Proc. ACM-BCB'11 Conf. Bioinformatics, Computational Biology and Biomedicine*, Chicago, Aug. 2011.

30. Peterson C, Anderson JR, Neural networks and NP-complete optimization problems; a performance study on the graph bisection problem, *Complex Syst.* **2**(1):59–89 (1988).

31. Puig O, Caspary F, Rigaut G, Rutz B, Bouveret E, Bragado-Nilsson E, Wilm M, Séraphin B, The tandem affinity purification (TAP) method: A general procedure of protein complex purification, *Methods* **24**(3):218–229 (2001).

32. Ramadan E, Osgood C, Pothen A. The architecture of a proteomic network in the yeast. *Proc. CompLife2005, Lecture Notes in Bioinformatics*, vol. 3695, pp. 265–276 2005.

33. Rao MR, Cluster analysis and mathematical programming, *J. Am. Stat. Assoc.* **66**(335):622–626 (1971).

34. Reed BA, A gentle introduction to semi-definite programming, in *Perfect Graphs*, Wiley, Chichester, UK, 2001, pp. 233–259.

35. Seok SC, *Multilevel Clustering Algorithms for Documents and Large-Scale Proteomic Networks*, PhD thesis, University of Iowa, 2007.

36. Shi J, Malik J, Normalized cuts and image segmentation, *IEEE Trans. Pattern Anal. Machine Intell.* **22**(8):888–905 (Aug. 2000).

37. Spirin V, Mirny LA, Protein complexes and functional modules in molecular networks, *Proc. Natl. Acad. Sci. USA* **100**(21):12123–12128 (Oct. 2003).

38. Stewart GW, *Building an Old-Fashioned Sparse Solver*, Technical Report CS-TR-4527/UMIACS-TR-2003-95, Univ. Maryland, Sept. 2003.

39. Vazirani V, A theory of alternating paths and blossoms for proving correctness of the $O(\sqrt{V} E)$ general graph maximum matching algorithm, *Combinatorica* **14**(1):71–109 (1994).

40. Wang J, Li M, Deng Y, Pan Y, Recent advances in clustering methods for protein interaction networks, *BMC Genomics* **11**(S3):S10 (2010).

41. Yan JT, Hsiao PY, A fuzzy clustering algorithm for graph bisection, *Inform. Process. Lett.* **52**(5):259–263 (1994).

42. Zhang C et al, Fast and accurate method for identifying high-quality protein-interaction modules by clique merging and its application to yeast, *J. Proteome Res.* **5**(4):801–807 (2006).

CHAPTER 19

IDENTIFYING PROTEIN COMPLEXES FROM PROTEIN–PROTEIN INTERACTION NETWORKS

JIANXIN WANG, MIN LI, and XIAOQING PENG

19.1 INTRODUCTION

Protein complexes are groups of proteins that interact with each other at the same time and place, forming a single multimolecular machine, such as the anaphase promoting complex, RNA splicing and polyadenylation machinery, and protein export and transport complexes. Protein complexes can be classified into obligate and nonobligate types according to whether a protein of a complex can form a stable crystal structure of its own. If it can, (without any other associated protein) *in vivo*, then a complex formed by such proteins is called a *nonobligate protein complex*. On the other hand, some proteins can't be found to create a crystal structure independently, but can be found as part of a protein complex that does create a stable crystal structure. Such a protein complex is called an *obligate protein complex* [1]. Protein complexes also can be divided into two classes: transient protein complexes and permanent complexes. Transient protein complexes form and break down transiently in *vivo*, whereas permanent complexes don't show such behavior but are typically dissociated by proteolysis [1]. Many protein complexes are well understood, particularly in the model organism *Saccharomyces cerevisiae* (a strain of yeast, e.g., baker's yeast). For this relatively simple organism, the study of protein complexes is now being performed genomewide, and the elucidation of most protein complexes of the yeast is continuing. Identification of protein complexes has significant meaning in mining and analyzing function of modules in a protein network, as it reveals protein function and explains the mechanism of a particular biological process. One

Algorithmic and Artificial Intelligence Methods for Protein Bioinformatics. First Edition.
Edited by Yi Pan, Jianxin Wang, Min Li.
© 2014 John Wiley & Sons, Inc. Published 2014 by John Wiley & Sons, Inc.

method that is commonly used for identifying the members of protein complexes is immunoprecipitation. Computation methods are also used to predict protein complexes from prior knowledge of known complexes.

19.2   DENSITY-BASED AND LOCAL SEARCH METHODS

A protein–protein interaction network (PPI network) is represented as a undirected graph $G(V,E)$, where the vertices represent proteins and edges represent interactions. A graph is unweighted if the relationship between two proteins can be the simple binary values 1 or 0, where 1 denotes that the two proteins interact and 0 denotes that they do not interact. Sometimes, a graph is weighted if the edges of graph G are weighted with a value between 0 and 1, and the weight represents the probability that this interaction is a true positive. Clustering in PPI networks consists in grouping the proteins into sets (clusters) that demonstrate greater similarity among proteins in the same cluster than in different clusters. In PPI networks, the clusters correspond to two types of module: protein complexes and functional modules; however, there is no clear distinction between them. The clusters predicted by the clustering methods discussed in this chapter are considered as protein complexes.

Assumpting that the members in the same protein complex strongly bind each other, a cluster can be referred to as a *densely connected subgraph* within a PPI network. The key idea in identifying a protein complex is to detect highly connected subgraphs (clusters) that have more interactions among themselves and fewer with the rest of the graph. A fully connected subgraph, or clique that is not a part of any other clique is an example of such a cluster. In general, clusters are not required to be fully connected; instead, the density of connections in the cluster is measured by the parameter $d = 2m/(n(n-1))$, where n is the number of proteins in the cluster and m is the number of interactions between them. Many algorithms have been developed to identify clusters of sufficiently high d in a PIN.

Spirin and Mirny [2] present three methods for identifying clusters with high d.

1. Identifying all fully connected subgraphs (cliques) by complete enumeration. To find cliques of size n, one needs to enumerate only the cliques of size $n-1$. However, the use of cliques was too constraining given the incompleteness in the PPI data.
2. Assigning a *spin* to each node in the graph. Each spin can exist in several (more than two) states. Spins belonging to connected nodes have the lowest energy when they are in the same state. The concept behind this method is that spins belonging to a highly connected cluster fluctuate in a correlated fashion. By detecting correlated spins, the algorithm can identify nodes belonging to a highly connected area of the graph.
3. Formulating the problem of finding highly connected sets of nodes as an optimization problem. We find a set of n nodes that maximizes the function

$d(m,n) = 2m/(n(n - 1))$, where m is the number of interactions between n nodes. The parameter $(0 \leq d \leq 1)$ characterizes the density of a cluster. For a fully connected set of nodes, $d = 1$, and for a set not connected to one another, $d = 0$. The optimization Monte Carlo (MC) procedure begins with a connected set of n nodes randomly selected on the graph and proceeds by causing selected nodes to move along the edges of the graph to maximize Q. Moves are accepted according to Metropolis criteria. Their experiment shows MC performed better than SPC for clusters that share common nodes and for high-density graphs, whereas SPC has an advantage in identifying clusters that have very few connections to the rest of the graph. The MC algorithm has a drawback in that the size of the predicted clusters needs to be predefined by users.

Algorithms for finding clusters, or locally dense regions, of a graph are an ongoing research topic in computer science. To find locally dense regions of a graph, MCODE [3] used a vertex weighting scheme based on the core clustering coefficient. It consists of three stages: vertex weighting, complex prediction, and optionally postprocessing. The first stage of MCODE, vertex weighting, weights all the vertices on the basis of the core clustering coefficient. Different from the clustering coefficient, the core clustering coefficient of a vertex v is defined as the density of the highest k core of the immediate neighborhood of v (vertices connected directly to v) including v. A k core is a graph of minimal degree k [graph G, for all v in G, $\deg(v) > = k$]. The second stage, molecular complex prediction, takes as input the vertex weighted graph, seeds a complex with the highest weighted vertex, and recursively moves outward from the seed vertex, including vertices in the complex whose weight is above a given threshold, which is a given percentage away from the weight of the seed vertex. In this way, the densest regions of the network are identified. The vertex weight threshold parameter defines the density of the resulting complex. A threshold that is closer to the weight of the seed vertex identifies a smaller, denser network region around the seed vertex. In the postprocessing step, MCODE filters or adds proteins according to connectivity criteria.

The aim of many density-based algorithms is to detect the densely connected subgraphs. However, ensuring density alone is not sufficient to achieve this objective. An algorithm DPClus [4] is based on the combination of density and periphery to mine dense subgraphs. Similar to MCODE, DPClus also weights all the vertices in its first step and starts at a highest weighted vertex. In DPClus, a vertex's weight is defined as the sum of the weights of the edges connected to the vertex and the weight of an edge (u,v) is the number of the common neighbors of the vertices u and v. DPClus takes the highest weighted vertex as an initial cluster and extends the cluster gradually by adding vertices from its neighbors. All neighbors are sorted according to their priorities. A neighbor's priority within a cluster is determined by the sum of the weights and the number of the edges between the neighbor and the vertices in the cluster. DPClus uses two parameters—d_{in}(a value of minimum density) and CP_{in} (a minimum value for cluster property)—to determine whether a neighbor i should be added to the cluster n. For a given cluster n with density d_n, the cluster property CP_{in} of any vertex i is defined as $CP_{in} = |E_{in}|/(k \times d_n)$, where $|E_{in}|$ is the total number of edges between the vertex i and the vertices of cluster n and k is the number of vertices in cluster n. Once a cluster is generated, DPClus removes it from the graph. Then, the weights of all the vertices in the remaining graph are recomputed and the next cluster is formed in the remaining graph. The process continues until no edge remains in the remaining graph. In such cases, DPClus can generate only nonoverlapping clusters. To generate overlapping clusters, DPClus extends the nonoverlapping clusters by adding their neighbors in the original graph (rather than in the remaining graph).

Li et al. [5] found out that most protein complexes have a very small diameter and a very small average vertex distance when investigating the structures of known protein complexes in MIPS, and proposed an algorithm abbreviated IPCA [5] to identify protein complex from PPI networks by combining vertex distance and subgraph density. IPCA consists of four stages: weighting vertex, selecting seed, extending cluster, and extending-judgment. IPCA uses diameter (or average vertex distance) and interaction probability IN_{vk} to determine whether a neighbor v should be added to a cluster k. For a cluster k, the interaction probability IN_{vk} of a vertex v to it is defined as $IN_{vk} = |E_{vk}|/n$. IPCA can generate overlapping clusters directly and does not need to consider the identified clusters' neighbors in the original graph.

Besides the typical methods discussed above, a number of other methods based on dense and local research have also been proposed to detect protein complex in PPI networks. Bu et al. [6] proposed a quasiclique algorithm to find clusters. Their key idea is that the proteins corresponding to absolutely larger components tend to form a quasiclique for each eigenvector with a positive eigenvalue. In addition to quasicliques, Bu et al. also detected the quasibipartites as clusters. Cui et al. [7] also developed an efficient algorithm for finding cliques and near-cliques in protein interaction networks and showed that a quasiclique as well as a clique often represented a biologically meaningful unit such as functional module or protein complex. Xiong et al. [8] applied an association pattern discovery method to find the *hypercliques* in the yeast protein interaction network as protein complexes.

19.3 HIERARCHICAL CLUSTERING METHODS

Hierarchical clustering is one of the most common methods of classification used in PPI networks to detect protein complexes or functional modules. Generally, the hierarchical clustering algorithms can represent the hierarchy of a complex network as a tree. According to the difference between the processes of the tree's construction, hierarchical clustering algorithms can be divided into two classes: agglomerative algorithms and divisive algorithms. *Agglomerative algorithms* start at the bottom of the tree and iteratively merge vertices, whereas *divisive algorithms* begin at the top and recursively divide a graph into two or more subgraphs. For merging vertices or separating the graph, various heuristic rules have been used, such as betweenness centrality [9–11], clustering coefficient, and minimum cut.

Many studies have shown that PPI networks are composed of communities that are densely connected within themselves but sparsely connected with the rest of the network [9–13]. As the number of edges that connect communities is small and all shortest paths between different communities must traverse one of these edges, the edges that connect communities will have higher edge betweenness than those in communities. The edge betweenness of an edge e is defined as follows [10,11]

$$BC(e) = \sum_{s,t \in V, \ s \neq t} \frac{\sigma_{st}(e)}{\sigma_{st}} \tag{19.1}$$

where $\sigma_{st}(e)$ denotes the total number of shortest paths between s and t that pass through edge e.

On the basis of the analysis above, Girvan–Newman (GN) algorithm [10] was proposed to detect community structures in complex networks by removing edges with highest betweenness from the original graphs. As the original GN algorithm does not include a clear definition of module, it does not formally determine which parts of the tree are modules. To break through the limitation, Radicchi et al. proposed two new module definitions: strong module and weak module [14]. The community C in graph G is a *strong module* if

$$k^{in}(i, C) > k^{out}(i, C), \quad \forall i \in C \tag{19.2}$$

where $k^{in}(i,C)$ is the number of edges that connect vertex i to other vertices in C and $k^{out}(i,C)$ is the number of edges that connect vertex i to other vertices in the rest of the graph G. The community C in graph G is a *weak module* if

$$\sum_{i \in C} k^{in}(i, C) > \sum_{i \in C} k^{out}(i, C) \tag{19.3}$$

By combining the GN division process with the two new module definitions, Radicchi gave a new self-contained algorithm to identify modules from a network [14]. The main difference between Radicchi's algorithm and the GN algorithm is that when a graph or subgraph is split into two subgraphs, the two subgraphs are not split in Radicchi's algorithm if they are all modules.

Luo et al. modified the definition of a weak module by extending the concept of degree from a single vertex to a subgraph and developed an agglomerative algorithm MoNet [15]. MoNet initialed each vertex as a cluster and then assembled the clusters into modules by gradually adding edges to the clusters in the reverse order of deletion using the GN algorithm.

More definitions and modifications of modules and betweenness were proposed on the basis of Girvan, Newman's and Radicchi's work. The hierarchical algorithms were also extended in weighted PPI networks. More details are given by Wang et al. [16].

An alternative formulation of betweenness-based decomposition [17], which was based on vertex betweenness instead of edge betweenness, was proposed to allow vertices to be presented in multimodules, since most of the betweenness-based clustering algorithms grouped vertices into separated clusters. This algorithm guaranteed detection of overlapping modules by dividing the graph at the vertices with the highest betweenness and copying such vertices into the divided subgraphs.

Betweenness-based clustering approaches are computationally expensive because they require the repeated evaluation for each edge in the graph, and there have been many at tempts to speed up these algorithms. To develop a fast hierarchical clustering algorithm, Radicchi et al. [14] and Li et al. [18] used the local quantity (edge clustering coefficient) instead of the global quantity (betweenness). The clustering coefficient of an edge $e(u,v)$ is [14]

$$C_{u,v}^{(3)} = \frac{Z_{u,v}^{(3)}}{\min[(k_u - 1), (k_v - 1)]} \tag{19.4}$$

where $Z_{u,v}^{(3)}$ is the number of triangles built on that edge $e(u,v)$ and min $[(k_u - 1),(k_v - 1)]$ is the minimum possible degree of u and v. The idea behind the definition is that many triangles exist in clusters and the edges between different clusters are seldom included in triangles. Thus, edges with small values of $C_{u,v}^{(3)}$ tend to lie between different clusters.

Li et al. calculated the common neighbors instead of the triangles or high-order cycles and defined the clustering oefficient of an edge $e(u,v)$ as [18,19]

$$ECV(u, v) = \frac{|N_u \cap N_v|^2}{|N_u| \times |N_v|} \tag{19.5}$$

where N_u is the set of neighbors of vertex u and N_v is the set of neighbors of vertex v, respectively. $N_u \cap N_v$ is the set of common neighbors of vertex u and vertex v. Moreover, the edge clustering coefficient can be extended to a weighted PPI network [19,20]

$$Cc_{u,v} = \frac{\sum_{k \in I_{u,v}} w(u, k) \cdot \sum_{k \in I_{u,v}} w(v, k)}{\sum_{s \in N_u} w(u, s) \cdot \sum_{t \in N_v} w(v, t)} \tag{19.6}$$

where $w(u,v)$ denotes the weight of edge $e(u,v)$ and $I_{u,v}$ denotes the set of common vertices in N_u and N_v (i.e., $I_{u,v} = N_u \cap N_v$).

Li et al. also extended the *weak module* to the λ *module* [18,19]. The community C in an unweighted graph G is a λ *module* if

$$\sum_{i \in C} k^{\text{in}}(i, C) > \lambda \sum_{i \in C} k^{\text{out}}(i, C) \tag{19.7}$$

Similarly, the community C in a weighted graph G is a λ *module* if [23,24]

$$\sum_{i \in C} k_w^{\text{in}}(i, C) > \lambda \sum_{i \in C} k_w^{\text{out}}(i, C) \tag{19.8}$$

where $k_w^{\text{in}}(i,C)$ is the sum of weights of edges connecting vertex i to other vertices in C and $k_w^{\text{out}}(i,C)$ is the sum of weights of edges connecting vertex i to other vertices in the remainder of the graph G. Using the definitions of edge clustering coefficient and λ module, Wang et al proposed a fast agglomerative algorithm HC-PIN [19] that can be used in both weighted an unweighted PPI networks.

More recently, Wang et al. [21] combined the local metric (clustering coefficient, also termed *commonality*) and the global metric (betweenness) to generate clusters for balance and consistency.

Besides the two typical metrics discussed above, a number of other metrics have also been suggested for use in hierarchical clustering algorithms. Hartuv and Shamir [22] used the minimum cut to remove edges recursively and developed a divisive algorithm for the discovery of highly connected subgraphs (HCS). Arnau et al. [23] developed a hierarchical clustering algorithm, named UVCLUSTER, based on the shortest path between any two vertices in protein interaction networks. Lu et al. [24] suggested a simple graphical measure to depict the relationship between proteins and extracted the topological information of the network, such as quasicliques and spokelike modules, into a clustering tree. Several similarity measures, such as diffusion kernel similarity, shortest-path-based similarity, and adjacency matrix–based similarity, are evaluated by Wang et al. [25]. They proposed a nonnegative matrix factorization (NMF)-based method with the usage of diffusion kernel similarity for clustering complex networks and biological networks.

The definition of similarity metric or distance measure is a crucial step in hierarchical clustering. How to evaluate the metrics is another challenge in hierarchical clustering. Two evaluation schemes suggested by Lu et al. based on the depth of hierarchical tree and width of ordered adjacency matrix, may be useful. Moreover, Chen et al. [26] presented a formal definition of similarity metric and discussed the relationship between similarity metric and distance metric; they also presented general solutions to normalizing a given similarity metric or distance metric, which have provided a theory basis for constructing metrics.

The hierarchical clustering approach can present the hierarchical organization of protein interaction networks. Its drawback is that it cannot generate overlapping clusters, except that special preprocessing or other strategies are used. In addition, the hierarchical clustering approaches are known to be sensitive to the noisy data in protein interaction networks [27].

19.4   FINDING OVERLAPPING CLUSTERS

More recently, much attention has been focused on the clustering algorithms for finding overlapping clusters. Most proteins have more than one biological function; thus each protein may be involved in multiple complexes or functional modules. In this section, we mainly discuss some representative algorithms that have been proposed for the purpose of finding overlapping clusters. Roughly, these algorithms can be classified into three groups:

1. *Algorithms Based on Cliques.* Typical algorithms include CPM [28], LCMA [29], CMC [30], and EAGLE [31]. A *clique percolation method* (CPM) [28] generates overlapping clusters by finding k-clique percolation communities. A k clique is a complete subgraph of size k. Two k cliques are considered adjacent if they share exactly $k-1$ vertices. A cluster is defined as a union of all k cliques that can be reached from each other through a series of adjacent k cliques. Although it has many attractive characters, CPM also has several limitations: (a) its results are highly correlated to the value of parameter k and (b) the proteins not included in any k cliques are neglected. To overcome the disadvantages of CPM, people often adopt some preprocessing or postprocessing when using it. Instead of finding all the maximal cliques, Li et al. [29] proposed LCMA to detect the local cliques for each protein and then merge the detected local cliques according to their affinity. The affinity between two identified clusters is determined by their intersection sets and each cluster's size. Two clusters are more similar and have larger affinity if they have larger intersection sets and similar sizes. The CMC algorithm [30] identifies protein complexes from the weighted PPI network. It first generates a weighted PPI network by an iterative scoring method. Then, it identifies protein complexes by removing or merging highly overlapped maximal cliques in this weighted PPI network on the basis of their interconnectivity. Unlike the CPM, LCMA, and CMC algorithms, EAGLE [31] is a hierarchical clustering algorithm. Its initial cluster set consists of all maximal cliques and the remaining vertices in the network. As some maximal cliques overlap each other, EAGLE can generate a dendrogram of overlapping modules by gradually merging the pair of clusters with the maximum similarity. To determine the place of the cut in the dendrogram, EAGLE extends a quality function of modularity (EQ) to judge the quality of network's cover and to output the best cover with the maximum value of EQ. Compared with the three algorithms described above, EAGLE can identify both overlapping and hierarchical functional modules.

2. *Algorithms Based on the "Seed Expand" Method.* The methods based on this concept—MCODE [3], DPClus [4], and IPCA [5]—are discussed in Section 19.2.

3. *Algorithms Based on Local Fitness.* The typical algorithm is NFC [32]. This method searches for the natural modules of each node by expanding it until it reaches the local maximal of a fitness function. During the procedure, nodes can be visited many times. Thus, overlapping modules are naturally discovered.

Besides the three types of algorithms, described above, other methods, such as core attachment [33], MCL [34,35], and fuzzy clustering [36], can also be used in PPI networks to find overlapping functional modules. Core attachment identifies the cores and attachments of functional modules in PPI networks separately. MCL (Markov cluster algorithm) has been proved to be a very successful clustering procedure. It constructs a stochastic Markovian matrix representing the transition probabilities between all pairs of vertices and simulates random walks on networks, by alternating two operations: expansion and inflation. As MCL is fast and scalable, it has been applied to find functional modules.

19.5 IDENTIFICATION OF PROTEIN COMPLEXES BY INTEGRATING MULTIPLE BIOLOGICAL SOURCES

The methods discussed above for identifying clusters are based mostly on graph-theoretic properties solely and require only protein interaction data. However, to some extent, a precise protein interaction network is more important than clustering methods, which not only contain less false-positive information but also can largely determine the accuracy of protein complex detection.

Other than the adoption of preprocessing, several researchers have suggested developing robust clustering algorithms by integrating data from multiple sources, such as genomic data, structure information, gene expression, and gene ontology (GO) annotations. The approaches differ in the way the sources are combined.

Zhang et al. [37] developed another multistep but easy-to-follow framework for the detection of protein complexes that estimated the affinity between each pair of proteins according to their copurification patterns derived from MS data. Jung et al. [38] presented a method for detecting protein complexes on the basis of integration of protein–protein interaction (PPI) data and mutually exclusive interaction information drawn from structural interface data of protein domains. By excluding interaction conflicts, Jung extracted cooperative sets of proteins such as the simultaneous protein interaction cluster (SPIC) from the protein interaction network.

Owing to the attribute that members in a cluster typically perform a specific biological function [39], several clustering algorithms have been proposed with a combination of PPI data and gene expression data. For example, Jansen et al. [40] related whole-genome expression data with PPIs and scored expression activity in complexes. Hanisch et al. [41] proposed a coclustering methodology by using a distance function based on the similarity of gene expression profiles with network topology. Ideker et al. [42] developed a clustering algorithm for the discovery of active subnetworks that showed significant changes in expression over a particular subset of the conditions. More recently, Ulitsky and Shamir [43] transformed the high-throughput expression data into similarity values, from which they found clusters, termed *jointly active connected subnetworks* (JACSs), that manifested high similarity. Ulitsky and Shamir [44] presented another novel confidence-based method for extracting functionally coherent coexpressed gene sets, named *coexpression zone analysis using networks* (CEZANNE), by using expression profiles and confidence-scored protein interactions.

With the availability of PPI data for most species (yeast, fly, worm, etc.), it has become feasible to use cross-species analysis to derive protein complex detection based on the evolution of the PPI networks. Sharan and coworkers proposed a series of methods for comparative analysis in two or more species. They used these methods for conserved pathway detection [45], protein function analysis [46], and conserved protein complex detection [47–49]. Basically, to detect the conserved protein complexes in two species, an orthology graph is constructed, whose nodes correspond to pairs of putative orthologous proteins (a protein may appear in multiple nodes with different orthologs), and whose edges correspond to protein interactions. The edges of the graph are assigned weights with probabilistic meaning, so that high-weight subgraphs correspond to conserved protein complexes. Then, a practical method is used to search the orthology graph for complexes of densely interacting proteins, which is based on forming high-weight seeds and extending them using local search.

Network alignment is also applied on conserved protein complex detection in two or more networks. Koyuturk et al. [50] proposed local alignment algorithm termed MaWISh, based on the duplication/divergence models that focus on understanding the evolution of protein interactions. The algorithm constructs a weighted global alignment graph and tries to find a maximum induced subgraph in it. The Graemlin algorithm developed by Flannick et al. [51] scored a possibly conserved module between different networks by computing the log ratio of the probability that the module is subject to evolutionary constraints and the probability that it is under no constraints, considering the phylogenetic relationships between species whose networks are being aligned. Dutkowski et al. [52] also proposed an evolution-based framework to detect conserved protein complexes across multiple species. First, all the proteins from different species are clustered by MCL with BLAST E scores as pairwise similarity. The proteins from each cluster are homologous and thus believed to have a common ancestral protein. Next, a gene tree is built for each protein group and reconciled with a common species tree. Then, the interactions between ancestral proteins are assigned weights based on the interactions observed in the input PPI networks and on the sequence of evolutionary events (duplications, speciations, and deletions) extracted from the reconciled gene trees. Finally, after removal of the edges with weights lower than an appropriate threshold in the conserved ancestral PPI network, the connected components are considered as conserved protein complexes.

With the rapidly expanding resource of microarray data and other biological information, such as structure profiles and phylogenetic profiles, combining multiple biological sources is believed to be an intriguing method for solving the problem of unreliable interaction data when clustering in protein interaction networks.

19.6   IDENTIFYING PROTEIN COMPLEXES FROM DYNAMIC PPI NETWORK

Cellular systems are highly dynamic and responsive to cues from the environment. Their response to external stimuli is regulated by networks with diverse molecular interactions, such as protein–protein interactions and protein–DNA interactions. Despite the availability of large-scale biological network data, gaining a system-level understanding of the dynamic nature of cellular activity remains a difficult and frequently overlooked task. Since there rarely is any direct information available on the temporal dynamics of these network interactions, the majority of molecular interaction network modeling and analysis has focused solely on static properties. A static PPI network obtained from yeast two-hybrid experiments can be viewed as a comprehensive graph with edges (interactions) that eventually may occur under the set of tested conditions. Thus, it is not guaranteed that all interactions can occur simultaneously, and this may lead to inaccuratey protein complex identification. To address this issue, a number of researchers have attempted to model and analyze interactions and network dynamics [53–61]. A real protein interaction network in the cell changes over time, environments and different stages of the cell cycle [54]; this fluctuation is called *dynamics*. In the methods described [53–61], static protein interaction networks provide a scaffold by integrating other dynamic information, such as gene expression data and subcellular localization. Gene expression data under different conditions or different stages in cellular cycles can reflect the dynamics of the presence of protein. Some investigators [55] found out that most proteins interact with few partners, whereas a small but significant proportion of proteins, the *hubs*, interact with many partners. They further revealed that there are two types of hub: "party" hub, where proteins interact with most of their partners simultaneously, and "date" hub, in which proteins bind their different partners at different times or locations. Focused on the dynamic formation of protein complex, De Lichtenberg et al. [56] constructed time-dependent PPIN by integrating PPIN and gene expression. By analyzing the dynamics of protein complexes during the yeast cell cycle, they discovered that most complexes consist of both periodically and constitutively expressed proteins, suggesting a mechanism of just-in-time assembly. Other methods [57] combined gene expression data with PPI networks to classify dynamic proteins that are present (expressed) periodically and static proteins that are present (expressed) all the time, and further identified dynamic modules and static modules on static PPI networks. Tang et al. [60] split the original PPI network into timecourse subnetworks, by giving a potential threshold value in the gene expression data to determine whether a protein is expressed at this timepoint. The difference among these subnetworks is assumed to depict the dynamic changes of protein expression. Wang et al. [61] also tried to distinguish the key point of dynamics of protein interaction networks. They pointed out that the dynamic changes of protein activity are more meaningful than the dynamic changes of protein presence, and therefore proposed an active protein interaction network model. The active protein interaction network is extracted from PPI and gene expression data, by adopting a 3σ principle to identify active information of each protein. It is desirable that the dynamic protein interaction network combined with more biological information depict the real network more vividly, and make the analysis result more helpful for biologists. However, at the very beginning of dynamic network modeling, this method will be fraught with many problems. The first issue is whether a graph-based model is suitable for modeling a dynamic network. A new model might be needed to represent dynamic network.

19.7   CHALLENGES AND FUTURE RESEARCH

In the postgenomic era, an important challenge is to analyze biological systems from the network level, in order to understand the topological organization of protein interaction networks, identify protein complexes and functional modules, discover functions of uncharacterized proteins, and obtain more exact networks. While some clustering approaches have been applied successfully in the discovery of protein complexes or functional modules, methods for clustering and analyzing protein interaction networks are less mature.

The main challenges for clustering protein interaction networks include: how to define the quality of a cluster and develop robust algorithm in the presence of noisy protein interaction networks; how heavily two clusters should overlap each other, and whether, it is computationally difficult for most current clustering algorithms to accurately identify protein complexes or functional modules from large-scale protein interaction networks, especially to discover mesoscale clusters. There is little a priori knowledge on clustering protein interaction networks, such as cluster number and cluster size. How to discriminate between complex and dynamic protein interaction networks is also a very difficult task.

The methods for distinguishing complex from dynamic protein interaction networks are in a nascent stage. Furthermore, techniques and methods for developing both robust and fast clustering algorithms are directions for further research. Moreover, it will be important to determine whether there is any relationship between the two properties of overlap and hierarchical organization among clusters, as these two issues were usually considered separately. Some research has been performed on complex networks, such as word association networks and scientific collaboration networks [31], to detect both the overlapping and hierarchical properties of a community structure. Do these properties also apply in protein interaction networks? Additionally, integration of multiple resources will help to detect clusters more accurately and will continue to attract interest.

REFERENCES

1. Amoutzias G, Van de Peer Y, Single-gene and whole-genome duplications and the evolution of protein-protein interaction networks, *Evolut. Genomics Syst. Biol.* 413–429 (2010).

2. Spirin V, Mirny LA, Protein complexes and functional modules in molecular networks, *Proc. Natl. Acad. Sci. USA* **100**:12123–12128 (2003).

3. Bader GD, Hogue CW, An Automated method for finding molecular complexes in large protein interaction networks, *BMC Bioinformatics*, **4**:2 (2003).

4. Altaf-Ul-Amin M, Shinbo Y, Mihara K, et al., Development and implementation of an algorithm for detection of protein complexes in large interaction networks, *BMC Bioinformatics* **7**:207 (2006).

5. Li M, Chen J, Wang JX, et al., Modifying the DPClus algorithm for identifying protein complexes based on new topological structures, *BMC Bioinformatics* **9**:398 (2008).

6. Bu D, Zhao Y, Cai L, et al., Topological structure analysis of the protein-protein interaction network in budding yeast, *Nucleic Acids Res.* **31**(9):2443–2450 (2003).

7. Cui G, Chen Y, Huang DS, Han K, An algorithm for finding functional modules and protein complexes in protein-protein interaction networks, *J. Biomed. Biotechnol.* **1**:10 (2008).

8. Xiong H, He X, Ding C, et al., Identification of functional modules in protein complexes via hyperclique pattern discovery, *Proc. Pacific Symp. Biocomputing*, 2005, vol. **10**, pp. 221–232.

9. Narayanan S, *The Betweenness Centrality of Biological Networks*, MS in Computer Science, Virginia Polytechnic Inst. and State Univ., Sept. 16, 2005.

10. Girvan M, Newman M, Community structure in social and biological networks, *Proc. Natl. Acad. Sci. USA* **99**:7821–7826 (2002).

11. Newman M, Girvan M, Finding and evaluating community structure in networks,. *Phys Rev. E* **69**(2):1–16 (2004).

12. Rives AW, Galitski T, Modular organization of cellular networks, Proc. *Natl. Acad. Sci. USA* **100**(3):1128–1133 (2003).

13. Barabasi A, Oltvai Z, Network biology: Understanding the cells's functional organization, *Nat. Rev. Genet.* **5**(2):101–113 (2004).

14. Radicchi F, Castellano C, Cecconi F, Defining and identifying communities in networks, *Proc Natl. Acad. Sci. USA* **101**(9):2658–2663 (2004).

15. Luo F, Yang Y, Chen CF, et al., Modular organization of protein interaction networks, *Bioinformatics* **23**(2):207–214 (2007).

16. Wang J, Li M, Deng Y, Pan Yi, Recent advances in clustering methods for protein interaction networks, *BMC Genomics* **11**(Suppl 3):S10 (2010) doi:10.1186/1471-2164-11-S3-S10.

17. Pinney J, Westhead D, Betweenness-based decomposition methods for social and biological networks, in Barber S, Baxter PD, Mardia KV, Walls RE, eds., *Interdisciplinary Statistics and Bioinformatics*, Leeds Univ. Press, 2006, pp. 87–90.

18. Li M, Wang JX, Chen J, et al., A fast agglomerate algorithm for mining functional modules in protein interaction networks, *Proc. 2008 Int. Conf. Biomedical Engineering and Informatics*, IEEE Press, 2008, pp. 3–7.

19. Wang J, Li M, Chen J, Pan Y, A fast hierarchical clustering algorithm for functional modules discovery in protein interaction networks, *IEEE/ACM Trans. Comput. Biol. Bioinform.* **8**(3):607–620 (2011).

20. Li M, Wang JX, Chen J, Pan Y, Hierarchical organization of functional modules in weighted protein interaction networks using clustering coefficient, *Proc. ISBRA2009*, Lecture Notes in Bioinformatics (LNBI) Series, Vol. 5542, 2009, pp. 75–86.

21. Wang C, Ding C, Yang Q, Holbrook SR, Consistent dissection of the protein interaction network by combining global and local metrics, *Genome Biol.* **8**:R271 (2007).

22. Hartuv E, Shamir R, A clustering algorithm based graph connectivity, *Inform. Process. Lett.* **76**:175–181 (2000).

23. Arnau V, Mars S, Marín I: Iterative cluster analysis of protein interaction data, *Bioinformatics* **21**:364–378 (2005).

24. Lu H, Zhu X, Liu H, Skogerbo G, Zhang J, Zhang Y, et al., The interactome as a tree: An attempt to visualize the protein-protein interaction network in yeast, *Nucleic Acids Res.* **32**(16):4804–4811 (2004).

25. Wang RS, Zhang SH, Wang Y, et al., Clustering complex networks and biological networks by nonnegative matrix factorization with various similarity measures, *Neurocomputing* **72**:134–141 (2008).

26. Chen S, Ma B, Zhang K, On the similarity metric and the distance metric, *Theor. Comput. Sci.* **410**:2365–2376 (2009).

27. Cho YR, Hwang W, Ramanmathan M, Zhang AD, Semantic integration to identify overlapping functional modules in protein interaction networks, *BMC Bioinformatics* **8**:265 (2007).

28. Palla G, Dernyi I, Farkas I, et al., Uncoverring the overlapping community structure of complex networks in nature and society, *Nature* **435**(7043):814–818 (2005).

29. Li XL, Tan SH, Foo CS, et al., Interaction graph mining for protein complexes using local clique merging, *Genome Informatics*, **16**:260–269 (2005).

30. Liu G, Wong L, Chua HN, Complex discovery from weighted PPI networks, *Bioinformatics* **25**(15):1891–1897 (2009).

31. Shen H, Cheng X, Cai K, Hu MB, Detect overlapping and hierarchical community structure in networks, *Physica A* **388**:1706–1712 (2009).

32. Lancichinetti A, Fortunato S, Kertesz J, Detecting the overlapping and hierarchical community structure in complex networks, *New J. Phys.* **11**:1–17 (2009).

33. Leung HCM, Xiang Q, Yiu SM, Chin FYL, Predicting protein complexes from PPI data: A core-attachment approach, *J. Comput. Biol.* **16**(2):133–144 (2009).

34. Dongen S, *Graph Clustering by Flow Simulation*, PhD dissertation, Centers for Mathematics and Computer. Science, Univ. Utrecht, 2000.

35. Enright AJ, Van Dongen S, Ouzounis CA, An efficient algorithm for large-scale detection of protein families, *Nucleic Acids Res.* **30**(7):1575–1584 (2002).

36. Zhang S, Wang RS, Zhang XS, Identification of overlapping community structure in complex networks using fuzzy c-means clustering, *Physica.* **374**(1):483–490 (2007).

37. Zhang B, Park BH, Karpinets T, Samatova NF, From pull-down data to protein interaction networks and complexes with biological relevance, *Bioinformatics* **24**(7):979–986 (2008).

38. Jung SH, Jang W, Hur H, Hyun B, Han D, Protein complex prediction based on mutually exclusive interactions in protein interaction network, *Genome Informatics* **21**:77–88 (2008).

39. Hartwell LH, Hopfield JJ, Leibler S, Murray AW, From molecular to modular cell biology, *Nature* **402**(6761 Suppl) C47–C52 (1999).

40. Jansen R, Greenbaum D, Gerstein M, Relating whole-genome expression data with protein-protein interactions, *Genome Res.* **12**:37–46 (2002).

41. Hanisch D, Zien A, Zimmer R, Lengauer T, Co-clustering of biological networks and gene expression data, *Bioinformatics* **18**:S145–S154 (2002).

42. Ideker T, Ozier O, Schwikowski B, Siegel AF, Discovering regulatory and signalling circuits in molecular interaction networks, *Bioinformatics* **18**:S233–S240 (2002).

43. Ulitsky I, Shamir R, Identification of functional modules using network topology and high-throughput data, *BMC Syst. Biol.* **1**:8 (2007).

44. Ulitsky I, Shamir R, Identifying functional modules using expression profiles and confidence-scored protein interactions, *Bioinformatics* **25**:1158–1164 (May 1, 2009).

45. Kelley RM, Sharan R, Karp RM, Sittler T, Root DE, Stockwell BR, Ideker T, Conserved pathways within bacteria and yeast as revealed by global protein network alignment, *Proc. Natl. Acad. Sci. USA* **100**(20):11394–11399 (2003).

46. Sharan R, Suthram S, Kelley RM, Kuhn T, McCuine S, Uetz P, Sittler T, Karp RM, Ideker T, Conserved patterns of proteininteraction in multiple species, *Proc Natl. Acad. Sci. USA* **102**(6):1974–1979 (2005).

47. Sharan R, Ideker T, Kelley BP, Shamir R, Karp RM, Identification of protein complexes by comparative analysis of yeast and bacterial protein interaction data, *Proc RECOMB Conf.*, 2004, pp. 282–289.

48. Hirsh E, Sharan R, Identification of conserved protein complexes based on a model of protein network evolution, *Bioinformatics* **23**(2):e170–e176 (2006).

49. Dost B, Shlomi T, Gupta N, Ruppin E, Bafna V, Sharan R, QNet: A tool for querying protein interaction networks, *Proc. RECOMB Conf.*, 2007, pp. 1–15.

50. Koyuturk M et al., Pairwise alignment of protein interaction networks, *J. Comput. Biol.* **13**:182–199 (2006).

51. Flannick J et al., Graemlin: General and robust alignment of multiple large interaction networks, *Genome Res.* **16**:1169–1181 (2006).

52. Dutkowski J, Tiuryn J, Identification of functional modules from conserved ancestral protein-protein interactions, *Intell. Syst. Mol. Biol.* (Suppl. *Bioinformatics*) **23**(13):149–158 (2007).

53. Bulashevska S, Bulashevska A, Eils R, Bayesian statistical modelling of human protein interaction network incorporating protein disorder information, *BMC Bioinformatics* **11**:46 (2010).

54. Teresa MP, Mona S, Donna KS, Toward the dynamic interaction: It's about time, *Brief. Bioinformatics* 15–29 (Jan. 8, 2010).

55. Han JJ, Bertin N, Hao T, Evidence for dynamically organized modularity in the yeast protein-protein interaction network, *Nature* **430**:88–93 (2004).

56. De Lichtenberg U, Jensen LJ, Brunak S, et al., Dynamic complex formation during the yeast cell cycle, *Science* **307**:724–727 (2005).

57. Komurov K, White M, Revealing static and dynamic modular architecture of the eukaryotic protein interaction network, *Mol. Syst. Biol.* **3**:110 (2007).

58. Jin R, McCallen S, Liu CC, Xiang Y, Almaas E, Zhou XJ, Identifying dynamic network modules with temporal and spatial constraints, *Proc. Pacific Symp. Biocomputing* 2009, pp. 203–214.

59. Bossi A, Lehner B, Tissue specificity and the human protein interaction network, *Mol. Syst. Biol.* **5**:260 (2009).

60. Tang X, Wang J, Liu B, Li M, Chen G, Pan Y, A comparison of the functional modules identified from time course and static PPI network data, *BMC Bioinformatics* **12**:339 (2011).

61. Wang J, Peng X, Li M, Luo Y, Pan Y, Active protein interaction network and its application in protein complex detection, *Proc. IEEE Conf. Bioinformatics and Biomedicine (BIBM)*, 2011, pp. 37–42.

CHAPTER 20

PROTEIN FUNCTIONAL MODULE ANALYSIS WITH PROTEIN–PROTEIN INTERACTION (PPI) NETWORKS

LEI SHI, XIUJUAN LEI, and AIDONG ZHANG

The inherent, dynamic, and structural behaviors of complex biological networks in a topological perspective have been widely studied. These studies have attempted to discover hidden functional knowledge on a system level since biological networks provide insights into the underlying mechanisms of biological processes and molecular functions. A functional modules can be identified from biological networks as a subnetwork whose components are highly associated with each other through links. Conventional graph-theoretic algorithms had a limitation on accuracy of functional modules detection because of complex connectivity and overlapping modules. Whereas partition-based or hierarchical clustering methods produce pairwise disjoint clusters, density-based clustering methods that search densely connected subnetworks are able to generate overlapping clusters. However, they are not applicable to identifying functional modules from a biological network that is generally sparse. A more recently proposed functional influence-based approach effectively handles the complex but sparse biological networks, generating large overlapping modules. A better understanding of higher-order organizations in biological networks reveals functional behaviors of molecular components, and can be utilized in practical biomedical applications, such as drug development and disease diagnosis [37].

20.1 INTRODUCTION

Since the sequencing of the human genome was brought to fruition [19,35], the field of genetics now stands on the threshold of significant theoretical and

Algorithmic and Artificial Intelligence Methods for Protein Bioinformatics. First Edition.
Edited by Yi Pan, Jianxin Wang, Min Li.
© 2014 John Wiley & Sons, Inc. Published 2014 by John Wiley & Sons, Inc.

practical advances. Crucial to furthering these investigations is a comprehensive understanding of the expression, function, and regulation of the proteins encoded by an organism. This understanding is the subject of the discipline of proteomics. Proteomics encompasses a wide range of approaches and applications intended to explicate how complex biological processes occur at a molecular level, how they differ in various cell types, and how they are altered in disease states.

In particular, the elucidation of protein function has been, and remains, one of the most central problems in computational biology. Proteins are macromolecules that serve as building blocks and functional components of a cell, and account for the second largest fraction of the cellular weight after water. Proteins are responsible for some of the most important functions in an organism, such as constitution of the organs (structural proteins), the catalysis of biochemical reactions necessary for metabolism (enzymes), and the maintenance of the cellular environment (transmembrane proteins). Thus, proteins are the most essential and versatile macromolecules of life, and knowledge of their functions is a crucial link in the development of new drugs and better crops, and even the development of synthetic biochemicals such as biofuels [37].

More recently, the high-throughput biotechniques have provided additional opportunities for inference of protein functions. Protein–protein interaction (PPI) data, enriched by high-throughput experiments, including yeast two-hybrid analysis [20,34], mass spectrometry [10,16], and synthetic lethality screen [10], have provided important clues of functional associations between proteins. The protein interaction network can be described as a complex system of proteins linked by interactions. Examples of complex systems include social networks, the World Wide Web, and biological systems such as metabolic networks, gene regulatory networks, and protein interaction networks. Biological networks contain the information of biochemical reactions or biophysical interactions between molecular components under certain environmental conditions. Since molecular functions are performed by a sequence of such reactions and interactions, biological networks are valuable resources for predicting functions of unknown genes or proteins and discovering functional pathways. Systematic analysis of biological networks has thus become a primary issue in bioinformatics research [37].

A *module* (also called a *functional module*) is defined as a maximal set of molecules that participate in the same function [15]. It can be identified from biological networks as a subnetwork whose components are highly associated with each other through links. More recent studies have revealed that the biological networks are typically modular in topology [3]. Identifying such functional modules in PPI networks is very important for understanding the structure and function of these fundamental cellular networks. Therefore, developing an effective computational approach to identify functional modules should be highly challenging but indispensable.

A wide range of graph-theoretic algorithms have been applied to biological networks for identifying functional modules. However, their accuracy and efficiency were limited by critical challenges such as the following:

- Biological networks are structured by complex connectivity, which results from the existence of numerous crosslinks between modules. Classical graph-theoretic algorithms are inappropriate for handling such complexity because of inefficiency.
- There is a one-to-many correspondence between molecular components and functions because a molecule may perform several different functional activities under different environmental conditions.

In this chapter, we propose an *ant colony optimization* (ACO)-based algorithm with the topology of the network for the functional module detection. In computer science and operations research, the ACO algorithm is a probabilistic technique for solving computational problems that can be reduced to finding good paths through graphs. This algorithm is a member of the ant colony algorithms family, in swarm intelligence methods, and it constitutes some metaheuristic optimizations. Initially proposed by Marco Dorigo in 1992 in his PhD thesis [8], the first algorithm attempted to search for an optimal path in a graph, based on the behavior of ants seeking a path between their colony and a source of food. The original idea has since diversified to solve a wider class of numerical problems, and as a result, several problems have emerged, drawing on various aspects of the behavior of ants. Here we use ACO-based algorithm to solve the function module detection problem in PPI networks.

The remainder of this chapter is organized as follows:

1. We will introduce the properties of protein protein interaction networks.
2. The previous graph clustering methods that can be applied to functional module identification from biological networks will be introduced.
3. We will introduce a method to build a weighted PPI network.
4. An ACO-based clustering algorithm will be explained in detail.
5. We conclude the chapter by presenting experimental results that illustrate the effectiveness of the proposed method.

20.2   PROPERTIES OF PPI NETWORKS

The term *protein–protein interaction* (PPI) *network* refers to the sum of PPIs occurring among a set of related proteins. Such networks are typically represented by graphs, in which a set of nodes represents proteins and a set of edges, representing interactions, connects the nodes. Many much of the more recent research has involved both empirical and theoretical studies of these PPI networks. Graph theories have been successfully applied to the analysis of PPI networks, and many graph and component measurements specific to this field have been introduced. This section explores the basic terms and measurements used to characterize the graphical representation of PPI networks properties.

20.2.1 Representation of PPI Networks

The computational investigation of PPI network mechanisms begins with a representation of the network structure. As mentioned above, the simplest representation takes the form of a mathematical graph consisting of nodes and edges [36].
Proteins are represented as nodes in such a graph; two proteins that interact
physically are represented as adjacent nodes connected by an edge. We will first
discuss a number of fundamental properties of these graphic representations prior
to an exploration of the algorithms.

20.2.1.1 Graph   Proteins interact with each other to perform a specific cellular function or process. These interacting patterns form a PPI network that is
represented by a graph $G = (V, E)$ with a set of nodes V and a set of edges E,
where $E \subseteq V \times V$:

$$V \times V = \{(v_i, v_j)|v_i \in V, \quad v_j \in V, \quad i \neq j\} \tag{20.1}$$

An edge $(v_i, v_j) \in E$ connects two nodes v_i and v_j. The vertex set and edge
set of a graph are denoted by $V(G)$ and $E(G)$, respectively. Graphs can be
directed or undirected. In directed graphs, each directed edge has a source and a
destination vertex. In undirected graphs, the order of the incident vertices of an
edge is immaterial, since the edges have no direction. Graphs can be weighted
or unweighted; in the latter, each edge can have an associated real-value weight.

20.2.2 Basic Concepts

20.2.2.1 Degree   In an undirected graph, the degree (or connectivity) of a
node is the number of other nodes with which it is connected [3]. This is the
most elementary characteristic of a node. For example, in the undirected network
shown in Figure 20.1, node A has degree $k = 5$. Let $N(v_i)$ denote the neighbors

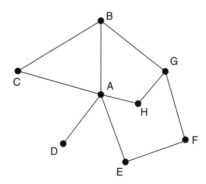

Figure 20.1   A graph in which node A has a degree of 5. (*Source:* Adapted by permission
from Macmillan Publishers Ltd: *Nature* [3], copyright 2004).

of node v_i, that is, the set of nodes connected to v_i. The degree $d(v_i)$ of v_i is then equivalent to the number of neighbors of v_i, or $|N(v_i)|$.

In directed graphs, the outdegree of $v_i \in V$, denoted by $d^+(v_i)$, is the number of edges in E that have origin v_i. The indegree of $v_i \in V$, denoted by $d^-(v_i)$, is the number of edges with destination v_i. For weighted graphs, all these concepts can be represented as the summation of corresponding edge weights.

20.2.2.2 *Distance Path, Shortest Path, and Mean Path*   Many relationships within a graph can be envisioned by means of conceptual walks and paths. A *walk* is defined as a sequence of nodes in which each node is linked to its succeeding node. A *path* is a walk in which each node in the walk is distinct. In the path that starts from v_i, passes through v_k, and ends with v_j, $\langle v_i, v_k, v_j \rangle$, v_i and v_j are termed the *source node* and *target node*, respectively. The set of paths with source node v_i and target node v_j is denoted by $P(v_i, v_j)$. The length of a path is the number of edges in the sequence of the path. A shortest path between two nodes is the minimum-length path connecting the nodes. $SP(v_i, v_j)$ denotes the set of the distinct shortest paths between v_i and v_j. The distance between two nodes v_i and v_j is the length of the shortest path between them and is denoted by $\mathrm{dist}(v_i, v_j)$.

A graph $G' = (V', E')$ is a subgraph of the graph $G = (V, E)$ if $V' \subseteq V$ and $E' \subseteq E$. A *vertex-induced subgraph* is a vertex subset V' of a graph G together with any edges in edge subset E' whose endpoints are both in V'. The induced subgraph of $G = (V, E)$ with vertex subset $V' \subseteq V$ is denoted by $G[V']$. The *edge-induced subgraph* with edge subset $E' \subseteq E$, denoted by $G[E']$, is the subgraph $G' = (V', E')$ of G, where V' is the subset of V that are incident vertices of at least one edge in E'.

20.2.2.3 *Degree Distribution*   Graph structures can be described according to numerous characteristics, including the distribution of pathlengths, the number of cyclic paths, and various measures to compute clusters of highly connected nodes [36]. Barabasi and Oltvai [3] introduced the concept of degree distribution $P(k)$ to quantify the probability that a selected node will have exactly k links. $P(k)$ is obtained by tallying the total number of nodes $N(k)$ with k links and dividing this figure by the total number of nodes N. Different network classes can be distinguished by the degree distribution. For example, a random network follows a Poisson distribution. By contrast, a scale-free network has a power-law degree distribution, indicating that a few hubs bind numerous small nodes. Most biological networks are scale-free, with degree distributions approximating a power law, $P(k) \sim k^{-\gamma}$. When $2 \leq \gamma \leq 3$, the hubs play a significant role in the network [3].

20.3   PREVIOUS MODULE DETECTION APPROACHES

Previous graph clustering methods can be categorized into three groups: partition-based clustering, hierarchical clustering, and density-based clustering.

The *partition-based clustering* approaches explore the best partition which divides the graph into several subgraphs. The *hierarchical clustering* approaches iteratively merge two subgraphs that are the most similar (or closest), or recursively divide the graph or subgraph by disconnecting the weakest links. The *density-based* approaches search the densely connected subgraphs. They are able to detect overlapping clusters consistent with real functional modules, but exclude sparsely connected vertices, which are typically abundant in a biological network, from the clusters identified. The previous methods in these three categories will be summarized in the following text.

20.3.1 Partition-Based Clustering

King et al. [22] proposed a cost-based local search algorithm modeled called *restricted neighborhood search clustering* (RNSC) on the metaheuristic search. The process begins with a list of random or user-specific clusters, and calculates the cost of initial clusters by the cost function defined below. It then iteratively moves each node on the border of a cluster to an adjacent cluster in a random manner to find a lower cost. It finally detects the partition with the minimum cost.

The cost function is determined by the number of invalid connections. An invalid connection incident with a vertex v is a connection that exists between v and a vertex in a different cluster, or, alternatively, a connection that does not exist between v and a vertex in the same cluster as v. Let α_v be the number of invalid connections incident with v. The naive cost function of a cluster C in a graph G is then defined as follows:

$$C_n(G,C) = \frac{1}{2} \sum_{v \in V} \alpha_v \tag{20.2}$$

For a vertex v in G, let β_v be the size of the following set: v itself, any vertex connected to v, and any vertex in the same cluster as v. The scaled cost function of C is then defined as follows:

$$C_n(G,C) = \frac{|V|-1}{3} \sum_{v \in V} \frac{\alpha_v}{\beta_v} \tag{20.3}$$

This measure reflects the size of the area that v influences in the cluster. Both cost functions seek to define a clustering scenario in which the vertices in a cluster are all connected to one another and there are no other connections between two clusters. Since the RNSC is randomized, different runs on the same input data will generate different clustering results. As another weakness, this method requires the prior knowledge of the exact number of clusters existing in a network.

This method has been applied to finding protein complexes from protein interaction networks [22]. However, they needed to filter the output modules to find true protein complexes according to cluster size, cluster density, and functional homogeneity. Only the clusters that satisfy these three criteria have been considered as predicted functional modules.

20.3.2   Hierarchical Clustering

The bottom–up hierarchical clustering approaches start from single-vertex clusters and iteratively merge the closest vertices or clusters into a supercluster. For the iterative merging, the similarity or distance between two vertices or two clusters should be measured, for example, the similarity using the reciprocal of the shortest path distance between two vertices [30] and the similarity from the statistical significance of common interacting partners [12,31]. Other advanced distance metrics such as Czekanovski–Dice distance [4] have also been used for this task. The Czekanovski–Dice distance D between two vertices i and j is described as

$$D(i,j) = \frac{|\text{Int}(i)\Delta\text{Int}(j)|}{|\text{Int}(i) \cup \text{Int}(j)| + |\text{Int}(i) \cap \text{Int}(j)|} \tag{20.4}$$

where $\text{Int}(i)$ denotes the set of neighbor vertices directly connected to i including the vertex i itself, and Δ represents the operator for symmetric difference between two sets.

Two subgraphs to be merged can be selected by an optimization process. The similarity or distance can be measured in two steps to improve the accuracy. The UVCLUSTER algorithm [1] first uses the shortest-path distances as primary distances to apply the agglomerative hierarchical clustering. Next, on the basis of the clustering results, it calculates the secondary distances. As a greedy optimization algorithm, two subgraphs to be merged can be found on each iteration by searching the best modularity. In this work, the modularity Q of a graph is defined as

$$Q = \sum_i (e_{ii} - (\textstyle\sum_j e_{ij})^2 \tag{20.5}$$

where e_{ii} is the number of intraconnecting edges within a cluster i and e_{ij} is the number of interconnecting edges between two clusters i and j. The superparamagnetic clustering (SPC) method [33] is another example of iterative merging. The most similar pair of vertices can be selected from the identical ferromagnetic spins.

These approaches are appealing for real biological applications because biological functions are also described by hierarchical ordering in general. Despite the advantage of building the potential hierarchy of molecular components, these approaches may not have a meaningful guidance of the halting point of the merging process to yield true functional modules.

The top–down hierarchical clustering approaches have the opposite procedure, starting from one cluster including all vertices in a graph and recursively dividing it. The recursive minimum-cut algorithm [14] is a typical example in this category. However, it is computationally expensive to find the minimum number of cuts in a complex system. Thus, the vertices or edges to be removed for the graph division can be selected in alternative ways. For example, they can be iteratively found using the betweenness measure [27], which gives a high score to the edge located between potential modules. The betweenness C_B of an edge e is calculated by the fraction of shortest paths passing through the edge, as

$$C_B(e) = \sum_{s \neq t \in V, e \in E} \frac{|\rho_{st}(e)|}{|\rho_{st}|} \qquad (20.6)$$

where $\rho_{st}(e)$ is the set of the shortest paths between two vertices s and t, which are passing through the edge e, and ρ_{st} is the set of all shortest paths between s and t. Iterative elimination of the edges with the highest betweenness divides a graph into two or more subgraphs, and the iteration proceeds recursively into each subgraph to detect final clusters [11]. While the betweenness assesses the global connectivity pattern for each vertex or edge, the local connectivity can be considered to select the interconnecting edges to be cut. For instance, the edge is selected by the lowest rate of common neighbors between two ending vertices.

These approaches can reveal the global view of the hierarchical structure. Previously, the betweenness-based hierarchical method was popularly used in biological network analysis [9,17]. However, finding the correct dividing points is the most crucial and time-consuming process for the application to large, complex biological networks. In addition, as a critical shortcoming, these top–down hierarchical clustering approaches are sensitive to noisy data, which frequently occurr in real biological networks.

20.3.3 Density-Based Clustering

Molecular complex detection (MCODE) [2] is an effective approach for detecting densely connected regions in large biological networks. This method weights a vertex by local neighborhood density, chooses a few seeds with a high weight, and isolates the dense regions according to given parameters. The MCODE algorithm operates in three steps: vertex weighting, protein complex (cluster) generation, and an optional postprocessing step to filter or add vertices to the resulting clusters according to certain connectivity criteria.

In the first step, all vertices are weighted on the basis of their local density using the highest k core of the vertex neighborhood. The k core of a graph is defined as the maximum subgraph if every vertex has at least k links. It is obtained by pruning all the vertices with a degree less than k. Thus, if a vertex v has degree d_v and it has n neighbors with degree less than k, then the degree of v becomes $d_v - n$. It will also be pruned if $k > (d_v - n)$. The core clustering coefficient of a vertex v is defined as the density of the highest k core of the vertices connected directly to v, together with v itself. Compared with the traditional clustering coefficient, the core clustering coefficient amplifies the weighting of heavily interconnected graph regions while removing the many less connected vertices. For each vertex v, the weight of v is

$$w = k \times d \qquad (20.7)$$

where d is the density of the highest k-core graph from the set of vertices including all the vertices directly connected with v and the vertex v itself.

The second step of the algorithm is the cluster generation. With a vertex-weighted graph as an input, a subgraph with the highest-weighted vertex is selected as the seed. Once a vertex is included, its neighbors are recursively inspected to determine whether they are a part of the cluster. The seed is then expanded to a cluster until it reaches a density threshold of the cluster. If a vertex is checked more than once, overlapping clusters can be yielded. This process stops when no additional vertices can be added to the cluster. The vertices included in the cluster are marked as having been examined. This process is repeated for the next-highest unexamined weighted vertex in the graph. In this manner, the densest regions of the graph are identified.

This method has been specifically devised to detect protein complexes in protein interaction networks [2]. In the experiment with the yeast protein interaction network, MCODE effectively located the densely connected regions as protein complexes based solely on the connectivity data.

20.4 WEIGHTED GRAPH MODEL OF PROTEIN INTERACTION NETWORKS

Many methods are based on the assumption that interacting proteins should share common functions. Table 20.1 shows the percentage of *function-relevant* interactions in three protein–protein interaction datasets: DIP, MIPS, and BioGrid (see Section 20.6 for detailed description). An interaction is considered to be *function-relevant* if the two proteins involved in the interaction have at least one function in common. In this test, we adopt FunCat (version 20070316) [26] in the MIPS database as our annotation categories. From Table 20.1, we can see that only 30–40% of the observed interactions are relevant in functions. In other words, few observed interactions share functions. Among those sharing function pairs, some share more functions than the others. Table 20.2 shows the percentage of *function-consistent* protein pairs observed to interact in the three datasets. Formally, we define two proteins P_1 and P_2 as being *function-consistent* if $|[F(P_1) \cap F(P_2)]/[F(P_1) \cup F(P_2)]| \geq \frac{1}{2}$, where $F(P_1)$ and $F(P_2)$ are functions of P_2 and P_2, respectively. As shown, only a small percentage

TABLE 20.1 Percentage of Function-Relevant Interactions in Three Protein Interaction Datasets

Dataset	Total Number of Interactions	Number of Function-Relevant Interactions	Percentage (%)
DIP	14,162	5,216	36.83
MIPS	13,877	4,189	30.18
BioGrids	117,675	36,446	30.97

TABLE 20.2   Percentage of Function-Consistent Protein Pairs that Interact in Protein Interaction Datasets

Dataset	Total Number of Interactions	Number of Function-Consistent Interactions	Percentage (%)
DIP	20,099	1283	6.38
MIPS	21,795	898	4.12
BioGrids	21,499	2718	12.64

of *function-consistent* protein pairs are observed to interact in the interaction datasets. These observations suggest two possibilities: (1) the protein interaction data may have many false interactions that need to be removed from protein interaction data or (2) a weighted graph needs to be built to show the reliability between two proteins and to show the *functional similarity* between two proteins. Since proteins with similar functions are likely to interact with each other in cells, we assume that the more reliable two proteins are, the more chance that they share common proteins.

We define a *weighted protein interaction network* [29] as follows. A weighted protein interaction network is a weighted undirected graph $G = (P, I, W)$, where P is a set of vertices, I is a set of edges between the vertices [$I \subseteq (u, v)|u, v \in P$], and W is a function making each edge in I to a real value in the range of $[0 \cdots 1]$. Each vertex $v \in P$ in the graph represents a protein. Each edge $(u, v) \in I$ represents an interaction between proteins u and v. For each edge (u, v), $w(u, v)$ is the weight of (u, v) that represents the probability of this interaction being a true positive. Figure 20.2 shows our weighted protein interaction network model.

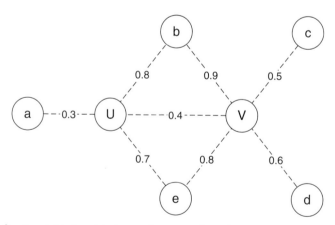

Figure 20.2   A weighted protein interaction network model. Nodes U and V are proteins. Node a, b, c, d, e are neighbors of U and V. The number on the edge between two nodes is the weight of the edge.

The nodes represent the proteins, the edges between nodes represent the interactions between proteins, and the numbers on the edges represent the weights between interacted proteins.

In this chapter, we use the following additional terminologies. A *neighbor* of a vertex v is a vertex adjacent to v, also called *direct neighbor*. *Level k neighbor* of vertex v is a vertex having k edges or steps to reach vertex v. The degree of a vertex v, denoted as $D(v)$, is the sum of weights of the edges connecting v: $D(v) = \sum_{(u,v)\in I} w(u,v)$. A *walk* is an alternating sequence of vertices and edges, where each edge is incident to the vertices immediately preceding and succeeding it in the sequence. A *path* is a walk with no repeated vertices.

Generally, there are two approaches to give a probability estimate for each interactions. We can use either the probability estimates of single interactions or the reliability estimates of interaction datasets. Here we choose the first one and use mainly the topological features of PPI networks to assign the weights. The method we used is called PathRatio, described in our previous paper [32].

The value of PathRatio reflects the reliability between two proteins in the network. In a protein interaction network, the closer two proteins, the more chances they should share common functions. Table 20.3 shows clearly that there are quite strong functional influence between level 1 and level 2 neighbors, still some influence for level 3 neighbors, but weaker influence for neighbors higher than 3 in the yeast protein interactions. So in this chapter, when we calculate the PathRatio between two vertices, we only calculate it up to the third level. The higher the value of PathRatio, the more reliable these two proteins are, that is, the higher the probability that these two proteins share common proteins. In this way, we changed this weighted graph to a *functional similarity* interaction network.

This new interaction network is different from the previous proposed methods in the following ways:

- The neighbors of one annotated protein include both direct neighbors and indirect neighbors up to level 3.
- These functional similarity–based weighted networks have the weight for each pair of neighbors, which suggests that they might have similar functions.

TABLE 20.3 Fraction of Annotated Yeast Proteins that Share Functions with Level 1, 2, 3, or 4 Neighbors Exclusively

Shared Functions with	Number of Corresponding Neighbors	Number of Sharing Common Functions	Proteins Fraction
Level 1 neighbors	4,812	1,136	23.61
Level 2 neighbors	203,574	40,275	19.78
Level 3 neighbors	1,381,525	185,182	13.45
Level 4 neighbors	913,742	49,068	5.17

20.5 THEORIES AND METHODS

20.5.1 Traveling Salesperson Problem and Its Transformation

The *traveling salesperson problem* (TSP) is a classic problem in the field of graph theory and combinatorial optimization. The TSP can be described as follows: Given n cities where the distances between any two cities are known, a traveling salesperson wants to visit all n cities in a tour so that each city is visited exactly once and the total distance of traveling is minimal [23]. The TSP is NP-hard, and no polynomial algorithm has been found, but the optimal solutions can be approximated using methods like linear programming or heuristic searching [24]. Johnson and Zhang [21] pointed out that the rearrangement clustering problem is equivalent to TSP and can be solved optimally by solving the TSP. Thus, they transferred clustering a PPI network to rearrangement clustering problem and use a TSP solver to cluster the PPI network. However, this clustering method has some pitfalls, which have been illustrated by Climer and Zhang [7] and are discussed will in Section 20.6. In this section, we solve the TSP problem by ACO algorithm and clustering the PPI network on it.

20.5.2 Ant Colony Optimization (ACO) Algorithm for Traveling Salesperson Problem

The ACO algorithm is a probabilistic technique for solving computational problems that can be reduced to finding good paths through graphs. In ACO, a set of software agents called *artificial ants* search for good solutions to a given optimization problem. To apply ACO, the optimization problem is transformed into the problem of finding the best path on a weighted graph. The artificial ants (hereafter *ants*) incrementally build solutions by moving on the graph. The solution construction process is stochastic and is biased by a pheromone model, that is, a set of parameters associated with graph components (either nodes or edges) whose values are modified at runtime by the ants.

To apply ACO to the TSP, we consider the graph defined by associating the set of cities with the set of vertices of the graph. This graph is called a *construction graph*. Since it is possible to move from any given city to any other city in the TSP, the construction graph is fully connected and the number of vertices is equal to the number of cities. We set the lengths of the edges between the vertices to be proportional to the distances between the cities represented by these vertices, and we associate pheromone values and heuristic values with the edges of the graph. Pheromone values are modified at runtime and represent the cumulated experience of the ant colony, while heuristic values are problem-dependent values that, in the case of the TSP, are set to be the inverse of the lengths of the edges [25].

The ants construct the solutions as follows. Each ant starts from a randomly selected city (vertex of the construction graph). Then, at each construction step it moves along the edges of the graph. Each ant memorizes its path, and in subsequent steps it chooses among the edges that do not lead to vertices that it has already visited. An ant has constructed a solution once it has visited all the vertices of the graph. At each construction step, an ant probabilistically chooses the edge to follow among those that lead to yet unvisited vertices. The probabilistic rule is biased by pheromone values and heuristic information, the higher the pheromone and the heuristic value associated with an edge, the higher the probability that an ant will choose that particular edge. Once all the ants have completed their tour, the pheromone on the edges is updated. Each pheromone value is initially decreased by a certain percentage. Each edge then receives an amount of additional pheromone proportional to the quality of the solutions to which it belongs (there is one solution per ant) [25].

This procedure is repeatedly applied until a termination criterion is satisfied.

20.5.3   ACO-Based Algorithm Applied in PPI Networks

In this section, we describe the ACO-based algorithm for clustering proteins in PPI networks.

Similar to TSP, in the PPI network we are trying to find the shortest path to cover all the nodes in the network. So, when the ants travel from initial node and back, the ones moving in the shorter path returns earlier and the quantity of pheromone that is deposited in this path is apparently more than in the longer path. Other ants definitely will follow, moving in the shorter path, and will deposit their own pheromone. With increasing number of ants moving and depositing their pheromone in this path, the optimal path from initial node to the last node is established. The solution construction will terminate when all nodes are visited. By finding the optimal path in PPI network, we not only find the shortest path reaching all the nodes in PPI network but also find which nodes and edges are the most visited ones along the paths.

How the ants select the path are described as follows. Each ant selects the next node independently. The probability of an ant k moving from node i to node j is calculated by using the formula

$$p_{ij}^k(t) = \frac{[\tau_{ij}(t)]^\alpha \cdot [\eta_{ij}]^\beta}{\sum_{l \in N_i^k} [\tau_{il}(t)]^\alpha \cdot [\eta_{il}]^\beta} \tag{20.8}$$

where $\eta_{ij} = 1/d_{ij}$ is a heuristic value that is available a priori and α and β are two parameters that determine the relative influence of the pheromone trail and the heuristic information.

The pheromone trails of the ants must be updated to reflect the ant's performance and the quality of solutions found. This is very important for improving the future solutions. The pheromone trails are updated after all ants have constructed their tours. The updating consists of two processes: evaporation and depositing the pheromone.

The pheromone evaporation and deposit proceed according to the following equation

$$\tau_{ij}(t+1) = (1 - \rho) \cdot \tau_{ij}(t) + \sum_{k=1}^{m} \Delta \tau_{ij}^{k}(t) \tag{20.9}$$

where ρ is a parameter that controls the evaporation and $\Delta \tau_{ij}$ is the pheromone added to the trail.

This updating encourages the use of the shortest path and increases the probability that future paths will use the trail contained in the best solutions. This process is repeated for a predetermined number of iterations. All the iterations will produce the best solutions for this algorithm, and it definitely will contribute the optimal solutions (optimal path) for the clustering PPI network problem.

20.5.4 ACO-Based Functional Module Detection Method

We believe [18], that the bridging edges are capable of identifying edges that are located and connect subregions of the network. From the last step, we have already obtained the optimal path by applying an ACO-based algorithm. On the optimal path, those bridging edges are the ones that have smaller PathRatio or reliability, and they are also those that connect different functional modules in PPI networks. Thus, by removing those higher-ranking edges, we could generate the functional modules that are hidden in the complex PPI networks. An ACO-based functional module detection (ACO-FMD) method is introduced in Algorithm 20.1.

```
Input: the graph G(V,E)
Output: ModulesList, the list of final modules
 G': A clone of graph G
 topEdge: the edge with the highest rank
 densityThreshold: subgraph density threshold
 while G != empty do
   Calculate the ranking edges for all edges in graph G with
        ACO described above
   topEdge = The edge with the highest rank
   Remove topEdge
   if there is a new isolated module s then
     if Density(s,G') > densityThreshold then
     ModulesList.add(s)
     G.remove(s)
     end if
   end if
 end while
 Return ModulesList
```

Algorithm 20.1   ACO-FMD(G). A functional module detection algorithm based on ant colony optimization.

The iterative graph partitioning algorithm involves three sequential processes:

Process 1—compute the rank of all edges in graph G and select edge e with the highest rank.

Process 2—remove edge e.

Process 3—if some subgraph s is isolated from G and the density of s in the intact graph G' is greater than threshold, s will be as one of the final clusters and be removed from G.

20.6 EXPERIMENTAL RESULTS

20.6.1 Data Preparation

For our experiments, we used core protein interaction data of *Saccharomyces cerevisiae* from DIP [13]. It contains 2526 distinct proteins and 5949 interactions.

To evaluate the effectiveness of our method, we used FunCat as the functional annotations from MIPS database [26]. The scheme of FunCat is a tree-shaped hierarchical structure. To avoid overspecific annotations, we cut the scheme at the third level and obtained 259 functional categories.

20.6.2 Functional Module Detection

To test the performance of identifying specific functional modules, we compared the functional modules that we achieved to the MIPS functional categories. We extracted the proteins appearing in the level 4 functional categories, which are related to *cell cycle and DNA processing*. We thus used 452 distinct proteins

TABLE 20.4   Comparative Analysis[a]

Method	Number of Modules	Average Size of Modules	Node Discard Rate	Average p Score
ACO-FMD	129	30.17	36.7	16.80
Infor-Flow	115	34.70	34.8	18.27
Maximal Cliq	120	5.65	98.4	10.61
Quasi-Clique	103	11.17	80.8	11.5
Mincut	114	13.46	35	7.23
Neighbor-Merg	64	7.91	79.9	9.16
Interconnetion-Cut	180	10.26	21.0	8.19

[a]Performance of BridgeRemove method on the DIP PPI dataset is compared with six graph clustering approaches (Maximal Cliq, Quasi-Clique, Rives, Mincut, Markov clustering, Samanta). Column 2 shows the number of clusters detected. Column 3 shows the average size of each cluster. Column 4 represents the average F measure of the clusters for MIPS complex modules. The average F-measure value of detected modules was calculated by mapping each module to the MIPS complex module with the highest F-measure value. Column 5 indicates the Davies–Bouldin cluster quality index. Comparisons are performed on the clusters with four or more components.

TABLE 20.5   Additional Comparative Analysis[a]

Method	Number of Modules	Average Size of Modules	Node Discard Rate	Average p Score
Max-Min Ant	141	32.59	35.1	17.91
ACO-FMD	129	30.17	36.7	16.80
Elitist Ant System	113	25.9	53.8	13.62

[a]Performance of several different ACO-based algorithms are compared on the DIP PPI dataset. Column 2 lists the number of modules detected. Column 3 shows the average size of each module. Column 4 represents the discard rate of the nodes in the process of clustering. Column 5 indicates the average p score.

annotated on 18 different functional categories. Since a protein can perform multiple functions, the modules should overlap; in other words, several nodes may belong to several different modules simultaneously. In addition, we also use a p value from hypergeometric distribution to evaluate our output modules [6]. Low p indicates that the module closely corresponds to the function because the network has a lower probability to produce the module by chance.

We compared our approach to several previous state-of-the-art methods, including the Maximal-Cliq and Quasi-Clique methods [28] in density-based approaches, the Mincut, Neighbor-Merg, and Interconnection-Cut method [9] in hierarchical approaches, and the information flow method from our previous paper [6]. After dropping small modules whose size is <5, we computed the average (p value) [5]. The overall results are shown in Table 20.4. Although the clique-based method was able to find the overlapping clusters and the information flow (Infor-Flow) method uses the weighted network as an input, they generated numerous small clusters with a very few disproportionally large clusters, which caused low accuracy. The edge-betweenness cut method yielded a large number of clusters because all isolated subnetworks are considered as clusters. The number of disjoint clusters rendered this method inaccurate. It explicitly demonstrates that our ACO-FMD algorithm showed better performance than the other competing methods. It also shows that our ACO-FMD approach properly handled the complex connections by dynamic flow simulation. Moreover, the problem of false positive data, which frequently appear in biological networks, could also be resolved by this simulation.

To demonstrate flexibility of our proposed platform and to illustrate the different performance of several ACO algorithms, we compared several representative ACO algorithms applied in the DIP PPI network. In Table 20.5, we could see that the MaxMin Ant algorithm achieved the best performance by giving the hightest number of modules with relatively high average size and small discard rate.

20.7 CONCLUSION

The ACO algorithm has been applied to several combinatorial optimizations successfully [8]. In this chapter, we analyze and detect functional modules from protein–protein interaction networks with the ACO algorithm. By analyzing the topology of the PPI network, we build a more reliable weighted network. On that, instead of using traditional density-based or hierarchical clustering methods, we have shown that the combination of ACO with the TSP approach could be used to detect functional modules in PPI networks with a little transformation. We have successfully obtained the optimal path for the PPI network and the bridging nodes. In addition, we proposed an ACO-FMD method to cluster those functional modules. Through experimental comparison, we have shown that our proposed method is superior to the previous clustering methods in terms of p score and average modules size. Since ACO is still a relatively new algorithm, we can improve it in many ways. In the future, with the development of ACO algorithms and improvement of the reliability of PPI networks, we believe that the method we proposed could achieve even better results.

REFERENCES

1. Arnau V, Mars S, Marin I, Iterative cluster analysis of protein interaction data, *Bioinformatics* **21**(3):364–378 (2005).
2. Bader GD, Hogue CW, An automated method for finding molecular complexes in large protein interaction networks, *BMC Bioinformatics* **4**(2):(2003).
3. Barabasi A-L, Oltvai ZN, Network biology: Understanding the cell's functional organization, *Nat. Rev. Genet.* **5**:101–113 (2004).
4. Brun C, Herrmann C, Guenoche A, Clustering proteins from interaction networks for the prediction of cellular functions, *BMC Bioinformatics* **5**(95):(2004).
5. Cho Y-R, Hwang W, Ramanathan M, Zhang A, Semantic integration to identify overlapping functional modules in protein interaction networks, *BMC Bioinformatics* **8**(265):(2007).
6. Cho Y-R, Shi L, Zhang A, Functional module detection by functional flow pattern mining in protein interaction networks, *BMC Bioinformatics* **9**(Suppl. 10):O1 (2008).
7. Climer S, Zhang W, Rearrangement clustering: Pitfalls, remedies and applications, *J. Machine Learn. Res.* **7**:909–943 (2006).
8. Dorigo M, Maniezzo V, Colorni A, The ant system: Optimization by a colony of cooperating agents, *IEEE Trans. Syst. Man Cybernet. B* **26**(1):(1996).
9. Dunn R, Dudbridge F, Sanderson CM, The use of edge-betweenness clustering to investigate biological function in protein interaction networks, *BMC Bioinformatics* **6**(39): (2005).
10. Gavin A-C, et al, Functional organization of the yeast proteome by systematic analysis of protein complexes, *Nature* **415**:141–147 (2002).

11. Girvan M, Newman MEJ, Community structure in social and biological networks, *Proc. Natl. Acad. Sci. USA* **99**(12):7821–7826 (2002).

12. Goldberg DS, Roth FP, Assessing experimentally derived interactions in a small world, *Proc. Natl. Acad. Sci. USA* **100**(8):4372–4376 (2003).

13. Guimera R, Amaral LAN, Functional cartography of complex metabolic networks, *Nature* **433**:895–900 (2005).

14. Hartuv E, Shamir R, A clustering algorithm based on graph connectivity, *Inform. Process. Lett.* **76**:175–181 (2000).

15. Hartwell LH, Hopfield JJ, Leibler S, Murray AW, From molecular to modular cell biology, *Nature* **402**:c47–c52 (1999).

16. Ho Y et al, Systematic identification of protein complexes in *Saccharomyces cerevisiae* by mass spectrometry, *Nature* **415**:180–183 (2002).

17. Holme P, Huss M, Jeong H, Subnetwork hierarchies of biochemical pathways, *Bioinformatics* **19**:532–538 (2003).

18. Hwang W, Cho YR, Zhang A, Ramanathan M, Cascade: A novel quasi all paths-based network analysis algorithm for clustering biological interactions, *BMC Bioinformatics* **9**:64 (2008).

19. International Human Genome Sequencing Consortium, Initial sequencing and analysis of the human genome, *Nature* **409**:860–921 (2001).

20. Ito T, Chiba T, Ozawa R, Yoshida M, Hattori M, Sakaki Y, A comprehensive two-hybrid analysis to explore the yeast protein interactome, *Proc. Natl. Acad. Sci. USA* **98**(8):4569–4574 (2001).

21. Johnson O, Zhang W, A traveling salesman approach for predicting protein functions, *Source Code Biol. Med.* **1**:3 (2006).

22. King AD, Przulj N, Jurisica I, Protein complex prediction via cost-based clustering, *Bioinformatics* **20**(17):3013–3020 (2004).

23. Lawler EL, Lenstra JK, Rinnooy Kan AHG, Shmoys DB, *Traveling Salesman Problem: A Guided Tour of Combinatorial Optimization*, September, 1985 Wiley Interscience.

24. Lin S, Kernighan BW, An effective heuristic algorithm for the traveling salesman problem, *Oper. Res.* **21**:498–516, (1973).

25. Dorigo M, Ant colony opimization, *Scholarpedia* **2**(3):1461 (2007).

26. Mewes HW et al, MIPS: Analysis and annotation of proteins from whole genome in 2005, *Nucleic Acids Res.* **34**:D169–D172 (2006).

27. Newman MEJ, Scientific collaboration networks. II. Shortest paths, weighted networks and centrality, *Phys. Rev. E* **64**:016132(2001).

28. Palla G, Derenyi I, Farkas I, Vicsek T, Uncovering the overlapping community structure of complex networks in nature and society, *Nature* **435**:814–818 (2005).

29. Pei P, Zhang A, A topological measurement for weighted protein interaction network, *Proc. 16th IEEE Computational Systems Bioinformatics Conf. (CSB)*, 2005, pp. 268–278.

30. Rives AW, Galitski T, Modular organization of cellular networks, *Proc. Natl. Acad. Sci. USA* **100**(3):1128–1133 (2003).

31. Samanta MP, Liang S, Predicting protein functions from redundancies in large-scale protein interaction networks, *Proc. Natl. Acad. Sci. USA* **100**(22):12579–12583 (2003).

32. Shi L, Cho Y-R, Zhang A, Ann based protein function prediction using integrated protein-protein interaction data, *Proc. Joint Int. Conf. Bioinformatics, Systems Biology and Intelligent Computing*, 2009, pp. 271–277.

33. Tetko IV, Facius A, Ruepp A, Mewes HW, Super paramagnetic clustering of protein sequences, *BMC Bioinformatics* **6**(82):(2005).

34. Uetz P et al, A comprehensive analysis of protein-protein interactions in Saccharomyces cerevisiae, *Nature* **403**:623–627 (2000).

35. Venter JC et al, The sequence of the human genome, *Science* **291**:1304–1351 (2001).

36. Wagner A, How the global structure of protein interaction networks evolves, *Proc. R. Soc. Lond* **270**:457–466 (2003).

37. Zhang A, *Protein Interaction Networks: Computational Analysis*, Cambridge Univ. Press, 2009.

CHAPTER 21

EFFICIENT ALIGNMENTS OF METABOLIC NETWORKS WITH BOUNDED TREEWIDTH

QIONG CHENG, PIOTR BERMAN, ROBERT W. HARRISON, and ALEXANDER ZELIKOVSKY

21.1 INTRODUCTION

The accumulation of results of thousands of experiments, as well as high-throughput genomic, proteomic, and metabolic data, allows for increasingly accurate modeling and reconstruction of biological molecular interactions in the form of metabolic, regulatory, and signal transduction networks that are critical to understanding of vital cellular processes. With the growth of identified biological networks stored in several public collections of databases (e.g., KEGG [17] and BioCyc [6]), the development of efficient computational tools for assessing, comparing, and curating the wealth of data has become essential.

Many such needs can be addressed by a network alignment approach that can be used for comparing biological networks between different species to reveal evolutionary conservation of most vital life processes. We investigate a general network alignment problem—a pathway forms a pattern, and a cellular network (usually from another species) forms the text, and we want to find the best correspondence between the text and the pattern. Existing approaches suffer from low scalability even when applied to usually sparse graphs.

The authors in this chapter develop a computationally much more efficient approach based on homomorphisms and homeomorphisms, allowing toleration of the divergence within the alignment of metabolic pathways. Although metabolic pathways may exhibit fairly complex structures, their analysis of existing databases shows that corresponding graphs have very restricted treewidth for

Algorithmic and Artificial Intelligence Methods for Protein Bioinformatics. First Edition.
Edited by Yi Pan, Jianxin Wang, Min Li.
© 2014 John Wiley & Sons, Inc. Published 2014 by John Wiley & Sons, Inc.

which very efficient alignment algorithms can be developed. They present the first polynomial time algorithm for optimal alignment of metabolic pathways with bounded treewidth. In particular, the optimal alignment from pathway P to pathway T can be found in time $O(|V_P\|V_T|^{\alpha+1})$, where V_P and V_T are the vertex sets of pathways and α is the treewidth of P. They implemented the algorithm for alignment of metabolic pathways of treewidth 2 with arbitrary metabolic networks. The authors also demonstrate how to apply the network alignment to identifying inconsistency, inferring missing enzymes, and finding potential candidates for filling the holes.

The remainder of the chapter is organized as follows. In the next section the authors give a brief overview of current state-of-the-art methods in metabolic pathway/network alignment and how they can be used in automatic data curating. The generalized network alignment problem is formulated in Section 21.3, and tree decomposition–based solution is described in Section 21.4. Finally, Section 21.5 describes application of our network alignment algorithm to finding and filling holes in metabolic networks.

21.2 AN OVERVIEW OF METABOLIC NETWORK ALIGNMENT AND MINING APPROACHES

A metabolic network is a union of pathways, each representing a flow of consecutive enzymatic reactions that take specific metabolites (also called *substrates*) as an input to yield specific products. In such pathways, a substrate is converted into a product by the first enzyme in the pathway, and the product of the first reaction then becomes the substrate for the next reaction. Although simple pathways can frequently be represented as chains, complex pathways can exhibit a complex topological structure. When comparing metabolism of different organisms, it is preferred to align their entire metabolic networks rather than just pathways so that alternative pathways will be not missed.

Let the *pattern* be an incomplete metabolic network or its part for which one is searching homologous parts in the text, that is, the known metabolic network of a different species. Usually, alignment of the pattern and the text requires establishing a partial correspondence between vertices and directed edges of the pattern and the text such that paths and edges can be matched and certain parts of both the pattern and the text can be completely deleted. In general, insertions and deletions as well as label mismatches (i.e., when matched vertices are labeled with different enzymes) increase the alignment cost.

21.2.1 Previous Work on Metabolic Network Alignment

Existing approaches to subgraph iso- and homeomorphism restrict the size [25,31] or topology of the pattern [14,15,22,24,29] or use heuristics and approximation algorithms. GraphMatch [25] allows deletion of disassociated vertices of the query network and then aligns its remainder to the target network by subgraph isomorphism. However, stating the problem as subgraph iso/homeomorphism does not meet the requirement of gene duplication. Therefore, homomorphism approach suggested by Cheng et al. [22] and its generalization in this chapter better reflect the underlying metabolic model.

A naive enumeration algorithm used to obtain network alignment is exponential. The early studies focused only on similarities between vertices such as proteins or genes composing pathways disregarding topology [14,15]. Later Kelley et al. [31] took into account the nonlinearity of protein network topology and reduced it to a problem of finding the highest-score path of length L in an acyclic graph. The runtime of their procedure is practical if the pathlength L is restricted to 6. Pinter et al. [29] also keeps network topology intact but requires pattern and text graphs to be trees. The runtime of their algorithm is

$$O \left(\frac{|V_P|^2 |V_T|}{\log |V_P|} + |V_P||V_T| \log |V_T| \right).$$

However, subgraph iso/homeomorphism does not capture the widespread evolution machinery of gene duplication that results in vertex copying [30]. Yang et al. [25] proposed path matching and graph matching algorithms. Path matching finds a best homeomorphic alignment from path to graph, which allows the operations of vertex insertions and deletions. Their graph matching allows deletion of disassociated vertices or induced subnetwork in query network and then aligns its remainder to target network by subgraph isomorphism.

An eigenvalue-based approach due to Ay et al. [4] simultaneously aligns different types of entity, such as enzymes, reactions, and compounds. It creates and solves an eigenvalue problem for each entity type. They enforce the consistency while combining the alignments of different entity types by considering the reachability sets of entities. This method is capable of discovering alternative pathways but too coarse to be used for data curation.

Our 2007 paper [22] considers the case when the pattern topology is restricted to polytrees and no vertex deletion in the pattern is allowed, that is, where the edges of the homomorphic image of the entire tree pattern should be subdivided by degree 2 vertices to obtain a graph isomorphic to a subgraph of the text. It is shown that the network alignment problem admits an $O(|V_T||E_T| + |V_T|^2|V_P|)$ exact algorithm, where V_P and V_T are vertex sets of the pattern and text, respectively, and E_T is the edge set of the text. In another paper [21] we presented a formulation that also incorporated pattern vertex deletion and an efficient algorithm for finding optimal network alignment of a pattern network with a limited size of the feedback vertex set into an arbitrary network. Unfortunately, the metabolic pathways may have very large feedback vertex set, thus restricting application of the algorithm in practice.

Dost et al. [7] formulated the problem as an optimal homomorphism problem. Authors employed a color coding technique to find the optimum mapping of a pattern with treewidth w. They first randomly colored V_T with $|V_P|$ colors. Then they ran a dynamic programming to find colorful matches of subpatterns of

P, where a match is colorful if each pattern node is mapped to a text node of a different color. The dynamic programming takes $O(2^{|V_P|}|V_T|^{w+1})$ time, and it has to be repeated roughly $O(e^{|V_P|})$ times (to ensure that the optimum homomorphism may, indeed, be colorful).

More recently, Bruckner et al. [32] proposed an approach of network querying that disregards the topology of the query. Instead they merely require that the image of the query set (together with inserted nodes) be connected in the text graph. This formulation is well motivated for mapping protein complexes into a protein–protein interaction network, and it allows handle deletions and insertions, while performing queries much faster than optimal homomorphism queries, namely, in time $3^{|V_P|} \times |E_T|i)$, where i is the number of allowed insertions.

21.2.2   Mining Metabolic Networks Using Alignment

Most of the high-throughput genomic, proteomic data are not catalogued or processed directly by hand but by computational technologies. Because of the noise [12], all of them require data curation. For BioCyc, only a part of pathway data have received person-decades of literature-based curation and are the most accurate [16]. Inspecting the existing pathways can help resolve the ambiguity of databases. Network alignment can help to identify potential inconsistency and partially identified enzymes. Similarly, it can be used to predict potential candidates for certain enzymes that may be partially annotated or completely missing (pathway holes).

A similar approach to pathway hole prediction and filling has been proposed [19,20]. It uses available structure of the metabolic network to enhance the predictive capability of the expression data. It is based on DNA homology, which is less effective than using amino acid sequence homology since amino acids may be coded by multiple codons. A Bayesian method for identifying missing enzymes in predicted metabolic pathway databases was proposed by Green and Karp [16]. Their method uses a set of sequences encoding the required activity in other genomes to identify candidate proteins in the genome of interest, and then evaluates each candidate by using a simple Bayesian classifier for the desired function. This method has been cross-validated showing 71% precision on known reactions.

21.3   GENERALIZED NETWORK ALIGNMENT PROBLEM

In this chapter the authors define network alignment that allows mismatches, insertions, and deletions of vertices-enzymes as well as aligning not only the entire pattern but also any of its subnetworks.

In order to allow restricting alignment to a subnetwork, we should allow deletion of an arbitrary vertex. Therefore, we distinguish two kinds of vertex deletions: (1) *bypass deletion*, corresponding to the replacement of a few consecutively acting enzymes with a single multifunctional enzyme or enzyme using

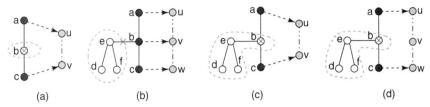

(a)   (b)   (c)   (d)

Figure 21.1 (a) Bypass deletion of a patten vertex b of degree 2. The cost of alignment is $\Delta(a, u) + \Delta(b, \mathbf{b}) + \Delta(c, v)$ (b) Strong deletion of three pattern vertices d, e and f. The cost of alignment is $\Delta(a, u) + \Delta(b, v) + \Delta(c, w) + \Delta(d, \mathbf{d}) + \Delta(e, \mathbf{d}) + \Delta(f, \mathbf{d})$; (c) composition of strong and bypass deletions. The cost of alignment is $\Delta(a, u) + \Delta(b, \mathbf{b}) + \Delta(c, w) + \Delta(d, \mathbf{d}) + \Delta(e, \mathbf{d}) + \Delta(f, \mathbf{d})$. (d) Composition of strong and bypass deletions with a vertex insertion (v is inserted). The cost of alignment is $\Delta(a, u) + \Delta(b, \mathbf{b}) + \Delta(c, w) + \Delta(d, \mathbf{d}) + \Delta(e, \mathbf{d}) + \Delta(f, \mathbf{d}) + \lambda$. In structures (a), (c), and (d) (a, c) is a mapped path.

an alternative catalysis; and (2) *strong deletion*, symbolizing the matching of a properly connected subgraph of the pattern network (see Fig. 21.1). Intuitively, we can simplify the pattern with a sequence of deletions (see Fig. 21.1c) and then map it into the text inserting some new vertices if necessary. A strong deletion of a vertex v involves removal of arbitrary vertex v together with all its incoming and outgoing edges (in the formal definition, we will map v into $\mathbf{d}$.) A bypass deletion can be applied only to a vertex v with a single incoming and a single outgoing edge (possibly, after earlier strong deletions); it replaces a path (u, v, w) with a single edge (u, w) (in the formal definition, we will map v into $\mathbf{b}$.) A vertex insertion is inverse to bypass deletion—it corresponds to replacement of a single multifunctional enzyme with a few consecutively acting enzymes or simply addition of extra enzymes for additional intermediate reactions. Graphically, vertex insertion corresponds to mapping of an edge (u, v) into a longer path by adding intermediate vertices (see Fig. 21.1d).

Our formal definition below requires network alignment to map a part of the pattern into the text such that each mapped pattern path is mapped into some text path. Let graphs $P = (V_P, E_P)$ and $T = (V_T, E_T)$ represent pattern and text metabolic networks, respectively. Let $f : P \to T$ map every vertex in V_P to $V_T \cup \{\mathbf{b}, \mathbf{d}\}$. A pair of pattern vertices $u, v \in V_P$ is a *mapped path* if $f(u), f(v) \in V_T$ and either $(u, v) \in V_P$ or there exists a u–v path in P whose all-intermediate vertices are bypass deleted. Let E_P^f be the set of all mapped paths defined by f. The mapping f is called a *network alignment* if

1. For each mapped u–v path in P we have $f(u) \neq f(v)$ and there exists a $f(u)$–$f(v)$ path in T.
2. Given $f(w) = \mathbf{b}$, then there exists exactly one mapped path through w.
3. The set of mapped paths E_P^f is connected.

Uniqueness in condition 2 is required to ensure that if two paths intersect in P, their images (if they exist) should also intersect in T. Since the image of a mapped $u-v$ path is a $f(u)-f(v)$ path, all intermediate vertices in the $f(u)-f(v)$ path do not have a preimage and are penalized as insertions. We define $\sigma(f(u), f(v))$ as the minimum number of insertions, that is, the number of intermediate vertices on the shortest $f(u)-f(v)$ path.

The alignment should be penalized for (1) mismatches between aligned enzymes, (2) strong deletions, (3) bypass deletions, and (4) insertions. Thus we obtain the following cost function

$$\text{Cost}(f) = \sum_{u \in V_P} \Delta(u, f(u)) + \lambda \sum_{(u,v) \in E_P^f} \sigma(f(u), f(v)) \tag{21.1}$$

where $\Delta(u, f(u))$ is the penalty for a mismatch between enzymes corresponding to u and $f(u)$ [22,25,29]; $\Delta(u, \mathbf{d})$ and $\Delta(u, \mathbf{b})$ are penalties for strong and bypass deletions of u, respectively; and λ is the penalty per single enzyme insertion. The cost function (21.1) is a generalization of the cost functions first introduced by Pinter et al. [29] when any connected part of the pattern pathway is allowed to map (they [29] suggested that the entire pattern pathway should be mapped). Minimizing introduced penalty for strong deletions is equivalent to finding the largest common motif present in the pattern and the text. Several examples of computing alignment costs are given in Figure 21.1.

We now can formulate the main problem.

Problem 21.1   Generalized Metabolic Network Alignment. Given two metabolic networks, the pattern P and the text T, find the network alignment f from P to T of minimum cost according to (21.1).

21.4   A GENERALIZED DYNAMIC PROGRAMMING ALGORITHM

Efficient dynamic programming algorithms exist for polytree patterns (a *polytree* is a directed graph that becomes a tree if all its edges are stripped of directions) and arbitrary texts [22]. Also, in cases when the number of cycles in the pattern graph is not large, we have proposed the use of an efficient algorithm [21]. In this chapter we address how to handle patterns of the most general structure that can have a large number of disconnected cycles.

We wish to identify graph-theoretic parameters that are bounded for metabolic networks (and thus distinguish them from general graphs) and whose restriction allows polynomial time solutions for the metabolic network alignment problem. The natural candidate for such a parameter would be the size of the feedback vertex set (minimum number of vertices whose deletion makes graph acyclic), but it is not good enough since the metabolic networks have a large number of nonintersecting cycles. Instead, we consider a treewidth of a graph defined in terms of a tree decomposition [27]. A tree decomposition represents the vertices

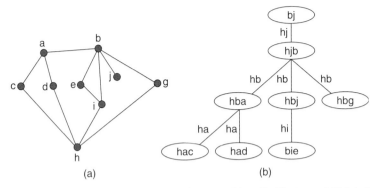

Figure 21.2   Pattern graph P and its tree decomposition D. Vertices of D labeled with the same vertex of P form a connected subtree of D.

of the given graph P as subtrees of a tree D, in such a way that vertices of P are adjacent only when the corresponding subtrees intersect (see Fig. 21.2). Each node u (edge e) of D is labeled with the P vertices whose subtrees contain node u (edge e). The label of a D edge forms a vertex separator of P. The width of a tree decomposition D is the maximum number of P vertices in a label of a D node minus 1. The treewidth of P is the minimum width of a tree decomposition of P.

A decomposition tree can be normalized by collapsing the adjacent nodes with identical labels. Because an edge label is the intersection of the label of the nodes that it is connecting, after the normalization, edge labels are smaller than the node labels; hence, they are not larger than the treewidth.

The graphs with bounded treewidth look attractive since they may contain any number of nonintersecting cycles and many important NP-hard graph problems can be solved efficiently for them [1,5,8–10,13].

Moreover, several biological models of metabolic network evolution, including retrograde evolution [18], patchwork evolution [28], duplication [3], and hierarchical [2] models, imply that the evolution adds/deletes enzymes into existing pathways and also adds alternative pathways. Such modifications of a graph will not increase the treewidth beyond 2. Moreover, duplication of genes and increase in the specificity of the enzymes also may result in decreasing treewidth. All this implies that we would rarely see metabolic networks with a treewidth of >2. Indeed, our analysis shows that for B. *subtilis* out of 159 recorded pathways, only one has treewidth 2 or 1, and in E. *coli* 6 pathways out of 256 have treewidth 3. Similarly, treewidth 3 has only in 1 out of 59 pathways in *Halobacterium* and 9 out of 179 in S. *cerevisiae*. An example of a pathway whose treewidth is 3 is given on Figure 21.3. Note that duplication of genes and increase of the specificity of the enzymes may split one of the enzymes from the set {6.3.1.5, 2.7.7.18, 3.6.1.22} into two so that the resulting pathway will decrease its treewidth to 2. The entire metabolic networks of E. *coli*, B. *subtilis*, S. *cerevisiae* and *Halobacterium* have treewidth 3.

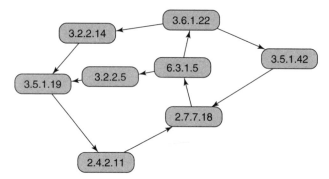

Figure 21.3   A part of a pathway (pyridine nucleotide cycling in *S. cerevisiae*) that has treewidth 3.

Such observations imply that we can focus only on graphs with treewidth 1, 2, and 3. The graphs with treewidth 1 are polytrees for which efficient dynamic programming has already been implemented [23]. The graphs with treewidth 2 are called *series-parallel graphs*, which means that all graphs cannot be contracted to a complete graph on four vertices K_4, (graph P in Fig. 21.2 is a series-parallel graph).

The main steps of the proposed algorithm for series-parallel patterns are as follows:

1. Finding all shortest-path distances in the text graph—to quickly compute the cost of a mapped path in terms of vertex insertions.
2. Finding tree decomposition of the pattern—a minimum treewidth decomposition can be found in linear time if the treewidth has a constant bound [9].
3. Filling dynamic programming table—each table row will correspond to an edge in the decomposition tree D.

Our dynamic programming corresponds to a divide-and-conquer method that we can perform using α-vertex separators of P, where α is the treewidth of P. Each dynamic programming table entry corresponds to an optimal solution of the following subproblem: where to map P nodes that are present in a subtree of the decomposition tree D rooted at a node s to minimize the cost so far, or *local cost*. We fill the dynamic programming table in a bottom–up manner along the tree decomposition D, so when we need to find optimal mapping of the nodes in the label set of s, we already know where all downstream labels are mapped, that is, we are mapping them having *assumptions* (i.e., images of downstream nodes). (As we will see further in one case, it is necessary to have limited assumptions about the solution outside the subtree.)

To simplify the algorithm description, we can assume that the label set of every node in the decomposition tree D has $(\alpha + 1)$ P nodes except for an added extra root node that has a label set of size α, and that every edge label has size α.

Letting s be an arbitrary nonroot vertex of D, we further use the following notations. The label set of the edge that connects s with the parent is denoted by S_s. Also, the (only) node of the label set of s that is not in S_s is denoted u_s. As S_s is a node separator whose deletion will disconnect the graph, we consider a partition of $V_P - S_s$ into S_s^{up} and S_s^{down}, where S_s^{down} are the nodes in the labels of the subtree rooted by s and S_s^{up} is its complement to $V_P - S_s$.

First, our assumptions will fix $f(u)$ for each $u \in S_s$ (recall that S is a vertex separator). However, we also need to know a bit more to ensure that f is a network alignment and to compute the local cost of extending f to S_s^{down}. We need to ensure that the following three conditions are satisfied:

1. The set Def of all P nodes not mapped to **d** form a connected subgraph.
2. The restrictions of bypass deletion are satisfied.
3. The replacement and insertion costs are computed correctly.

To ensure condition 1, we will know on assume the partition of $\text{Def} \cap S_s$ between the connected components of $\text{Def} \cap (S_s^{down} \cup S_s^{up})$. A separate consideration requires the case when $f(u) = \mathbf{d}$ for each $u \in S_s$. Then we need to know if all nondeleted nodes are in S_s^{up} or in S_s^{down}. In both cases the consequences are obvious, and we will omit them in further discussion.

The algorithm tries every possible $f(u_s)$, and iterates through the list of children of s (this iteration obviously takes zero steps if s is a leaf). The new assumption of $f(u_s)$ determines the local cost: replacement cost $\Delta(u_s, f(u_s))$, and insertion costs that we will discuss later (because they involve the extra assumptions we make to properly handle the bypass deletions). The new assumption also determines how $\text{Def} \cap (S_s \cup \{u_s\})$ is partitioned between the connected components of $\text{Def} \cap (S_s^{down} \cup \{u_s\} \cup S_s^{up})$ (because we have determined whether $u_s \in \text{Def}$ and we know edges between u_s and S_s).

When we consider a child c, we make every possible assumption consistent with our knowledge so far, we look up the respective cost in the dynamic programming table, and thus we derive a possible cost of a new assumption. Consider a pair v, w of P nodes from the label set of s. If either of them is not in Def, the connectivity requirement does not concern them, and if they are assumed to be in the same connected component, the requirement is already satisfied for this pair. If we select an assumption for c that does not connect v and w, then this solution for c has to connect them, so we will further assume that v, w are connected. Conversely, if we select an assumption for c that does connect v and w, then this solution does not have to connect them within the subtree of c, so we we will further assume that v, w are not connected. In this fashion, for every possible connectivity assumption that we can have after considering c, we will obtain a certain cost that we can maintain in a table.

After considering all children, the only acceptable final assumption is that every pair in $\text{Def} \cap (S_s \cup \{u_s\})$ is connected, and we computed the minimum cost of assuring this assumption. If this is not possible, then we assign infinity to that cost.

Ensuring condition 2 means that if $f(v) = \mathbf{b}$, then there exists v', v'' such that $v' \neq v''$, pattern P contains the directed path (v', v, v''), and the set of neighbors of v that are in Def is equal to $\{v', v''\}$. We can say that v' is an in-neighbor of v and v'' is an out-neighbor. Thus we need *bypass* assumptions that answer the questions: for $v \in S_s$ such that $f(u) = \mathbf{b}$, are in- and out-neighbors in $S_s^{\text{up}} \cup S_s$?

We can observe that bypass assumptions can eliminate certain values for $f(u_s)$; for example, if $v \in S_s$, $f(u) = \mathbf{b}$, and the in-neighbor of v is in $S_s \cup S_s^{\text{up}}$ and P contains the direct edge (u_s, v), then we must have $f(u_s) = \mathbf{d}$. We apply the bypass assumptions similarly to connectivity assumptions; namely, a valid solution to an instance must ensure the desired final effect. Hence we maintain a table of bypass assumptions for $S_s \cup \{u_s\}$ and when the loop for children terminates, all bypass assumptions must have positive answers.

Condition 3 requires that when we determine a mapped path, such as (v, w) mapped to $(f(v), f(w))$, then we can locally increment the local cost by $\lambda \times \sigma(f(v), f(w))$. If (v, w) is a single-hop path (i.e., an edge in P), then this is straightforward; we use the convention that node s determines direct edges between u_s and S_s, and when we fill a table entry for s, we have assumptions as to what $f(u_s)$ is and what $f(v)$ is.

We will now consider the case when (u, v) is a multihop path through bypass-deleted vertices. Filling a table entry starts with the assumption on $f(S_s)$ and the connectivity pattern in $S_s \cup S_s^{\text{up}}$. In the current iteration, we consider how to extend this assumption to $f(u_s)$. When we loop through the children of s, we maintain a table of possible accumulated assumptions on the connectivity patterns in $S_s \cup \{u_s\}$ that consider the connections through S_s^{up} and, for each child c already processed, through S_c^{down}. Thus at any step we have a set of P nodes included in connectivity assumptions, so at some step a mapped path becomes contained in this set. We describe the connectivity assumptions for bypass deletions below.

The assumptions concern the label set of the edge that connects s with the parent S_s and when we are maintaining a table to fill a table entry $S_s \cup \{u_s\}$. A node v in the interface set that has $f(v) = \mathbf{b}$ is on a longer mapped path, and we need to assume the status of this path. We need to compute the minimum local cost for the following four possible cases and assumptions:

1. The path extends into another branch of the tree; we can represent this assumption as $f(v) = \mathbf{b}$.

2. Connecting to a node $w \in S_s^{\text{down}}$ such that $f(w) \in V_T$ completes the path [we need to have the assumption on $f(x)$ where x is the other end of the mapped path, and we do not need an assumption on the actual identity of x].

3. Connecting to another w in the interface set that has $f(w) = \mathbf{b}$ completes a mapped path (we need to know where the path endpoints that correspond to v and w are mapped).

4. Connecting to two nodes in S_s^{down} such that $f(w) \in V_T$ completes the path (this is a combination of two assumptions of the types described above).

When we define $f(u_s)$, we are constrained by the assumptions (decisions) about S_s as they may restrict the value of $f(u_s)$ to **d** or **b**; if we cannot consistently define $f(u_s)$, then we assign infinite cost to the respective table entry. If we complete a bypass path, then the assumptions include the images $f(w)$ and $f(w')$ for the endpoints of that path and we add $\lambda \times \sigma(f(w), f(w'))$ to the cost of the table entry.

One can see that we can find a solution in time $O((d+1)|V_T|)$, where d is the number of children of s. Because the average number of children of tree node is below 1, this means that the average time needed to compute an entry in the dynamic programming table is $O(|V_T|)$, while we have $O(|V_P||V_T|^\alpha)$ such instances. Hence the time needed for dynamic programming is $O(|V_P||V_T|^{\alpha+1})$. Because this time is longer than the time needed to solve all-pairs shortest paths for the text graph, we conclude that we can find a minimum cost network alignment in time $O(|V_P||V_T|^{\alpha+1})$ for series-parallel patterns. Thus we proved the following

Theorem 21.1 The generalized network alignment problem can be solved in time $O(|V_P||V_T|^{\alpha+1})$, where α is the treewidth of the pattern graph $P = (V_P, E_P)$ and $|V_T|$ is the number of vertices in the text graph $T = (V_T, E_T)$.

As a corollary we obtain the following result

Corollary 21.1 The generalized network alignment problem for series-parallel patterns can be solved in time $O(|V_P||V_T|^3)$, where $|V_P|$ and $|V_T|$ are the numbers of vertices in the pattern graph $P = (V_P, E_P)$ and the text graph $T = (V_T, E_T)$, respectively.

Allowing pattern vertex deletion allows better alignments. Table 21.1 illustrates advantage of the network alignment (HH) over homomorphisms H (network alignment without vertex deletion). The number of mismatches and number of gaps are the measures of how well the pattern is matched to the text network. For both characteristics—number of mismatches and number of gaps—the former significantly outperform the latter.

TABLE 21.1 Alignment of Tree Pathways from Different Species with Optimal Homomorphisms (H) and Optimal Network Alignment (HH)[a]

	E. coli→T. thermophilus		E. coli→B. subtilis		E. coli→H. NRC1		E. coli→S. cerevisiae	
	Mismatches	Gaps	Mismatches	Gaps	Mismatches	Gaps	Mismatches	Gaps
HH	0.58	0.04	0.23	0.03	1.60	0.10	0.22	0.04
H	0.76	0.07	0.38	0.06	2.31	0.12	0.22	0.05

[a]The average number of mismatches and gaps is reported on common statistically significant matched pathways.

21.4.1 Data

The genome-scale metabolic network data in our studies were drawn from BioCyc [6,11,26], the collection of 260 pathway/genome databases, each of which describes metabolic pathways and enzymes of a single organism. We have chosen metabolic networks of *E. coli*, the yeast *S. cerevisiae*, the eubacterium *B. subtilis*, the archeabacterium *T. thermophilus* and the halobacterium *H. NRC1* to cover major lineages Archaea, Eukaryotes, and Eubacteria. The bacterium *E. coli* with 255 pathways is the most extensively studied prokaryotic organism. *T. thermophilus*, with 149 pathways, belongs to Archaea. *B. subtilis*, with 172 pathways, is one of the best understood Eubacteria in terms of molecular biology and cell biology. *S. cerevisiae*, with 175 pathways is the most thoroughly researched eukaryotic microorganism. *H. NRC1* with 58 pathways has been extensively used for postgenomic analysis.

21.4.2 Statistical Significance of Mapping

Although the cost of network alignment reflects the similarity of pathways, it alone cannot assure us that such cost is not obtained by chance. Only statistically significant cost values can be taken into account. Statistical significance is measured by the *p*-value, that is, the probability of the null hypothesis that the cost value is obtained by pure chance.

We followed two standard randomization procedures:

1. *Reshuffling Edges.* We randomly permute pairs of edges (u, v) and (u', v') if no other edges exist between these four vertices u, u', v, v' in the text graph by reconnecting them as (u, v') and (u', v). This allows us to keep the incoming and outgoing degrees of each vertex intact.
2. *Reshuffling Nodes.* We randomly permute the labels of vertices, which only keep the conserved degree distribution of the whole graph.

We further developed two random graph generators: (1) reshuffling only the vertices with the same degree (same indegree and outdegree), which allows us to keep the same degree and degree distribution; and (2) generating a random spanning tree first and then adding random edges until the required number of edges is reached. In the procedure of random tree generation, we start with $|V|$ partial trees $Tree = \{t_1, t_2, \ldots, t_{|V|}\}$, where each t_i consists of a single vertex $v_i \in V$. Every tree and every vertex in the tree have the following parameters such as original indegree, original outdegree, unsatisfied indegree, and unsatisfied outdegree, denoted respectively as *indegree, outdegree, −indeg,* and *−outdeg* on a vertex or a tree. We randomly choose two partial trees t_i and t_j satisfying $outdegree(t_j)$-$outdeg(t_i) \geq 0$ or $indegree(t_j) - indeg(t_i) \geq 0$; we connect the chosen trees by randomly choosing two vertices from the trees (satisfying the same rule on vertex as on the tree) and linking the vertices, and change the parameters of the vertices and the corresponding partial trees. The iterative procedure terminates when all the V nodes are included in the final tree.

We find the minimum-cost network alignments from the pattern graph into the fully randomized text graph and check to determine whether its cost is at least as low as the minimum cost before randomization of the text graph. We say that the alignment is statistically significant with $p < 0.01$ if we found at most nine better costs in 1000 randomization of the text graph.

For simplicity, we have evaluated our randomized p-value computation for the four random graph generator on the trees. We extracted 156 tree pathways from *E. coli* and 100 tree pathways from *yeast*. We ran all-against-all alignment from *E. coli* to *yeast* and *yeast* and *E. coli* and observed the distribution of alignment pairs under different p-values. We have developed an alignment tool called MetNetAligner that supports different alignment algorithms. The web service is coded by JAVA, and its embedded alignment programs are coded by ANSI C.

21.4.3 Experiments

We ran all-against-all alignment among four species (*B. subtilis*, *E. coli*, *T. thermophilus*, and *S. cerevisiae*). For each pair of them, using our algorithm we find the minimum-cost network alignment from each pathway of one species to each pathway of the other and check to determine whether this biological homology is statistically significant. The experiments were run on a Pentium 4 processor, 2.99-GHz clock with 1.00 GB RAM. The total runtime was 2.5 h for the input/output of pathways and computing the optimal pattern-to-text mapping and its p value for every pair of pathways (there are in total 654,481 pattern–text pathway pairs).

Our approach uses EC encoding and the tight reaction property classified by EC. The EC number is expressed with a four-level hierarchical scheme. The four-digit EC number, $d_1.d_2.d_3.d_4$, represents a sub-sub-subclass indication of biochemical reaction (see examples in Fig. 21.3). If the $d_1.d_2$ of two enzymes are different, their similarity score is infinite; if d_3 of two enzymes are different, their similarity score is 10; if d_4 of two enzymes are different, their similarity score is 1; otherwise the similarity score is 0. The corresponding penalty scores are 0.5 and 0 individually for pattern vertex deletion and text vertex deletion, respectively. Additionally, we allow pattern partially identified enzymes to be mapped to any enzyme in text without any penalty, but in a sequence that is the reverse of that for partially identified enzymes as occurs in text, a 0.1 score as mismatch penalty will apply during mapping by any enzyme in pattern. Our implementation also provides a previously known enzyme similarity score [29], but that score scheme results in biochemically fewer relevant pathway matches.

21.4.4 Results

For alignments from *Thermus thermophilus* to *B. subtilis*, there are in total 2968 statistically significant mapped pairs; 87 of 149 *T. thermophilus* pathways have statistically significant aligned images in *B. subtilis* and 143 out of 172 *B. subtilis* pathways have statistically significant preimages. For alignments from *E. coli* to *S. cerevisiae*, there are in total 5418 statistically significant mapped pairs; 109 out of 255 *E. coli* pathways have statistically significant aligned images in *S. cerevisiae*, and 153 out of 175 *S. cerevisiae* pathways have statistically significant homomorphic preimages. We find more statistically significant pathway alignments than in Pinter et al. [29] (52,703 vs. 13,110 out of total 654,481 pattern–text pathway pairs).

21.5 PREDICTING PATHWAY HOLES AND RESOLVING ENZYME AMBIGUITY

The metabolic network alignment is proposed for applications such as predicting and filling holes in existing pathway descriptions. As discussed in previous sections, given a pattern pathway in question, we align it to all known pathways and find a statistically significant alignment score. Then we can check where the unknown enzymes in the pattern are mapped to. We also can check all inconsistencies that may indicate incorrect enzyme assignment or absence of certain enzymes. We distinguish two types of pathway hole:

Type 1. A hole representing an enzyme with partially or completely unknown EC notation (e.g., EC 1.2.4.—or .—.) in the currently available pathway description. This type of hole is caused by ambiguity in identifying a gene and its product in an organism.

Type 2. A hole representing an enzyme that is completely missing from the currently available pathway description. This type of hole occurs when the gene encoding an enzyme is not identified in an organism's genome.

An example of pathway hole of type 1 and how that hole can be filled using alignment is illustrated in Figure 21.4. For two enzymes in the pattern we find plausible candidates. Figure 21.5 illustrates a type 2 hole. The shaded enzyme is completely missing from the pattern.

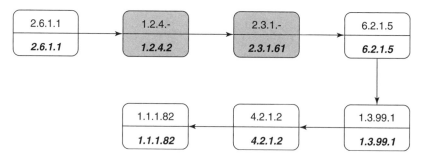

Figure 21.4 The type 1 hole. Alignment of glutamate degradation VII pathways from *T. thermophilus* and *B. subtilis* ($p < 0.01$). The shaded node reflects enzyme homology.

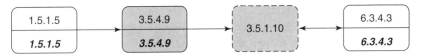

Figure 21.5   The type 2 hole. Alignment of formaldehyde oxidation V pathway in *B. subtilis* with formyl THF biosynthesis pathway in *E. coli*.

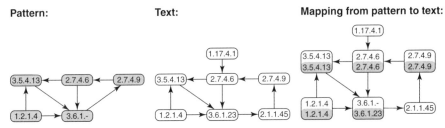

Figure 21.6   Partial pathway in de novo biosynthesis of pyrimidine deoxyribonucleotides from *Bacillus subtilis* with ambiguity introduced in one label and a hole instead of another enzyme. Alignment with the original pathway allows restoration of the label and detection and filling the hole.

Figure 21.6 illustrates applications of our implementation. We pick up a pathway, named de novo biosynthesis of pyrimidine deoxyribonucleotides, from the *Bacillus subtilis* species, randomly change a vertex label with the dashedline label so that a label is fuzzed, or delete a single enzyme. By aligning the modified graph with the original one, we find the potential holes and even potential candidates to fill them.

We propose the following three-level framework for filling pathway holes. The holes are identified as the enzymes (EC notations) present in the text organism, but absent or ambiguous in the pattern organism. The framework first extracts the text organism's sequences for enzymes appearing as holes in the pattern. The 1 level search is conducted by querying the database for the enzymes that appear as holes in the pattern organism, and their sequences are extracted. Pairwise alignment is done between the sequences for pattern and text. Accession numbers for alignments showing >50% identity are selected as fillings.

At level 2, sequences for left and right neighbors in the pattern organism are extracted. Pairwise alignment is conducted between text sequences for the hole and the left and right neighboring enzymes in the pattern pathway. Significant alignments (identity >50%) are reported as recommended fillings.

At the third level, sequences for the group neighbors (EC notation $d.d.d.x$) for the pattern organism are extracted. Pairwise alignment of the group neighbors is done with text sequence, and significant alignments are reported as alternative pathways. A user-defined value of x is taken to extract the number of group neighbor sequences. Prosite matching is done between the text enzyme and all the proteins with >50% identity. Proteins showing the highest prosite matching score are selected as candidate fillings. The P value is calculated for fillings on the basis of the sequence similarity score.

Our experiments show that the proposed three-level framework efficiently finds enzymes that have been intentionally removed from *E. coli* pathways.

REFERENCES

1. de Fluiter BLE, Bodlaender HL, Parallel algorithms for treewidth two. *LNCS*, **1335**:157–170 (1997).

2. Ravasz E, Somera AL, Mongru DA, Oltvai ZN, Barabsi AL, Hierarchical organization of modularity in metabolic networks science, *Science* **297**(5586):1551–1555 (2002). doi:10.1126/science.1073374.

3. Chung F, Lu L, Dewey G, Galas D, Duplication models for biological networks, *J. Comput. Biol.* **10**:677–687 (2003).

4. Ay F, Kahveci T, de Crecy-Lagard V, A fast and accurate algorithm for comparative analysis of metabolic pathways, *J. Bioinformatics Comput. Biol.* **7**(3):389–428 (2009).

5. Woeginger G. H, Exact algorithms for np-hard problems: A survey, in *Combinatorial Optimization*, Edmonds Festschrift, LNCS Series Vol. 2570, 2003, pp. 185–207.

6. See http://www.biocyc.org/.

7. Dost B, Shlomi T, Gupta N, Ruppin E, Bafna V, Sharan R, Qnet: A tool for querying biological networks. *J. Comput. Biol.* **15**(7):913–925 (2008). doi: 10.1089/cmb.2007.0172.

8. Bodlaender H, Hagerup T, Parallel algorithms with optimal speedup for bounded treewidth, *SIAM J. Comput.* **27**(6):1725–1746 (1998).

9. Bodlaender H, Koster A, Combinatorial optimization on graphs of bounded treewidth, *Comput. J.* **51**(3):255–269 (2008).

10. Bodlaender H, de Fluiter B, Parallel algorithms for series parallel graphs, *ESA*, 277–289 (1996).

11. Keeler IM, Collard VJ, Gama CS, Ingraham J, et al, EcoCyc: A comprehensive database resource for *Escherichia coli*, *Nucleic Acids Res.* **33** (database issue):D334–D337 (2005).

12. Han J-DJ, Understanding biological functions through molecular networks, *Cell Res.* **18**:224–237 (2008).

13. Valdes J, Tarjan R, Lawler E, The recognition of series parallel digraphs, *SIAM J. Comput.* **11**(2):298–313 (1982).

14. Chen M, Hofestaedt R, Pathaligner: Metabolic pathway retrieval and alignment, *Appl. Bioinformatics* **3**(4):241–252 (2004).

15. Chen M, Hofestaedt R, An algorithm for linear metabolic pathway alignment, *In Silico Biology* **5**(2):111–128 (2005).

16. Green ML, Karp PD, A bayesian method for identifying missing enzymes in predicted metabolic pathway databases, *BMC Bioinformatics* **5**:76 (2004). doi:10.1186/1471-2105-5-76.

17. Kanehisa M, Goto S, Hattori M, Aoki-Kinoshita KF, Itoh M, Kawashima S, Katayama T, Araki M, Hirakawa M, From genomics to chemical genomics: New developments in kegg, *Nucleic Acids Res.* **34**:D354–D357 (2006).

18. Horowitz NH, On the evolution of biochemical syntheses., *Proc Natl Acad Sci USA* **31**(6):153–157 (1945).

19. Kharchenko P, Chen L, Freund Y, Vitkup D, Identifying metabolic enzymes with multiple types of association evidence, *BMC Bioinformatics* **7**:177 (2006). doi: 10.1186/1471-2105-7-177 [PMCID: PMC1450304].

20. Kharchenko P, Vitkup D, Church GM, Filling gaps in a metabolic network using expression information, *Bioinformatics* **20**(Suppl. 1):i178–185 (2004).

21. Cheng Q, Berman P, Harrison R, Zelikovsky A, Fast alignments of metabolic networks, *Proc. IEEE Int. Conf. Bioinformatics and Biomedicine (BIBM)*, Philadelphia, PA 2008, pp. 147–152.

22. Cheng Q, Harrison R, Zelikovsky A, Homomorphisms of multisource trees into networks with applications to metabolic pathways, *Proc. IEEE Int. Conf. Bioinformatics and Bioengineering (BIBE)*, Boston, MA 2007, pp. 350–357.

23. Cheng Q, Harrison R, Zelikovsky A, Metnetaligner: A web service tool for metabolic network alignments, *Bioinformatics* **25**(15):1989–1990 (2009).

24. Cheng Q, Kaur D, Harrison R, Zelikovsky A, Homomorphisms of multisource trees into networks with applications to metabolic pathways. *Proc. RECOMB Satellite Conf. Systems Biology*, 2007.

25. Yang Q, Sze S-H, Path matching and graph matching in biological networks, *J. Comput. Biol.* **14**(1):56–67 (2007).

26. Caspi R, Foerster H, Fulcher CA, Hopkinson R, et al, Meta-Cyc: A microorganism database of metabolic pathways and enzymes, *Nucleic Acids Res.* **34** (database issue):D511–D516 (2006).

27. Diestel R, *Graph Theory*, Springer, Berlin, 2005.

28. Jensen RA, Enzyme recruitment in evolution of new function, *A Innu. Rev. Microbiol.* **30**:409–425 (1976).

29. Pinter RY, Rokhlenko O, Yeger-Lotem E, Ziv-Ukelson M, Alignment of metabolic pathways, *Bioinformatics* **21**(16):3401–3408 (Aug. 2005).

30. Sharan R, Ideker T, Modeling cellular machinery through biological network comparison, *Nat. Biotechnol.* **24**(4):427–433 (2006).

31. Sharan R, Suthram S, Kelley RM, Kuhn T, McCuine S, Uetz P, Sittler T, Karp RM, Ideker T, Conserved patterns of protein interaction in multiple species, *Proc. Natl. Acad. Sci.* **102**:1974–1979 (2005).

32. Bruckner S, Huffner F, Karp RM, Shamir R, Sharan R, Topology-free querying of protein interaction networks, *Proc. 13th Annual Int. Conf. Research in Computational Molecular Biology (RECOMB '09)*, 2009.

CHAPTER 22

PROTEIN–PROTEIN INTERACTION NETWORK ALIGNMENT: ALGORITHMS AND TOOLS

VALERIA FIONDA

22.1 INTRODUCTION

Biological processes regulating cell lifecycle are determined from complex interactions among cell constituents (e.g., proteins); thus, cell behavior and functions can be better understood by analyzing complex protein interaction patterns than individual proteins. Starting from this observation, many techniques for properly mining protein interaction data and revealing possibly new, useful biological information, have been developed.

These tools leverage protein–protein interaction (PPI) networks as a formal model to encode protein interaction data. At its most basic abstraction level, the PPI network of a given organism can be represented as a graph, the nodes of which represent the proteins belonging to that organism, and an edge between two proteins encodes the fact that these two proteins interact.

Several tools have been proposed to perform the topological and functional analysis of PPI networks. Such techniques are able, by exploiting some specialized algorithms, to infer new information about cellular activity and evolutive processes of the species. These specialized algorithms are often based on the comparison of two or more PPI networks of different organisms with the aim of transferring biological knowledge from one species to another (or, possibly, more) species, thus allowing us to better characterize some previously inadequately characterized organisms.

Algorithmic and Artificial Intelligence Methods for Protein Bioinformatics. First Edition.
Edited by Yi Pan, Jianxin Wang, Min Li.
© 2014 John Wiley & Sons, Inc. Published 2014 by John Wiley & Sons, Inc.

Generally speaking, there are several ways to compare PPI networks, but network alignment and network querying are two of the most signicant ones [25].

Network querying techniques search a whole PPI network to identify conserved occurrences of a given query module from another or possibly the same species [9,10]. Since the query generally encodes a well-characterized protein functional module, its occurrences in the queried PPI network suggest that the latter (and then the corresponding organism) features the function encoded by the former.

Network alignment is the process of globally comparing two or more PPI networks of different species in order to identify similarity and dissimilarity regions. Network alignment is commonly applied to detect conserved subnetworks, which are likely to represent common protein functional modules [22,23,28].

The knowledge that can be inferred through the application of PPI network alignment techniques covers several biological aspects. Indeed, the results of a PPI network alignment algorithm can be, among other things, used to (1) predict the functions of a protein functional module, (2) predict protein functions and functional annotations, (3) validate protein interactions, (4) predict protein–protein interactions, (5) detect orthology, and (6) reconstruct phylogenetic trees.

However, although very useful, the problem of aligning PPI networks is intrinsically difficult. Indeed, two important issues must be taken into account: (1) that subgraph isomorphism checking, which is a subproblem of network alignment, is well known to be NP-complete [15]; and (2) that any effective approach should look for approximated, rather than exact, corresponding (sub)networks, to accurately factor in the possible modifications determined by the evolutive processes of the species [5] and the high number of both false positive and false negative interaction data currently available.

The problem of aligning PPI networks has been studied by several researchers [1,4,6–9,11–14,16–24,26–32]. However, there is still room for improvement in terms of both efficiency and biological relevance of the results obtained. Indeed, since PPI network alignment involves the subgraph isomorphism calculation that is computationally hard, in general there is a tradeoff between the efficiency of an alignment algorithm and the quality of the results that it yields. Indeed, exhaustive search, able to single out the top-scoring alignments, according to a given scoring schema, is often impractical because of the size of involved PPI networks. Thus, the research area concerning the design and development of computational techniques for PPI network alignment is still open and worth investigating.

In this context, the goal of this chapter is to review the state of the art and analyze and compare various aspects of available PPI network alignment algorithms. In particular, the following facets will be considered: (1) adopted network model, (2) similarity measures exploited to assess protein similarity, (3) *local* versus *global* PPI network alignment, (4) *pairwise* versus *multiple* PPI network alignment, (5) additional biological information exploited (e.g., phylogenetic information), (6) validation method, and (7) data used for the evaluation.

Some relevant data pertaining to the comparisons carried out in this chapter are listed in Table 22.1 (concerning points 1–5) and Table 22.2 (concerning points 6 and 7).

The remainder of this chapter is organized as follows. The next section starts by providing some background information. Moreover, a basic comparison of the PPI network alignment techniques, focusing on points 1–4, is developed. Section 22.3 briefly describes the algorithms and tools and compares them on point (5). In Section 22.4, a coarse-grain comparison is carried out with respect to points (6) and (7). Finally, Section 22.5 discusses the strengths and weaknesses of the approaches considered and draws some conclusions.

22.2 PRELIMINARIES

This section starts by providing some background information on how PPI networks can be modeled and on the different types of PPI network alignment. Hence, PPI network alignment algorithms will be compared along the following directions:

1. Adopted network model
2. Similarity measures exploited to assess protein similarity
3. *Local* versus *global* PPI network alignment
4. *Pairwise* versus *multiple* PPI network alignment

Some relevant data pertaining the comparison carried out in this section are listed in Table 22.1.

22.2.1 Biological Network Modeling (Point 1)

A protein–protein interaction network of a given organism is commonly represented by an undirected graph $G = (P, I)$ (see Fig. 22.1), in which the set of nodes P denotes the set of proteins of that organism and the edge set I encodes the set of interactions between pairs of proteins. In the most general definition, each edge $e \in I$ takes the form of a triplet $e = \langle p_i, p_j, w_{i,j} \rangle$, where $p_i, p_j \in P$ are the interacting proteins and $w_{i,j} \in [0, 1]$ denotes the reliability for that interaction to be actually held under the particular experimentally measured conditions. Realiability scores usually depend on the number and type of experiments in which the interaction has been observed. This modeling of PPI networks has been adopted in all of the approaches reviewed, but only in some of them [9,11,12,14,17,23,28,29] the edge labels have actually been used to incorporate reliability information. Techniques that do not take into account reliability information can be assumed to manage graphs with all the edge weights set to 1.

TABLE 22.1   Comparison Summary[a]

Algorithm or Tool	Edge Weights (1)	Node Similarity (2)	Local versus Global (3)	Pairwise versus Multiple (4)	Biological Information (5)
PathBlast [19]	No	Sequence	Local	Pairwise	—
NetworkBlast [27]	No	Sequence	Local	Multiple (3 species)	—
NetworkBlast-M [18]	No	Sequence	Local	Multiple	Phylogenetic information
Sharan et al. [26]	No	Sequence	Local	Pairwise	—
Graemlin [14]	Yes	Nonoverlapping homologous groups	Local	Pairwise	Phylogenetic information
Graemlin 2.0 [13]	No	Sequence	Local	Multiple	Phylogenetic information
Bandyopadhyay et al. [4]	No	Inparanoid clusters	Local	Pairwise	—
MaWish [20]	No	Sequence	Local	Pairwise	—
Hirsh and Sharan [17]	Yes	Sequence	Local	Pairwise	—
IsoRank [28]	Yes	Sequence	Global	Pairwise	—
IsoRankM [29]	Yes	Sequence	Global	Multiple	—
Isorank-N [23]	Yes	Sequence	Global	Multiple	—
Dutkowski and Tiuryn [7]	No	Nonoverlapping homologous groups	Local	Multiple	Phylogenetic information
Bi-Grappin [12]	Yes	Sequence	Local	Pairwise	—
Sub-Grappin [11]	Yes	Sequence	Local	Pairwise	—
QSim [8]	No	Inparanoid clusters, sequence	Local	Pairwise	—
Zaslavskiy et al. [32]	No	Inparanoid clusters	Global	Pairwise	—
Domain [16]	No	—(edge similarity)	Local	Pairwise	Domain composition of proteins
Ali and Deane [1]	No	Sequence and functional (GO)	Local	Pairwise	—
HopeMap [30]	No	KEGG orthologous groups	Local	Pairwise	—
Towfic et al. [31]	No	Sequence	Global	Pairwise	—
PISwap [6]	No	Sequence	Global	Pairwise	—
GRAAL [21]	No	Topological	Global	Pairwise	—
H-GRAAL [24]	No	Topological	Global	Pairwise	—
MI-GRAAL [22]	No	Sequence and topological	Global	Pairwise	—
ABINET [9]	Yes	Sequence	Global	Paiwise	—

[a]Points 1–7, in column headings in this table and Table 22.2, are described at the end of Section 22.1.

TABLE 22.2   Evaluation and Results Validation

Algorithm or Tool	Validation Method (6)	Analysed Organisms (7)	Databases (7)
PathBlast [19]	Statistical significance, MIPS and TIGR categories	S. cerevisiae, H. pylori	DIP
Network Blast [27]	Cross-validation, MIPS complexes, GO annotations	S. cerevisiae, C. elegans, D. melanogaster	DIP
Network Blast-M [18]	GO annotations	S. cerevisiae, C. elegans, D. melanogaster, and 10 microbial networks	DIP and generated via SRINI algorithm
Sharan et al. [26]	Jaccard distance, MIPS complexes	S. cerevisiae, H. pylori	DIP
Graemlin [14]	KEGG orthologous groups, GO annotations	10 microbial networks	Generated via SRINI algorithm
Graemlin 2.0 [13]	KEGG complexes	S. cerevisiae, C. elegans, D. melanogaster, M. musculus, H. sapiens	DIP, IntAct, Stanford NetDB
Bandyopadhyay et al. [4]	Cross-validation	S. cerevisiae, D. melanogaster	DIP
MaWish [20]	Statistical significance	S. cerevisiae, C. elegans, D. melanogaster	BIND, DIP
Hirsh and Sharan [17]	MIPS complexes, GO annotations	S. cerevisiae, D. melanogaster	DIP
IsoRank [28]	Manually case-by-case	S. cerevisiae, D. melanogatser	GRID, DIP
IsoRankM [29]	GO annotations	S. cerevisiae, C. elegans, D. melanogaster, M. musculus, H. sapiens	—
Isorank-N [23]	GO and KEGG annotations	S. cerevisiae, C. elegans, D. melanogaster, M. musculus, H. sapiens	BioGRID, DIP, HPRD
Dutkowski and Tiuryn [7]	MIPS categories	S. cerevisiae, C. elegans, D. melanogaster	DIP
Bi-Grappin [12]	Manually case-by-case	S. cerevisiae, C. elegans, D. melanogaster	DIP
Sub-Grappin [11]	Manually case-by-case	S. cerevisiae, D. melanogaster	DIP, MINT
QSim [8]	GO annotations	S. cerevisiae, D. melanogaster	DIP
Zaslavskiy et al. [32]	Orthologous groups of HomoloGene	S. cerevisiae, D. melanogaster	DIP

(Continued)

TABLE 22.2 *(Continued)*

Algorithm or Tool	Validation Method (6)	Analysed Organisms (7)	Databases (7)
Domain [16]	MIPS complexes, GO annotations	*S. cerevisiae, C. elegans, D. melanogaster*	DIP
Ali and Deane [1]	MIPS complexes, GO annotations	*S. cerevisiae, C. elegans, D. melanogaster, H. sapiens*	DIP, HPRD
HopeMap [30]	KEGG orthologous groups, GO annotations	*S. cerevisiae, E. coli, S. crescentus, D. melanogaster, S. typhimurium*	DIP, Stanford NetDB
Towfic et al. [31]	GO annotations	*S. cerevisiae, D. melanogaster, M. musculus, H. sapiens*	DIP
PISwap [6]	Orthologous groups of HomoloGene, GO annotations	*S. cerivisiae, C. elegans, D. melanogaster*	—
GRAAL [21]	Statistical significance, GO annotations, sequence similarity	*S. cerevisiae, H. sapiens*	—
H-GRAAL [24]	Statistical significance, GO annotations, sequence similarity	*S. cerevisiae, H. sapiens*	—
MI-GRAAL [22]	GO annotations	4 bacteria	—
ABINET [9]	GO annotations	*S. cerevisiae, E. coli, D. melanogaster, H. pylori, H. sapiens*	BioGRID, DIP

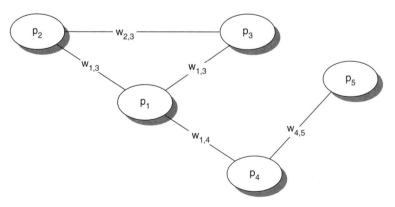

Figure 22.1 An example of protein–protein interaction network graph.

22.2.2 Node Similarity Computation (Point 2)

Generally, the similarity between pairs of proteins (nodes) is computed by exploiting some properties of the two proteins. A common way to compute protein similarity is to consider the score obtained by aligning their amino acid sequences. The alignment of two protein amino acid sequences is a way of arranging the two sequences in order to identify similarity regions (deriving from functional, structural, or evolutionary relationships between the sequences). One of the most widely used programs to align protein sequences is BLAST (basic local alignment search tool) [2]. The output of a BLAST alignment is an expectation value (the so called *E-value*). The lower the *E-value* is, the more significant the alignment is. Several of the techniques reviewed [1,6,8,9,11–13,17–20,22,23,26–29,31] exploit the results obtained from protein sequence alignments for computing node similarity scores.

Another way to compute protein similarity, used by some of the approaches discussed here [4,7,8,14,30,32], is the exploitation of orthologous groups. An orthologous group contains proteins that have evolved from a common ancestor protein and may perform similar functions. Thus, two proteins belonging to the same orthologous group can be considered similar.

One of the approaches reviewed, QSim [8], computes the node similarity on the bases of both the previous information. Indeed, it assigns a similarity value equals to 1 to protein pairs belonging to the same orthologous group and a value computed exploiting the sequence similarity otherwise.

Protein similarity can also be computed on the basis of protein functional information and, in this respect, protein gene ontology (GO) annotations [3] can be used. GO is a standardized classification scheme that categorizes protein functions into cellular component, molecular function, and biological process. GO functional annotations of a protein can refer to one or more of such categories. Some of the algorithms proposed to align PPI networks [1] exploit protein functional similarity either alone or in combination with sequence similarity.

Only one [16] out the 26 approaches computes edge similarity, on the basis of protein functional domain composition, instead of node similarity.

Only few of the proposed algorithms [21,22] do not exploit any kind of biological information to compute node similarity but make use of only information about the structure of the PPI networks involved in the alignment process.

22.2.3 Local versus Global PPI Network Alignment (Point 3)

The ultimate goal of network alignment is to identify an alignment among the input PPI networks, which corresponds to a mapping among their nodes. These mappings may be partial or complete, and this distinction led to the definition of two classes of alignment algorithms:

- *Local PPI Network Alignment (LNA) Algorithms.* These algorithms attempt to discover similar subnetworks between two (or possibly more) PPI networks and require neither that the discovered similar subnetworks cover all the nodes in the input networks nor that they do not overlap.

- *Global PPI Network Alignment (GNA) Algorithms.* These algorithms attempt to find a unique, major alignment among the whole input networks and require that all the nodes of the input networks have to be involved in the alignment.

Thus, GNA algorithms aim at finding a single consistent mapping while LNA algorithms attempt to identify several smaller mappings. Initially, researchers focused only on the LNA problem and developed several tools capable to face it [1,4,7,8,11–14,16–20,26,27,30]. Only after some time has the GNA problem has been introduced along with tools able to solve it [6,9,21–24,28,29,31,32].

22.2.4 Pairwise versus Multiple PPI Network Alignment (Point 4)

Another interesting line of comparison among the algorithms proposed for aligning PPI networks is the distinction among those designed to align a pair of PPI networks and those able to align more than two PPI networks.

In a first stage, the developed algorithms were pairwise alignment algorithms; thus, the majority of alignment techniques currently available belong to this category [1,4,6,8,9,11,12,14,16,17,19–22,24,26,28,30–32]. Then, as a natural evolution, more sophisticated techniques able to deal with multiple PPI networks were introduced, some of them efficient enough to align three PPI networks simultaneously [27] and others efficient enough to handle several PPI networks in a reasonable amount of time and using a reasonable amount of resources [7,13,18,23,29].

22.2.5 Approximation Handling

Protein–protein interaction network alignment algorithms try to align two or more PPI networks to identify *similar* portions that probably, were conserved during the evolution. This means that the aligned (sub)networks contain proteins performing similar functions that have similar interaction patterns. The keyword in this context is *similar*. Indeed, algorithms suitable for PPI network alignment should look for approximated rather than exact alignments. Approximation handling is necessary to deal with the events that, during evolution, can modify the structure of PPI networks and also to take into account the high number of both false negative and false positive interaction data currently available.

The most important events that can modify the structure of a PPI network are *gene duplication*, which causes the addition of new nodes (proteins), and *link dynamics*, corresponding to gain or loss of interactions (edges) through mutations in proteins [5]. Hence, to handle these biological events, different types of approximation should be taken into account: (1) *node insertions*, corresponding to the addition of nodes in one of the input PPI networks; (2) *node mismatch*, corresponding to a pair of proteins characterized by low similarity, but sharing

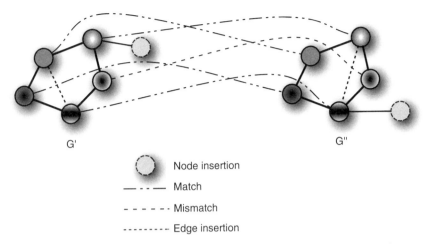

Figure 22.2   An example of approximated alignment of two PPI networks.

similar characteristics (e.g., proteins sharing similar interaction patterns); and
(3) *edge insertions*, corresponding to the addition of interactions in one of the
input PPI networks. As a result, some of the nodes of one network may not
correspond to any node of the other network(s), some corresponding nodes may
have low similarity, and some interactions may be missed in the alignment (see
Fig. 22.2 for an example).

Given a set of input PPI networks, alignment algorithms usually associate a
score with each possible alignment (mapping of the nodes) of the input networks
and try to find the alignment having the maximum score. Of course, in this
respect, approximations occurring in a particular alignment should penalize the
ranking of this alignment in the overall set of alignments.

22.3   METHODS (Point 5)

The problem of aligning PPI networks has been studied by several researchers.
Hence, several tools [1,4,6–9,11–14,16–24,26–32] have been made available.
These tools are briefly discussed in the remainder of this section.

22.3.1   Local PPI Network Alignment Algorithms

The first approach proposed to align PPI networks is PathBlast [19]. PathBlast
is able to identify the conserved pathways across a pair of input networks. The
method starts by building a global alignment graph, where each node represents
a pair of similar proteins, one from each input network, and edges represent
either conserved interactions or gaps (corresponding to both node insertions and
deletions) or mismatches. The method is based on a linear time (in terms of the

number of edges of the alignment graph) procedure, that makes usage of dynamic programming, for the identification of conserved pathways. PathBlast has been extended into NetworkBlast [27], a tool for discovering conserved pathways and complexes across more than two PPI networks. Such an extension is based on the idea that each node of the alignment graph identifies a group of homologous proteins, instead of only a pair of them. NetworkBlast, in turn, has been subsequently extended to NetworkBLAST-M [18], which is based on a particular representation of the alignment graph that has linear size with respect to the size of the input PPI networks, obtained by avoiding the explicit representation of every set of potentially orthologous proteins, thus gaining in efficiency. NetworkBLAST-M is based on progressive alignments and uses phylogenetic information in order to guide the alignment.

Sharan et al. [26] proposed a probabilistic method, based on a probabilistic model, for the local paiwise alignment of PPI networks. In particular, the input PPI networks are combined for obtaining an *orthology graph* in which nodes are pairs of orthologous proteins and the edges, representing interactions, are weighted using the probabilistic model. In this way, the alignment problem is translated into the problem of identifying high-weight complexes of densely interacting proteins.

Graemlin [14] is an algorithm for multiple network alignment that introduces a probabilistic formulation of the topology matching problem. According to the algorithm formulation, the groups of aligned proteins have to be disjoint and represent homologous groups. To search for alignment between two input networks, Graemlin generates a set of seeds from each input network, where each seed is a set of close proteins, in order to cut search space. Then, by enumerating the seeds between the two networks, it tries to transform each of them, in turn, into an high-scoring alignment. When applied to multiple networks, Graemlin uses a phylogenetic tree and successively aligns the closest pairs of networks. After each stage of the alignment, it obtains several new networks, each of which is placed as a parent of the two aligned networks. The method iterates this process until all the networks are at the root of the tree. Graemlin has been extended by Graemlin 2.0 [13], which introduces a novel scoring function and an algorithm that automatically learns the scoring function's parameters and that is able to align multiple networks in linear time.

Bandyopadhyay et al. [4] proposed a strategy to identify functionally related proteins supplementing sequence-based comparisons with information on conserved protein–protein interactions. The idea is that the probability of functional orthology of a pair of proteins is influenced by the probability of functional orthology of their neighbor proteins. This method first aligns two PPI networks using only sequence similarities, and in particular by using Inparanoid clusters for pairing the proteins of the two input networks, and then perform probabilistic inference to identify pairs of proteins that are likely to retain the same function.

MaWIsh [20] is a tool that implements a duplication divergence model to carry out pairwise network alignment. In particular, this system merges the two input networks into a single alignment graph, formulates network alignment as a maximum-weight-induced subgraph problem, and proposes several heuristics to solve it. The duplication/divergence model is used to accurately identify and interpret conservation of interactions, complexes, and modules across species. Indeed, this model allows to discover alignments that take into account conjectures about the structure of the network of the common ancestor.

Hirsh and Sharan [17] proposed a new probabilistic model for aligning the PPI networks of two species, based on a model describing the evolution of the identified protein complexes from an ancestral species. First, this technique builds the alignment graph [19,27], by using sequence similarity information, and identifies clusters of conserved interactions. Then, the identified protein complexes are scored according to their fit to the model with respect to the likelihood that they arise at random.

Dutkowski and Tiuryn proposed an approach [7] based on the phylogenetic history of proteins and a stochastic evolutionary model of interaction emergence, loss, and conservation. The first stage of the approach is the reconstruction of the conserved ancestral PPI (CAPPI) network. In more detail, it concerns the reconstruction of the hypothetical sequence of evolutionary events (duplications, deletions, and speciations), by which the proteins of the input PPI networks evolved from their counterparts in the common ancestral network. In the second step, the posterior probabilities of interactions between proteins at each stage of evolution are determined using a stochastic model. The topology of the ancestral network (and of each network at each stage of evolution) is determined by the most probable interactions. Finally, conserved ancestral interactions in the CAPPI network are identified and are projected back onto the input networks to determine the alignment.

Bi-Grappin [12] is a tool proposed for aligning two PPI networks by identifying proteins that share both significant sequence similarity and similar neighbor topologies. It starts from initial similarity values based only on sequence similarity and for each pair of possibly matching proteins (that share a sequence similarity above a certain threshold). It then refines their similarity by comparing their neighborhoods at different distances. The greater the distance of the compared neighborhoods is, the lower the influence of their similarity or dissimilarity is on the protein pairs. Bi-Grappin has been subsequently exploited as a module for a local pairwise alignment algorithm called sub-Grappin [11] that iterates (i) an application of Bi-Grappin for obtaining refined node similarity values that incorporate topological information and (ii) an execution of a procedure called Collapse that recursively merges pairs of nodes in progressively larger corresponding subgraphs.

QSim [8] is a tool proposed to align two PPI networks that recall the same idea as Bi-Grappin according to which two proteins are similar if they both share a significant sequence similarity and their neighborhoods are similar. QSim has been obtained by an adaptation of an existing algorithm for network simulation. The peculiarity of this tool is that it performs an asymmetric alignment in the sense that it searches for local matches of one network into the other. This translate in the fact that, in contrast to Bi-Grappin, when computing the maximum matching between two neighborhoods, it allows the same protein of the second network to correspond to more than one protein in the first network. QSim starts by computing an initial similarity value for each pair of proteins and then refines the initial similarities by estimating the similarity of protein neighborhoods. It stops when the estimated similarity values converge to a unique global optimum.

Domain [16] is a tool for domain-oriented alignment of PPI networks. It follows a *direct edge alignment* paradigm that is alternative to the common *node-than-edge* one. According to this paradigm, the peculiarity of Domain is that it does not explicitly identify homologous proteins, but directly aligns PPIs across species by decomposing them in terms of their constituent domain–domain interactions (DDIs). In more detail, Domain consists of three stages:

1. Construction of a complete set of alignable pairs of edges (APE). A pair of edges is said to be alignable if there exists a DDI that can plausibly mediate the two associated PPIs.
2. Building of an APE graph, an undirected weighted graph, where nodes correspond to the identified APEs, and edges correspond to evolutionary relationships.
3. Exploitation of a heuristic search to identify high-scoring non-redundant subgraphs from the resultant APE graph.

Ali and Deane [1] proposed a method for aligning PPI networks that exploits a protein functional similarity measure based on protein GO annotations. Four scores are assigned to each edge (representing an interaction) to take into account different contributions. The first two contributions are obtained by two alignments of the input networks according to sequence and functional similarity only. The two alignments provide, for each edge, two different alignment scores, one from the sequence-based alignment and the other from the function-based alignment. The third score is a graph-based score computed by mixing a cluster coefficient, that is, a local network measure of how close a node and its neighbors are to being a clique, and a normalized edge betweenness value, which factors in, for each edge, the number of shortest paths between its ends. Finally, the fourth score encompasses the information obtained from coexpression data. These four scores are combined to obtain a single edge weight. Starting from the so built graph, the algorithm extracts a set of modules that potentially correspond to conserved functional modules.

HopeMap [30] is an iterative connected components–based algorithm with linear running time for pairwise network alignment. HopeMap is based on the observation that the number of true homologs across species is relatively small compared to the total number of proteins in all species. Thus, HopeMap starts by picking up highly homologous groups and then searches for maximal conserved interaction patterns according to a generic scoring schema. The tool uses the results of homologous clustering to build a network alignment graph, where nodes represent sets of homologous proteins and edges represent conserved protein–protein interactions. This network alignment graph is searched for the strongly connected components (clusters), which are ranked by combining genomic similarity scores, interaction conservation, and functional coherence.

22.3.2 Global PPI Network Alignment Algorithms

IsoRank [28] is an algorithm for pairwise global alignment of PPI networks aiming at finding a correspondence between nodes and edges of the input networks that maximizes the overall match between the two networks. IsoRank works in two stages: (1) it associates a score with each possible match between nodes of the two networks, and (2) it constructs the mapping for the global network alignment by extracting mutually consistent matches according to a bipartite graph-weighted matching performed on the two entire networks. IsoRank has been extended to an approach for multiple network alignment, called IsoRank-M [29]. IsoRank-M is based on the exploitation of an approximate multipartite graph-weighted matching. IsoRank-M was subsequently extended to IsoRankN (IsoRank-Nibble) [23], which relies on spectral clustering on the induced graph of pairwise alignment scores. As it is based on spectral methods, IsoRankN is both error-tolerant and computationally efficient.

Zaslavskiy et al. proposed an approach [32] to globally align PPI networks by reformulating the PPI alignment problem as a graph matching problem. Two problems have been considered in this work. The first problem considers strict constraints on the sequence similarity of matching proteins, while the second one aims at finding an optimal compromise between sequence similarity and interaction conservation in the alignment. In particular, the authors investigate the applicability of modern state-of-the-art exact and approximate methods for solving the two types of graph matching problems.

Towfic et al. [31] proposed a class of algorithms that align PPI networks by subdividing them into subgraphs and recursively aligning this subgraphs (according to the divide-and-conquer paradigm). The subgraphs are compared and scored using graph kernels. In more detail, their algorithm is based on the two following steps: (1) decomposing each input PPI network into smaller subnetworks and (2) computing the alignments of the two networks in terms of the optimal alignments of their subnetworks. The choice of the method for decomposing the two networks and the choice of the scoring function to use for measuring subnetwork similarity defines the particular alignment algorithm within the class.

PISwap [6] is an algorithm for computing the global alignment of two PPI networks based on local optimization. The algorithm starts from an initial alignment based only on sequence information and proceeds by refining this alignment exploiting information about interaction conservation in order to take also into account information about network topology. The refinement phase is based on the progressive swapping of edge pairs for maximizing the total matching score.

Kuchaiev et al. proposed an algorithm called GRAAL [21] that does not exploit any kind of biological information but is based on the topology of the two input networks only. GRAAL exploits a cost function based solely on a measure of network topological similarity. In particular, GRAAL starts with some seed node pairs that have topologically similar neighborhoods and tries to iteratively extend the alignment. GRAAL has been extended into H-GRAAL [24], which utilizes maximum bipartite matching for computing the best alignment between a pair of PPI networks instead of the seed-and-extend approach. H-GRAAL has been subsequently extended to consider any number and type of node similarity measures (topological, sequence-based, functional, etc.), thus obtaining MI-GRAAL [22].

ABINET [9] is a tool for the global alignment of two PPI networks having the peculiarity of computing an asymmetric alignment. Indeed, it uses one of the two input networks as master and the other as slave. The *master* network is the one that guides the alignment, in the sense that the algorithm prefers to maintain the topological characteristics of the *master* network rather than the *slave* one. ABINET works by generating from the *master* network an alignment model, that is, a finite-state automaton in which state transitions are guided by a linearization of the slave network. Matching subgraphs are finally extracted by using the Viterbi algorithm.

22.4 COARSE-GRAIN COMPARISON

In the previous sections, network alignment tools were compared with respect to (1) adopted network model, (2) similarity measures exploited to asses protein similarity, (3) *local* versus *global* PPI network alignment, (4) *pairwise* versus *multiple* PPI network alignment, and (5) additional biological information exploited (e.g., phylogenetic information). In this section a comparison will be carried out along the following further directions: (6) validation of results and (7) data used for the evaluation.

Some relevant data pertaining the comparison carried out in this section are listed in Table 22.2.

22.4.1 Validation of Results (Point 6)

Various methods are used to validate the results obtained during the experimental evaluation of the PPI network alignment algorithms.

Some algorithms exploit as a basic measure of the *goodness* of the results obtained, some measures borrowed from other fields: (1) the statistical significance of the results [19–21,24], that is, the probability that the same results would not be obtained on random data; (2) some clustering coefficients as the Jaccard distance [26]; and (3) some well-known data mining techniques such as cross-validation [4].

As for the biological validation of results, a very basic method of validation, adopted by some approaches [11,12,28], is the manual case-by-case analysis for checking the presence of well-known functional modules.

For those algorithms that considered no biological information but only topological information during the alignment process [21,24], a good parameter for estimating biological significance is the sequence similarity of aligned proteins.

Some basic validation methods exploit annotations to the Munich Information Center for Protein Sequences (MIPS), KEGG or gene ontology (GO), or information about orthologous groups (e.g., HomoloGene, Inparanoid). These methods are based on checking the portion of aligned pairs of proteins that share some common annotation or that are in the same orthologous group [8,9,21,22,24,32].

Some researchers, to assess the biological significance of results, used the functional enrichment or coherence computed for the obtained aligned complexes with respect to some functional categories of MIPS [16,19], the Institute for Genomic Research (TIGR) [19], GO annotations [1,6,14,16–18,23,27,28,30,31], and KEGG annotations [23]. Functional enrichments identify the set of annotations that annotate a group of proteins with a significant p-value. The functional coherence of a complex, on the other hand, is computed as the average pairwise functional coherence of the aligned protein pairs (the *functional coherence* of a protein pair is the median of the portion of GO terms to which both proteins are annotated).

More sophisticated measures are related to the *specificity* and the *sensitivity* of the alignment techniques. In this respect, the *purity* of an identified complex is computed as the portion of proteins that are annotated to the same category [7,16,17,19]. A complex is considered *pure* if (1) it has at least three annotated proteins and (2) the portion of proteins annotated to the same category exceeds a given threshold (the threshold can be 50% [19] or 75% [16,17]).

The *specificity* has been defined in several ways:

- The percentage or portion of identified complexes that are functionally coherent [18]
- The portion of identified complexes that have purity ≥ 0.5 [26]
- The number of enriched aligned complexes [14]
- The average, over all aligned complexes, of the fraction of aligned proteins in each complex that also belong to the same KEGG pathway [13]
- The portion of aligned complexes with significant match in MIPS [16,17].

The *sensitivity* has been also defined, by the different research groups, in different ways:

- The number of distinct annotation categories covered [18]
- The number of identified complexes for which there is a MIPS category containing at least half of its proteins, divided by the number of MIPS category with at least three annotated proteins [26]
- The number of KEGG pathways that are correctly aligned in the two species [14]
- The average, over all KEGG pathways, of the portion of proteins in each KEGG pathway that are also in the same aligned complexes [13]
- The portion of MIPS complexes that have a significant match with respect to the aligned complexes [16,17].

22.4.2   Data Used for the Evaluation (Point 7)

The approaches developed for aligning PPI networks were tested by their developers on the networks of different organisms, and the interaction data used for the evaluation have been extracted from several databases.

The best characterized organism is *Saccharomyces cerevisiae*, which is a common species of yeast. *S. cerevisiae* was the first eukaryotic genome that was completely sequenced; it is very well characterized, and many yeast proteins and protein complexes are annotated to functional categories. Indeed, for example, many proteins important in human biology were first discovered by studying their homologs in yeast. For these reasons, *S. cerevisiae* is a good benchmark for assessing the biological relevance of the results obtained by an alignment algorithm and, indeed, several approaches for PPI network alignment have been evaluated using this organism [1,4,6–9,11–13,16–21,23,24,26–28,30–32].

The first database in which the interaction data among the proteins of different organisms have been collected is DIP (Database of Interacting Proteins); hence, it has been the most widely used one during the experimental campaign of the PPI network alignment tools [1,4,7–9,11–13,16–20,23,26–28,30–32]. In subsequent years, a large number of further databases storing PPI data have been created and used for obtaining PPI data, such as IntAct [13], Stanford NetDB [13,30], BIND [20], GRID [28], BioGRID [9,23], HPRD [1,23] and MINT [11].

22.5   CONCLUDING REMARKS

This chapter has presented a comparative review of the methods developed for the problems encountered in both *local* and *global* alignment of protein–protein interaction networks. Hopefully, this investigation has been useful for identifying missing requirements in current PPI network alignment solutions and has opened paths of research in this context.

Indeed, even if in the last few years several tools have been developed and some of them are efficient and effective, none of them seems to be yet sufficiently consistent with all the requirements of any biologists. In fact, some of the tools do not yet exploit all the additional available information (e.g., protein annotations or interaction reliability coefficients) that might improve the quality of results.

However, despite these limitations, the results obtained by these techniques are surprising and biologically meaningful, thus making this area a promising field for future investigative research. Indeed, the comparative analysis, and thus the alignment, of PPI networks can help in significantly improving our knowledge of biological data and mechanisms on the basis of life processes.

REFERENCES

1. Ali W, Deane CM, Functionally guided alignment of protein interaction networks for module detection, *Bioinformatics* **25**(23):3166–3173 (2009).

2. Altschul SF, Gish W, Miller W, Myers EW, Lipman DJ, Basic local alignment search tool, *J. Mol. Biol.* **215**(3):403–410 (1990).

3. Ashburner M, Ball C, Blake J, Botstein D, Butler H, Cherry M, Davis A, Dolinski K, Dwight S, Eppig J, Gene ontology: Tool for the unification of biology, *Nat. Genet.* **25**(1):25–29 (2000).

4. Bandyopadhyay S, Sharan R, Ideker T, Systematic identification of functional orthologs based on protein network comparison, *Genome Res.* **16**(3):428–435 (2006).

5. Berg J, Lassig M, Wagner A, Structure and evolution of protein interaction networks: A statistical model for link dynamics and gene duplications, *BMC Evolut. Biol.* **4**(1):51FF. (2004).

6. Chindelevitch L, Liao C-S, Berger B, Local optimization for global alignment of protein interaction networks, *Proc. Pacific Symp. Biocomputing*, 2010, pp. 123–132.

7. Dutkowski J, Tiuryn J, Identification of functional modules from conserved ancestral protein-protein interactions, *Intell. Syst. Mol. Biol./Eur. Conf. Comput. Biol. (ISMB/ECCB)* (*Bioinformatics* Suppl.) **23**(13):149–158 (2007).

8. Evans P, Sandler T, Ungar LH, Protein-protein interaction network alignment by quantitative simulation, *Proc. IEEE International Conference on Bioinformatics and Biomedicine*, 2008, pp. 325–328.

9. Ferraro N, Palopoli L, Panni S, Rombo SE, Asymmetric comparison and querying of biological networks, *IEEE/ACM Trans. Comput. Biol. Bioinform.* **8**(4):876–889 (2011).

10. Fionda V, Palopoli L, Panni S, Rombo SE, Protein-protein interaction network querying by a "focus and zoom" approach, *Proc. International Conference on Bioinformatics Research and Development*, 2008, pp. 331–346.

11. Fionda V, Palopoli L, Panni S, Rombo SE, Extracting similar sub-graphs across ppi networks, *Proc. International Symposium on Computer and Information Sciences*, 2009, pp. 183–188.

12. Fionda V, Palopoli L, Panni S, Rombo SE, A technique to search for functional similarities in protein-protein interaction networks, *Int. J. Data Mining Bioinformatics* **3**(4):431–453 (2009).

13. Flannick J, Novak A, Do CB, Srinivasan B, Batzoglou S, Automatic parameter learning for multiple local network alignment, *J. Comput. Biol.* **16**(8):1001–1022 (2009).

14. Flannick J, Novak A, Srinivasan B, McAdams HH, Batzoglou S, Graemlin: General and robust alignment of multiple large interaction networks, *Genome Res.* **16**(9):1169–1181 (2006).

15. Garey MR, Johnson DS, Computers and Intractability: *A Guide to the Theory of NP-Completeness*, Mathematical Sciences Series, Freeman, 1979.

16. Guo X, Hartemink AJ, Domain-oriented edge-based alignment of protein interaction networks, *Bioinformatics* **25**(12):i240–i246 (2009).

17. Hirsh E, Sharan R, Identification of conserved protein complexes based on a model of protein network evolution, *Bioinformatics* **23**(2):170–176 (2007).

18. Kalaev M, Bafna V, Sharan R, Fast and accurate alignment of multiple protein networks, *J. Comput Biol.* **16**(8):989–999 (2009).

19. Kelley BP, Sharan R, Karp RM, Sittler T, Root DE, Stockwell BR, Ideker T, Conserved pathways within bacteria and yeast as revealed by global protein network alignment, *Proc. Natl. Acad. Sci. USA* **100**(20):11394–11399 (2003).

20. Koyutürk M, Kim Y, Topkara U, Subramaniam S, Szpankowski W, Grama A, Pairwise alignment of protein interaction networks, *J. Comput Biol.* **13**(2):182–199 (2006).

21. Kuchaiev O, Milenkovic T, Memisevic V, Hayes W, Przulj N, Topological network alignment uncovers biological function and phylogeny, *J. R. Soc. Interface* **7**(50):1341–1354 (2010).

22. Kuchaiev O, Przulj N, Integrative network alignment reveals large regions of global network similarity in yeast and human, *Bioinformatics* **27**(10):1390–1396 (2011).

23. Liao C-S, Lu K, Baym M, Singh R, Berger B, Isorankn: Spectral methods for global alignment of multiple protein networks, *Bioinformatics* **25**(12):i253–i258 (2009).

24. Milenković T, Ng Leong WL, Hayes W, Przulj N, Optimal network alignment with graphlet degree vectors, *Cancer Informatics* **9**:121–137 (2010).

25. Sharan R, Ideker T, Modeling cellular machinery through biological network comparison, *Nat. Biotechnol.* **24**(4):427–433 (2006).

26. Sharan R, Ideker T, Kelley B, Shamir R, Karp RM, Identification of protein complexes by comparative analysis of yeast and bacterial protein interaction data, *J. Comput. Biol.* **12**(6):835–846 (2005).

27. Sharan R, Suthram S, Kelley RM, Kuhn T, McCuine S, Uetz P, Sittler T, Karp RM, Ideker T, Conserved patterns of protein interaction in multiple species, *Proc. Natl. Acad. Sci. USA* **102**(6):1974–1979 (2005).

28. Singh R, Xu J, Berger B, Pairwise global alignment of protein interaction networks by matching neighborhood topology, *Proc. Annual International Conference on Research in Computational Molecular Biology*, 2007, vol. **4453**, pp. 16–31.

29. Singh R, Xu J, Berger B, Global alignment of multiple protein interaction networks with application to functional orthology detection, *Proc. Natl. Acad. Sci. USA* **105**(35):12763–12768 (2008).

30. Tian W, Samatova NF, Pairwise alignment of interaction networks by fast identification of maximal conserved patterns, *Proc. Pacific Symp. Biocomputing*, 2009, pp. 99–110.

31. Towfic F, West Greenlee MH, Honavar V, Aligning biomolecular networks using modular graph kernels, *Proc. Workshop on Algorithms for Bioinformatics (WABI)*, 2009, pp. 345–361.

32. Zaslavskiy M, Bach FR, Vert J-P, Global alignment of protein-protein interaction networks by graph matching methods, *Bioinformatics* **25**(12):i259–i267 (2009).

PART V

APPLICATION OF PROTEIN BIOINFORMATICS

CHAPTER 23

PROTEIN-RELATED DRUG ACTIVITY COMPARISON USING SUPPORT VECTOR MACHINES

WEI ZHONG and JIEYUE HE

23.1 INTRODUCTION

At present, combinatorial chemistry can produce millions of new molecules at a time. However, this high level of production cannot exhaust the trillions of potential combinations within a few thousand years. The quantitative structure–activity relationship (QSAR) analysis is required to restrict the search space to avoid produce and test every possible molecular combination. QSAR analysis is very important for understanding the correlation between the molecule's activities and structure. Intelligent machine learning techniques are important tools for QSAR analysis. As a result, these techniques are integrated into the drug production process. The effective intelligent computational model can reduce the cost of drug design significantly by producing the sublibrary of molecular combination derived from a much larger library. This survey compares the performance of several popular machine learning technique for drug activity. The machine learning techniques introduced in this chapter are used to predict activity of pyrimidines and triazines based on the structure–activity relationship of these compounds. Pyrimidines and triazines are two important inhibitors of *Escherichia coli* dihydrofolate reductase (DHFR). Analysis and prediction of activities of these two inhibitors is very important for finding potential treatment agents for malaria, bacterial infection, and other serious disease. This chapter focuses especially on granular kernel trees (GKTs). GKTs are designed to include previous domain knowledge and voting schemes in order to optimize the performance of the SVM kernels and reduce the training time substantially.

Algorithmic and Artificial Intelligence Methods for Protein Bioinformatics. First Edition.
Edited by Yi Pan, Jianxin Wang, Min Li.
© 2014 John Wiley & Sons, Inc. Published 2014 by John Wiley & Sons, Inc.

23.2 RELATED STUDIES FOR PYRIMIDINES DRUG ACTIVITY COMPARISON

Combinatorial chemistry has helped produce hundreds, thousands, and even millions of new molecular compounds at a time [3]. This high-throughout production cannot exhaust the trillions of potential combinations within a few thousand years. Consequently, much faster searching process is required to produce and test thousands of molecular combinations in a short amount of time. quantitative structure–activity relationship (QSAR) analysis has been increasingly applied to the drug production process [3]. QSAR is one of the most important techniques in reducing the search space for new drugs. An effective intelligent system based on QSAR analysis for drug screening can produce significant economic benefit. The assumption of QSAR is that the variation of biological activity among a group of molecular compounds is closely related to the variation of their respective structural and chemical features. QSAR tries to search a set of rules or functions that can predict a molecule's activity using its physicochemical descriptors. QSAR focuses on chemical reactivity, biological activity, and toxicity [3]. This kind of analysis is needed to study the relationship between attributes of a finite number of compounds and a known target activity. The dataset in the QSAR analysis usually contains few compounds with many attributes, which are difficult for standard statistical approaches. The solution of the QSAR analysis can be used to design the combinatorial library in the initial stage of the production process. Because the number of potential molecular combinations from existing databases is huge, the search space for potentially useful combinations must be reduced greatly. During the virtual screening, QSAR analysis can distinguish molecules that potentially produce a desired effect on synthesis. Consequently, QSAR analysis can help the drug designer construct a small sub-library containing suitable molecules selected from a large and more diverse library [3]. This combinatorial sublibrary is important to identify an interesting molecule, which might potentially lead to drug discovery.

The intelligent computational system has become an important tool for QSAR analysis. After the compounds having diverse biological and chemical activities and functionality are discovered using this system, detailed QSAR analysis is conducted to analyze their relationship. Finally, the predictive rules are used to predict activity of the molecules according to their chemical and physical properties and to discern the relationships among biological activities of compounds. During the analysis process, the biological and chemical activities are evaluated by the log function defined by $\log(1/C)$, where C is the constant value for the inhibitory growth concentration [5].

Many machine learning techniques, including the genetic algorithm (GA) [1], inductive logic programming (ILP) [2], and support vector machines (SVMs) [3], have been proposed for QSAR analysis and drug activity comparison. In these work, one type of *E. coli* dihydrofolate reductase (DHFR) called *pyrimidines* is closely studied [5]. These inhibitors are potential therapeutic agents for treating malaria, bacterial infection, toxoplasma, and cancer.

Hirst and his colleagues compared neural networks (NNs), ILP, and linear regression for modeling activities of pyrimidines using QSAR analysis [2]. They use cross-validation methods in order to conduct a statistically rigorous evaluation of the prediction performance of various methods. The training set and testing set are chosen randomly, and the performances of different methods are developed on the basis of the same training dataset. Molecules in the ILP analysis are represented by features instead of Hansch parameters [2]. Hirst's study used 74 pyrimidines. Biological activities are evaluated by the association constant defined by log (K_i). The dataset used in this study has been widely studied by other QSAR methods. Furthermore, the results generated by the QSAR model are compared with the X-ray stereochemistry of interaction [2]. This particular study used the fivefold cross-validation test. Each of the 55 pyrimidines in the cross-validation study shows up only once in one of the test sets [2]. This study applies neural networks for linear regression. The neural network includes a large number of basic computational units that are connected to one another. Each computational unit performs a weighted sum of incoming signals. The neural networks are organized into several layers including an input layer, hidden layers, and an output layer. In these layers, the signal is propagated forward from the input layers to the output layer through any number of hidden layers. The neural network is modeled to study the mapping function between input and output signals. By updating the weights in well-defined manners based on the learning rules, the sum of the squared error between the target signal and training signals is minimized. Besides the neural network, this work also useds inductive logic programming (ILP) for drug design problems since ILP can be specially designed to discern the relationship between different molecule structures. The logical relationship between different objects can be expressed by a subset of predicate calculus [2]. The ILP program needs three types of facts: (1) positive, (2) negative, and (3) background. The positive facts are the paired example of greater activity [2]. The negative facts are the paired example of lower activity. The ILP program needs both positive and negative facts to generate the balanced results. The background facts consist of the chemical structures of the drugs and the properties of the substituent. The fivefold cross-validations include 2198 background facts, 1394 negative facts, and 1394 positive facts.

Their studies revealed that neural networks and ILP have better performance than linear regression using the attribute representation. ILP analysis can also generate rules for explaining the relationship between the inhibitors' activities and their chemical structures. Rule generation provides better interpretation of the biological activity of the inhibitors and their chemical structure. The study also shows that neural networks tend to overfit on the basis of attribute representation. Hidden units cannot improve the performance of neural networks for QSAR analysis. Experiential results generated from the linear regression and the neural network indicate that the 5-substituent should have a low metabolic rate (MR) value. In contrast, the 3-substituent has a high MR value. The neural network often produced different sets of important attributes as compared to regression analysis. For small datasets, full capability of neural networks may not be fully utilized [2].

Burbride et al. [3] compared several learning algorithms for structure–activity relationship (SAR) analysis, which can be used to reduce the search for new drugs since the different molecular combinations can be studied using the intelligent system. The effective solution for drug search can provide significant economic benefit by accelerating the search process substantially. The goal of SAR analysis is to find a rule that predicts a molecule's biological activities from its physicochemical attributes. In this particular study, they are interested in predicting qualitative biological activity for drug design, using a publicly downloadable dataset [3]. Machine learning techniques are used to study the relationships between different known target activities with respect to the attributes of a finite number of compounds. SAR analysis is used to study many areas of modern drug design. For example, the system developed by this study can be applied to design combinatorial libraries in the early stage of the production process. SAR analysis can be used to search for appropriate molecules for the sublibrary selected from a larger and more diverse library [3]. The datasets used in this study are obtained from the UCI Data Repository. The machine learning techniques are applied to predict the inhibition ability of dihydrofolate reductase using pyrimidines. The QSAR system generally tries to solve the regression problem by learning the posterior probability of the target, given some predictive features. There are three positions of possible substitution in each drug. Each substitution position has several important descriptors, including polarity, size, flexibility, and hydrogen bond donor and acceptor. The system can be used to generate the classification rule. Each rule can be used to predict which of two unseen compounds can potentially perform greater activities. In this study, several machine learning algorithms, including neural networks, the decision tree, and the support vector machine are compared [2]. In the experiment, the prediction performance of SVM for the inhibition of dihydrofolate reductase by pyrimidines is compared with that of several other popular machine learning algorithms. The experimental results show that the prediction performance of SVM is significantly better than that of the artificial neural networks, a radial basis function (RBF) network, and a C5.0 decision tree.

23.3   FEATURE GRANULES AND HIERARCHICAL KERNEL DESIGN

Support vector machines (SVMs) have been extensively applied to many data mining applications with strong generalization capabilities. The training complexity of SVM is highly related to the size of the training sample. For many drug-related studies, the size of the molecule combination is usually potentially very large. How to shorten the SVM training time for a large dataset remains one of the most challenging problems in SVM research. In order to explore the SVM's capacity for drug design and reduce the training time significantly, we focus on the hierarchical kernel design proposed by Jin [5] for drug activity comparison. The principle of the hierarchical kernel design is applied to produce powerful and flexible structures called *granular kernel trees* (GKTs).

The construction of the GKT is divided into four phases:

Phase 1. The feature granules are generated by grouping related features, together on the basis of chemical and biological properties such as molecular structure, feature relationships, or functional similarity [5]. These features can be grouped together by an automatic learning model such as the genetic algorithm.

Phase 2. Granular SVM kernels are chosen from the traditional kernels such as RBF kernels and polynomial kernels. These traditional kernels have shown good performance in many real-world problems. Some special-purpose kernels can be designed to solve some particular problems.

Phase 3. A suitable number of layers, nodes, and connections are selected to construct the tree structure.

Phase 4. The GKT's parameters are optimized by the genetic algorithm (GA). Based on the concept of chromosome, the GAs evaluate the performance of SVMs using the fitness functions. The roulette wheel method is used to select individual chromosome for the new generation. The crossover operation can be performed between two chromosomes to exchange genetic material between two parents. Some of genes in randomly selected chromosomes can be replaced by random values produced in a specified range.

All GKTs take advantage of biological and chemical properties of molecules to optimize kernels effectively. The GKT model can be easily parallelized to reduce the training time significantly. For the GKT model, the input vectors are decomposed into several feature granules according to the possible substituent locations. As a result, each pyrimidine drug pair has six feature granules, each of which has nine features. Two GKT variants, GKT1 and GKT2, are used to model drug activity for pyrimidines [5]. The structures for GKT1 and GKT2 are shown in Figures 23.1, 23.2 and 23.3. GKT1 is a two-layer kernel tree with all granules fused by a sum operation. Each granule pair of GKT2 is represented by a two-layer subtree.

Both GKT1 and GKT2 models use 55 drugs in the pyrimidines dataset [5]. Each drug has three possible substitution positions (R_3, R_4, and R_5). Each substitution position includes nine chemical and biological features. These nine features include polarity, size, flexibility, hydrogen bond donor, and acceptor, π donor and π acceptor, polarizability, and σ effect [5]. Figure 23.4 shows the structure of pyrimidines. Each substituent is represented by nine chemical properties features including polarity, size, flexibility, hydrogen-bond donor, hydrogen-bond acceptor, π donor, π acceptor, polarizability and σ effect. The substituent is used to identify drug activities. Each input vector represents features of two drugs in a specific order. The vector is labeled as positive if the activity of the first drug is higher than that of the second one. Otherwise, it is labeled as negative. The features of input vectors are shown in Figure 23.5. The total number of features for

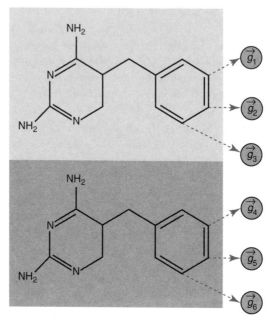

Figure 23.1 Feature granules in the pyrimidine drug pair [5].

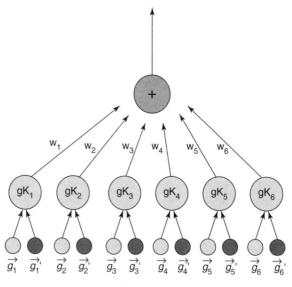

Figure 23.2 GKTs-1 [5].

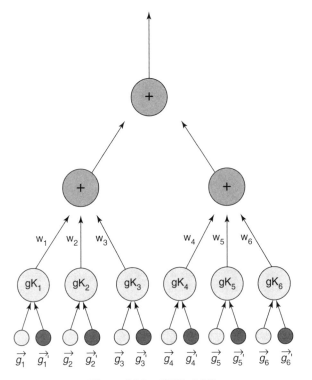

Figure 23.3 GKTs-2 [5].

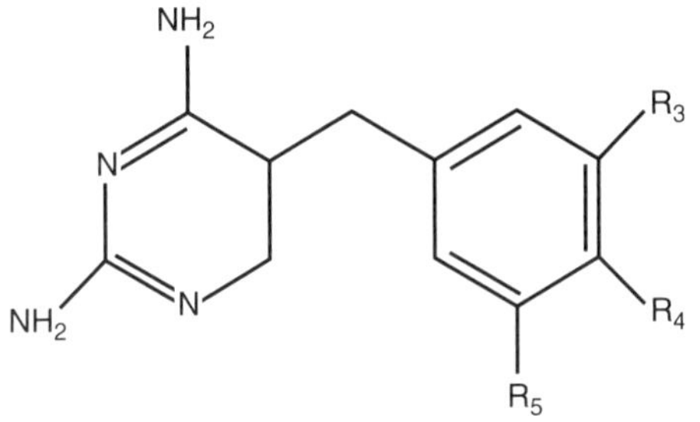

Figure 23.4 Structure of pyrimidines [5].

label	drug1			drug2		
+	9	9	9	9	9	9

	drug2			drug1		
−	9	9	9	9	9	9

Figure 23.5 Sample input vector [5].

each vector is 54. The pyrimidine–dataset is randomly divided into the training set and testing set in the proportion of 4:1. The training set has 44 compounds, and the testing set has 11 compounds.

23.4 EXPERIMENTAL RESULTS FOR DIFFERENT MACHINE LEARNING MODELS

Burbidge compared the performance of SVMs, neural networks, RBF networks, and decision trees on this dataset [3]. Table 23.1 indicates that the prediction accuracy of SVMs is much better than that of other learning algorithms.

Bo discusses performance comparison for SVM, granular kernel trees (GKTs), and evolutionary granular kernel trees (EGKTs) [5]. The RBF kernel functions are selected for SVM training. Fivefold cross-validation is adopted for the pyrimidine training set. For the GA optimization, the probability of crossover is 0.7 and the mutation rate is 0.5 [5]. Performance rates of SVM and three other types of kernel machines are compared in Table 23.2 [5]. This table shows that SVMs combined with GKTs outperform SVMs by 3% and 3.3% on the testing dataset. Furthermore, the fitness values of SVMs using GKTs-1 and GKTs-2 have also improved compared with SVMs. The testing accuracy of SVMs with GKTs-1 is higher than that of SVMs with GKTs-2 [5].

TABLE 23.1   Performance Comparison of SVMs, MLP, RBF Networks, and C5.0 on the Pyrimidine Dataset

Algorithm	Testing Accuracy (%)
SVMs + RBF	87
MLP	86
Pruned neural network	84
Dynamic neural network	85
RBF network	77
C5.0	81

Source: Jin [5].

TABLE 23.2   Performance Comparison for SVMs, GKT1, and GKT2 on the Pyrimidine Dataset

Parameter	SVMs + RBF + Gas (%)	SVMs + GKT1 + Gas (%)	SVMs + GKT2 + Gas (%)
Fitness	84.5	86.6	88.5
Training accuracy	96.8	96.8	98.8
Testing accuracy	88.4	91.7	91.4

Source: Jin [5].

SUMMARY

In this chapter, we have surveyed several machine learning models for drug activity comparison. In particular, we have discussed SVMs and the more advanced model GKT in detail. Since the SVM is a robust and highly accurate intelligent classification model, the kernel of SVM can be customized for QSAR analysis. The comparative study for the sample dataset demonstrates that the GKT1 and GKT2 models outperform several of the most frequently used learning algorithms [5]. The experimental results also demonstrate that the MLP model can achieve similar prediction accuracy but that the training period required for this model is an order of magnitude longer [2]. This becomes a serious issue when using QSAR on a large number of molecular compounds. The performance of other machine techniques such as an RBF network or decision tree is far inferior to that of the SVM [3]. However, since the SVM is a deterministic learning algorithm, it can produce reproducible and verifiable results. During the optimization process, SVM converges to the global, rather than local, optimum, which is a significant advantage as compared to other machine learning techniques. Our survey shows that the SVM has a great potential for application to QSAR analysis in the future.

REFERENCES

1. Devillers J, *Neural Networks and Drug Design*, Academic Press, 1999.
2. Hirst JD, King RD, Sternberg MJE, Quantitative structure-activity relationships by neural networks and inductive logic programming. I. The inhibition of dihydrofolate reductase by pyrimidines, *J. Comput. Aided Mol. Design* **8**(4):405–432 (1994).
3. Burbidge R, Trotter M, Buxton B, Holden S, Drug design by machine learning: Support vector machines for pharmaceutical data analysis, *Comput. Chem.* **26**(1):4–15 (2001).
4. Newman DJ, Hettich S, Blake CL, Merz CJ, *UCI Repository of Machine Learning Databases*, Dept. Information and Computer Science, Univ. California, Irvine, 1998.
5. Bo J, *Evolutionary Granular Kernel Machines*, PhD dissertation, Georgia State University, 2007.

CHAPTER 24

FINDING REPETITIONS IN BIOLOGICAL NETWORKS: CHALLENGES, TRENDS, AND APPLICATIONS

SIMONA E. ROMBO

24.1 INTRODUCTION

For many years, analysis of biological sequences (also termed *biosequences*) associated with proteins and genomes played a key role in understanding the mechanisms inside the cell [7,47,49]. After the genome coding of several organisms was completed [13], significant attention began to focus on studying how cellular components interact with each other to accomplish the biological functions of the cell [59].

While biosequences are usually represented by strings defined on a finite alphabet, where symbols are associated with amino acids or nucleotides, interaction data can be instead modeled by graphs, called *biological networks*, where nodes represent components and edges their interactions. The set of all the protein–protein interactions (PPIs) of a specific organism represents its *interactome*.

Despite the different models adopted to analyze biological data, there is a common peculiarity characterizing them; this is termed their intrinsic *repetitiveness*. The presence of repetitions can be considered biologically *interesting* in many cases, for example, when the presence of repeted elements is discovered among cells belonging to different organisms, or if a specific feature appears several times in the same cell. Often suitable statistical indices can be usefully exploited in order to characterize the significativeness of the repetitions found [51].

Algorithmic and Artificial Intelligence Methods for Protein Bioinformatics. First Edition.
Edited by Yi Pan, Jianxin Wang, Min Li.
© 2014 John Wiley & Sons, Inc. Published 2014 by John Wiley & Sons, Inc.

Searching for common substrings in a set of biosequences can help classify them and predict their biological function [36]. On the other hand, the presence of repeated modules across biological networks was also shown to be very relevant. Indeed, several studies proved that biological networks can often be understood in terms of coalitions of basic repeated building blocks [40,44]. Discovering similar subnetworks in the interactome of different organisms is useful in revealing complex mechanisms at the basis of evolutionary conservations, and to infer the biological meaning of groups of interacting cellular components, possibly belonging to organisms not yet well characterized [53].

The problem of finding interesting repetitions in biological data can be formulated according to different perspectives. In general, if S is a suitable data structure storing the specific biological data under consideration (e.g., a string or a graph), we can distinguish the following three main classes of problems:

1. Given a substructure Q (e.g., a substring or a subgraph), where some elements can also be unspecified, find all portions of S that are *similar* to Q, according to some specific similarity function.

2. Find a set of significative objects $\{P_1, P_2, \ldots, P_n\}$, not specified a priori, such that each p_i *is repeated* in S a number of times over a fixed threshold. A limited number of mismatches are usually allowed in the repetitions.

3. Given a set $\{S_1, S_2, \ldots, S_m\}$ of data structures; find a set of significative objects $\{P_1, P_2, \ldots, P_n\}$, not specified a priori, such that each P_i is *repeated* (but for possible mismatches) in k of the S_j, with k over a fixed threshold.

In both the second and the third formulations of the problem, instead of considering as a gauge of interestingness the frequency of repetitions, other statistical evaluations, such as expectation or Z score, can be suitably exploited as well.

From sequences to networks, the difficulty in solving the problems listed above increases. While most exact algorithms searching for repetitions in biosequences need polynomial time (despite the number of repetitions that can be generated), the case of biological networks is much more complicated, often involving subgraph isomorphism checking, which is known to be NP-complete [27]. Therefore, using exact algorithms to search for repetitions in biological networks is seldom feasible, except in a few cases, for which fixed-parameter tractability (FPT) algorithms were designed [e.g., 6,15]. However, such exact approaches are suitable only for specific contexts, where the most general techniques are based on approximate and heuristic approaches [e.g., 38,56].

The main goal of this chapter is to analyze how the general problem of finding repetitions in biological data evolved from sequences to networks data, by focusing on the open challenges and specific applications in biological networks.

In particular, we first recall some basic notions about the domain under consideration, that is, biological networks (Section 24.2). Then, in Section 24.3, we describe in detail how the three problem formulations listed above can be specialized in both the biological sequence and network domains, and we also provide an overview of the main applications in biological networks (Section 24.4). Finally, in Section 24.5 we draw our conclusive remarks.

24.2 THE BIOLOGICAL NETWORKS DOMAIN

Since the 1990s, both high-throughput experimental techniques [28,34] and computational methods [43,59] have contributed to collection of cellular component interactions, stored in public databases [e.g., 8,30,42]. To model such biological information, suitable networks where interacting components are linked together have been exploited.

Three main types of biological networks have been studied in the literature: *protein–protein interaction* (*PPI*) *networks*, *metabolic networks*, and *gene regulatory networks*. All these networks may be represented as graphs $G = \langle N, E \rangle$, where N is a set of nodes and E is a set of (directed/indirect) edges.

In the following sections, we briefly recall the main characteristics of each kind of biological network.

24.2.1 Protein–Protein Interaction Networks

Proteins are the basic constituents of living beings. It has been shown that studying how proteins interact inside the cell is necessary to understanding the biological processes in which they are involved [59]. Many PPIs have been discovered in the last years [28,34,43].

The set of all the PPIs of a given organism is its *interactome*, usually modeled by an indirect graph, called a *protein–protein interaction network* (PPI network), where nodes represent involved proteins and edges encode their interactions. Figure 24.1 illustrates such a representation for a small portion of the *Saccharomyces cerevisiae* interactome.

Often, a PPI network is represented by its *adjacency matrix*, that is, a binary matrix M where both rows and columns are associated with the proteins in the network, such that $M[i,j] = 1$ if protein i interacts with protein j, and $M[i,j] = 0$ otherwise.

24.2.2 Metabolic Networks

Metabolic networks model the whole set of metabolic and physical processes on the basis of the physiological and biochemical properties of the cell, such as the chemical reactions of metabolisms and the corresponding regulatory interactions. Metabolic networks are often employed to simulate and understand the molecular mechanisms that regulate the organisms, often correlating the genome with aspects of molecular physiology [25,58].

A metabolic network is often modeled by a bipartite graph, where the two types of nodes represent, respectively, reactions and chemical compounds (see Fig. 24.2). Alternatively, a metabolic network can be represented by a compound

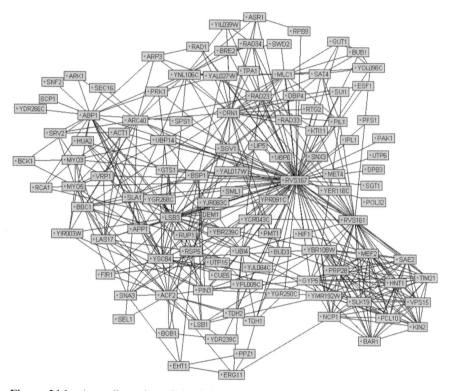

Figure 24.1 A small portion of the *Saccharomyces cerevisiae* interactome, drawn by using PIVOT [45].

graph, that is, a compact version of the bipartite graph where only compound vertices are retained and information on the reactions is stored as edge labels. The reaction graph is the symmetric representation of a compound graph (i.e., reaction vertices are retained and information on the compounds is stored as edge labels). When directed versions of these graphs are considered, the direct edges express the reversibility/irreversibility of some reactions.

24.2.3 Gene Regulatory Networks

Gene regulatory networks denote the genes expressed in the cell in response to biological signals. Gene regulatory networks are also called *transcription regulation networks*, since they describe the interactions between transcription factor proteins and the genes that they regulate [9,37]. Transcription factors respond to biological signals and accordingly change the transcription rate of genes, allowing cells to produce the proteins they need at the appropriate times and amounts [41].

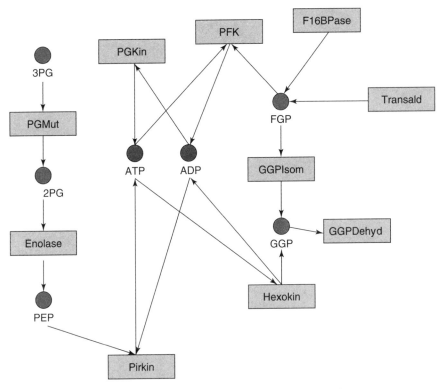

Figure 24.2 An example of a metabolic network.

A gene regulatory network can be represented as a directed graph, in which nodes represent proteins, their corresponding mRNAs, and protein–protein complexes (see Fig. 24.3). In particular, the nodes of a gene regulatory network are also associated with genes, by referring to the DNA sequences that are transcribed into the mRNAs that translate into proteins. Edges between nodes represent individual molecular reactions, the protein–protein and protein–mRNA interactions through which the products of one gene affect those of another one. When interactions are *inductive* (i.e., meaning that an increase in the concentration of one component leads to an increase in the other one), they are represented by arrowheads; when interactions are inhibitory (i.e., when an increase in one component leads to a decrease in the other one), then they are represented by filled circles. A series of edges indicates a chain of such dependences, with cycles corresponding to feedback loops.

A gene regulatory network may also be represented as a *connectivity matrix M*, such that $M_{ij} = 1$ if the component associated with node j encodes a transcription factor regulating the component associated to node i, and $M_{ij} = 0$ otherwise.

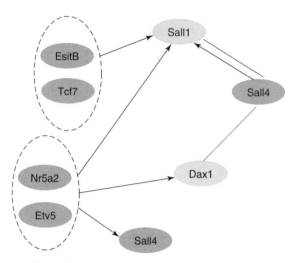

Figure 24.3 A small portion of the gene regulatory network in mouse embryonic stem cells [63].

24.3 PROBLEM FORMULATION

We now consider some technical details concerning the problem of searching for *repetitions* in biological data.

Let S be a complex structure (e.g., a string or a graph) containing basic elements (e.g., characters or nodes). We suppose that all the basic elements in S can be represented as suitable symbols. Let Σ be the finite alphabet containing all such symbols. The following definition is important to understand when substructures of the same kind of S are repeated in S, or in a set of structures like S.

Definition 24.1: Occurrence Let $\mathcal{P}$ be a complex structure of the same type as S, and Σ' be the finite alphabet containing all the symbols associated with the basic elements in $\mathcal{P}$, such that $\Sigma' \cap \Sigma \neq \emptyset$. Furthermore, let $\mathcal{F}$ be a function having two complex structures as its arguments and returning as output their distance, according to some specific formula depending on the context under consideration. A substructure $S' \subset S$ is an *occurrence* of $\mathcal{P}$ iff

$$\mathcal{F}(\mathcal{P}, S') \leq t_h$$

where t_h is a suitable threshold value fixed a priori.

In the biosequences domain, suitable distances that can be adopted are for example the Hamming and the Levenshtein distances. When S is a graph modeling a biological network, the concept of *distance* is less immediately defined. Indeed, the concept of similarity between subgraphs is always to be related to the subgraph isomorphism check, which is a difficult task, as mentioned earlier [27]. Furthermore, several distinct aspects can be taken into account, for example, the focus can be on the similarity between nodes, rather than between edges and structures, according to the specific biological problem under consideration.

Accordingly, different formulations of the problem of finding repetitions in biological data can be provided.

Formulation 24.1: Matching a Query   Let $\mathcal{P}$ be a complex structure, called *query*, of the same type as S, such that the size of $\mathcal{P}$ is much less than the size of S, and let Σ' be the finite alphabet containing all the symbols associated with the basic elements in $\mathcal{P}$, such that $\Sigma' \cap \Sigma \neq \emptyset$. The problem of *matching $\mathcal{P}$ in* S consists in finding all the occurrences of $\mathcal{P}$ in S.

In biosequences analysis, Formulation 24.1 is the analog of string pattern matching, where approximate occurrences can be handled by allowing wild-cards and/or gaps [26]. As an example, let S be a string $s = abccacccbaaa$ $bcbacaabcaaabcccccc$ defined on the finite alphabet $\Sigma = \{a, b, c\}$ and let $\mathcal{P}$ be the string $p = abc \cdot \cdot c$, defined on $\Sigma' = \{a, b, c, \cdot\}$. If $t_h = 2$ and the Hamming distance is considered, it is easy to see that p has three occurrences in s, thus matching p in s the output result set is $\{abccac, abcbac, abccc\}$.

In biological networks analysis, matching a query consists in analyzing an input network, called the *target* network, searching for possible subnetworks that are similar to a query subnetwork of interest. Such a problem, also known as *network querying* [20,62], "is aimed at transferring biological knowledge within and across species" [53]. The so-found subnetworks may indeed correspond to cellular components involved in the same biological processes or performing similar functions than components in the query.

When approximate occurrences are searched for, mismatches possibly including both node/edge insertions and deletions can be allowed as well. The following example clarifies how Formulation 24.1 can be applied to biological networks.

Example 24.1   Consider the query and target networks shown in Figure 24.4. Let Q be the query network and suppose that, given a subnetwork T' of the target network T, the chosen function $\mathcal{F}$ returns to output the number of "differences" between Q qnd T' defined as follows. Let $E_Q = \{\langle q_1, q_2 \rangle, \langle q_1, q_3 \rangle, \ldots, \langle q_h, q_k \rangle\}$ and $E_{T'} = \{\langle t'_1, t'_2 \rangle, \ldots, \langle t'_m, t'_n \rangle\}$ be two sets of pairs individuating the (possibly directed) edges in Q and T', respectively. Then, $\mathcal{F}$ returns the size of the set $E_Q \setminus \{E_Q \cap E_{T'}\}$. Note that $\mathcal{F}$ is equal to zero for pairs of identical subgraphs, such that both nodes and edges overlap.

If $t_h = 2$, the two subgraphs highlighted by a green circle in the target network, together with the subgraph circled by a dashed red line, indicate occurrences of Q in T with respect to $\mathcal{F}$.

Now consider a different distance; that is, for each edge $\langle q_i, q_j \rangle$ in Q, assume that an edge $\langle t'_k, t'_l \rangle$ in T' is searched for such that q_i is equal to t'_k and q_j is equal to t'_l, respectively. For each edge of Q such that the corresponding edge in

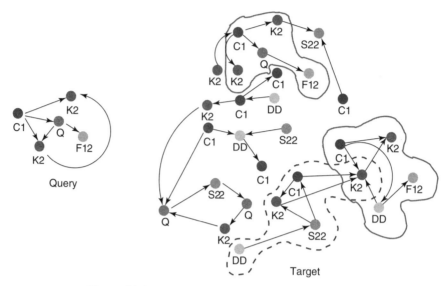

Figure 24.4   Matching a query on biological networks.

T' according to this rule is missing, the distance between Q and T' is increased by one. For each direct path of length 2 in Q, another direct path of length 2 is searched for in T', such that the first node and the last node in the path are equal. For each of such paths in Q that is missed in T', the distance between Q and T' is increased by one.

With this new distance, and by considering a threshold value $t_h = 2$, analogously to the previous case, it is easy to see that the subgraph highlighted by the dashed red line in T' is no longer an occurrence of Q.

Formulation 24.2: Discovering Repetitions in a Single Structure   Let S be a complex structure defined on the finite alphabet Σ of basic elements. *Discovering repetitions in a single structure* corresponds to finding a set of significative substructures $\{P_1, P_2, \ldots, P_n\}$, not specified a priori, such that the number of occurrences of each P_i satisfies some specific constraints making P_i worth to be considered *interesting*.

Formulation 24.2 is related to the concept of *motif*, which has been exploited in different applications of computational biology [3,47]. Depending on the context, *what is a motif* may assume sensibly different meanings. In general, motifs are always associated to repetitive objects. For example, a repeated substring can be considered a motif when its frequency is greater than a fixed threshold, or instead when it is much different from that expected [2].

Also in the context of biological networks, a motif can be defined according to its *frequency* or to its *statistical significance* [12]. In the first case, a motif is a subgraph that appears more often than a given threshold number of times in an input network; in the second case, a motif is a subgraph that appears more (or less) often than expected. In particular, to measure the statistical significance of the motifs, many works compare the number of appearances of the motifs in the biological network with the number of appearances in a number of randomized networks [17], by exploiting suitable statistical indices such as the *p value* or the *z score* [44].

Despite the similarity with sequences, network motifs present important differences with respect to string motifs, the main important of which concerns the computational complexity of the problem of motif extraction, which is polynomial for strings and exponential (in the size of the input structure) for networks.

Figure 24.5 shows two of the most frequent network motifs, called *brick* and *feedforward loop*, respectively.

Formulation 24.3: Discovering Repetitions in Multiple Structures   Let $\{S_1, S_2, \ldots, S_n\}$ be a set of complex structures defined on the finite alphabet Σ of basic elements. *Discovering repetitions in multiple structures* corresponds to finding a set of significant substructures $\{P_1, P_2, \ldots, P_n\}$, not specified a priori, such that each P_i has an occurrence in at least k (e.g., two) S_i.

As is Formulation 24.2, Formulation 24.3 is also related to the concept of *motif*. However, in this case the repetitions to be searched for occur in different structures, rather than in a single one.

Searching for common substrings repeated in a set of biosequences can be useful for classifying them. For example, if there are m amino acid sequences and k of them present one or several similar subsequences, the corresponding proteins most likely belong to the same protein family. In sequence analysis, alignment is often performed to arrange the biosequences in such a way as to identify regions of similarity that may be a consequence of functional, structural, or evolutionary relationships between them. The so-aligned biosequences are usually represented as rows within a matrix. Gaps may also be inserted between the characters, so that identical or similar characters are aligned in successive columns and individuating common subsequences is then simpler.

When biological networks are considered, discovering repetitions in multiple structures consists in finding a set of conserved edges across the input networks, that is, a set of conserved subgraphs.

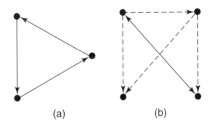

(a)   (b)

Figure 24.5   (a) Brick; (b) feedforward loop.

For both sequences and networks Formulation 24.3 can be performed by aligning pairs of structures (sequences or networks) or more than two structures at a time. Multiple alignments are often useful to individuate evolutionary conservations, but they are computationally difficult to produce. Furthermore, two different cases can be distinguished:

1. For each pair P_i, P_j of extracted repetitions, P_i and P_j cannot overlap; that is, they have no common elements. This is a case of *global alignment*.
2. For each pair P_i, P_j of extracted repetitions, P_i and P_j may overlap; that is, they have common elements. This is a case of *local alignment*.

24.3.1 Global Alignment

Global sequence alignment consists in aligning every character in every input sequence, and it is useful when the sequences in the query set are similar and of roughly equal size.

Global network alignment aims at finding a unique (possibly the best one) overall alignment between the input networks, in such a way that all the nodes of the networks are mapped.

Global sequence alignment is often used to compare genomic sequences to understand variations between species. Analogously, global network alignment may be used, for example, to compare interactomes and to understand cross-species variations. In contrast to global sequence alignment, global network alignment may also be useful when the input networks have significantly different sizes.

In greater detail, the output of global network alignment is a set of tuples $\langle P_1, P_2, \ldots, P_k \rangle$ where each P_i is a subgraph of one of the input networks that is similar to the other subgraphs in the same tuple. In terms of repetition, we can see such a tuple as the set of occurrences of the same motif, occurring in k of the input networks. The peculiarity of global alignment as opposed to the local one is that each P_i cannot share common nodes with any other P_j of the same input network that is involved in a different output tuple.

24.3.2 Local Alignment

Local sequence alignment aims at identifying regions of similarity within long sequences that are often widely divergent overall. Local sequence alignment is useful to analyzing dissimilar sequences, for which are suspected to contain regions of similarity or similar sequence motifs within their larger sequence context.

Local network alignment instead consists in finding similar motifs between two or several networks, and the mappings corresponding to different motifs may also be mutually inconsistent. The objective is to find multiple unrelated regions of isomorphism among the input networks, with each region implying a mapping independently of the others. Local network alignment may be applied, for example, to search for a known functional component (e.g., pathways, complexes) in a new species.

The output of local network alignment is, again, a set of tuples $\langle P_1, P_2, \ldots, P_k \rangle$, similar to the case of global network alignment. However, in this case, each P_i can share common nodes with some other P_j of the same input network, involved in a different output tuple.

24.4 METHODS

In this section we summarize the more recent applications for each formulations presented in the previous section with respect to the problem of searching repetitions in biological networks.

24.4.1 Matching a Query

Many approaches presented in the literature that aim at searching for small query subnetworks repeated in a target network focus on queries that are not general graphs, but paths or trees. As an example, Kelley et al. proposed PathBLAST [31], an approach to align two PPI networks by combining interaction topology and protein sequence similarity in order to identify conserved interaction pathways and complexes. Their algorithm searches for high-scoring pathway alignments involving two paths, one for each network, in which proteins of the first path are paired with putative homologs occurring in the same order in the second path. This is achieved by generating a network alignment graph where each node consists of a pair of sequence-similar proteins, each belonging to a different species; thus, links between pairs of nodes may be associated with conserved protein interactions between the corresponding proteins. As a byproduct, the authors use PathBLAST also for network querying by designating one of the two networks in input as the query for the other one.

Pinter et al. [48] proposed MetaPathwayHunter, an algorithm to query metabolic networks, where the queries are multisource trees. In particular, these query trees are directed acyclic graphs for which the correspondent undirected graphs are trees such that some of the nodes may present both incoming and outgoing edges. MetaPathwayHunter searches the networks for approximated matching, allowing node insertions (only one node), whereas no deletions are allowed.

QPath and QNet were proposed by Shlomi et al. [55] and Dost et al. [15], respectively. QPath queries a PPI network by a query pathway consisting of a linear chain of interacting proteins belonging to another organism. The algorithm works similarly to sequence alignment, by aligning the query pathway to putative pathways in the target network, so that proteins in analogous positions have similar sequences. PPI networks interactions reliability scores are considered, and insertions and deletions are allowed. QNet is an extension of QPath in which the queries are trees or graphs with limited treewidth.

GenoLink [16] is a system able to integrate data from different sources (e.g., databases of proteins, genes, organisms, chromosomes) and to query the resulting data graph by graph patterns with constraints attached to both vertices and edges; a query result is the set of all the subgraphs of the target graph that are sufficiently similar to the query pattern and satisfy the constraints.

Yang and Sze [60] considered the two problems of path matching and graph matching. In particular, they present an exact algorithm to search for subgraphs of arbitrary structure in large graph, grouping related vertices in the target network for each vertex in the query. Although their algorithm is accurate and also efficient enough to be considered exact, the authors state that it is practical for queries having ≤ 20 nodes, and its performance improves if the query is a sparse graph.

Ferro et al. [19] present an approach called NetMatch, a Cytoscape plugin for the network querying allowing for an approximated query, such that certain parts of the subgraph query may be left unspecified. A query for NetMatch is a graph in which some nodes are specified and others are wildcards (which can match an unspecified number of elements). Ferro et al. [19] focus mainly on the topological similarity between the query and target graphs, without taking into account information about node similarities.

Fionda et al. [21] modeled PPI networks through labeled graphs in order to factor in the reliability of interactions, allowing for a more accurate analysis, and a proposed a technique is based on maximum-weight matching of bipartite graphs.

Rombo et al. [50] present an efficient framework based on hidden Markov models that can be used for finding homologous pathways in a network of interest. Given a query path, the method identifies the top k matching paths in the network, which may contain any number of consecutive insertions and deletions. The authors apply their method on PPI networks.

Blin et al. [6] propose an algorithm for matching a query in the shape of graphs, based on dynamic programming and the color coding technique. To transform graphs queries into trees without loss of information, they use a feedback vertex set coupled to a node duplication mechanism. The resulting algorithm is FPT for querying graphs with a bounded size of their feedback vertex set, by giving an alternative to the treewidth parameter, which can be better or worse for a given query. The approach has been successfully applied to retrieve human query networks in the shape of graphs into the fly PPI network.

Ferraro et al. [18] propose AbiNet, an approach for aligning and querying biological networks according to an *asymmetric* comparison, allowing utilization of differences in the characterization of organisms. They exploit finite automatons suitably coupled with the Viterbi algorithm and use the best characterized organism (*master*) as a fingerprint to guide the alignment process to the second input network (*slave*). AbiNet allows for two different uses of the network querying mode: set the network query as the master and the target one as the slave, if attention is focused on finding the pairwise interactions of a specific module (the query) that are conserved in a specific organism (the target). The opposite master/slave arrangement is appropriate when, instead, the objective is to individuate possible diversifications of a module in a more complex target organism.

24.4.2   Discovering Repetitions in a Single Structure

The search of significant repetitions in a single biological network was pioneered by Shen-Orr et al. [54], who defined *network motifs* as "patterns of interconnections that recur in many different parts of a network at frequencies much higher than those found in randomized networks." They [54] studied the transcriptional regulation network of *Escherichia coli*, by searching for small motifs composed by three or four nodes. In particular, three highly significant motifs characterizing such network have been discovered; the most famous is the *feedforward loop*, shown in Figure 24.5b, whose importance has been shown in further studies [39,40].

The technique presented by Shen-Orr et al. [54] laid the foundations for different extensions, mainly of three proposed in 2004 and 2008 [5,10,61].

Yeger-Lotem et al. [61] identified composite motifs consisting of two kinds of interaction by exploiting edges of different colors in the network modeling. The authors identified an integrated cellular interaction network by two types (colors) of edges, representing protein–protein and transcription–regulation interactions, and developed algorithms for detecting network motifs in such networks with multiple types of edges. Such a study may be considered as a basic framework for detecting the building blocks of networks with multiple types of interaction.

In another study [5], topological motifs derived from families of mutually similar, but not necessarily identical, patterns were discussed and extracted from the gene regulatory network of *E. coli*. The authors developed a search algorithm to extract topological motifs called *graph alignment*, in analogy to sequence alignment, that is based on a scoring function. They observed that, in biological networks, functionally related motifs do not need to be topologically identical; thus, they discussed motifs derived from families of mutually similar but not necessarily identical patterns.

In yet another study [10], *n*-node "bridge" and "brick" motifs were searched for in complex networks, and the presence of such motifs was associated with network topology, but not with network size. The authors proposed a method for performing simultaneously the detection of global statistical features and local connection structures, and the location of functionally and statistically significant network motifs.

All these approaches [5,10,54,61] relate the concept of *motif* only to network topology, without considering possible properties shared by network nodes in terms of their mutual similarity. According to such a definition of motifs, subgraphs containing the same number of nodes and presenting similar topology may be recognized as motifs, although their nodes are associated with components presenting significant differences (e.g., proteins with very low sequence homology).

Lacroix et al. [35], observed biological networks (e.g., metabolic networks) where a purely topological definition of motifs seems to be inappropriate, as similar topologies can give rise to very different functions. Thus, they [35] introduce a new definition of motifs in the context of metabolic networks, such that the components of the network play a central role and the topology can be added only as a further constraint.

Similarly to the Lacroix et al. study [35], Parida [46] related the concept of motif is to both graph structure and node similarity. In particular, the author presents a three-step exact approach based on the application of the notion of maximality, used extensively in strings, to graphs.

Both works [35,46] open the way for definition of new, exact, or approximate, approaches for motif extraction, taking into account not only the network topology but also the biological properties of the interacting components.

24.4.3   Discovering Repetitions in Multiple Structures

We consider at first the case of global network alignment, which was proposed for the first time by Singh et al. [56]. In particular, the authors present IsoRank, an algorithm for pairwise global alignment of PPI networks working in two stages: (1) associating a score with each possible match between nodes of the two networks, and then (2) constructing the mapping for the global network alignment by extracting mutually consistent matches according to a bipartite graph weighted matching performed on the two entire networks. IsoRank was extended in Singh's later paper [57], where a multiple alignment among five PPI networks is illustrated. To this aim, the authors exploited an approximate multipartite graph weighted matching.

Liao et al. [38] proposed the IsoRankN (IsoRank-Nibble) tool, which is a global multinetwork alignment tool based on spectral clustering on the induced graph of pairwise alignment scores. As it is based on spectral methods, IsoRankN is both error-tolerant and computationally efficient.

A graph-based maximum structural matching formulation for pairwise global network alignment was introduced [32]. On the basis of such formulation, an approach exploiting the Lagrangian relaxation technique combined with a branch-and-bound method to perform global network alignment is proposed.

In another paper [11] the algorithm PISwap is presented for computing global pairwise alignments of protein interaction networks. The approach is based on a local optimization heuristic that has previously demonstrated its effectiveness for a variety of other NP-hard problems, such as the traveling salesperson problem (TSP). PISwap begins with a sequence-based network alignment and then iteratively adjusts the alignment by incorporating network structure information.

The already discussed AbiNet [18] performs an *asymmetric* global alignment on pairs of biological networks. It is able to return biologically meaningful associations that a symmetric approach (such as IsoRank) does not find, as shown by an experimental campaign performed on yeast, fly, humans, and two bacteria.

Local network alignment was pioneered by Kelley et al. [31] with Pathblast, whose main characteristics were described in Section 24.4.1. Pathblast has been extended [52] for comparison with several PPI networks. In particular, such an extension is based on the generation of a network alignment graph where each node consists of a group of sequence-similar proteins, one for each species, and each link between a pair of nodes represents a conserved protein interaction between the corresponding protein groups.

In another study [33], a pair of PPI networks are considered as input and a technique using duplication/divergence models through definition of duplications, matches, and mismatches in a graph-theoretic framework is presented. In particular, the alignment problem is reduced to a graph optimization problem, and efficient heuristics are proposed to solve this problem.

Bandyopadhyay et al. [4] proposed a strategy to identify functionally related proteins supplementing sequence-based comparisons with information on conserved protein–protein interactions. The technique first aligns two PPI networks using only sequence similarities, and then performs probabilistic inference (based on Gibbs sampling) to identify pairs of proteins that are likely to retain the same function. The approach has been specifically applied to resolve ambiguous functional orthology relationships in PPI networks.

Functional orthology detection was been considered in another study [23], where Bi-GRAPPIN, a method based on maximum-weight matching of bipartite graphs, is presented. In particular, the bipartite graphs result from comparing the adjacent nodes of pairs of proteins occurring in the input networks. The basic idea is that proteins belonging to different networks should be matched in terms of not only their own sequence similarity but also the similarity of proteins with which they significantly interact with. Bi-GRAPPIN has been exploited [22] as a preliminary step in applying a node collapsing–based technique to extract similar subgraphs from two input networks.

Flannick et al. [24] presented an algorithm for multiple network alignment, named Graemlin. Graemlin aligns an arbitrary number of networks to individuate conserved functional modules, greedily assigning the aligned proteins to nonoverlapping homology classes and progressively aligning multiple input networks. The algorithm also allows searching for different conserved topologies defined by the user. It can be used either to generate an exhaustive list of conserved modules in a set of networks (network-to-network alignment) or to find matches to a particular module within a database of interaction networks (query-to-network alignment).

In another study [14] the algorithm C3Part-M, based on a nonheuristic approach exploiting a correspondence multigraph formalism to extract connected components conserved in multiple networks, is presented and applied on PPI networks. C3Part-M is compared with NetworkBlast-M [29], another technique more recently proposed on the basis of a novel representation of multiple networks that is linear only with respect to their size.

24.5 CONCLUDING REMARKS

In both biosequences and biological networks, the presence of repetitions is usually associated with biologically significant conservations. Thus several techniques have been proposed in the literature to extract interesting repetitions from biological data, and different formulations of such a problem are possible, as we showed in this chapter.

When biological networks are considered, the extraction of interesting similarities involves the subgraph isomorphism problem, which is known to be NP-complete [27]. For this reason, some of the approaches, described [e.g., 48,55] search for repeated structures simpler than graphs, such as trees or paths. Furthermore, the number of existing approximate techniques is notably greater than the number of exact methods. In particular, exact approaches have been proposed when the size of the subgraphs to search for can be fixed a priori, such as in the case of querying and motif extraction. If exact algorithms are exploited, the size of subgraphs has to be restricted to only few nodes.

Some of the approaches reviewed in this chapter focus only on the topological similarity between the conserved subgraphs. Others also factor in information about node similarities in the process of extracting conserved regions, often relaxing topology constraints. Only a few methods have been presented that also apply edge information, such as reliability or different kinds of interaction. Considering both node and edge information seems to be a successful approach for analysis of biological networks. Indeed, in contrast to the biosequences domain, biological interaction data are often affected by noise because much information is retrieved by computational and high-throughput experimental techniques [28,34].

A major challenge in biological networks analysis is the need to define more efficient algorithms capable of detecting significant repetitions occurring in a large number of networks. Indeed, the amount of available interaction data is increasing exponentially, and searching for common motifs in different networks could be useful in classifying the corresponding interactomes and identifying similar functional groups across species. While multiple sequence alignment has been massively exploited, multiple network alignment is still in its infancy, because such a task is computationally difficult for networks with thousands of nodes and interactions.

Finally, we point out that, although there has been some attempt to define statistical indices in the biological network domain [44], a general and universally accepted methodology for measuring the biological significance of the repetitions detected is still lacking.

REFERENCES

1. Alon U, Network motifs: Theory and experimental approaches, *Nature* **8**:450–461 (2007).

2. Apostolico A, Bock ME, Lonardi S, Monotony of surprise and large-scale quest for unusual words, *J. Comput. Biol.* **10**(2/3):283–311 (2003).

3. Apostolico A et al, Finding 3d motifs in ribosomal rna structures, *Nucleic Acids Res.* **37**(4):e29 (2008).

4. Bandyopadhyay S, Sharan R, Ideker T, Systematic identification of functional orthologs based on protein network comparison, *Genome Res.* **16**(3):428–435 (2006).

5. Berg J, Lassig M, Local graph alignment and motif search in biological networks, *Proc. Natl. Acad. Sci. USA* **101**(41):14689–14694 (2004).

6. Blin G, Sikora F, Vialette S, Querying graphs in protein-protein interactions networks using feedback vertex set, *IEEE/ACM Trans. Comput. Biol. Bioinformatics.* **7**:628–635 (2010).

7. Brazma A et al, Approaches to the automatic discovery of patterns in biosequences, *J. Comput. Biol.* **5**(2):277–304 (1998).

8. Chatraryamontri A et al, MINT: The molecular interaction database, *Nucleic Acids Res.* **35**(database issue):D572–D574 (2006).

9. Cheadle C et al, Control of gene expression during t cell activation: Alternate regulation of mrna transcription and mrna stability, *BMC Genomics* **6**(1):75 (2005).

10. Cheng C-Y, Huang C-Y, Sun C-T, Mining bridge and brick motifs from complex biological networks for functionally and statistically significant discovery, *IEEE Trans. Syst. Man Cybernet. B* **38**(1):17–24 (2008).

11. Chindelevitch L, Liao C-S, Berger B, Local optimization for global alignment of protein interaction networks, *Proc. Pacific Symp. Biocomputing*, 2010, pp. 123–132.

12. Ciriello G, Guerra C, A review on models and algorithms for motif discovery in protein-protein interaction network, *Brief. Funct. Genomics Proteomics* **7**(2):147–56 (2008).

13. International Human Genome Sequencing Consortium, Finishing the euchromatic sequence of the human genome, *Nature* **431**(7011):931–945 (2004).

14. Denielou Y-P, Boyer F, Viari A, Sagot M-F, Multiple alignment of biological networks: A flexible approach, *Proc. Combinatorial Pattern Matching'09*, 2009, pp. 263–273.

15. Dost B et al, Qnet: A tool for querying protein interaction networks, *Proc. RECOMB'07*, 2007, pp. 1–15.

16. Durand P et al, GenoLink: A graph-based querying and browsing system for investigating the function of genes and proteins, *BMC Bioinformatics* **7**(21):(2006).

17. Erdos P, Renyi A, On the evolution of random graphs, *Publ. Mater. Inst. Hung. Acad. Sci.* **5**:17–61 (1960).

18. Ferraro N, Palopoli L, Panni S, Rombo S, Asymmetric comparison and querying of biological networks, *IEEE/ACM Trans. Comput. Biol. Bioinformatics* **8**:876–889 (2011).

19. Ferro A et al, Netmatch: A cytoscape plugin for searching biological networks, *Bioinformatics* **23**(7):910–912 (2007).

20. Fionda V, Palopoli L, Biological network querying techniques: Analysis and comparison, *J. Comput. Biol.* **18**(4):595–625 (2011).

21. Fionda V, Palopoli L, Panni S, Rombo SE, Protein-protein interaction network querying by a "focus and zoom" approach, *Bioinformatics Res. Devel.* **13**:331–346 (2008).

22. Fionda V, Panni S., Palopoli L, Rombo SE. Extracting similar sub-graphs across ppi networks, *Proc. Int. Symp. Computing and Informatics Sciences*, 183–188 (2009).

23. Fionda V, Panni S, Palopoli L, Rombo SE, A technique to search functional similarities in ppi networks, *Int. J. Data Mining Bioinformatics*, **3**(4):431–453 (2009).

24. Flannick J et al, Graemlin: General and robust alignment of multiple large interaction networks, *Genome Res.* **16**(9):1169–1181 (2006).

25. Francke C, Siezen RJ, Teusink B, Reconstructing the metabolic network of a bacterium from its genome, *Trends Microbiol.* **13**(11):550–558 (2005).

26. Galil Z, Giancarlo R, Data structures and algorithms for approximate string matching, *J. Complex.* **4**(1):33–72 (1988).

27. Garey M, Johnson D, *Computers and Intractability: A Guide to the Theory of NP-completeness*, Freeman, New York, 1979.

28. Ito T et al, A comprehensive two-hybrid analysis to explore the yeast protein interactome, *Proc. Natl. Acad. Sci. USA* **98**(8):4569–4574 (2001).

29. Kalaev M, Bafna V, Sharan R, Fast and accurate alignment of multiple protein networks, *Proc. RECOMB'08*, 2008.

30. Karp PD et al, Expansion of the BioCyc collection of pathway/genome databases to 160 genomes, *Nucleic Acids Res.* **19**:6083–6089 (2005).

31. Kelley BP et al, Conserved pathways within bacteria and yeast as revealed by global protein network alignment, *Proc. Natl. Acad. Sci. USA* **100**(20):11394–11399 (2003).

32. Klau GW, A new graph-based method for pairwise global network alignment, *BMC Bioinformatics* **10**(Suppl. 1):S59 (2009).

33. Koyuturk M et al, Pairwise alignment of protein interaction networks, *J. Comput. Biol.* **13**(2):182–199 (2006).

34. Krogan NJ, Cagney G, et al, Global landscape of protein complexes in the yeast *Saccharomyces cerevisiae*, *Nature* **440**(7084):637–643 (2006).

35. Lacroix V, Fernandes CG, Sagot M-F, Motif search in graphs: Application to metabolic networks, *IEEE/ACM Trans. Comput. Biol. Bioinformatics* **3**(4):360–368 (2006).

36. Lesk A, *Introduction to Protein Science Architecture, Function, and Genomics*, Oxford Univ. Press, 2004.

37. Levine M, Davidson EH, Gene regulatory networks for development, *Proc. Natl. Acad. Sci. USA* **102**:4936–4942 (2005).

38. Liao C-S et al, Isorankn: Spectral methods for global alignment of multiple protein networks, *Bioinformatics* **25**:i253–i258 (2009).

39. Mangan S, Alon U, Structure and function of the feed-forward loop network motif, *Proc. Natl. Acad. Sci. USA* **100**(21):11980–11985 (2003).

40. Mangan S, Itzkovitz S, Zaslaver A, Alon U, The incoherent feed-forward loop accelerates the response-time of the *gal* system of *Escherichia coli*, *J. Mol. Biol.* **356**(5):1073–1081 (2005).

41. Matys V et al, Transfac and its module transcompel: Transcriptional gene regulation in eukaryotes, *Nucleic Acids Res.* **34**:D108–D110 (2006).

42. Mewes HW et al, MIPS–a database for protein sequences, homology data and yeast genome information, *Nucleic Acids Res.* **25**:28–30 (1997).

43. Miller JP et al, Large-scale identification of yeast integral membrane protein interactions, *Proc. Natl. Acad. Sci. USA* **102**(34):12123–12128 (2005).

44. Milo R et al, Network motifs: Simple building blocks of complex networks, *Science* **298**(5594):824–827 (2002).

45. Orlev N, Shamir R, Shiloh Y, PIVOT: Protein interaction visualization tool, *Bioinformatics* **20**(3):424–425 (2004).

46. Parida L, Discovering topological motifs using a compact notation, *J. Comput. Biol.* **14**(3):46–69 (2007).

47. Parida L, *Pattern Discovery in Bioinformatics, Theory and Algorithms*, Chapman & HAll/CRC, 2008.

48. Pinter R et al, Alignment of metabolic pathways, *Bioinformatics* **21**(16):3401–3408 (2005).

49. Posada D, *Bioinformatics for DNA Sequence Analysis*, Humana Press, 2009.

50. Qian X, Sze S-H, Yoon B-J, Querying pathways in protein interaction networks based on hidden markov models, *J. Comput. Biol.* **16**(2):145–57 (2009).

51. Rombo SE, Utro F, Giancarlo R, Basic statistical indices for SeqAn, in Gogol-Döring A, Reinert K, *Biological Sequence Analysis Using the SeqAn C++ Library*, Chapman&Hall/CRC Mathematical & Computational Biology Series, 2009, pp. 249–260.

52. Sharan R et al, From the cover: Conserved patterns of protein interaction in multiple species, *Proc. Natl. Acad. Sci. USA* **102**(6):1974–1979 (2005).

53. Sharan R, Ideker T, Modeling cellular machinery through biological network comparison, *Nat. Biotechnol.* **24**(4):427–433 (2006).

54. Shen-Orr SS, Milo R, Mangan S, Alon U. Network motifs in the trascriptional regulation network of *Escherichia coli*, *Nature* **31**:64–68 (2002).

55. Shlomi T et al, Qpath: A method for querying pathways in a protein-protein interaction network, *BMC Bioinformatics* **7**: (2006).

56. Singh R, Xu J, Berger B, Pairwise global alignment of protein interaction networks by matching neighborhood topology, *Proc. Res. Comput. Mol. Biol.*, pp 16–31, (2007).

57. Singh R, Xu J, Berger B, Global alignment of multiple protein interaction networks, *Proc. Pacific Symp. Biocomputing*, pp. 303–14, (2008).

58. Stelling J, Klamt S, Bettenbrock K, Schuster S, Gilles ED. Metabolic network structure determines key aspects of functionality and regulation, *Nature* **420**:190–193 (2002).

59. von Mering D, Krause C, et al., Comparative assessment of a large-scale data sets of protein-protein interactions, *Nature* **417**(6887):399–403 (2002).

60. Yang Q, Sze S-H, Saga: A subgraph matching tool for biological graphs, *J. Comput. Biol.* **14**(1):56–67 (2007).

61. Yeger-Lotem E et al., Network motifs in integrated cellular networks of transcription regulation and protein protein interaction, *Proc. Natl. Acad. Sci. USA* **101**(16):5934–5939 (2004).

62. Zhang S, Zhang X-S, Chen L, Biomolecular network querying: A promising approach in systems biology, *BMC Syst Biol.* **2**:5 (2008).

63. Zhou Q, Chipperfield H, Melton DA, Wong WH, A gene regulatory network in mouse embryonic stem cells, *Proc. Natl. Acad. Sci. USA* **104**(42):16438–16443 (2007).

CHAPTER 25

MeTaDoR: ONLINE RESOURCE AND PREDICTION SERVER FOR MEMBRANE TARGETING PERIPHERAL PROTEINS

NITIN BHARDWAJ, MORTEN KÄLLBERG, WONHWA CHO, and HUI LU

25.1 INTRODUCTION

Cell signaling is a complex system of communication that governs basic cellular activities and coordinates cell actions. The process involves complex arrays of inter-molecular interactions, including protein–protein, protein–lipid, protein–carbohydrate, protein–nucleic acid, and protein–small molecule interactions [1]. As a part of this highly organized process, many proteins are redistributed within the cell to various cellular compartments [2]. A large majority of these dynamic proteins target various cellular membranes by recognizing specific lipids and/or proteins. These proteins, collectively known as *peripheral proteins* [3], are different from integral membrane proteins in that they interact with membranes mostly reversibly in response to specific signals. Peripheral proteins also play crucial roles in other cellular processes, including membrane trafficking, cell motility, apoptosis, viral infection, and cell metabolism. Many of these peripheral proteins have been implicated in major human diseases, such as cancer [4] and AIDS [5].

Most peripheral proteins interact with cell membranes via one or more modular domains, known either as *membrane targeting domains* (MTDs) or as *lipid binding domains* (LBDs), which are specialized in lipid binding [6,7]. The MTDs and LBDs are referred to the same class of domains; for simplicity, we will refer to them as MTDs. Since the discovery that the C1 (protein kinase C conserved *1*) domain could bind phorbol ester [8] and diacylglycerol [9], the list of MTDs has rapidly grown. MTDs now include C1 [10,11], C2 (protein kinase C conserved 2) [10,12,13], PH (pleckstrin homology) [14,15], FYVE (Fab1/YOTB/Vac1/EEA1)

Algorithmic and Artificial Intelligence Methods for Protein Bioinformatics. First Edition.
Edited by Yi Pan, Jianxin Wang, Min Li.
© 2014 John Wiley & Sons, Inc. Published 2014 by John Wiley & Sons, Inc.

[16], PX (phox) [17], ENTH (Epsin *N*-terminal homology) [18], ANTH (AP180 *N*-terminal homology) [18], BAR (Bin/Amphiphysin/Rvs) [19], FERM (four-point one-ezrin-radixin-moesin) [20], and tubby domains [21]. Because of the immense significance of MTDs in diverse cellular processes, they have received much attention since 2002 or so from both experimentalists and computational biologists. Three-dimensional (3D) structures of many MTDs and host proteins have been solved, and biophysical studies by EPR, X-ray reflectivity, and fluorescence techniques have elucidated the diverse membrane binding mechanisms of these domains. Also, various microscopic techniques have been used to study their cellular dynamics and localization. De spite their importance, however, a dedicated web-based resource that provides comprehensive information about MTDs has been lacking. The *Orientation of Protein in Membranes* (OPM) database contains some information about MTDs but focuses primarily on the integral membrane proteins [22]. This is in contrast to abundant resources dedicated to proteins involved in other interactions such as protein–protein [23,24], protein–DNA [25], and protein–ligand interactions [26]. We therefore created MeTaDoR as a comprehensive resource solely dedicated to MTDs.

This chapter describes the navigation through MeTaDoR to demonstrate how the resource could be used to obtain various types of information about MTDs. MeTaDoR integrates all the essential information about MTDs at a publicly available platform (Fig. 25.1). Included are sequences, structures, membrane binding

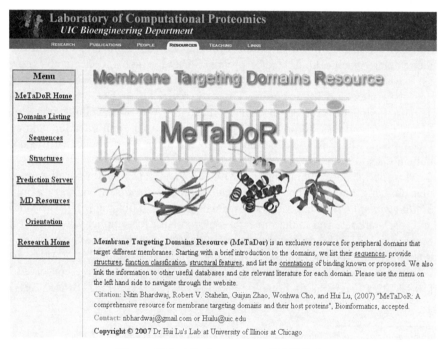

Figure 25.1 The homepage of MeTaDoR.

modes of MTDs, manually curated classification of proteins into membrane binding/nonbinding and a search function. It also provides two more services beyond the standard collection of data: (1) molecular dynamics resources, including forcefield parameters of nonstandard lipids that are necessary for the molecular dynamics-based studies; and (2) an online prediction server for MTD identification. MeTaDoR has been and will be updated regularly so as to include new information about MTDs.

25.2 RESOURCE CONTENT

25.2.1 Domain Listing

The MeTaDoR menu begins with the listing of all known MTDs with links to more detailed descriptions about individual domains (Fig. 25.2). So far, nine domain families have been reported to bind lipids and target membranes. These include BAR, C1, C2, ENTH, FERM, FYVE, PH, PX, and Tubby domains. Newly discovered MTDs include the PDZ domain [27], which will be listed in MeTaDoR as more biophysical data become available. The description of each domain (Fig. 25.3) begins with a brief introduction of the function and occurrences of a prototype domain and the listing of some of its host proteins. It is followed by a 3D structure, preferentially as a complex with a lipid molecule (or metal ions). Also listed is the subcellular localization of the domain determined under various physiological conditions. For each MTD, the relevant literature is provided with at least one recent review article.

25.2.2 Sequences

The next menu, *sequences*, lists the sequences of all the MTDs in Prosite format [28]. It also provides a more condensed tab-delimited format that can be easily parsed to retrieve other information along with sequences, such as function and subcellular location. These sequences were collected after searching the entire Prosite database with the name of each domain as the keyword and including all well-annotated hits. Not all MTDs are known to be directly involved in recruiting the host protein to the membranes; some are implicated in protein–protein interactions, and others may play a structural role for the host protein. To provide clear distinction among such cases, we also provide classification for each specific domain as membrane binding or nonbinding (Fig. 25.4). This classification was manually curated by examining each domain for its binding property, function, and subcellular localizations, among other information.

25.2.3 Structures

Under the *structures* menu, the PDB [29] IDs of all the domains whose structures have been solved are listed for each MTD. An initial list of these structures was

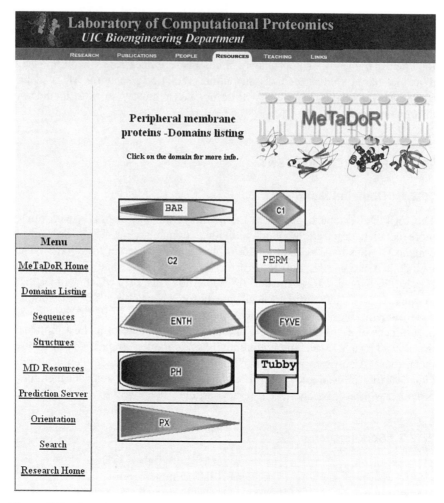

Figure 25.2   Domains listing in MeTaDoR. All currently known peripheral domains are included.

obtained by searching the PDB database with the name of each domain family as the keyword. To remove structures that are not related to these domains, the title of each structure file from the initial list was then checked manually. These IDs have been linked to the corresponding Pfam [30] entry as well (Fig. 25.5).

25.2.4   Orientations

The membrane-bound orientations of MTDs provide critical insight into how these proteins achieve optimal interactions with membrane lipids and how these

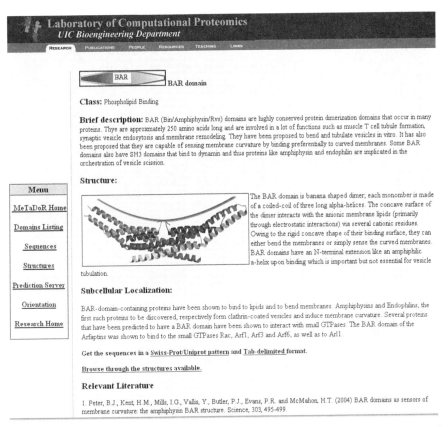

Figure 25.3 Domain description with BAR domain as an example. It includes a brief description, key structural features, subcellular locations, and relevant literature.

interactions are regulated. MeTaDoR provides the reported binding orientations of MTDs relative to the membrane in the *Orientation* menu (Fig. 25.6). These orientations were obtained by extensively searching the literature related to MTDs. Because of the technical difficulties involved in determining the membrane-bound orientation of proteins experimentally, only limited data are available in the literature. A clear distinction is therefore made between hypothetical and experimentally determined orientations. All the instances of known orientation have also been linked to the original article(s). Those proteins whose depth of membrane penetration is experimentally determined are also indicated. Apart from the corresponding PDB IDs, a brief *Remarks* section is included that describes the residues that are involved in lipid interaction, the mechanism and the nature of this interaction, and the role of metallic ions in the interaction (if any). MeTaDoR has also been crosslinked to another database, OPM [22], whenever similar data are found in both resources.

Protein Name	Species	Binding/Non-Binding	Function	Subcellular Location	Primary Sequence
AMPH_CHICK	Others	1	May participate in mechanisms of regulated	Synaptic vesicle; synaptic vesicle membr	VLQKLGKADETKDEQFEEYVQNFKRC
AMPH_HUMAN	Human	1	May participate in mechanisms of regulated	Synaptic vesicle; synaptic vesicle membr	VLQKLGKADETKDEQFEEYVQNFKRC
AMPH_MOUSE	Mouse	1	May participate in mechanisms of regulated	Synaptic vesicle; synaptic vesicle membr	VLQKLGKADETKDEQFEEYVQNFKRC
AMPH_RAT	Others	1	May participate in mechanisms of regulated	Synaptic vesicle; synaptic vesicle membr	VLQKLGKADETKDEQFEEYVQNFKRC
SH3G1_HUMAN	Human	1	May play a regulatory role in synaptic vesicle	Cytoplasm (By similarity). Membrane; pe	SEKVGGAEGTKLDDDFKEMEKKVDV1
SH3G1_MOUSE	Mouse	1	May play a regulatory role in synaptic vesicle	Cytoplasm. Membrane; peripheral membr	SEKVGGAEGTKLDDDFKEMEKKVDV1
SH3G1_RAT	Others	1	May play a regulatory role in synaptic vesicle	Cytoplasm. Membrane; peripheral membr	SEKVGGAEGTKLDDDFREMEKKVDIT:
SH3G2_HUMAN	Human	1	Plays a role in synaptic vesicle recycling, in	Cytoplasm. Membrane; peripheral membr	SEKVGGAEGTKLDDDFKEMERKVDV1
SH3G2_MOUSE	Mouse	1	Plays a role in synaptic vesicle recycling, in	Cytoplasm (By similarity). Membrane; pe	SEKVGGAEGTKLDDDFKEMERKVDV1
SH3G2_RAT	Others	1	Plays a role in synaptic vesicle recycling, in	Cytoplasm. Membrane; peripheral membr	GDDCNFGPALGEVGEAMRELSEVKD:
SH1LB1_HUMAN	Human	1	Exhibits lysophosphatidic acid acyltransfera	Cytoplasm. Membrane; peripheral membr	EEKLGQAEKTELDAHLENLLSKAECTK
SH1LB1_MOUSE	Mouse	1	Exhibits lysophosphatidic acid acyltransfera	Cytoplasm. Membrane; peripheral membr	EEKLGQAEKTELDAHLENLLSKAECTK
BIN1_HUMAN	Human	1	May be involved in regulation of synaptic ves	Isoform BIN1: Nucleus. Isoform IIa: Cytop	VLQIKLGKADETKDEQFEQCVQNFNKC
BIN1_MOUSE	Mouse	1	May be involved in regulation of synaptic ves	Cytoplasm (By similarity). Nucleus (By si	VLQIKLGKADETKDEQFEQCVQNFNKC
BIN1_RAT	Others	1	May be involved in regulation of synaptic ves	Cytoplasm (By similarity). Nucleus (By si	VLQIKLGKADETKDEQFEQCVQNFNKC
DNMBP_HUMAN	Human	1	Scaffold protein that links dynamin with actin	Cytoplasmic. Localized to synapses and	LKHLTGFAPQIKDEVFEETEKNFRMQE
DNMBP_MOUSE	Mouse	1	Scaffold protein that links dynamin with actin	Cytoplasmic. Localized to synapses and	LKHLTGFAPQIKDEVFEETEKNFRMQ(
RV161_YEAST	Yeast	1	Component of a cytoskeletal structure that is required for the formation of endocytic ve	HSVIIKNVDKTIDKEYDMEERRYKVLQF
RV167_YEAST	Yeast	1	Component of a cytoskeletal structure that is required for the formation of endocytic ve	FRGKFYQMGEQTEDDPVYEDAERRFQEI
SH3G3_HUMAN	Human	1	May play a regulatory role in synaptic vesicle	SEKISGAEGTKLDEEFLNMERKKDITN
SH3G3_MOUSE	Mouse	1	May play a regulatory role in synaptic vesicle recycling (By similarity).	SEKISGAEGTKLDEEFLNMERKKDTSK
SH3G3_RAT	Others	1	May play a regulatory role in synaptic vesicle recycling.	YLQRNPAYRAKLGMLNTMSKLRGDV
3BP1_HUMAN	Human	1	Binds differentially to the SH3 domains of certain proteins of signal transduction pathw	SLGRTPETAEFLGEDLLQVEQRLEPAH
3BP1_MOUSE	Mouse	1	Binds differentially to the SH3 domains of certain proteins of signal transduction pathw	MAESFKELDPDSSMGKALEMTCAIQN
BIN3_HUMAN	Human	0	Involved in cytokinesis and septation where it has a role in the localization of F-actin	GQPIKKQIVPKTVERDFEREYGKLQQLI
BIN3_MOUSE	Mouse	0	Involved in cytokinesis and septation where it has a role in the localization of F-actin	(B GQPIKKQIVSKTVERDFEREYGKLQQLI
BIN3_RAT	Others	0	Involved in cytokinesis and septation where it has a role in the localization of F-actin	(B GQPIKKQIVSKTVERDFEREYGKLQQLI
BIN3_XENLA	Others	0	Involved in cytokinesis and septation where it has a role in the localization of F-actin	(B GQPIKKQIVPKTVERDFEREYGKLQQLI
HOB1_SCHPO	Yeast	0	Has a role in DNA damage signaling as a part of stress response processes.	LRSIKFNVGEITKDPIYEDAGRRFKSLE1
HOB3_SCHPO	Yeast	0	Involved in cytokinesis and septation where it has a role in the localization of F-actin.	VMMKTGHVERTVDREFETEERRYRTN
P29_ECHGR	Others	0			GELVNKNEKTSYPTRTSDLHEIDQMK/
SH1LE2_HUMAN	Human	0		Cytoplasm.	EEKFGQAEKTELDAHFENLLARADSTH
SH1LE2_MOUSE	Mouse	0		Cytoplasm (By similarity).	EEKFGQAEKTELDAHFENLLARADSTH

Figure 25.4 A snapshot of the tab-delimited sequence page that allows easy parsing of the important information. It also provides the classification of each instance into binding and nonbinding.

25.2.5 MD Resources

A large number of MTDs specifically recognize and interact with lipids. For example, C1 domains specifically recognize diacylglycerols [10], whereas various PH domains specifically target phosphoinositides [31]. The mechanisms by which MTDs interact with membranes containing these specific lipids, thereby causing downstream effects, including protein activation and membrane deformation, have been a subject of many molecular dynamics studies [32–36]. For the purpose of these simulations, the force-field parameters of lipids are required. Despite the wealth of experimental data on lipids, these parameters are not available for many lipids, including key signaling lipids such as phosphoinositides, phosphatidylserine, and diacylglycerols. We have developed and tested the force-field parameters for many of these lipids and provide these parameters under the *MD resources* menu to facilitate the molecular dynamics study of MTDs. We also provide links to appropriate tutorials that describe how these parameters can be used to start the simulations. These parameters were developed and refined carefully after repeated testing through the simulation of the bilayers containing these lipids. PDBs of some preequilibrated membrane systems have also been provided (Fig. 25.7). We have used these forcefield parameters to obtain detailed mechanistic information about how MTDs interact with membranes [37].

25.2.6 Prediction Server

We have linked MeTaDoR to the online membrane binding protein prediction server (*prediction server* menu) that has been in operation since 2007 and has received numerous submissions from users around the world. Users can freely submit either a structure file of their protein or the PDB ID of the protein.

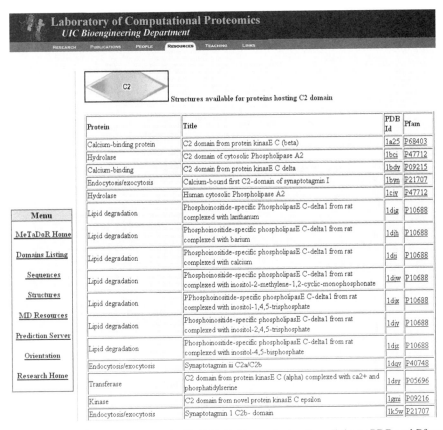

Figure 25.5   The structure page in MeTaDoR. For each structure, links to PDB and Pfam are provided.

The prediction strategy is based on a machine learning protocol that we developed earlier and has been shown to achieve a high success rate [38]. To the best of our knowledge, it is currently the only publicly available prediction algorithm to identify membrane binding proteins. More specifically, the prediction is based on a number of properties calculated from the structures of several MTDs. We use the propensity of the 20 amino acids to be found on the surface of the domain structure, and the overall charge and electrostatic properties of the domain (i.e., the size of the first few largest cationic patches) as descriptors. Using a dataset consisting of 230 nonbinding domains and 40 experimentally verified MTDs, we have trained and evaluated the classifier, achieving 91.6% accuracy with a good balance between sensitivity and specificity [38]. The protocol is constantly being improved and updated on the server. Figure 25.8 shows the submission form for the prediction server. The user will need to submit the name and the institutional affiliation (1) as well as the email address (2) that the result should be returned to. Finally, a choice is given between submitting a PDB ID or a structure (in PDB format) of user's choice (3).

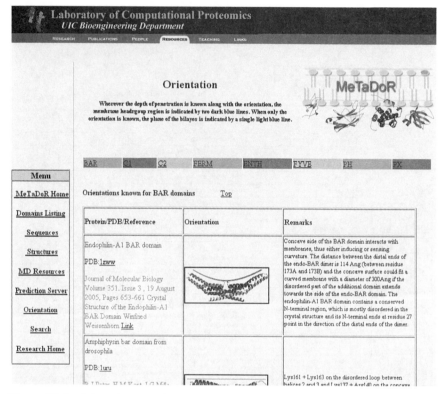

Figure 25.6   Orientation page in MeTaDoR. The page provides the PDB IDs, the literature proposing or establishing the orientation, and some remarks about the orientation.

25.2.7   Search Function

A search menu is provided to search the database for specific proteins/domains (Fig. 25.9). The user can search the database by querying the database with a Boolean combination of the fields of domain name, species, class, Swiss-Prot ID, host–protein name, and keywords in function and location description. Four different search fields can be used in a single run for a refined and advanced search. A sequence homology search for a specific sequence or subsequence can also be performed that has been implemented using BLAST [39].

25.3   SUMMARY AND CONCLUSION

Protein–membrane interactions play a key role in many cellular events, including cell signaling and membrane trafficking. Peripheral membrane proteins that mediate most of these interactions are cytosolic proteins that recognize and bind various membranes mostly in a reversibly manner. The majority of these proteins contain modular domains, generally known as *membrane targeting domains*

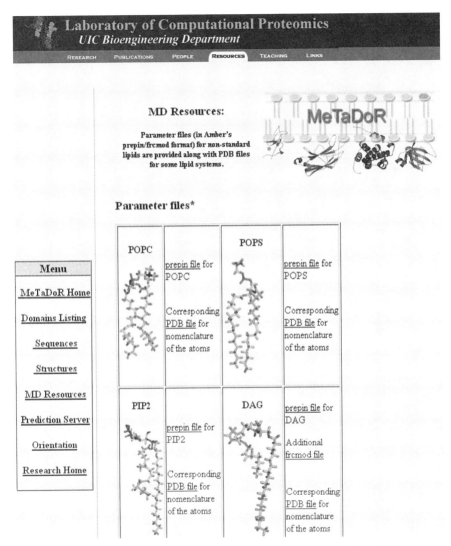

Figure 25.7 MD resources provided in MeTaDoR that include the forcefield parameter files and PDB of some lipid systems to facilitate MD studies of these protein–lipid systems.

(MTDs) or *lipid binding domains*, which are specialized in recognizing specific lipids and are responsible for driving peripheral proteins to the membranes. Considering the significance of these domains, we have created a comprehensive resource dedicated to MTDs, MeTaDoR (*membrane targeting domains resource*). MeTaDoR provides comprehensive structural and functional information about these domains. Beginning with a short introduction to all major MTDs, it briefly lists their subcellular localization and structural features that define their lipid

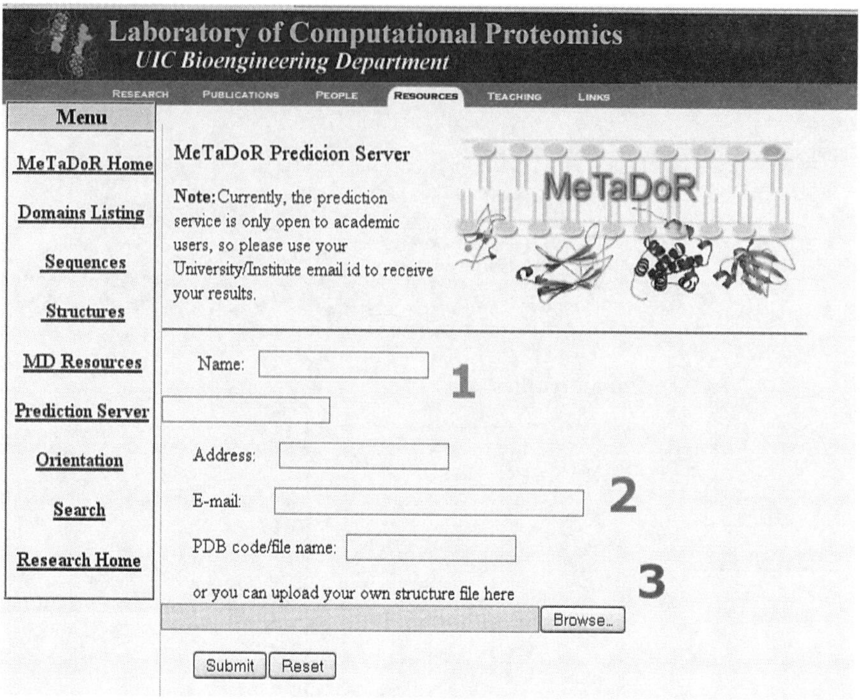

Figure 25.8   The submission form for the prediction server. The user will have to submit name and institutional affiliation (1), the email to which the results should be sent (2), and the PDB ID or the file of the domain on which the prediction should be made (3).

binding properties. Next in the menu, it lists the sequences of all known MTDs in two formats: standard Prosite format and an easy-to-parse tab-delimited format. As not all MTDs are known to be involved in direct membrane targeting, in the latter format, we also provide a manually curated classification of these domains into membranebinding or nonbinding. Also, structures of all MTDs and their host proteins, whenever available, are provided along with corresponding links to PDB and Pfam databases. Experimentally determined or proposed membranebinding orientations of these proteins are also listed with links to the appropriate literature. To facilitate molecular dynamics studies to understand how these domains interact with membranes, the forcefield parameters for many nonstandard lipids that commonly interact with these domains are also provided. Finally, a search function with various search fields and an online server for predicting membrane binding properties of proteins are included. The resource is updated on a regular basis and is publicly available at the URL http://proteomics.bioengr.uic.edu/metador.

MeTaDoR represents the first dedicated and comprehensive resource for MTDs providing all the essential information about these domains and their host proteins (Table 25.1). MeTaDoR provides the sequences and other information about

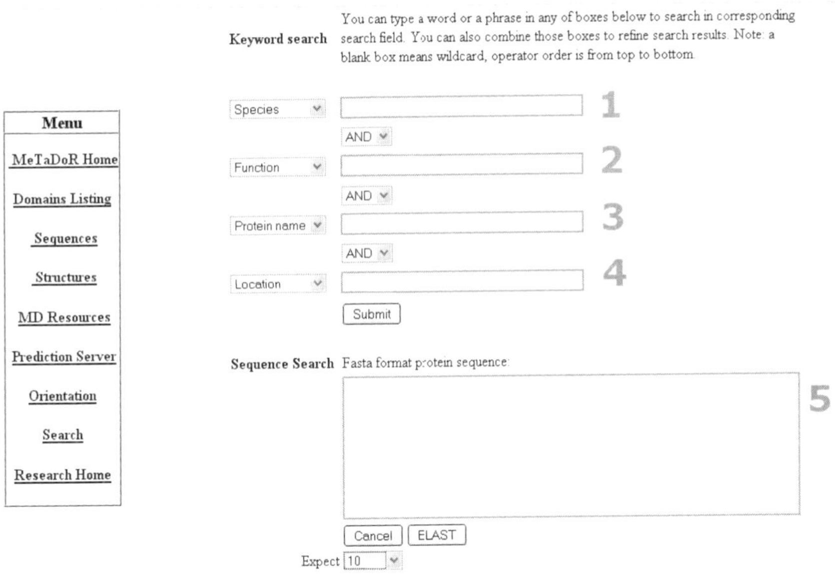

You can type a word or a phrase in any of boxes below to search in corresponding
Keyword search search field. You can also combine those boxes to refine search results. Note: a
blank box means wildcard, operator order is from top to bottom.

Menu
MeTaDoR Home
Domains Listing
Sequences
Structures
MD Resources
Prediction Server
Orientation
Search
Research Home

Species [ ] **1**
AND

Function [ ] **2**
AND

Protein name [ ] **3**
AND

Location [ ] **4**
Submit

Sequence Search Fasta format protein sequence:

5

Cancel   ELAST
Expect 10

Figure 25.9 The user is able to search the database backing MeTaDoR by several different means. The database can be queried using a Boolean combination of the field's species, function keywords (host) protein name, location, Swiss-Prot ID, and class (fields 1–4). Furthermore, the user has the option of submitting a protein sequence in FASTA format in order to obtain homologous MTDs as defined by the scoring function defined in the BLAST algorithm (field 5).

TABLE 25.1   Current Statistics as of August 2008 for Each Domain Family in the Database

Domain	Number of Sequences	Number of Structures	Number of Orientations
BAR	40	5	3
C1	166	14	2
C2	339	39	2
ENTH	51	10	1
FERM	109	19	1
FYVE	81	9	1
PH	542	77	3
PX	157	10	2
Tubby	10	4	—

MTDs in an easy-to-use format. It lists all known structures and membrane binding orientations of these domains with appropriate links. To facilitate their molecular dynamics studies, the force-field parameters for commonly interacting lipids are also provided. MeTaDoR is also coupled with an online prediction server for identifying membrane binding domains, and a search function is also provided. Finally, MeTaDoR will be maintained and updated on a regular basis to incorporate new structural and functional information about MTDs. Overall, integration of essential information about these important domains in a readily available and user-friendly format makes MeTaDoR a useful and powerful resource for the research community.

ACKNOWLEDGMENT

This work was supported by NIH Grants P01AI060915 (HL), GM52598 (WC), GM68849 (WC), and GM76581 (WC) and by the CBC catalyst award (WC and HL).

REFERENCES

1. Teruel MN, Meyer T, Translocation and reversible localization of signaling proteins: A dynamic future for signal transduction, *Cell* **103**(2):181–184 (2000).

2. Pawson T, Scott JD, Signaling through scaffold, anchoring, and adaptor proteins, *Science* **278**(5346):2075–2080 (1997).

3. Hurley JH, Membrane binding domains, *Biochim Biophys. Acta* **1761**(8):805–811 (2006).

4. Vivanco I, Sawyers CL, The phosphatidylinositol 3-kinase AKT pathway in human cancer, *Nat. Rev. Cancer* **2**:489–501 (2002).

5. Saad JS, Miller J, Tai J, Kim A, Ghanam RH, Summers MF, Structural basis for targeting HIV-1 Gag proteins to the plasma membrane for virus assembly, *Proc Natl. Acad. Sci. USA* **103**(30):11364–11369 (2006).

6. Cho W, Stahelin RV, Membrane-protein interactions in cell signaling and membrane trafficking, *Annu. Rev. Biophys. Biomol. Struct.* **34**:119–151 (2005).

7. DiNitto JP, Cronin TC, Lambright DG, Membrane recognition and targeting by lipid-binding domains, *Sci. STKE (Signal Transduct. Knowl. Environ.)* **2003**(213):re16 (2003).

8. Ono Y, Fujii T, Igarashi K, et al, Phorbol ester binding to protein kinase C requires a cysteine-rich zinc- finger-like sequence, *Proc. Natl. Acad. Sci. USA* **86**(13):4868–4871 (1989).

9. Oancea E, Teruel MN, Quest AF, Meyer T, Green fluorescent protein (GFP)-tagged cysteine-rich domains from protein kinase C as fluorescent indicators for diacylglycerol signaling in living cells, *J. Cell. Biol.* **140**(3):485–498 (1998).

10. Cho W, Membrane targeting by C1 and C2 domains., *J. Biol. Chem.* **276**(35): 32407–32410 (2001).

11. Yang C, Kazanietz MG, Divergence and complexities in DAG signaling: looking beyond PKC, *Trends Pharmacol. Sci.* **24**(11):602–608 (2003).

12. Nalefski EA, Falke JJ, The C2 domain calcium-binding motif: structural and functional diversity, *Protein Sci.* **5**(12):2375–2390 (1996).

13. Rizo J, Sudhof TC, C2-domains, structure and function of a universal Ca^{2+}-binding domain. *J. Biol. Chem.* **273**(26):15879–15882 (1998).

14. Ferguson KM, Kavran JM, Sankaran VG, et al, Structural basis for discrimination of 3-phosphoinositides by pleckstrin homology domains, *Mol. Cell.* **6**(2):373–384 (2000).

15. Lemmon MA, Ferguson KM, Signal-dependent membrane targeting by pleckstrin homology (PH) domains., *Biochem. J.* **350**(Pt. 1):1–18 (2000).

16. Stenmark H, Aasland R, Driscoll PC, The phosphatidylinositol 3-phosphate-binding FYVE finger, *FEBS Lett.* **513**(1):77–84 (2002).

17. Xu Y, Seet LF, Hanson B, Hong W, The Phox homology (PX) domain, a new player in phosphoinositide signalling, *Biochem J.* **360**(Pt. 3):513–530 (2001).

18. De Camilli P, Chen H, Hyman J, Panepucci E, Bateman A, Brunger AT, The ENTH domain, *FEBS Lett.* **513**(1):11–8 (2002).

19. Habermann B, The BAR-domain family of proteins: a case of bending and binding? *EMBO Reports* **5**(3):250–255 (2004).

20. Bretscher A, Edwards K, Fehon RG, ERM proteins and merlin: integrators at the cell cortex, *Nat. Rev. Mol. Cell Biol.* **3**(8):586–599 (2002).

21. Carroll K, Gomez C, Shapiro L, Tubby proteins: The plot thickens, *Nat. Rev. Mol. Cell Biol.* **5**(1):55–63 (2004).

22. Lomize MA, Lomize AL, Pogozheva ID, Mosberg HI, OPM: Orientations of proteins in membranes database, *Bioinformatics* **22**(5):623–625 (2006).

23. Mewes HW, Frishman D, Mayer KF, et al, MIPS: Analysis and annotation of proteins from whole genomes in 2005, *Nucleic Acids Res*. **34**(database issue):D169–D172 (2006).

24. Salwinski L, Miller CS, Smith AJ, Pettit FK, Bowie JU, Eisenberg D, The Database of Interacting Proteins: 2004 update, *Nucleic Acids Res.* **32**(database issue):D449–D451 (2004).

25. Kumar MD, Bava KA, Gromiha MM, et al, ProTherm and ProNIT: Thermodynamic databases for proteins and protein-nucleic acid interactions, *Nucleic Acids Res*. **34**(database issue):D204–D206 (2006).

26. Puvanendrampillai D, Mitchell JB, L/D Protein Ligand Database (PLD): Additional understanding of the nature and specificity of protein-ligand complexes, *Bioinformatics* **19**(14):1856–1857 (2003).

27. Wu H, Feng W, Chen J, Chan LN, Huang S, Zhang M, PDZ domains of Par-3 as potential phosphoinositide signaling integrators, *Mol. Cell* **28**(5):886–898 (2007).

28. Hulo N, Bairoch A, Bulliard V, et al, The PROSITE database, *Nucleic Acids Res*. **34**(database issue):D227–D230 (2006).

29. Berman HM, Battistuz T, Bhat TN, et al, The Protein Data Bank, *Acta Crystallogr. D Biol. Crystallogr*. **58**(Pt. 6, No. 1):899–907 (2002).

30. Bateman A, Coin L, Durbin R, et al, The Pfam protein families database, *Nucleic Acids Res.* **32**(database issue):D138–D141 (2004).

31. Lemmon MA, Membrane recognition by phospholipid-binding domains, *Nat. Rev. Mol. Cell Biol.* **9**(2):99–111 (2008).

32. Gumbart J, Wang Y, Aksimentiev A, Tajkhorshid E, Schulten K, Molecular dynamics simulations of proteins in lipid bilayers, *Curr. Opin. Struct. Biol.* **15**(4):423–431 (2005).

33. Scott HL, Modeling the lipid component of membranes, *Curr. Opin. Struct. Biol.* **12**(4):495–502 (2002).

34. Jaud S, Tobias DJ, Falke JJ, White SH, Self-induced docking site of a deeply embedded peripheral membrane protein, *Biophys. J*, **92**:517–524 (2006).

35. Sansom MS, Models and simulations of ion channels and related membrane proteins, *Curr Opin. Struct. Biol.* **8**(2):237–244 (1998).

36. Blood PD, Voth GA, Direct observation of Bin/amphiphysin/Rvs (BAR) domain-induced membrane curvature by means of molecular dynamics simulations, *Proc. Natl. Acad. Sci. USA* **103**(41):15068–15072 (2006).

37. Manna D, Bhardwaj N, Vora MS, Stahelin RV, Lu H, Cho W, Differential roles of phosphatidylserine, PtdIns(4,5)P2 and PtdIns(3,4,5)p3 in plasma membrane targeting of C2 domains: Molecular dynamics simulation, membrane binding, and cell translocation studies of the PKCalpha c2 domain, *J. Biol. Chem*. **293**:26047–26058 (2008).

38. Bhardwaj N, Stahelin RV, Langlois RE, Cho W, Lu H, Structural bioinformatics prediction of membrane-binding proteins, *J. Mol. Biol.* **359**(2):486–495 (2006).

39. Altschul SF, Gish W, Miller W, Myers EW, Lipman DJ, Basic local alignment search tool, *J. Mol. Biol.* **215**(3):403–410 (1990).

CHAPTER 26

BIOLOGICAL NETWORKS–BASED ANALYSIS OF GENE EXPRESSION SIGNATURES*

GANG CHEN and JIANXIN WANG

26.1 INTRODUCTION

Diagnostic and prognostic gene signatures for complex diseases is a major step toward better personal medicine. A gene signature is a group of genes whose expression pattern represents the status of a gene expression disease [1]. Identification of the gene signatures of disease subtypes, risk stratification, pathologic parameters, and clinical outcomes has the potential to help physicians and surgeons find a personal optimized treatment, avoid unnecessary medication, and reduce costs [2,3].

Various gene signatures are developed for various complex diseases, especially cancer. Since researchers found that gene expression signatures were able to predict clinical outcome of breast cancer in 2002 [4,5], this method has become a hot topic and attracted the attention of both biologists and oncologists. Signatures for various phenotypes, such as poor prognosis [5], invasiveness [6], recurrence [7], and metastasis [8,9], have been experimentally derived from patient groups and biological hypotheses. MammaPrint, a fully commercialized microarray-based 70-gene signature for breast cancer that was developed by Agendia (http://www.agendia.com/), was approved by FDA [10] in 2009. Because of rapid development of high-throughput tecniques, such as microarry, the number of gene signatures has grown quite rapidly.

*This work is supported in part by the National Natural Science Foundation of China under Grants 61003124 and 61073036

Algorithmic and Artificial Intelligence Methods for Protein Bioinformatics. First Edition.
Edited by Yi Pan, Jianxin Wang, Min Li.
© 2014 John Wiley & Sons, Inc. Published 2014 by John Wiley & Sons, Inc.

495

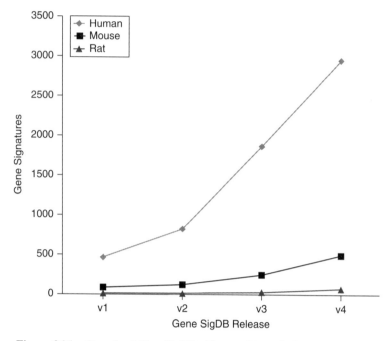

Figure 26.1   Growth of GeneSigDB. (*Source*: From Culhane et al. [11]).

The first release of GeneSigDB [11], published in August 2009, contained only 575 gene signatures. In the latest release, GeneSigDB contains 3515 gene signatures for more than 50 tissues, and diseases of three species are collected from 1604 published articles. Figure 26.1 shows the growth of gene signatures in the GeneSigDB. Because of space limitation, we cannot list them one by one. Details of these gene signatures can be found in GeneSigDB (http://compbio.dfci.harvard.edu/genesigdb/).

However, as pointed out in several articles, distinct signatures share very few genes, even though they paradoxically occupy a common prognosis space [12–14]. For both cancer biologists and oncologists, there are two critical problems: (1) how to explain the lack of overlap among gene signatures for a common diseases and (2) whether these disjoint genetic signatures can provide a unified insight into the relationship between gene expression and clinical outcome.

Meanwhile, biological networks, such as protein interaction networks and gene coexpression networks, are becoming popular in many studies, including the study of gene signatures of complex diseases. Computational biologists have developed many methods to identify gene signatures by combining gene expression profiles, biological networks, and other related data. Using data on biological networks, researchers also want to integrate different gene signatures by considering the interactions among genes.

The rest of this chapter is organized as follows: a brief introduction of gene signatures is provided in Section 26.2; biological network–based identification of gene signatures is described in Section 26.3; in Section 26.4, we discuss protein interaction network–based integration of different gene signatures; and discussion and conclusion are provided in the Section 26.5.

26.2 GENE EXPRESSION SIGNATURES

26.2.1 Identification of Gene Signatures

Analysis of the gene signatures in GeneSigDB release 4 reveals that the most common array platforms were Affymetrix platforms, particularly u133a and u133plus2 arrays. However, the computational methods used to select genes from the experimental results to construct gene signatures are vary significantly in different studies. Basically, as shown in Figure 26.2, these different methods can be divided into two classes, top–down (data-driven) approaches and the 'bottom–up' (hypothesis-driven) approaches [14]:

1. *Data-Driven Approach.* Also known as an *unsupervised approach*, this method tries to seek gene expression profiles that are associated or correlated with clinical outcome without any a priori biological assumption. Gene signatures identified by this type of approach include the 70-gene signature and 76-gene signature developed Netherlands Cancer Institute in Amsterdam with Rosetta Informatics-Merck, and the Erasmus MC in Rotterdam together with Veridex, respectively [4,9]. Although these signatures were built using a different microarray platform and had only a small gene overlap, a feature common to the gene signatures developed by data-driven approaches is that they correctly identified high-risk patients while also identifying a higher number of low-risk patients not needing treatment in comparison to the clinical guidelines. A flaw of data-driven approach is the gene signatures that identified by this kind of approach need more analysis to be interpreted.

2. *Hypothesis-Driven Approach.* Also known as a *supervised approach*, this method attempts to derive gene expression signature based on some biological hypothesis. Gene signatures developed by such approaches include the 97-gene signature of breast cancer developed by Sotiriou et al. [15] and the 96-gene signature of invasive potential in metastatic melanoma cells developed by Jeffs et al. [16]. By incorporating a priori biological knowledge, one can easily interpret the gene signatures identified by the hypothesis-driven apparoach are easy to interpret from a biological perspective. The protein interaction network represents the complicate relationship among proteins and genes. We will focus on the methods that incorporate protein interaction networks.

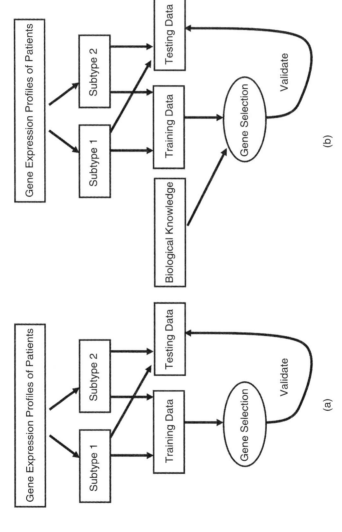

Figure 26.2 Overview of data-driven (a) and hypothesis-driven (b) approaches.

26.2.2 Low Overlap among Signatures

As mentioned elsewhere [12–14,17], there is very small overlap among different gene signatures. To validate this observation, we obtained 94 human breast cancer gene signatures from the GeneSigDB release 2. Because of the different generation methods and the various purposes of these signatures, the size of these signatures are very different. The largest signature contains 3260 genes, and the smallest signature contains only 4 genes. The median size of these signatures is 46.

To evaluate the similarity among these gene signatures, we analyze the overlap among the 94 gene signatures (see Table 26.1). The analysis result is very consistent with the results reported in previous literature. A very small overlap is found among different signatures. While 4143 (58.6% of the total number) genes are found in only one signature, only 24(0.4%) genes overlapped among 10 or more signatures, and none of the genes overlapped among all 94 signatures. The lack of overlap is an obstacle to biological intepretation of the gene signatures and also indicates that the gene signatures identified by most existing methods are not sufficiently stable.

26.2.3 Possible Explanation of Low Overlap

Obviously, complex heterogeneity of signatures is possibly caused by different probe design, different platforms, or inadequate patient samples, and becomes an obstacle in interpretation and integration of various signatures of complex

TABLE 26.1 Overlap among 94 Breast Cancer Gene Signatures

Frequency	Number of Genes
1	4143
2	1608
3	687
4	323
5	148
6	56
7	40
8	23
9	15
10	13
11	4
12	3
14	1
15	1
16	1
17	1

diseases. Gene ontology enrichment, pathway analysis, and some genome-scale methods are proposed to explain the lack of overlap [14,18,19]. Van Vliet et al. [18], list five possible explanations for the small overlap between signatures:

1. There may be heterogeneity in expression due to different platform technologies and references

2. There may be differences in supervised protocols with which signatures are extracted

3. Although the genes are not exactly the same, they represent the same set of pathways or function modules.

4. There may be differences in clinical composition between datasets (i.e., sample heterogeneity).

5. Small sample size problems may cause inaccurate signatures.

Through a large-scale analysis performed on 947 breast cancer samples from Affymetrix platform, Van Vliet et al. [18] conclude that the small signature overlap is most likely due to small sample size problem (explanation 5). However, the conclusion might be specific to the datasets and the specific techniques used in their work. By comparison of three prognostic gene expression signatures for breast cancer, Haibe-Kains et al. [14] suggested that the small overlap between the different prognostic gene signatures resulted because these different signatures represented largely overlapping biological processes (explanation 3). By taking into account the biological knowledge that exists among different signatures, Blazadonakis et al. [19] found that different signatures are similar at biological level, rather than gene level (explanation 3). Much work has been done in an effort to understand the small overlap between gene signatures, but so far there is no widely accepted explanation. Actually, explanation 3 indicates that the small overlap among gene signatures is caused by the complex interactions between genes and gene products. The interactions among genes and gene products can be represented as biological networks. Therefore, protein interaction networks can be used to identify stable gene signatures and interpret the relationship among them.

26.3   BIOLOGICAL NETWORK–BASED IDENTIFICATION OF GENE EXPRESSION SIGNATURES

As is well known, virtually no biological moleculars, such genes and proteins, can perform biological function individually. They always associate together to achieve some particular functions. Therefore, various moleculars probably associate together to influence the states and outcome of diseases. Biological networks consisting of biological molecules and the interactions among them allow us to uncover the functions of genes and proteins at network level. Therefore, by incorporating biological networks, gene expression profiles, and other clinical data, we can investigate the relationship between complex diseases and genes to find the gene signatures of complex diseases.

An important work in this field is that by Chuang et al. [6], who proposed a protein interaction network–based approach that identifies biomarkers to predict the likelihood of metastasis in unkonwn samples. In this study, they identified biomarkers not as individual genes but as subnetworks extracted from protein interaction databases. Protein interaction networks and gene expression profiles of different phenotypes are integrated in this study. First, they divided the protein interaction network into subnetworks. Then, each subnetwork was scored to assess its activity in each patient, defined by averaging its normalized gene expression values. Finally, the discriminative potential of each subnetwork was computed on the basis of the mutual information between its activity score and the metastatic/non-metastatic disease status over all patients. Significantly discriminative subnetworks were identified by comparing their discriminative potentials to those of random networks and used to classify the cancer patients. Compared with traditional analysis methods, the classification accuracy of metastasis of network-based method was higher. The subnetwork biomarkers identified by this network-based method are more informative and reproducible across datasets.

By integrating high-quality human protein interactions and a computationally derived phenotype similarity score, Lage et al. [20] performed a systematic, large-scale analysis of human protein complexes comprising gene products implicated in many different categories of human disease and created a phenome–interactome network. Using a phenomic ranking of protein complexes linked to human diseases, they developed a predictor for many complex diseases, such as retinitis pigmentosa, epithelial ovarian cancer, inflammatory bowel disease, amyotrophic lateral sclerosis, Alzheimer disease, type 2 diabetes, and coronary heart disease.

Taylor et al. [21] analyzed hub proteins in human protein interaction networks. They found signaling domains more often in intermodular hub proteins that are coexpressed with their interacting partners in a tissue-restricted manner and also more frequently associated with oncogenesis. By analyzing two breast cancer patient cohorts, they found that altered modularity of the human interactome may be useful as an indicator of breast cancer prognosis. They developed a prognostic gene signature of breast cancer that consists of the hub proteins whose relative expression with each of their interacting partners differed significantly between patients who survived versus those who died from disease.

By integrating protein interaction networks and gene–gene coexpression networks, Erik van den Akker et al. proposed a nongreedy method for dissecting the interaction network into a set of disjoint subnetworks that are functionally coherent to improve gene signatures for classifying breast cancer metastasis [22].

Since 2010, Guo et al. have developed a series of implication networks methods for identification of gene signatures of various complex diseases [23–30]. They [27,29] used implication networks based on prediction logic to construct genomewide coexpression networks for different disease states and then selected candidate genes that coexpressed with major disease signal hallmarks. Finally, they used the univariate Cox model and Relief algorithm to select the top genes that were most predictive of clinical outcome to construct the gene signature for non–small cell lung cancer. A 13-gene lung cancer prognosis signature with significant prognostic stratifications is identified by this method. To predict lung cancer risk and survival, they developed a smoking associated six-gene signature [28]. In this study, they developed an induction algorithm based on prediction logic to generate implication networks that were used to infer the relevance of signaling pathways in a set of selected genes associated with smoking and lung cancer survival.

As described above, biological networks, such as gene coexpression networks and protein interaction networks, are combined with gene expression profiles of patients with different disease status to identify gene signatures and achieved much success.

26.4 BIOLOGICAL NETWORK–BASED INTEGRATION OF GENE EXPRESSION SIGNATURES

As shown in Section 26.2.1, the overlap among different gene signatures is very limited. It is difficult to interpret the lack of overlap and integrate different signatures if we don't consider the functional and physical interactions among genes and proteins. The interactions among genes and proteins consist of biological networks. Therefore, many network-based explanations are proposed to explain the lack of overlap among gene signatures. Furthermore, on the basis of data on biological networks, researchers also want to integrate different signatures to provide a unifed insight to the relationship between gene expression and diseases.

By single-protein analysis of networks (SPAN [31]) and conservative permutation resampling, a small but more biologically significant breast cancer signature consisting of 54 genes is identified from a protein interaction network, including 250 cancer-related genes reported in the literatures [17,32].

By taking into account the biological knowledge that exists among different signatures, and applying it as a means of integrating the signatures and refining their statistical significance on the datasets, Blazadonakis et al. [19] derived a unified signature that is significantly improved over its predecessors in terms of performance and robustness. Their motive in this approach was to assess the problem of evaluating different signatures not in a competitive but rather in a complementary manner, where one is treated as a pool of knowledge contributing to a global and unified solution.

Wang et al. [12] proposed a graph centrality method to integrate different gene signatures of breast cancer. As shown in Figure 26.3, they constructed a context-constrained protein interaction network of breast cancer by integrating different gene signatures of breast cancer and protein interaction data. Then, they selected a given number of genes that have high graph centrality to construct the integrated gene signature. According to gene ontology and KEGG pathway enrichment analysis, the graph centrality gene signatures are closely related to

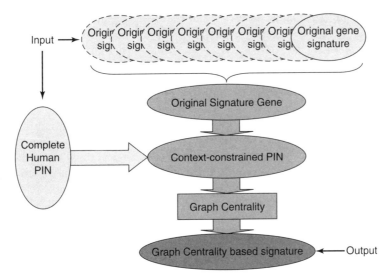

Figure 26.3 Overview of the graph centrality integration method proposed by Wang et al. [12].

cancers. Microarray datasets of breast cancer patients from the GEO database are used to validate the graph centrality gene signatures. According to the expression profiles of the gene signatures, the breast cancer patients are divided into two groups with different clinical parameters.

Frohlich [33] has developed an alogirthm to obtain a consensus gene signature from six different gene signatures for breast cancer. First, they clustered genes from different gene signatures based on their shortest-path distance in a protein interaction network. Then, for each cluster, they identified lowest common ancestors (LCAs), which are proteins that are commonly upstream of a set of proteins and thus may exhibit a certain regulatory influence. Finally, the set of LCAs and the set of genes appearing in the majority of signatures form their consensus gene signature.

As presented in Table 26.2, all these integration methods are based on breast cancer data. However, besides the interactions among genes and proteins, different cancers and diseases are also associated with each other. A unified

TABLE 26.2 Summary of Gene Signature Integration Methods

Disease	Original Signature	Method	Result Signature Size	Reference
Breast cancer	—	SPAN	54	32
Breast cancer	3	Fisher ratio	—	19
Breast cancer	94	Graph centrality	54	12
Breast cancer	6	Shortest-path distance	203	33

gene signature of similar diseases can be constructed by incorporating gene expression profiles, protein interaction networks, and the relationship among diseases.

26.5   DISCUSSION AND CONCLUSION

Biological networks are widely used in various biomedical researches, such as prediction of the function of biological moleculars, identification of protein complexes, and functional modules. More recently, biological networks such as gene coexpression networks and protein interaction networks have been used to identify and integrate gene signatures of complex diseases. Research reviewed in this chapter proves that biological networks are effeicient in identifying robust, informative, and reproducible gene signatures.

Although many successes have been made, many problems have to be solved. First, most existing gene signatures focus on one specific status of disease. By integrating various biological networks and clinical information, researchers need to develop gene signature of multistatus disease to provide a unified insight into the disease mechanism. In addition, most existing network-based gene signature identification and integration methods are designed for static biological networks. As is well known, biological networks are dynamic systems. Researchers can reconstruct dynamic biological networks by integrating various data, such as time series gene expression data. Gene signatures from such dynamic networks should be more informative. The last but also the most important issue is the fact that network-based gene signatures still lack overlap. Similar to traditional methods, gene signatures identified by different network-based methods are very different. Comprehensive analysis and novel methods are needed to solve these problems.

REFERENCES

1. Itadani H, Mizuarai S, Kotani H, Can systems biology understand pathway activation? Gene expression signatures as surrogate markers for understanding the complexity of pathway activation, *Curr. Genomics* **9**(5):349–360 (2008).

2. van't Veer LJ, Bernards R, Enabling personalized cancer medicine through analysis of gene-expression patterns, *Nature* **452**(7187):564–570 (April 2008).

3. Subramanian J, Simon R, Gene expression-based prognostic signatures in lung cancer: Ready for clinical use? *J. Natl. Cancer Inst.* **102**(7):464–474 (April 2010).

4. van 't Veer LJ, Dai H, van de Vijver MJ, et al, Gene expression profiling predicts clinical outcome of breast cancer, *Nature* **415**(6871):530–536 (Jan. 2002).

5. van de Vijver MJ, He YD, van 't Veer LJ, et al, A gene-expression signature as a predictor of survival in breast cancer, *New Engl. J. Med.* **347**(25):1999–2009 (Dec. 2002).

6. Chuang H-Y, Lee E, Liu Y-T, Lee D, Ideker T, Network-based classification of breast cancer metastasis, *Mol. Syst. Biol.* **3**:140 (2007).

7. Paik S, Shak S, Tang G, et al, A multigene assay to predict recurrence of tamoxifen-treated, node-negative breast cancer, *New Engl. J. Med.* **351**(27):2817–2826 (Dec. 2004).

8. Minn AJ, Gupta GP, Siegel PM, et al, Genes that mediate breast cancer metastasis to lung, *Nature* **436**(7050):518–524 (July 2005).

9. Wang Y, Klijn JGM, Zhang Y, et al, Gene-expression profiles to predict distant metastasis of lymph-node-negative primary breast cancer, *Lancet* **365**(9460):671–679 (2005).

10. Slodkowska EA, Ross JS, Mammaprint 70-gene signature: Another milestone in personalized medical care for breast cancer patients, *Expert Rev. Mol. Diagn.* **9**(5):417–422 (July 2009).

11. Culhane AC, Schrder MS, Sultana R, Picard SC, Martinelli EN, Kelly C, Haibe-Kains B, Kapushesky M, St Pierre AA, Flahive W, Picard KC, Gusenleitner D, et al, Genesigdb: A manually curated database and resource for analysis of gene expression signatures, *Nucleic Acids Res.* **40**(1):D1060–D1066 (Jan. 2012).

12. Wang J, Chen G, Li M, Pan Y, Integration of breast cancer gene signatures based on graph centrality, *BMC Syst. Biol.* **5**(Suppl. 3):S10 (2011).

13. Gnen M, Statistical aspects of gene signatures and molecular targets, *Gastrointest. Cancer Res.* **3**(2 Suppl.):S19–S21 (March 2009).

14. Haibe-Kains B, Desmedt C, Piette F, Buyse M, Cardoso F, van't Veer L, Piccart M, Bontempi G, Sotiriou C, Comparison of prognostic gene expression signatures for breast cancer, *BMC Genomics* **9**:394 (2008).

15. Sotiriou C, Wirapati P, Loi S, Harris A, Fox S, Smeds J, Nordgren H, Farmer P, Praz V, Haibe-Kains B, Desmedt C, Larsimont D, Cardoso F, Peterse H, et al, Gene expression profiling in breast cancer: Understanding the molecular basis of histologic grade to improve prognosis, *J. Natl. Cancer Inst.* **98**(4):262–272 (Feb. 2006).

16. Jeffs AR, Glover AC, Slobbe LJ, Wang L, He S, Hazlett JA, Awasthi A, Woolley AG, Marshall ES, Joseph WR, Print CG, Baguley BC, Eccles MR, A gene expression signature of invasive potential in metastatic melanoma cells, *PLoS One* **4**(12):e8461 (2009).

17. Chen J, Sam L, Huang Y, et al, Protein interaction network underpins concordant prognosis among heterogeneous breast cancer signatures, *J. Biomed. Informatics* **43**(3):385–396 (2010).

18. van Vliet MH, Reyal F, Horlings HM, et al, Pooling breast cancer datasets has a synergetic effect on classification performance and improves signature stability, *BMC Genomics* **9**:375 (2008).

19. Blazadonakis ME, Zervakis ME, Kafetzopoulos D, Complementary gene signature integration in multiplatform microarray experiments, *IEEE Trans. Inform. Technol. Biomed.* **15**(1):155–163 (Jan. 2011).

20. Lage K, Karlberg EO, Størling ZM, et al, A human phenome-interactome network of protein complexes implicated in genetic disorders, *Nat. Biotechnol.* **25**(3):309–316 (March 2007).

21. Taylor IW, Linding R, Warde-Farley D, Liu Y, Pesquita C, Faria D, Bull S, Pawson T, Morris Q, Wrana JL, Dynamic modularity in protein interaction networks predicts breast cancer outcome, *Nat. Biotechnol.* **27**(2):199–204 (Feb. 2009).

22. van den Akker EB, Verbruggen B, Heijmans BT, Beekman M, Kok JN, Slagboom PE, Reinders MJT, Integrating protein-protein interaction networks with gene-gene co-expression networks improves gene signatures for classifying breast cancer metastasis, *J. Integrative Bioinformatics* **8**(2):188 (2011).

23. Mettu RKR, Wan Y-W, Habermann JK, Ried T, Guo NL, A 12-gene genomic instability signature predicts clinical outcomes in multiple cancer types, *Int. J. Biol. Markers* **25**(4):219–228 (Nov. 2010).

24. Wan Y-W, Qian Y, Rathnagiriswaran S, Castranova V, Guo NL, A breast cancer prognostic signature predicts clinical outcomes in multiple tumor types, *Oncol. Reports* **24**(2):489–494 (Aug. 2010).

25. Wan Y-W, Sabbagh E, Raese R, Qian Y, Luo D, Denvir J, Vallyathan V, Castranova V, Guo NL, Hybrid models identified a 12-gene signature for lung cancer prognosis and chemoresponse prediction, *PLoS One* **5**(8):e12222 (2010).

26. Wan Y-W, Beer DG, Guo NL, Signaling pathway-based identification of extensive prognostic gene signatures for lung adenocarcinoma, *Lung Cancer* **76**(1):98–105 (April 2012).

27. Wan Y-W, Bose S, Denvir J, Guo NL, A novel network model for molecular prognosis, in *Proc. 1st ACM Int. Conf. Bioinformatics and Computational Biology (BCB'10)*, Assoc. Computing Machinery, New York, 2010, pp. 342–345.

28. Guo NL, Wan Y-W, Pathway-based identification of a smoking associated 6-gene signature predictive of lung cancer risk and survival, *Artif. Intell. Med.* **55**(2):97–105 (Feb. 2012).

29. Guo NL, Wan Y-W, Bose S, Denvir J, Kashon ML, Andrew ME, A novel network model identified a 13-gene lung cancer prognostic signature, *Int. J. Comput. Biol. Drug Design* **4**(1):19–39 (2011).

30. Wan Y-W, Xiao C, Guo NL, Network-based identification of smoking-associated gene signature for lung cancer, *Proc. IEEE Int. Bioinformatics and Biomedicine (BIBM) Conf.*, 2010. pp. 479–484.

31. Lee Y, Yang X, Huang Y, Fan H, et al, Network modeling identifies molecular functions targeted by mir-204 to suppress head and neck tumor metastasis, *PLoS Comput. Biol.* **6**(4):e1000730 (2010).

32. Chen JL, Li J, Stadler WM, Lussier YA, Protein-network modeling of prostate cancer gene signatures reveals essential pathways in disease recurrence, *J. Am. Med. Inform. Assoc.* **18**(4):392–402 (July 2011).

33. Frohlich H, Network based consensus gene signatures for biomarker discovery in breast cancer, *PLoS One* **6**(10):e25364 (2011).

INDEX

Algorithmic and Artificial Intelligence Methods for Protein Bioinformatics. First Edition.
Edited by Yi Pan, Jianxin Wang, Min Li.
© 2014 John Wiley & Sons, Inc. Published 2014 by John Wiley & Sons, Inc.

Wiley Series on

Bioinformatics: Computational Techniques and Engineering

Bioinformatics and computational biology involve the comprehensive application of mathematics, statistics, science, and computer science to the understanding of living systems. Research and development in these areas require cooperation among specialists from the fields of biology, computer science, mathematics, statistics, physics, and related sciences. The objective of this book series is to provide timely treatments of the different aspects of bioinformatics spanning theory, new and established techniques, technologies and tools, and application domains. This series emphasizes algorithmic, mathematical, statistical, and computational methods that are central in bioinformatics and computational biology.

Series Editors: **Professor Yi Pan** and **Professor Albert Y. Zomaya**
pan@cs.gsu.edu   zomaya@it.usyd.edu.au